ENDOMETRIOSIS TODAY
Advances in research and practice

THE INTERNATIONAL CONGRESS,
SYMPOSIUM AND SEMINAR SERIES

VOLUME 13

I·C·S·S

ISSN: 0969-2622

ENDOMETRIOSIS TODAY

Advances in research and practice

The Proceedings of the Vth World Congress on Endometriosis
Yokohama, Japan, October 1996

Edited by

H. Minaguchi
Yokohama City University School of Medicine, Yokohama, Japan

and

O. Sugimoto
Osaka Medical College, Kyoto, Japan

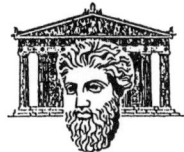

The Parthenon Publishing Group
International Publishers in Medicine, Science & Technology

NEW YORK   LONDON

British Library Cataloguing in Publication Data
Endometriosis today : advances in research and practice.
(The international congress symposium and seminar
series ; v. 13)
1. Endometriosis – Congresses
I. Minaguchi, H. II Sugimoto, O.
618.1

ISBN 1-85070-901-7

Library of Congress Cataloging-in-Publication Data
World Congress on Endometriosis (5th : 1996 :
Yokohama-shi, Japan)
    Endometriosis today : advances in research and
practice / edited by H. Minaguchi and O. Sugimoto.
    p. cm. (The International congress, symposium, and
seminar series ISSN 0969-2622 : v. 13)
    Includes bibliographical references and index.
    ISBN 1-85070-901-7
    1. Endometriosis – Congresses. I. Minaguchi, H.
II. Sugimoto, Osamu. III. Title. IV. Series.
    [DNLM: 1. Endometriosis – congresses. W1 IN736I
v. 13 1997 / WP 390 W927e 1997]
    RG483.E53W69 1996
    618.1 – dc21
    DNML/DLC
    for Library of Congress   97-15483
                                            CIP

Published in the UK by
The Parthenon Publishing Group
Casterton Hall, Carnforth
Lancs. LA6 2LA, England.

Published in the USA by
The Parthenon Publishing Group Inc.
One Blue Hill Plaza
PO Box 1564, Pearl River
New York 10965, USA.

Copyright © 1997 Parthenon Publishing Group Ltd

First Published 1997

No part of this book may be reproduced in any form
without permission from the publishers, except for the
quotation of brief passages for the purposes of review.

Composition by Speedlith, Manchester, UK.

Printed and bound by Butler & Tanner Ltd,
Frome & London, UK.

Contents

List of principal contributors		xi
Foreword		xvii

Section 1: Etiology and natural history of endometriosis

1	The uterus and menstruation in history and evolution C.A. Finn	3
2	Do all women have endometriosis? Reflections on pathogenesis J.L.H. Evers	14
3	New insights into adolescent endometriosis Y.T. Lim	21
4	The onset and progression of endometriosis in humans T. Fukaya, T. Murakami, J. Sugawara, H. Yoshida, A. Yajima and H. Hoshiai	28
5	The ovarian endometrioma I.A. Brosens	33
6	Rectovaginal septum adenomyotic nodule: a distinct entity J. Donnez, M. Nisolle and F. Casanas-Roux	35
7	Large ovarian endometriomas: new perspectives on histogenesis M. Nisolle, F. Casanas-Roux and J. Donnez	42
8	Deep endometriosis D.C. Martin, P.R. Koninckx, R.E. Batt and R. Smith	50
9	Natural history of endometriosis in baboons T.M. D'Hooghe	58

Section 2: The physiology of the endometrium, uterus and endometriosis

10	Endometrium in endometriosis M. Wingfield, A. Macpherson, P.A.W. Rogers and D.L. Healy	69
11	Endometriosis and pain: the role of prostaglandins K. Satoh, M. Tochigi and J.M. Teng	75

12	Uterine contractility in patients with endometriosis C. Bulletti, S. Rossi, A. Albonetti, V. Negrini, V. Polli, E. Giacomucci, D. De Ziegler and C. Flamigni	80
13	Growth factors in proliferative regulation of endometrium M. Taga, T. Takahashi and H. Minaguchi	85
14	Apoptosis in normal endometrium and adenomyosis Y. Otsuki, K. Ueki, M. Ueki, H. Yamashita, K. Matsumoto, E. Daikoku, Y. Fukuda, R. Hayashi, K. Nakamura, K. Nakao, O. Marukawa and Y. Ito	92
15	Heterotransplanted human endometrium in SCID mice in comparison with nude mice D. Aoki, Y. Katsuki, Y. Shibutani, Y. Udagawa, Y. Yoshimura and S. Nozawa	98

Section 3: Immunology

16	Immunomodulation of endometriotic implant growth and protein production W.B. Nothnick and M.W. Vernon	107
17	Endometrial immunology in endometriosis P. Miron, M.-H. Lachapelle and D.C. Roy	118
18	Peritoneal macrophages: a possible role in infertility associated with mild endometriosis R. Honda, K. Matsuura, Y. Fukumatsu, C. Onoda and H. Okamura	120
19	Effect of autoantibodies on embryo implantation W.P. Dmowski	123
20	Role of peritoneal inflammation in endometriosis associated with infertility J.K. Halme	132
21	Resident leukocytes in endometriosis C.A. Witz, N.A. Klein and R.S. Schenken	138
22	Cytokines in peritoneal fluid from women with active endometriosis T. Harada, F. Taniguchi, T. Iwabe, Y. Onohara, M. Tanikawa and N. Terakawa	144
23	Heat shock proteins and endometriosis H. Ota, S. Igarashi, J. Hatazawa and T. Tanaka	149

Section 4: Regulatory mechanisms, growth factors and cell adhesion molecules in the pathogenesis of endometriosis

24	Establishment of a permanent human endometriosis-derived cell line (FbEM-1) *J. Bouquet de Jolinière, M. Doussau, M. Canis, M. Levardon and J. Gogusev*	157
25	Expression of steroid receptors, vimentin and cytokeratin in endometriotic tissue *M. Nisolle, J. Donnez and F. Casanas-Roux*	165
26	Growth factor gene expression in endometriotic tissue *Y.M. Choi*	174
27	Potential implications of peritoneal fluid mitogens related to proteolysis of insulin-like growth factor binding protein-3 in the pathophysiology of endometriosis *A. Lemay, M. Koutsilieris, A. Akoum and R. Maheux*	181
28	Role of hepatocyte growth factor and its receptor *c-met* in pathogenesis of endometriosis *J. Sugawara, T. Fukaya, T. Murakami, H. Yoshida and A. Yajima*	191
29	Progesterone and transforming growth factor-β co-mediate matrix metalloproteinase expression in a model of endometriosis *K.G. Osteen, K.L. Bruner, L.I. Gold and E. Eisenberg*	200
30	The role of matrix metalloproteinases in the development of adenomyosis in humans and pituitary-grafted mice *M. Fujii, S. Mori, Y. Liao, T. Suzuki, M. Koizumi, T. Saito, T. Endo, S. Sagae and R. Kudo*	210
31	Endometriosis and infertility: insights with integrins used as markers of uterine receptivity *B.A. Lessey, J. Sun and J.E. Harris*	216
32	Expression of ICAM-1 in eutopic and ectopic endometrial cells *P. Viganò, B. Gaffuri, E. Somigliana, E. Iurlaro, A.M. Di Blasio and M. Vignali*	225
33	The role of cell adhesion molecules in the pathogenesis of endometriosis *G.A.J. Dunselman, P.J.Q. van der Linden, A.F.P.M. de Goeij and J.L.H. Evers*	231

Section 5: Classification

34	Do we need a classification for endometriosis? *M. Canis, A. Wattiez, J.L. Pouly, G. Mage and M.A. Bruhat*	239

| 35 | Anatomic and functional considerations in the development of a classification for endometriosis for pelvic pain and infertility
B.S. Hurst and J.A. Rock | 250 |
| 36 | Classification of endometriosis
D.K. Tran, J. Belaisch, J. Berthet, Y. Darbois, J.L. Leroy, M. Mintz, D. Querleu, C. Racinet and R. Trevoux | 259 |

Section 6: Surgical treatment

37	Operative endoscopy and videolaparoscopy: a 20th century surgical revolution *C. Nezhat, F. Nezhat, C.H. Nezhat and S. Tazuke*	271
38	Radical laparoscopic surgery for treatment of endometriosis *C. Wood*	289
39	Comparison of laser laparoscopic treatment of endometriosis with no treatment at all in the management of pain and infertility *C.J.G. Sutton*	297
40	Laparoscopic management of infertile patients with endometriosis *K. Okuda, M. Saeki and O. Sugimoto*	303
41	Office microlaparoscopy under local anesthesia for endometriosis *S.F. Palter*	309
42	Meta-analysis and evidence-based guidelines for treating endometriosis-associated infertility *G.D. Adamson*	315

Section 7: Medical treatment

43	The anticipated results from expectant management *A.F. Haney*	325
44	Effects of medical treatment on active lesions of peritoneal endometriosis *N. Terakawa and T. Harada*	329
45	Treatment of endometriosis with mifepristone (RU486) *L.M. Kettel*	334
46	Fundamental and phase I clinical study of YM511, a new aromatase inhibitor *H. Shigeta, H. Minaguchi, H. Kudoh, K. Noguchi, M. Ikeda and N. Nakamura*	339

Section 8: GnRH agonists

47	Development of LHRH analogs: past, present and future B. Lunenfeld	347
48	Role of GnRH agonist type and formulation in the management of endometriosis M. Filicori	354
49	GnRH analogs in the management of endometriosis K.-W. Schweppe	357
50	Treatment of symptomatic endometriosis with leuprolide in a 3-monthly versus a monthly depot formulation P.G. Crosignani, W. Vegetti, L. De Cecco, A. Sémino, A. Gastaldi, P. La Commare, P.L. Venturini, P. Vercellini and S. Oldani	360
51	Use of leuprolide acetate in combination with surgical treatment for women with endometriosis C.A. Winkel and M. Bray	365
52	Dose-related effects of leuprorelin acetate depot on the endocrinological changes and clinical improvement in women with endometriosis Y. Taketani, T. Uemura, H. Hoshiai and N. Terakawa	370

Section 9: Danazol

53	Analysis of danazol action K. Kato, K. Kato and N. Wake	381
54	Danazol decreases estrogen receptor (ER) and ER mRNA levels in peripheral monocytes due to suppression of the transcription rate of the ER gene J. Fujimoto, S. Ichigo, M. Hori, R. Misao, R. Hirose, Y. Nakanishi, H. Sakaguchi and T. Tamaya	386
55	Effects of danazol pretreatment for patients with endometriosis on their *in vitro* fertilization and embryo transfer outcomes N. Suganuma, T. Moriwaki, T. Ando, O. Narita, M. Osawa, T. Tanaka, H. Saito, M. Seki, O. Tsutsumi, H. Kanzaki, A. Hoshiai, S. Yamano, Y. Nagata, K. Matsuura and H. Okamura	392

Section 10: GnRH antagonists

56	Antagonistic analogs of LHRH in oncology and gynecology A.V. Schally, A.M. Comaru-Schally, D. Gonzalez-Barcena, T. Reissmann and J. Engel	401

57	GnRH analogs in gynecology: agonists and antagonists *R. Felberbaum and K. Diedrich*	414
58	Future possibilities for endometriosis treatment with GnRH antagonists *E.W. Bergink and H.J.T. Coelingh Bennink*	424
59	Development of an LHRH antagonist *T. Uemura, H. Minaguchi, H. Mori and Y. Taketani*	434

Section 11: *In vitro* fertilization

60	The place of *in vitro* fertilization in the treatment of endometriosis-related infertility *J.L. Pouly, M. Canis, L. Janny, P. Vye-Pouly, R. Zambrano, H. Laurichesse, R. Botroshvilli and C. Boyer-Medeville*	443
61	Assisted reproductive technologies, endometriosis and decision making *I.S. Tummon, B. Bany and J. Martin*	455
62	*In vitro* fertilization in patients with endometriosis *H. Saito, K. Nakahara, T. Saito, M. Ito, N. Ohta, T. Takahashi, N. Tezuka, N. Sakai and M. Hiroi*	461
63	The role of assisted reproductive techniques in endometriosis *S.C. Ng and S. Chew*	467
	Index	475

List of principal contributors

G.D. Adamson
Fertility Physicians of Northern California
540 University Avenue, Suite 200
Palo Alto
CA 94301
USA

D. Aoki
Department of Obstetrics & Gynecology
School of Medicine
Keio University
35 Shinano-machi
Shinjuku-ku
Tokyo 160
Japan

J. Belaisch
36 rue de Tocqueville
75017 Paris
France

E.W. Bergink
NV Organon
Scientific Development Group
PO Box 20
5430 BH Oss
The Netherlands

I.A. Brosens
Leuven Institute for Fertility and Embryology
Tiensevest 168
B-3000 Leuven
Belgium

C. Bulletti
Unit of Special Pelvic Surgery, Operative
  Laparoscopy and Hysteroscopy
1st Institute of Obstetrics & Gynecology
University of Bologna
Via Massarenti, 13
40138 Bologna
Italy

M. Canis
Centre Hospitalier Universitaire
Department of Obstetrics, Gynecology and
  Reproductive Medicine
Polyclinique de l'Hotel Dieu
13 Bd Charles de Gaulle 63033 Clermont-Ferrand
Cedex 1
France

Y.M. Choi
Department of Obstetrics and Gynecology
College of Medicine, Seoul National University
28 Yungun-Dong, Chongno-Ku
Seoul 110-744
Korea

P.G. Crosignani
Clinica Ostetrica e Ginecologica
Università di Milano
Via Commenda 12
20122 Milano
Italy

T.M. D'Hooghe
Leuven University Fertility Center and
  Department of Obstetrics & Gynecology
University Hospital Gasthuisberg
Herestraat 49
B-3000 Leuven
Belgium

K. Diedrich
Clinic for Obstetrics and Gynecology
University of Lubeck
Ratzeburger Allee 160
D-23538 Lubeck
Germany

W.P. Dmowski
Grant Hospital of Chicago
550 West Webster Avenue
Chicago, IL 60614
USA

J. Donnez
Department of Gynecology
Catholic University of Louvain
Cliniques Universitaires St-Luc
Avenue Hippocrate 10
1200 Brussels
Belgium

G.A.J. Dunselman
Department of Obstetrics and Gynecology
Academisch Ziekenhuis Maastricht
PO Box 5800
6202 AZ Maastricht
The Netherlands

J.L.H. Evers
Department of Obstetrics and Gynecology
Academisch Ziekenhuis Maastricht
PO Box 5800
6202 AZ Maastricht
The Netherlands

M. Filicori
Reproductive Endocrinology Center
Department of Obstetrics & Gynecology
University of Bologna
Bologna
Italy

C.A. Finn
Department of Veterinary Preclinical Sciences
The University of Liverpool
Leahurst
Chester High Road
Neston
Cheshire L64 7TE
UK

M. Fujii
Department of Obstetrics and Gynecology
Sapporo Medical University School of Medicine
South 1 West 17, Chuo-Ku
Sapporo 060
Japan

J. Fujimoto
Department of Obstetrics and Gynecology
Gifu University School of Medicine
40 Tsukasa-machi
Gifu 500
Japan

T. Fukaya
Department of Obstetrics and Gynecology
Tohoku University School of Medicine
1-1 Seiryomachi
Aoba-ku
Sendai 980-77
Japan

J. Gogusev
I.N.S.E.R.M. Unite 90
Hopital Necker-Enfants Malades
161 Rue de Sevres
75743 Paris Cedex 15
France

J.K. Halme
North Carolina Center for Reproductive Medicine
400 Ashville Avenue, Suite 200
Cary
NC 27511
USA

A.F. Haney
Division of Reproductive Endocrinology
 & Infertility
Duke University Medical Center
Box 2971
Durham
NC 27710
USA

T. Harada
Department of Obstetrics and Gynecology
Tottori University School of Medicine
Yonago 683
Japan

D.L. Healy
Monash University
Department of Obstetrics and Gynecology
Monash Medical Centre
Level 5, 246 Clayton Rd
Clayton, Victoria 3168
Australia

R. Honda
Department of Obstetrics and Gynecology
Kumamoto University School of Medicine
1-1-1 Honjo
Kumamoto 860
Japan

List of principal contributors

B.S. Hurst
Department of Obstetrics and Gynecology
University of Colorado Health Sciences Centre
4200 East Ninth Avenue
Box B198
Denver, Co 80262
USA

K. Kato
Department of Reproductive Endocrinology
Medical Institute of Bioregulation
Kyushu University
4546 Tsurimihara
Beppu, Oita 874
Japan

L.M. Kettel
San Diego Fertility Center
4150 Regents Park Row
Suite 325
La Jolla
CA 92075
USA

A. Lemay
Département d'Obstétrique et Gynécologie
Université Laval
Centre Hospitalier Universitaire de Québec
Pavillon St-Francois d'Assise
10, de l'Espinay
Québec G1L 3L5
Canada

B.A. Lessey
Department of Obstetrics and Gynecology
The University of North Carolina
   at Chapel Hill, School of Medicine
CB 7570, Old Clinic Building
Chapel Hill
NC 27599-7570
USA

Y.T. Lim
Department of Obstetrics and Gynecology
Kang Nam St Mary's Hospital
Catholic University Medical College
505 Banpodong Seochoku
Seoul 137-040
Korea

B. Lunenfeld
Department of Life Sciences
Bar-Ilan University
Ramat Gan 52900
Israel

D.C. Martin
University of Tennessee, Memphis
1717 Kirby Parkway, Suite 100
Memphis, TN 38120-4331
USA

H. Minaguchi
Department of Obstetrics and Gynecology
Yokohama City University School of Medicine
3-9 Fukuura
Kanazawa-ku
Yokohama 236
Japan

P. Miron
Montreal Institute for Reproductive Medicine
   (Bio-IMRM R&D Inc)
1100 Beaumont Avenue, Suite 305
Ville Mont-Royal
Québec H3P 3H5
Canada

H. Mori
Department of Obstetrics and Gynecology
Teikyo University School of Medicine
2-11-1 Kaga
Itabashi-ku
Tokyo 173
Japan

C. Nezhat
Stanford Endoscopy Center for Training &
   Technology (S.E.C.T.T.)
Stanford University School of Medicine
Medical School Office Building, Suite X340
Stanford, CA 94305-5408
USA

S.C. Ng
University Department of Obstetrics & Gynecology
National University Hospital
Lower Kent Ridge Road
Singapore 119074
Republic of Singapore

M. Nisolle
Department of Gynecology
University of Louvain
Cliniques Universitaires St-Luc
Avenue Hippocrate 10
1200 Brussels
Belgium

W. Nothnick
Department of Obstetrics and Gynecology
Division of Reproductive Endocrinology
University of Kentucky
800 Rose Street
Lexington
Kentucky 40536-0084
USA

K. Okuda
Department of Obstetrics and Gynecology
Osaka Medical College
2-7 Daigaku-cho
Takatsuki
Osaka 569
Japan

K.G. Osteen
Reproductive Medicine Research Laboratory
Department of Obstetrics and Gynecology
C-1100 Medical Center North
Vanderbilt University School of Medicine
Nashville, TN 37232-2515
USA

H. Ota
Department of Obstetrics and Gynecology
Akita University School of Medicine
1-1-1 Hondo
Akita City
Akita-ken 010
Japan

Y. Otsuki
Department of Anatomy and Biology
Osaka Medical College
2-7 Daigaku-machi
Takatsuki, Osaka 569
Japan

S.F. Palter
Yale Office Laparoscopy Program
Department of Obstetrics & Gynecology
Yale University School of Medicine
PO Box 208063
New Haven, CT 06520-8063
USA

J.L. Pouly
Department of Gynecology, Obstetrics and Reproductive Medicine
Polyclinique de l'Hôtel-Dieu
BP 69 Centre Hospitalier Universitaire
13 Boulevard Charles de Gaulle
63003 Clermont-Ferrand
France

J.A. Rock
Department of Gynecology and Obstetrics
Emory University School of Medicine
Woodruff Memorial Research Building
1639 Pierce Drive, Room 4208 WMB
Atlanta, GA 30322
USA

H. Saito
Department of Obstetrics and Gynecology
Yamagata University School of Medicine
2-2-2 Iidanishi
Yamagata 990 23
Japan

K. Satoh
Department of Obstetrics and Gynecology
Nihon University School of Medicine
30-1 Oyaguchi-kamimachi
Itabashi-ku
Tokyo 173
Japan

A.V. Schally
Department of Medicine
Tulane Medical Center
Section of Experimental Medicine
1430 Tulane Avenue
New Orleans
LA 70112-2699
USA

R.S. Schenken
Department of Obstetrics and Gynecology
University of Texas
Health Science Center at San Antonio
7703 Floyd Curl Drive
San Antonio
TX 78284-7836
USA

K.-W. Schweppe
Department of Obstetrics and Gynecology
KKH Ammerland, Academic Teaching Hospital
University of Göttingen
Am Flutter 47
D-26655 Westerstede
Germany

List of principal contributors

H. Shigeta
Department of Obstetrics and Gynecology
Yokohama City University
School of Medicine
3-9 Fukuura
Kanazawa-ku
Yokohama 236
Japan

N. Suganuma
Department of Obstetrics and Gynecology
Nagoya University School of Medicine
65 Tsurumai-cho
Showa-ku
Nagoya 466
Japan

J. Sugawara
Department of Obstetrics and Gynecology
Tohoku University School of Medicine
1-1 Seiryomachi
Aobaku
Sendai 980-77
Japan

O. Sugimoto
Osaka Medical College
28-1 Ishida Moriminami-cho
Fushimi-ku
Kyoto 601-13
Japan

C.J.G. Sutton
Waterden Road Clinic
8 Waterden Road
Guildford
Surrey GU1 2AW
UK

M. Taga
Department of Obstetrics & Gynecology
Yokohama City University School of Medicine
3-9 Fukuura
Kanazawa-ku
Yokohama 236
Japan

Y. Taketani
Department of Obstetrics and Gynecology
Faculty of Medicine
University of Tokyo 7-3-1
Hongo
Bunkyo-ku
Tokyo

N. Terakawa
Department of Obstetrics and Gynecology
Tottori University School of Medicine
86 Nishimachi
Yonago 683
Japan

I.S. Tummon
Department of Gynaecology & Reproductive Medicine
London Health Sciences Centre
University Hospital Campus
339 Windermere Road
London, Ontario N6A 5A5
Canada

T. Uemura
Department of Obstetrics and Gynecology
Yokohama City University School of Medicine
3-9 Fukuura
Kanazawa-ku
Yokohama 236
Japan

P. Viganò
II Department of Obstetrics and Gynecology and IRCCS Centro Auxologico Italiano
University of Milan
Milan
Italy

M. Wingfield
Monash University
Department of Obstetrics and Gynecology
Monash Medical Center
Level 5, 246 Clayton Road
Clayton, Victoria 3168
Australia

C.A. Winkel
Department of Obstetrics and Gynecology
Jefferson Medical College
Thomas Jefferson University
834 Chestnut Street
Philadelphia
PA 19107
USA

C. Wood
Monash Univesity
Ashbutton
Clayton, Victoria 3168
Australia

Foreword

Endometriosis remains a mysterious and elusive disease. The definition and classification of the disease still needs international consensus, but it is thought to affect as many as 10–15% of all women of reproductive age. Although malignant transformation of the disease is rare, the nature of endometriosis itself is invasive and persistent, and some of the complications, such as bowel obstruction and inflammation, become life-threatening. Sterility caused by endometriosis has proved to be one of the major concerns in the fields of research in reproduction.

In the last decade the study of endometriosis has shown tremendous advances with the development of varied, innovative techniques, but still leaves much to be discovered. Helped by the valuable suggestions and recommendations of the International Scientific Committee, the 5th World Congress on Endometriosis in Yokohama, Japan, made every effort to organize a program which covers this recent progress. Thus, the meeting featured all of the latest information and insights regarding endometriosis, including etiology and natural history, physiology of the uterus and endometrium, immunology, classification, medical and surgical treatment, etc. Research on the pathogenesis of endometriosis was especially focused on a better understanding of the cellular mechanisms, which may provide important clues for future developments in the prevention and therapy of endometriosis.

We thank Professor I. Brosens and the many other outstanding scientists for their presentations and unlimited contributions offered to the Congress.

The first World Congress on Endometriosis was held in 1986 in Clermont-Ferrand, France, organized by Professor Maurice Bruhart and colleagues, and has been successfully followed every two years. The Yokohama meeting was the first convening in Asia; it was successful, attracting 920 delegates from 54 countries. Each of the five congresses has been successful in playing an important role in the exchange of knowledge, ideas and hope through stimulating presentations and active, instructive communication, with an ultimate goal of reducing the suffering and despair caused by endometriosis and improving health care for women worldwide.

The Sixth World Congress on Endometriosis is scheduled to be held in Quebec City, Canada, in 1998.

Hiroshi Minaguchi
Osamu Sugimoto
Coordinators of the 5th World Congress on Endometriosis

Section 1

Etiology and natural history of endometriosis

The uterus and menstruation in history and evolution

C.A. Finn

It has been suspected for a long time that endometriosis is associated with menstruation and it is now generally accepted that the cause of the disease is to be found in the retrograde discharge of menstrual fluid at the end of the ovarian cycle. An understanding of the origins and meaning of menstruation is therefore of concern in the study of endometriosis.

Menstruation in history

Interest in menstruation goes back a very long time, in fact at the time of Aristotle menstrual fluid was a major plank in thinking about the origin of human life[1]. To philosophers at the time of Aristotle there were two secretions which came out of the human reproductive organs: semen from the penis of the male and menstrual fluid from the vagina of women. They must have known that the placing of the semen into the woman's vagina resulted in the birth of a baby, although exactly when this association was made is not known. Putting the known facts together, Aristotle proposed that the semen acted on the menstrual fluid inside the female to cause it to form into a baby. It was likened to the coagulation of milk by renin. The menstrual fluid provided the material on which the sperm acted.

That, then, the female does not contribute semen to generation [says Aristotle], but does contribute something, and that this is the matter of the cata-menia, or that which is analogous to it in bloodless animals, is clear from what has been said, and also from a general and abstract survey of the question. For there must needs be that which generates and that from which it generates, even if these be one, still they must be distinct in form and their essence must be different; and in those animals that have these powers separate in two sexes the body and nature of the active and passive sex also differ. If, then, the male stands for the effective and active, and the female, considered as female, for the pas-sive, it follows that what the female would contribute to the semen of the male would not be semen but material for the semen to work upon. This is just what we find to be the case, for the catamenia have in their nature an affinity to the primitive matter.

Not surprisingly, at that time the male was given the role of controller and designer of the process. This idea started in Greece, although it must have passed to India, where it gave rise to the unfortunate tradition of child brides. The Indians thought that as the menstrual fluid represented the material from which life was made, every time a woman menstruated a life was being wasted. It was therefore incumbent on a father to avoid this calamity by settling his daughter into the home and bed of a husband before she started to menstruate[1].

This idea, as strange as it may seem to us now, survived for over 1000 years, in fact until the time of Harvey[2], who showed from dissections of deer in Windsor Forest that there was no menstrual fluid in the uterus after copulation and therefore that the theory could not be correct. It is very interesting[3] to note that the deer which Harvey dissected would probably not have been pregnant, due to the fact that the males rutted a month earlier than ovulation in females, so he was lucky to have got the right answer, but probably for the wrong reason! During the 1000 years between Aristotle and Harvey, there were of course quite a lot of other ideas on menstruation. Galen for instance thought it was nature's way of getting rid of excess blood from the body and in one of his many medical books he gave very precise instruction on how blood was to be removed from women who failed to menstruate[4]. Isodore of Seville made some interesting observations on menstruation[5]. Isodore was Bishop of Seville in the 6th century. He proposed that infertility was due to the degree of thickness or thinness of either the semen or the menstrual fluid. Upon its thickness or thinness depended whether the resulting fluid stuck to the walls of the uterus. Isodore also made the interesting observation that 'women are the only menstrual animal', suggesting a good overall acquaintance with animals. Ettmuller[6] also commented on the fact that other animals do not menstruate. His explanation for this was that animals had so many offspring that there was no blood left over to waste by releasing it from the vagina. It is of course very relevant to remember that there were no compound microscopes around at that time and early workers could have had no idea of what was in either semen or the menstrual fluid. Isodore realized that menstrual fluid was no ordinary blood; according to him, 'On contact with this gore, crops do not generate, wine goes sour, trees lose their fruit, iron is corrupted by rust, copper is blackened. Should dogs eat any of it they go mad. Even bituminous glue which is dissolved neither by rain nor by (strong) water, polluted by this gore, falls apart by itself'.

Myths surrounding the process of menstruation have abounded right up to the present day. From the medical point of view, in spite of its primal role in the creation of babies, the fluid was considered to be unclean. Menstruating matrons were not able to enter the temples in Roman times, and to have intercourse during menstruation was considered to be a sin by the Catholic Church. Progress on understanding the true cause of procreation depended of course on the invention of the compound microscope and the discovery of the sperm and ovum. Much progress in understanding reproductive processes took place in the latter part of the 19th and early years of the 20th centuries. Estrous cycles and their hormonal control were worked out for many animals and the relationship between ovulation, copulation and pregnancy was soon apparent. In these post-Darwinian times it was assumed that what applied to animals must be true for humans. Unfortunately, this was not true. Some animals were known to bleed from the vagina and this was shown clearly to be associated with ovulation and estrus. Not many animals in fact do bleed at estrus to any great extent, but the one that does is of course man's oldest and closest ally, the dog. The discharge from the bitch's vagina must have been noticed frequently by both biologists and laymen, and it required no great feat of imagination to decide that proestrous bleeding in the bitch is equivalent to menstruation; even today many lay people believe this to be so. In fact some biologists fail to make the distinction. In a 20th century textbook of embryology it is stated that in some women there is a small menstrual flow (the 'Kleine Regel') at the time of ovulation[7]. The great Victorian biologists were convinced of the equivalence of the two processes, as can be seen clearly in the first edition of Marshall's famous work on *The Physiology of Reproduction*[8]. However, those who actually dealt with the condition – obstetricians, physicians and pathologists – were not so easily convinced and held to the view that menstruation was associated with the end of the ovarian cycle when an ovum had failed to implant[9]. As pointed out earlier, medical teaching since the time of Aristotle had associated menstruation with failure of pregnancy and the medical profession quite rightly did not yield this position. In fact, it soon became accepted that there is no relationship between proestrous bleeding in the bitch and menstruation in women, the former being due to diapedesis of red blood cells through the wall of the uterine blood vessels, and the latter being the result of breakdown of the wall of the uterus. It is interesting that, with the failure of this foray into menstruation, biologists have since showed very little interest in the subject and left it to the medical profession.

Consequently, whilst there has been a vast amount of work on the mechanisms of menstruation, not surprising in view of its clinical importance, there has been little on its biological significance. Since Darwin's time it has been assumed that any structure or physiological process must have some useful purpose, which would ensure its evolution. Therefore, during the last century, several authors put forward theories to explain why women menstruate. In the 1930s a Dr Ruddock[10] published a book on medical science called *Vitolagy*. In this he suggested that the purpose of menstruation was to give women vicarious sexual pleasure, thus preserving their virginity. He did, however, add that some authorities thought that menstruation was simply a way of getting rid of an unimplanted egg. Where he got his first suggestion from is anybody's guess!

More recently, there has been a serious suggestion that the reason menstruation has evolved, in spite of causing loss of blood (obviously not a desirable outcome), is that it is a method of getting rid of pathogens which are taken into the uterus attached to spermatozoa[11]. This theory can be criticized from several angles. The most common reason for the occurrence of menstruation is the absence of sperm; their presence is responsible for preventing menstruation taking place. It is difficult to see how menstruation could have evolved in response to something that causes it not to occur. Furthermore, if menstruation had evolved to combat infection associated with insemination, then all internal fertilizers (all mammals, birds and reptiles and many amphibia and fishes) should menstruate, which they do not.

Another recent theory is that menstrual fluid provides a signal to other members of the species indicating reproductive competence[12]. This does not seem very likely, in view of its occurrence at the end of the cycle. Many of the other primates give out sexual signals, but always during estrus; in fact there have been suggestions that women give out pheromones at the time of ovulation.

Another recent suggestion is that menstruation removes from the uterus blastocysts which have not implanted or failed to maintain their implantation[13]. This could well be a useful consequence of menstruation, but it is difficult to see why it should be confined to just a few primates.

There is also an argument as to whether it is valid to look for an explanation for menstruation based on natural selection. Most genetic changes and gene duplication on which selection is based (either beneficial or harmful), would be realized before an animal passed on its genes to the next generation. In the case of menstruation, however, the genes would in many cases be passed on before any deleterious effect became apparent, so that the chance of evolutionary pressures would be small.

If menstruation has not evolved in response to some direct selective pressure, then how has it evolved? To answer this question, it is useful to follow how the uterus has evolved.

The evolution of the uterus and menstruation

In mammals the uterus is a major organ of reproduction, forming the largest part of the female reproductive tract and, during pregnancy, occupying a large portion of the abdomen. However, in other orders it is considerably less prominent and in fact is not present in most animals, not even in all vertebrate species. An understanding of how the uterus evolved and the forces bringing about its evolution help us to appreciate its present form and function in mammals. The uterus did not suddenly appear as it is today, but has evolved gradually over millions of years.

As with other structures some indication of the evolution can be obtained from an examination of the embryology of the organ in mammals. The development of the reproductive tract in both the male and the female is intimately related to the development of the excretory organs (especially the mesonephros). The male reproductive tract takes over the mesonephric tubule system, and the mesonephric duct (Wolffian duct) forms the vas deferens, for the transport of sperm out of the animal. This, however, will only take place if androgen is present for a short critical period during fetal life. If androgen is not present at this time the mesonephric tubules and ducts involute. The female reproductive tract develops from tubes which form in association with the mesonephros and then grows caudally towards the urogenital sinus. These are the paramesonephric or Müllerian ducts. The ducts from either side in eutherians fuse caudally for varying lengths, depending on the species, and then open to the outside usually through a single opening. As development proceeds, the Müllerian duct differentiates into the oviduct, uterus, cervix and part of the vagina, the latter forming largely from the ectoderm of the urogenital sinus. The growth and differentiation of the female tract does not require the presence of hormone, but if anti-Müllerian hormone is secreted by the Sertoli cells of the male gonad at the critical period for reproductive tract development (this varies with species but is prenatal) then the Müllerian ducts fail to develop. The development of the female tract is thus the default condition. To obtain development of the male tract, the developing gonad must be male.

In eutherian mammals the uterus has evolved as a chamber in which the embryo and fetus can be nourished and protected. Its evolution was a necessary prerequisite for viviparity, but viviparity is not exclusive to mammals. Viviparous forms are found in many other classes, in fact among vertebrates the only classes not containing viviparous species are Cyclostomata and Aves, and among mammals not all orders are viviparous (monotremes lay eggs). Viviparity has evolved separately more than 100 times and it is likely that viviparity evolved independently in mammals from egg-laying reptiles. It is only in mammals that viviparity has become the norm. This will be discussed later. In following the evolution of the reproductive tract one has to rely heavily on observations of living species, which have themselves evolved to a greater or lesser extent from the primitive condition. Very little information about the reproductive tract can be obtained from fossils.

To trace the evolution of the uterus it is not very instructive to go further back than the chordates. Although species in other phyla have tubes for the transport of ova, these are not homologous to the structure which develops from the Müllerian duct. In fact the mesonephros as an organ of excretion first appears in vertebrates. Primitive chordates, like the amphioxus, have a different excretory system.

The ovaries of amphioxus are metameric and the ova are shed into the atrium (a cavity formed by a fold of skin over the gill slits). From there they pass to the outside through a pore, the atriopore. There is no duct system for the transport of ova, and fertilization is external. Clearly, the evolution of the mammalian uterus did not start in early chordates. The first appearance of the antecedent of the mammalian kidney is seen in primitive vertebrates, the cyclostomes (extant examples of which are lampreys and hagfish). This is the archinephros, with its archinephric duct. The former evolved into the mesonephros in cyclostomes and functions as an excretory organ, but there is no Müllerian duct and the mesonephric ducts are not used for the transport of gametes.

The gonads develop from mesoderm on the medial side of the archinephros, and in lampreys and hagfish the ova or sperm pass directly into the celom and then to the outside through a genital pore, which is closely associated with the opening of the archinephric duct to form a urogenital aperture. Fertilization is external.

A duct for the transport of ova first appeared in jawed fishes. Among the fishes there are many which still retain external fertilization and some (a few teleosts; family Salmonidae) in which the eggs pass into the celom and then escape through abdominal pores. Most teleosts, however, have an oviduct. This is formed from folds of peritoneum which also surround the ovary. The majority of teleosts have external fertilization, so the oviduct is used solely for the transport of ova to the outside, although it should be mentioned that in some modern teleosts embryos develop in the ovarian cavity, so that fertilization must have evolved to be internal in these.

The development of a tube between the ovary and the external environment was an essential first stage to internal fertilization. Most Elasmobranch fishes have internal fertilization and we see in these the forerunner of the Müllerian duct. This forms by splitting of the archinephric duct and acts as a duct for the transport of ova and sperm and a vessel in which fertilization can take place.

Amphibians have evolved away from fishes in many respects (respiration, locomotion) which allows them to live and move on land. However, as regards reproduction they have evolved little and they have to return to water to reproduce. Most of the anurans, for example, retain external fertilization, with the male depositing his sperm over the ova as they emerge from the female. Most urodeles have internal fertilization, although not with copulation. The sperm are laid by the male in small packets called spermatophores, which are then picked up by the female by muscular activity of the cloacal lips and deposited in specialized structures attached to the cloaca, the spermathecae. Ova can thus be fertilized on their way to the cloaca.

Internal fertilization was clearly a major step in the evolution of reproduction. It is of course a more efficient method of getting male and female gametes together and this was presumably the selective force ensuring it. However, of greater significance is the possibility that internal fertilization opens up of reproduction on dry land. External fertilization can only take place in water and it was therefore the evolution of the oviduct (Müllerian duct) which allowed the reptiles to conquer land. At the same time the presence of organisms of different genetic constitution, first the spermatozoa and then the zygote inside the mother, presented problems. This will be discussed later. A further consequence of internal fertilization was that the evolution of the embryo and the uterus had to proceed interdependently.

Many modern fishes have internal fertilization, but, as many amphibians do not, it is likely that the early amphibians evolved from externally fertilizing fishes. It is tempting to suggest that the move towards internal fertilization seen in urodele amphibians was critical in allowing the further evolution of vertebrates, leading to the age of reptiles.

Whilst intromission and internal fertilization were the first step in allowing reproduction on dry land, they were not in themselves sufficient. Survival and growth of the zygote on land requires a supply of nutrients, access to respiratory gases and protection of the embryo whilst it is developing, both against injury and against desiccation. The interrelated evolution of the Müllerian duct and the development of the embryonic membranes brings this about. A store of nutrients is added to the ova as they develop in the ovary, from material synthesized in the liver but processed in the ovarian follicle. After fertilization this yolk is surrounded by a membrane, the yolk sac, which allows it to be absorbed by the embryo. Several mechanisms evolved to protect the embryo against desiccation and damage. Initially there was the formation of the amnion around the embryo, so that it could grow in an aqueous constant-pressure environment. This is augmented by the laying down of protective coverings around the zygotes as they pass down the oviduct. The most obvious of these in reptiles and birds are a layer of albumen, shell membrane and shell. Albumen plays an important role in protection against desiccation, and the shell prevent physical damage. These layers are added during the passage of the egg down the oviduct, which has now become specialized into distinct areas, each secreting and adding a separate layer to the egg. These divisions of the oviduct can be clearly seen in crocodiles[14].

With the embryo enclosed inside a shell (cleidoic egg), a new problem was presented. The metabolism of amino acids involved in the growth and development of the embryo leads to the production of nitrogenous waste products. Animals developing in water can easily get rid of these as urea, which is soluble in water. However, inside a closed shell the concentrations of urea would rapidly become toxic. To combat this the embryo evolved mechanisms for the conversion of urea to uric acid, which is insoluble, and then developed a sac from the gut in which to store the uric acid, the allantois[15]. It is interesting that the embryonic membranes that play such an important role in obstetrics originally evolved to allow reptiles to live on land.

Thus, in reptiles the oviduct has developed from a simple tube for the transport of ova and sperm to an active glandular organ to play an active part in the survival of the embryo. This protective role is taken a stage further in some reptiles, in which the egg is retained in the oviduct during part or all of the embryo's development (ovoviviparity). As with oviparous development, the mother's contribution to the nutrition of the embryo has come from the provision of yolk to the ova.

The next major step was for the embryo to spend a longer period in the Müllerian duct and to obtain not just protection but also nutrients. As mentioned earlier viviparity with retention of the embryo in the mother has evolved in all classes of vertebrates except birds. Viviparity confers obvious advantages on the embryo in terms of protection and food supply. However, in spite of this, the majority of modern fishes, amphibia and reptiles and all birds have retained egg laying, whereas mammals have adopted viviparity almost universally. It would appear, therefore, to confer some particular advantage on mammals. This is possibly related to the evolution of homeothermy. Maintenance of body temperature obviously allowed mammals to survive in colder environments and to be active regardless of the outside temperature. It would, however, present considerable problems with regard to the embryo, which would not develop mechanisms for maintaining and controlling its temperature until late in its development. Birds solved this problem by incubating their eggs in nests; this would have been a hazardous method for warm-blooded animals living on land. Of the egg-laying mammals, the duck-billed platypus solves it by putting the egg in a pouch of skin. It is only the spiny anteater that builds a burrow as an incubator in which to hatch its eggs. Keeping the embryo inside the body is probably the easiest way of maintaining it at the correct temperature and probably explains the almost universal adoption of viviparity in mammals. The obvious question then is why no birds have evolved to be viviparous. The usual answer given to this is that flying would be difficult with young inside. This teleological answer may be true, but bats fly, as do some very heavy birds and viviparous insects.

Furthermore, some birds live mostly on land or water. The whole order of ratites, which includes ostriches and emus, do not fly. Even if pregnancy had restricted movement and grounded birds during the latter part of pregnancy, it would surely be easier to feed and keep embryos warm in the uterus than in a nest. The simplest explanation is that viviparity has not evolved in birds, because the chance genetic changes necessary to set off its evolution did not occur. Without this the advantage or disadvantage would be irrelevant.

Viviparity first occurred in fishes, but it is likely that the mammal-like reptiles (therapsids) from which mammals evolved were oviparous. Some interesting adaptations of the oviduct have occurred to facilitate viviparity in amphibians and reptiles, but it is unlikely that these are on the line of evolution leading to the development of the mammalian uterus and are therefore not relevant to its evolution.

The most primitive mammals, the monotremes, lay eggs, and like other egg-laying vertebrates they get much of the nutrients for embryonic development from the yolk, synthesized in the liver and laid down in the ovary. However, unlike the others, a significant amount of nutrients is added to the yolk during a lengthy sojourn of the embryo in the oviduct[16]. This is in spite of the fact that a shell membrane is laid down in the upper part of the oviduct and a hard shell in the lower. It appears that substances secreted by glands in the oviduct are absorbed by the yolk sac, thus increasing the amount of nutrients contained in the yolk and thus available to the embryo.

In monotremes, the Müllerian duct, in addition to providing a duct for the conduction of ova and sperm and synthesis of the protective covering for the embryo, has taken on a further function, that of assisting in the nutrition of the embryo. This development was a crucial step in the evolution of the uterus. The glands in the lower part of the oviduct, which had previously been responsible for the synthesis of the shell, have now taken on an additional function, secreting food for the embryo (embryotrophe). This type of nutrition in which substances are synthesized in the uterine glands, passed into the uterine lumen and then absorbed by the trophoblast is called histotrophic. In marsupials, little yolk is laid down in the ovum, but an albuminous coating and a shell membrane forms around the ovum in the upper part of the oviduct. These soon disappear and histotrophic nutrition from the uterine glands forms the major part of embryonic nutrition before birth in most marsupials. The yolk sac fuses with the trophoblast, and material is absorbed from the uterus and passes into the vitelline blood vessels. However, there are a few marsupial species in which the next stage in the evolution of the uterus can be seen – the passage of materials directly between the maternal and fetal bloodstreams. This coincides with the further development of the allantois, which had previously acted mainly as a reservoir for excretory products. The allantois enlarges and grows towards the trophoblast, with which it joins to form the allantochorion. Fetal blood vessels vascularize the allantochorion, which becomes closely apposed to the uterine luminal epithelium. There is now sufficiently close contact between the blood vessels of the fetus and the mother to allow exchange of materials between the two systems. This is known as hemotrophic fetal nutrition. In most eutherian mammals this is the main method of providing nutrients to the embryo and fetus. Yolk plays little if any part, but histotrophic nutrition is still an important part of embryo nutrition in the early stages of pregnancy in many species.

Further evolution of the uterus has resulted in improvements in the intimacy of the contact between the fetus and mother (reviewed in reference 17). Initially this involved an increase in the surface area of contact between the allantochorion and uterine luminal epithelium. The trophoblast and uterus increased massively in size, while the uterine surface became covered with microvilli, to which the trophoblast was closely apposed. Thus the area of contact for exchange increased dramatically.

However, a few species evolved in a different direction. In these the blastocyst remained small but moved out of the uterine lumen to lie inside the wall of the uterus, thus getting the trophoblast into very close apposition to the maternal blood. One method of doing this is seen in rats and mice. In these the blastocyst initially locates itself on one side of the uterine lumen. This triggers a programmed cell death response in the uterine luminal epithelial cells abutting the trophoblast[18]. The dead epithelial cells are phagocytosed by the trophoblast, thus removing the epithelial cells and locating the blastocyst among the stromal cells. An alternative method, which has evolved to its peak in the human, is for the trophoblast to burrow actively through the uterine luminal epithelium. In both these processes there is increased participation of the trophoblast, which up to now has been largely concerned with the transfer of gases and nutrients. In rodents the trophoblast gives a signal that causes the uterine epithelium to die, and once this has happened it actively invades the stroma. The invasive potential of the trophoblast when the epithelial barrier is broken was shown by placing blastocysts in other tissues, such as the kidney or testis[19]. In women the trophoblast becomes very aggressive and by its own activity burrows through the epithelium (part of the trophoblast becomes a syncytium, which may assist in this). The trophoblast also starts taking an active role in the production of hormones involved in the maintenance of pregnancy.

Having the blastocyst inside the uterus was a major step in the evolution of the uterus. In the early stages of its evolution the Müllerian duct had simply been a duct to transport a genetically similar ovum; this presumably presented few problems with foreign bodies. With the advent of internal fertilization the oviduct first had to contend with foreign tissue (sperm) from a genetically distinct mate and then from a genetically distinct zygote. By this stage of evolution animals had evolved mechanisms to deal with problems associated with invasion by foreign objects, by mounting a leukocyte reaction. This can be seen in primitive vertebrates and in some invertebrates[20]. In the mammalian uterus after mating, there is a massive passage of leukocytes into the uterine lumen; these remove the majority of the sperm by phagocytosis.

The zygote presents another problem. It is of course genetically distinct from the mother. However, the initial stages of fertilization and development occur inside the zona pellucida, which is secreted by the ovum before fertilization. This presumably protects the sperm and then acts as an initial barrier to factors that would allow the fertilized ovum to be recognized as a foreign object. In most vertebrates this covering is then rapidly augmented by secretions of the uterus (albumen, shell membranes, shell), further increasing the barriers between the zygote and its mother's tissues. The secretion of albumen may be a modified response to a foreign body. In hens a piece of foreign tissue, if present in the oviduct, will be covered in albumen and shell. With eutherian mammals (and presumably some of the other viviparous vertebrates) the absence of tertiary egg membranes and the removal of the zona pellucida exposes the uterus to foreign antigens.

The immunological problems presented by this are immense and have been widely studied. However, the inflammation response, which is a much more primitive and non-specific response[20], would have to have been overcome first for the embryo to survive long enough for the immune response to be a problem. It appears that a major factor in suppressing the initial inflammatory reaction is the high level of progesterone present at the time when the zygote arrives in the uterus and removes its zona. This appears to be sufficient, at least initially, in animals in which the embryo remains inside the lumen of the uterus. How the progesterone works is not known, although it is similar in structure to the main anti-inflammatory steroids from the adrenal cortex. If the source of progesterone is removed in sheep[21] (which have non-invasive implantation) or mice[22] or guinea-pigs[23], then there is a massive leukocyte invasion. Progesterone is a major factor in the ability of the uterus to maintain the fetus within the uterus. The evolution of the corpus luteum as an endocrine organ has clearly been a major factor in the evolution of viviparity in mammals[24]. Callard and colleagues[24] proposed a dual role for progesterone in the evolution of viviparity: firstly, the inhibition of myometrial contractions and secondly, the inhibition of estrogen-induced vitellogenesis. The suppression of the inflammatory reaction would be a third role. The corpus luteum of ovulation is generally found in viviparous animals and forms from the granulosa and thecal cells of the follicle, which in egg-laying species are involved in the processing of yolk.

In animals in which the blastocyst actually embeds inside the wall of the uterus, further problems had to be overcome. Having passed through the endometrial epithelium, the blastocyst lies in the endometrial stroma. This presents a dual problem. Firstly, the uterus is at risk from the invasiveness of the trophoblast and secondly, the embryo is at a greater risk from an inflammatory reaction by the endometrium. This appears to be overcome in rodents by the decidual cell reaction in the stroma. In preparation for the arrival of the blastocyst the stromal cells proliferate under the influence of progesterone. In areas in which a blastocyst is present, changes take place in the stroma to produce the decidual cell reaction. Contact between the trophoblast and the uterine epithelium provides a trigger to the endometrium; this not only causes the adjacent epithelial cells to die (discussed earlier) but also stimulates differentiation of the stroma. This involves transformation of stromal fibroblasts into decidual cells, increased permeability of blood vessels leading to edema of the stroma and migration of cells from the bone marrow and their development into specialized granular cells. These later become localized in the metrial area to become the metrial gland. These changes in the endometrial stroma appear to protect the uterus by encasing the embryo in a solid mass of cells joined together by gap junctions[25]. They are only found in areas of the uterus where a blastocyst is present. Similar changes in which the stroma is clearly differentiated into three zones with massive development of blood vessels occur in the endometrium of women at the end of the menstrual cycle. Stromal fibroblasts around the blood vessels transform into decidual cells, granular cells pass from the blood and edema develops in the stroma. Similar changes are seen in apes and old world monkeys, although the information available is considerably less.

It is clear that the changes in humans and rodents are similar, except that in the human they occur at the end of every menstrual cycle and are dependent on the presence of ovarian hormones only, whereas in rodents, in addition to the correct hormone milieu, the presence of a blastocyst is required to trigger the final stages of stromal differentiation.

This differentiation of the endometrial stroma represents a further stage in the evolution of the uterus. It is tempting to think that the reaction of the endometrium to a blastocyst has evolved from the inflammation reaction that follows trauma or the presence of a foreign body[26]. Certainly in rodents the fact that trauma or the presence of oil or carrageenin in the uterus can trigger a reaction is reminiscent of an inflammation response, as is the increased vascular permeability and the migration of leukocytes. The similarity of decidual tissue to granulation tissue was noted many years ago[27] and it has been suggested that the decidual cell reaction has evolved from the granulation tissue response, which follows inflammation as a protective mechanism to protect the uterus against the trophoblast[26]. Recently several cytokines and proteases associated with inflammation have been shown to be present at implantation in the endometrium. If the above suggestions are valid, the presence of inflammatory cytokines in the uterus at the time of implantation is not surprising. What is not clear is whether they have been incorporated into the implantation reaction and perform an essential function in the process or are simply relics of a suppressed inflammation response. There have been suggestions that some may be involved in the uterine control of embryonic development. This would represent a very considerable step in the evolution of the Müllerian duct and should not be accepted without very good evidence, which is not at present available.

A problem with attempting to relate the implantation reaction seen in rodents and the premenstrual changes in the endometrium of women with an inflammation reaction is that in women the endometrial stroma undergoes differentiation at the end of the cycle, regardless of whether a blastocyst is present or not. There is edema, decidual cell formation and passage of leukocytes into the stroma. If the implantation reaction of mammals has evolved from the foreign body response to a blastocyst, then the differentiation of the endometrium at the end of the cycle in women must represent further evolution of the uterus to ensure a response in anticipation of a blastocyst. Such anticipatory changes do occur in other physiological systems. For example, increased heart rate in anticipation of muscular exercise, and increased secretion of insulin during a meal in anticipation of increased blood sugar levels. Anticipatory preparation of the endometrium may have been a necessary evolutionary change associated with increased aggressiveness of the trophoblast, which does not just trigger programmed cell death in the uterine epithelium (as in the rodent) but actively burrows through the epithelium. Once again it appears that the evolution of the trophoblast and the endometrium have gone hand in hand.

A consequence of the anticipatory development of the endometrium under the control of ovarian hormones is that at the end of the menstrual cycle, with the demise of the corpus luteum and the sudden drop in progesterone support, the differentiated tissue and blood vessels will break down, with hemorrhage and tissue desquamation (menstruation). Therefore, it is suggested that menstruation is a consequence of the evolution of the endometrium in response to evolutionary changes in the trophoblast, to enable it more readily to tap the blood supply of its mother.

With the removal of progesterone, the uterine reaction in anticipation of a blastocyst, which had been modified by the progesterone, takes on the nature of a full-blooded inflammation reaction, with tissue desquamation and bleeding. Mice do not menstruate, because they do not undergo the decidual cell reaction, except during pregnancy. However, if ovariectomized mice are treated with ovarian hormones to sensitize the endometrium for decidualization, they will respond to an intraluminal injection of oil with a decidual reaction. This is dependent on a continued supply of progesterone. If this is stopped, the decidual tissue breaks down, with bleeding in the endometrium[28]. This is similar to menstruation in women and provides experimental support for the suggested answer to the question: why do women menstruate?

References

1. Needham, J. (1959). *A History of Embryology*, 2nd edn. (Cambridge: Cambridge University Press)
2. Harvey, W. (1666). *Exercitationes de Generatione Animalium*. (Padua: P. Frambotti)
3. Short, R.V. (1977). The discovery of the ovaries. In Zuckerman, S. and Weir, B.J. (eds.) *The Ovary*, 2nd edn. (New York: Academic Press)
4. Trotula of Salerno (11th century). *The Diseases of Women*, translated by Elizabeth Mason-Hohl, 1940. (Los Angeles: Ward Ritchie)
5. Grant, E. (ed.) (1964). *A Source Book in Medieval Science*. (Cambridge, MA: Harvard University Press)
6. Ettmuller, M. (1696). *Opera Medica*. (Amsterdam: Rips)
7. Harrison, R.G. (1959). *A Textbook of Human Embryology*. (Oxford: Blackwell)
8. Marshall, F.H.A. (1910). *The Physiology of Reproduction*. (London, New York, Bombay and Calcutta: Longman's Green)
9. Grosser, O. (1910). The development of the egg membranes and the placenta: menstruation. In Keibel, F. and Mall, F.P. (eds.) *Manuals of Human Embryology*. (Philadelphia: Lippincott)
10. Ruddock, E.H. (1930). *Vitalogy*. (Chicago: Vitalogy Association)
11. Profet, M. (1993). Menstruation as a defense against pathogens transported by sperm. *Q. Rev. Biol.*, **68**, 335–81
12. Worthman, C.M. and Smith, E.O. (1992). Why do women menstruate? Paper given to *American Anthropological Association*, San Francisco, California

13. Clarke, J. (1995). The meaning of menstruation in the elimination of abnormal embryos. *Hum. Reprod.*, **9**, 1204–6
14. Palmer, B.D. and Guillette, L.J. (1992). Alligators provide evidence for the evolution of an archosaurian mode of oviparity. *Biol. Reprod.*, **46**, 39–47
15. Baldwin, E. (1970). *An Introduction to Comparative Biochemistry*. (Cambridge: Cambridge University Press)
16. Hughes, R.L. and Carrick, F.N. (1978). Reproduction in female monotremes. *Aus. Zool.*, **20**, 233–53
17. Finn, C.A. (1994). Implantation. In Lamming, G.E. (ed.) *Marshall's Physiology of Reproduction*, 4th edn, vol. 3, pp. 157–231. (London: Chapman & Hall)
18. Finn, C.A. and Lawn, A.M. (1968). Transfer of cellular material between the uterine epithelium and trophoblast during the early stages of implantation. *J. Reprod. Fertil.*, **15**, 333–6
19. Kirby, D.R.S. (1969). Development of mouse eggs beneath the kidney capsule. *Nature (London)*, **187**, 707–8
20. Rowley, A.F. (1996). The evolution of inflammatory mediators. *Mediat. Inflamm.*, **5**, 3–13
21. Staples, L.D., Heap, R.B., Wooding, F.B.P. and King, G.J. (1983). Migration of leucocytes into the uterus after acute removal of ovarian progesterone during early pregnancy in sheep. *Placenta*, **4**, 339–49
22. Finn, C.A. and Pope, M. (1986). Control of leucocyte infiltration into the decidualized mouse uterus. *J. Endocrinol.*, **110**, 93–6
23. Deanesly, R. (1972). Retarded embryonic development and pregnancy termination in ovariectomized guinea pigs: progesterone deficiency and decidual collapse. *J. Reprod. Fertil.*, **28**, 241–7
24. Callard, I.P., Fileti, L.A., Perez, L.E., Sorbera, L.A., Giannoukos, G., Klosterman, I.L., Tsang, P. and McCracken, J.A. (1992). Role of the corpus luteum and progesterone in the evolution of vertebrate viviparity. *Am. Zool.*, **32**, 264–75
25. Finn, C.A. and Lawn, A.M. (1967). Specialized junctions between decidual cells in the uterus of the pregnant mouse. *J. Ultrastruct. Res.*, **20**, 321–7
26. Finn, C.A. (1986). Implantation, menstruation and inflammation. *Biol. Rev.*, **61**, 313–28
27. Turner, W.M. (1983). Report on the progress of anatomy. *J. Anat. Physiol.*, **8**, 159–78
28. Finn, C.A. and Pope, M.D. (1984). Vascular and cellular changes in the decidualized endometrium of the ovariectomized mouse following cessation of hormone treatment: a possible model for menstruation. *J. Endocrinol.*, **100**, 295–300

Do all women have endometriosis? Reflections on pathogenesis

J.L.H. Evers

Introduction

The *condition* of endometriosis is by no means an infrequent clinical finding in reproductive medicine clinics, especially since the introduction in the early 1980s of excellent optical instruments for endoscopy, and since the increased awareness in the late 1980s of subtle, hitherto unrecognized, atypical lesions. The *disease* of endometriosis is far less common, fortunately. It gives rise to dysmenorrhea in 60–80% of patients, to pelvic pain in 30–50%, to infertility in 30–40%, to dyspareunia in 25–40% and to menstrual irregularities in 10–20%. Involvement of adjacent organs, such as the bladder and the rectosigmoid, is rare (1–2%), but may cause severe complaints, and may even become life-threatening.

Literature findings suggest that endometriosis in many patients is a self-limiting disease. The early, non-pigmented papules (with invasive activity into the extracellular matrix of the host tissue) evolve into well-vascularized, hyperemic, red lesions, and finally will be subdued by the peritoneal defense system and will develop into the familiar black and blue 'powder-burn' lesions, poorly vascularized, quiescent and surrounded by white fibrotic tissue. Given the fact that endometriosis can be diagnosed reliably only at laparoscopy, the true incidence of endometriosis in normal healthy women is difficult to determine. Endometriosis has been found at 4–24% of sterilization laparoscopies, and at 21–85% of infertility laparoscopies.

Physiology

Apart from a few subhuman primates, one bat and the elephant shrew, the human female is the only menstruating mammal[1]. In normal, cycling endometrium, glandular epithelium undergoes rapid growth and remodeling during the follicular phase of the cycle. Growth ceases during the luteal phase and, in the absence of the continued progesterone-dominated environment of pregnancy, the arteries supplying the superficial layer of the endometrium constrict during the late luteal phase of the menstrual cycle, in response to the failing progesterone drive. Glandular activity decreases and loss of interstitial fluid occurs. Eventually the feeding arteries close down, making the superficial zone ischemic. After some time the constricted arteries open up again, the walls of the damaged surface vessels burst to release blood into the stroma, and ultimately patches of tissue separate from the basal layer of the endometrium. Metalloproteinases of the stromelysin family, collagenase and the extracellular matrix-degrading enzyme matrilysin are expressed in endometrium. They probably play a role in endometrial growth, remodeling and breakdown, and possibly in the establishment of ectopic endometriotic tissue and in determining its invasive properties[2].

Comparative endometriology

Few people, even few medical doctors, recognize that menstruation is a rare event in the animal kingdom. Apart from humans, only a few subhuman primates and two non-primate species, the elephant shrew and the bat, have been found to menstruate. Little is known about their cyclic endometrial development. Finn, in a beautifully written monograph, recently has reviewed our knowledge of the phenomenon of menstruation and concluded that the decidual cell reaction in the uterine stroma is a human species-specific adaptation of the endometrial inflammatory response that allows the implanting blastocyst to develop safely inside the uterine tissues, where usually this inflammatory response would have been directed at removal and destruction of the invading foreign object[1]. The premenstrual condition in women whereby the uterus is prepared in advance so as to be able to withstand the invasion of the blastocyst is considered by Finn to represent the latest stage in the evolution of implantation, with menstruation being the price to pay for the fact that during the menstrual cycle the human endometrium goes a stage further in the preparation of the stroma for implantation than does the uterus of non-menstruating species. The decidual reaction of the endometrial stroma cells represents a stage of differentiation which does not allow them to return to their former undifferentiated state again. If cells cannot be maintained, they must be discarded. As a result, in order for our species to survive, monthly menstruation troubles its female members.

Pathology

Sampson, in 1927[3], was the first to note blood escaping from the fimbrial end of the Fallopian tubes when surgery was performed during the menstrual period. Whether the refluxed endometrium implants on the peritoneal lining of the pelvic organs (metastasis theory[3]) or whether it induces a local metaplastic response in the peritoneum, leading to the neogenesis of endometrial tissue by mesothelial metaplasia at the ectopic site (metaplasia theory[4]), is still an unsolved problem and a matter of arduous debate among distinguished endometriologists. Most students of endometriosis, however, favor the implantation theory nowadays as the most important explanation for the pathogenesis of endometriosis, although not all aspects of the disease may be explained by this theory. Endometrial metaplasia of the peritoneal serosa may constitute an additional (and not an opposing) explanation: endometrial cells or cell products may stimulate metaplasia after they have been transported to a susceptible site in the abdominal cavity. Merrill[5] implanted millipore filters containing vital endometrium tissue in the abdominal cavity of rabbits. This study offers suggestive evidence that subcellular substances from (even decaying) endometrium apparently are capable of inducing endometrial metaplasia in mesothelium.

The reflux implantation theory of Sampson[3] is supported by the distribution of lesions in the abdominal cavity, the demonstration of the viability of shed menstrual endometrium in tissue culture, the immunohistochemical characteristics of endometrium shed in a retrograde fashion and its similarities to *in situ* endometrium, endometrium shed in an antegrade fashion and endometriosis lesions in the peritoneal cavity, the capacity for adhesion and proliferation of peritoneal cells obtained from the peritoneal fluid during the early follicular phase of the cycle, the high prevalence of endometriosis in girls with congenital menstrual outflow tract obstruction and animal experiments in which endometriosis was induced by the creation of uteropelvic fistulas. The reflux implantation theory is based on the assumption that retrograde menstruation takes place, and that viable endometrial cells reach the abdominal cavity, attach to the peritoneal lining and implant. Goodall[6] observed the spillage of blood in about 50% of laparotomies performed during menstruation. Blumenkrantz and co-workers[7] reported that nine of 11 women undergoing peritoneal dialysis had blood in the dialysate during their periods. Halme and co-workers[8] found red discoloration of the peritoneal fluid in 90% of patients with patent tubes, laparoscoped during their menstrual periods. Blood was found by Liu and Hitchcock[9] in 76%. Van der Linden and co-workers found endometrial cells in the peritoneal fluid during the early follicular phase of the cycle in all of their (16) patients[10]. Kruitwagen and co-workers were able to demonstrate the presence of endometrial cells in 79% of their early follicular phase peritoneal fluid samples and showed these cells to be viable in culture[11].

We may conclude from these studies that viable endometrial cells reach the abdominal cavity via the Fallopian tubes during the menstrual period in most, if not all, women with patent tubes. The volume of regurgitated menstrual debris may be determined by anatomic–mechanical predispositions. Ayers and Friedenstab showed uterotubal junction hypotonia in endometriosis patients as compared to (infertile) controls[12]. Their findings seem to be corroborated by Bartosik and co-workers[13], who found that more endometrial cells reached the abdominal cavity during flushing of the tubes in endometriosis patients. Whether the sheer volume or also the tissue properties of the regurgitated menstrual debris determines that endometriosis will develop in some patients and not in others, and whether differences in their peritoneal defense system contribute to the problem, still remains to be elucidated.

Defense systems in the peritoneal cavity

In women with endometriosis a local, sterile inflammation occurs in the peritoneal cavity. On theoretical grounds this inflammation may be a response to menstrual debris, either regurgitated through the Fallopian tubes or shed locally by the endometriotic implants. Haney and co-workers[14] have shown the latter mechanism to be the least likely. Elicitation of a reactive inflammatory response may be considered the body's first line of defense against the development of endometriosis. If the defense mechanism fails or if the aggression is too voluminous or too strong, viable endometrial cells will implant and develop into clinical endometriosis. The association between the sterile inflammation of the peritoneal fluid and infertility remains to be elucidated.

The peritoneal response to the invasion of regurgitated menstrual debris is directed at incapacitation, destruction and removal of these cells. This should prevent the adhesion of viable endometrial cells to the peritoneal lining, and their subsequent development into endometriotic lesions. An adequate response of this defense mechanism has been suggested as a facilitating factor for the development of endometriosis. Immunological factors have been the subject of many studies in this respect, although it should be stressed that no increased occurrence of immunological disorders has been found in endometriosis patients.

Drake and co-workers have reported increased volumes of peritoneal fluid in women with endometriosis, and have interpreted this as a sign of inflammation[15].

Macrophages are involved in phagocytosis and, through their secretory products, in inflammatory reactions. They constitute the dominant cell type in the cell population of the peritoneal fluid[16]. Macrophages are involved in the initiation of the inflammatory response as antigen-presenting cells and in the active phase as tumoricidal and microbicidal cells. Upon stimulation, resident peritoneal macrophages produce factors that stimulate proliferation of monocytes in the bone marrow. These monocytes travel to the site of violation of homeostasis (i.e. the peritoneal cavity) to take part, as activated macrophages, in the inflammatory response and defense reaction. In this respect they may be considered to be the garbage collection and disposal system of the peritoneal cavity. Halme and co-workers[8] found increased activation of peritoneal macrophages in infertile women with mild endometriosis. Proteolytic enzymes, lysozyme, γ-interferon, interleukin-1 and -2, tumor necrosis factor (TNF) and growth factors are amongst the secretory products of activated macrophages.

Also, the other major cell types of the immune system, T lymphocytes, B lymphocytes and natural killer (NK) cells have been studied in the peritoneal fluid of endometriosis patients. All cells have the capacity to produce cytokines, and cytokines in turn activate T cells, B cells, NK cells and macrophages. Of particular interest in this regard is the finding by Dunselman and co-workers[16] that, although activated macrophages show increased *in vitro* phagocytosis of sheep red blood cells, their capability to show chemiluminescence after ingestion of zymosan is decreased. This suggests that, in endometriosis patients, macrophages may lack, even when activated in other respects, sufficient capacity to clear the pelvic cavity of regurgitated menstrual debris, i.e. of viable endometrial cells. This is in accordance with an immunological basis for the development of endometriosis, as suggested by Steele and co-workers, who found reduced cell-mediated cytotoxicity toward autologous endometrial cells[17]. More recently, Oosterlynck and co-workers[18] reported defective NK cell activity in endometriosis patients, also resulting in decreased cellular immunity.

From the isolated reports on defense mechanisms in the peritoneal cavity published to date, one may conclude that a highly reactive peritoneal inflammatory response exists in endometriosis patients which may lower cycle fecundity through interference with intra-abdominal and intratubal reproductive processes. On the other hand, indications exist that isolated defects in these activated immunocompetent cells may explain why endometrial cells may implant and develop into endometriotic lesions. Furthermore, the adhesion of viable endometrial cells may even be facilitated by secretory products of the activated macrophages, e.g. fibronectin, and their outgrowth stimulated by inflammatory cell-derived growth factors, e.g. epidermal growth factor (EGF), transforming growth factor (TGF)-α, TGF-β and insulin-like growth factor (IGF)-1[19].

The battle of the islands

Malignant tumor research has shown that, after separation of individual tumor cells or groups of tumor cells from the primary tumor, the three crucial steps of invasion are: adherence of the tumor cells to the host tissue cells, local proteolysis associated with breakdown of the extracellular matrix and migration into the colonized tissue[20]. Regurgitated endometrial cells possess the capacity to attach to the peritoneal lining, as was shown by van der Linden and co-workers[10]. These authors concluded from their work that the expression pattern of cell adhesion molecules indicates that the loss of cell adhesion properties may play a role in the shedding of endometrial tissue during menstruation and that integrins, and perhaps cadherins, may also be operative in attachment of endometrial tissue fragments to the peritoneum. The demonstration of the expression of cell adhesion molecules by cells in menstrual effluent, endometrium and peritoneal fluid, as well as in endometriosis lesions is no conclusive evidence that endometriosis originates from the endometrium by retrograde shedding of viable tissue fragments. However, all cells potentially involved in the pathogenesis of endometriosis possess the ability to express integrin and cadherin cell adhesion molecules during the menstrual phase of the cycle. Although the exact mechanism by which endometrial cells might attach to the peritoneal serosa is still not clear, and although the first endometrial cell making contact with the first serosal cell still has to be observed, it has been established that early endometriosis invades the peritoneal extracellular matrix: products of local proteolysis, e.g. the aminoterminal propeptide of type III collagen, accumulate in the peritoneal fluid of patients with endometriosis, especially those with early, active lesions. Van der Linden and co-workers[10] showed E-cadherin to be expressed in *in situ* endometrial epithelial cells of 16 of 16 women, but in only one of 16 samples of endometrial cells retrieved from their peritoneal fluid during the menstrual period. Similarity with the loss of E-cadherin expression in invasive breast cancer would suggest a potential role for cadherins in invasive endometriosis. After cell division will have resumed, the new endometrial implant soon reaches a critical tissue volume. From then onwards it has to rely on new vessel ingrowth for support of its further outgrowth and development. In an elegant series of experiments, Oosterlynck and co-workers[21] investigated the presence of angiogenic factors in peritoneal fluid from 24 endometriosis patients and compared the results to those in 24 controls. Angiogenesis was assayed by the placement of glass fiber filters impregnated with peritoneal fluid on the exposed chorioallantoic membrane of chicken embryos. The peritoneal fluid of endometriosis patients appeared to contain more angiogenic activity than did the peritoneal fluid of controls.

Endometriosis: a never ending story?

In 1987, David Redwine[22] drew our attention to the age-related evolution in the color appearance of endometriosis. He found the mean age of endometriosis patients to increase from 21.5 years for those with clear papules only, via 26.3 years for those with red lesions, and 29.5 years for those with white lesions, to 31.9 years for those with black lesions. The age range of patients with clear papules only was 17–26 years, the age range of patients with black plus any other lesions was 17–43 and that of patients with black lesions only was 20–52 years. No patient over the age of 31 was found to present clear lesions. These findings suggest that endometriosis in many patients is a self-limiting disease. The early, non-pigmented papules (with invasive activity into the extracellular matrix of the host tissue) evolve into well-vascularized, hyperemic, red lesions, and finally are subdued by the peritoneal defense system and develop into the familiar black and blue 'powder-burn' lesions – poorly vascularized, quiescent and surrounded by white fibrotic tissue. One wonders what the age range will have been of those (rare) patients who have been described in the literature who showed invisible, i.e. microscopic, lesions only.

The concept of spontaneous resolution of endometriosis is corroborated by the composition of the patient groups usually described in treatment studies. Typically, patients with American Fertility Society (AFS) stages I and II disease constitute the majority of cases, whereas the group of patients belonging to stages III and IV is usually much smaller, irrespective of whether only surgical or also medical treatment studies are considered.

Although several studies have suggested that medical treatment is effective in inhibiting the progression of endometriosis, other investigations have cast doubt upon this conclusion. If second-look laparoscopy is performed during medical suppression of endometriosis and the findings are compared to those at first-look laparoscopy (when the pelvic environment was moist and active, with productive endometriotic foci and their inherent hyperemia, hemorrhage, secretion and inflammatory reaction), one may erroneously conclude that the less active, and therefore less visible, foci in the dry, inactive pelvis reflect regression or even resolution of endometriosis. After suppression has been discontinued, however, the foci will become reactivated again and the disease will return to its original path of development[23]. The final answer to the question of whether endometriosis is a progressive disease will have to come from long-term prospective investigations studying spontaneous evolution of peritoneal lesions without therapeutic interference. This will require the performance of second-look laparoscopy in a patient who has not received any treatment in the interval since her first laparoscopy. It is obvious that such groups will be difficult to collect.

Treatment studies: what do they teach us?

We may learn something from the evolution of disease as detailed in the no-treatment or placebo groups of the few randomized controlled studies published so far. Thomas and Cooke[24] showed, in 17 placebo-treated patients who underwent laparoscopy before and after 6 months of placebo treatment, unchanged or even diminished endometriosis in 53%, but an increment in 47%. Similar figures were obtained by other investigators[25,26]. Mahmood and Templeton noted improvement among 27% of untreated patients, an increment in 64%, and an unchanged situation in 9%[16]. Many other studies give indirect evidence that endometriosis is progressive. D'Hooghe and co-workers studied the spontaneous evolution of endometriosis in baboons and reported a significant increase in the number of lesions at repeat laparoscopy at 10 months[27]. The new lesions were mainly subtle, atypical (67%) and localized on the uterine peritoneum. Progression of endometriosis, however, did not go beyond revised-AFS (r-AFS) stage I. Repeat laparoscopies in ten baboons with an initially normal pelvis showed endometriosis to be present in seven after 10–12 months. They concluded that endometriosis was moderately progressive in the baboon, but never beyond the borders of r-AFS stage I. Remodeling of endometriosis lesions within stage I took place within a period of several months.

Final remarks and conclusions

From all published evidence we may conclude that endometriosis appears to be a dynamic disease, especially in the early phase, with subtle, atypical lesions emerging and vanishing again. In the end, however, the peritoneal defense system will prevail and the disease will be contained in the majority of patients. When doing repeat laparoscopies in young patients, one should be prepared to encounter more advanced histological types of lesions, which do not necessarily indicate more advanced stages of the disease: the classical, blue and black 'powder-burn' spots and 'blueberry' lesions reflect the extinguishing phase of the dynamic endometriotic process, and herald its inactivated histological end-stage. The dynamic phase of the disease may involve a varying interval of each patient's life, and medical suppression of the activity of the implants during this interval may lead one to conclude erroneously that treatment has been effective. If, subsequently (after the end of medical suppression of the activity of the lesions), ovarian activity resumes and the lesions are stimulated again by ovarian steroids, their productive activity returns. Recurrence of disease may be diagnosed if, at that stage, laparoscopy is performed, whereas in reality only reactivation of temporarily obscured lesions occurred. The suppressed, dormant (but never absent) lesions produce mucus again, desquamation occurs and there is reaction by the surrounding tissue. The inflammatory response, the local hyperemia and the neogenesis of vessels accentuate the presence of previously invisible endometriosis lesions and make them visible again. Endometriosis resumes its temporarily halted natural course of development, tissue remodeling occurs again, the battle between the aggressor and the defense system resumes and waxing and waning of the several types of lesions – red, white and black – can be found again.

References

1. Finn, C.A. (1987). Why do women and some other primates menstruate? *Perspect. Biol. Med.*, **30**, 566–74

2. Rodgers, W.H., Osteen, K.G., Matrisian, L.M., Navre, M., Giudice, L.G. and Gorstein, F. (1993). Expression and localization of matri-

lysin, a matrix metalloproteinase, in human endometrium during the reproductive cycle. *Am. J. Obstet. Gynecol.*, **168**, 253–6
3. Sampson, J.A. (1927). Peritoneal endometriosis due to menstrual dissemination of endometrial tissue into the peritoneal cavity. *Am. J. Obstet. Gynecol.*, **14**, 422–69
4. Meyer, R. (1919). Ueber den Stand der Frage der Adenomyositis und Adenomyome in algemeinen und insbesondere ueber adenomyositis seroepithelialis und Adenomyometritis sarcomatosa. *Zbl. Gynaekol.*, **43**, 745–50
5. Merrill, J.A. (1966). Endometrial induction of endometriosis across millipore filters. *Am. J. Obstet. Gynecol.*, **94**, 780–9.
6. Goodall, J.R. (1943). *A Study of Endometriosis, Endosalpingosis, Endocervicosis, and Peritoneo-Ovarian Sclerosis: A Clinical and Pathologic Study.* (Philadelphia: J.B. Lippincot)
7. Blumenkrantz, M.J. Gallagher, N., Bashore, R.A. and Tenckhoff, H. (1981). Retrograde menstruation in women undergoing chronic peritoneal dialysis. *Obstet. Gynecol.* **57**, 667–70
8. Halme, J., Hammond, M.G., Hulka, J.F., Raj, S.G. and Talbert, L.M. (1984). Retrograde menstruation in healthy women and in patients with endometriosis. *Obstet. Gynecol.*, **64**, 151–4
9. Liu, D.T. and Hitchcock, A. (1986). Endometriosis: its association with retrograde menstruation, dysmenorrhoea and tubal pathology. *Br. J. Obstet. Gynaecol.*, **93**, 859–62
10. Van der Linden, P.J.Q., De Goeij, A.F.P.M., Dunselman, G.A.J., Van der Linden, E.P.M., Ramaekers, F.C.S. and Evers, J.L.H. (1994). Expression of integrins and E-cadherin in cells from menstrual effluent, endometrium, peritoneal fluid, peritoneum, and endometriosis. *Fertil. Steril.*, **61**, 85–90
11. Kruitwagen, R.F., Poels, L.G., Willemsen, W.N., de Ronde, I.J., Jap, P.H. and Rolland, R. (1991). Endometrial epithelial cells in peritoneal fluid during the early follicular phase. *Fertil. Steril.*, **55**, 297–303
12. Ayers, J.W.T. and Friedenstab, A.P. (1985). Utero-tubal hypotonia associated with pelvic endometriosis. *Am. Fertil. Soc. Ann. Meeting Abstracts*, Abstract no. 131
13. Bartosik, D., Jacobs, S.L. and Kelly, L.J. (1986). Endometrial tissue in peritoneal fluid. *Fertil. Steril.*, **46**, 796–800
14. Haney, A.F., Jenkins, S. and Weinberg, J.B. (1991). The stimulus responsible for the peritoneal fluid inflammation observed in infertile women with endometriosis. *Fertil. Steril.*, **56**, 408–13
15. Drake, T.S., Metz, S.A., Grunert, G.M. and O'Brien, W.F. (1980). Peritoneal fluid volume in endometriosis. *Fertil. Steril.*, **34**, 27–31
16. Dunselman, G.A.J., Hendrix, M.G.R., Bouckaert, P.X.J.M. and Evers, J.L.H. Functional aspects of peritoneal macrophages in endometriosis of women. *J. Reprod. Fertil.*, **82**, 707–10
17. Steele, R.W., Dmowski, W.P. and Marmer, D.J. (1984). Immunologic aspects of human endometriosis. *Am. J. Reprod. Immunol.*, **6**, 33–6
18. Oosterlynck, D.J., Meuleman, C., Waer, M., Vandeputte, M. and Koninckx, P.R. (1992). The natural killer activity of peritoneal fluid lymphocytes is decreased in women with endometriosis. *Fertil. Steril.*, **58**, 290–5
19. Zhang, R.J., Wild, R.A., Medders, D. and Gunupudi, S.R. (1991). Effects of peritoneal macrophages from patients with endometriosis on the proliferation of endometrial carcinoma cell line ECC-1. *Am. J. Obstet. Gynecol.*, **165**, 1842–6
20. Liotta, L.A. (1992). Cancer cell invasion and metastasis. *Sci. Am.*, **266**, 54–9, 63–4
21. Oosterlynck, D.J., Meuleman, C., Sobis, H., Vandeputte, M. and Koninckx, P.R. (1993). Angiogenic activity of peritoneal fluid from women with endometriosis. *Fertil. Steril.*, **59**, 778–82
22. Redwine, D.B. (1987). Age-related evolution in color appearance of endometriosis. *Fertil. Steril.*, **48**, 1062–3
23. Evers, J.L.H. (1987). The second-look laparoscopy for evaluation of the result of medical treatment of endometriosis should not be performed during ovarian suppression. *Fertil. Steril.*, **47**, 502–4
24. Thomas, E.J. and Cooke, I.D. (1987). Impact of gestrinone on the course of asymptomatic endometriosis. *Br. Med. J.*, **294**, 272–4
25. Telimaa, S. (1988). Danazol and medroxyprogesterone acetate inefficacious in the treatment of infertility in endometriosis. *Fertil. Steril.*, **50**, 872–5
26. Mahmood, T.A. and Templeton, A. (1990). The impact of treatment on the natural history of endometriosis. *Hum. Reprod.*, **5**, 965–70
27. D'Hooghe, T.M., Bambra, C.S. Isahakia, M. and Koninckx, P.R. (1992). Evolution of spontaneous endometriosis in the baboon (Papio anubis, Papio cynocephalus) over a 12-month period *Fertil. Steril.*, **58**, 409–12

New insights into adolescent endometriosis

3

Y.T. Lim

Introduction

Endometriosis is a progessive and recurrent disease, mainly affecting women of reproductive age. It is likely that endometriosis occurs in most women at some stage in their reproductive years. A major offending factor inciting endometriosis is menstrual regurgitation. Exposure to menstruation and estrogen with multiple growth factors in the pelvis are important etiologically[1]. There are numerous unsolved aspects regarding etiology, pathogenesis, pathophysiology, natural history and management. As for the definition of endometriosis, there are some opinions that many mild cases of endometriosis could be considered as a non-disease, and it is only considered a disease if the presence of implants can be found and severe endometriotic disease is present[2].

The earliest onset of endometriosis was estimated at 3–4 years after menarche. An unusual case of endometriosis of the Fallopian tube was associated with right hematosalpinx 1 month after menarche at the age of 10 years[3]. Many studies have implied that the incidence of adolescent endometriosis might be higher than expected. We do not have a clear picture of the natural history of adolescent endometriosis. Endometriosis in the adolescent age group can cause dysmenorrhea, pelvic pain or abdominal pain, and adnexal mass.

Possible endometriotic adolescents should receive laparoscopic surgery in order to confirm the correct clinical diagnosis of 'endometriosis'. Early surgical intervention might permit accurate staging of endometriosis, debulking of disease, restoring the pelvic anatomy and temporarily halting the disease process. But there are no available data concerning the benefits of the early diagnosis of endometriosis in adolescents although surgical ablation may prevent progression of endometriosis[4].

The recurrence rate of endometriosis in adolescents undergoing conservative surgery remains unknown. Frequent recurrences are the well-known clinical situations following the medical or surgical 'single agent' therapy, because of the presence of possible microscopic endometriosis, the multifocal nature of endometriosis, varying vascular supply or adhesions around endometriotic lesions, and inadequate initial treatment. Endometriosis cannot be eradicated from the pelvic cavity with conventional treatments. Therefore more conservative, disease-modifying and non-invasive management of adolescent endometriosis might be acceptable to gynecologists, parents and patients.

Prevalence

A recent report in the literature suggests that endometriosis may not be uncommon in the adolescent age group[3]. Adolescent endometriosis was first described in 1929. Retrospective studies based on data from the 1930s to 1960s placed the incidence at approximately 0.2–4% for teenagers when compared with all females undergoing laparotomy. These studies have flaws in that the data are retrospective and biased by the thinking that endometriosis was rare in this age group; in addition, laparoscopy for diagnosis was not available[4].

More recently, Redwine reported that of 132 patients undergoing either laparoscopy or laparotomy in which endometriosis was diagnosed, 14 (10.6%) were in the 16–20 age group[5]. A study by Houston and colleagues[6] reviewed the community records of white females diagnosed with pelvic endometriosis in Rochester, Minnesota, from 1970 to 1979. They determined that the age-specific rates of endometriosis were lowest for women from 15 to 19 years of age. Of the 171 females with histologically confirmed disease, five were in that age group. With a population of approximately 2900 in the 15–19 age range in Rochester over the years of the study, the age-specific incidence in this community of histologically confirmed endometriosis was about 0.2%. Others looked only at adolescents presenting with dysmenorrhea, chronic pelvic pain, or dysfunctional uterine bleeding. In 1973, Bullock and colleagues[7] reported on their series of 18 teenagers with dysmenorrhea who did not respond to management with analgesics or oral contraceptives. The patients were evaluated by culdoscopy or colpotomy, and nine of them, aged 17–19, had endometriosis.

Three studies published in the 1980s which also examined endometriosis in adolescent females were surprising in both the high incidence of this finding and the similarity of results. In 1980, Goldstein and associates[8] revealed that of 140 adolescents undergoing laparoscopy for chronic pelvic pain, 66 (47%) were found to have endometriosis alone. The youngest patient diagnosed in this study was 10.5 years of age, with menarche occurring at age 10. Chatman and Ward[9] published their data on 43 laparoscopies performed on black adolescents with disabling pelvic pain and/or abnormal vaginal bleeding. Of these, 65% were found to have endometriosis. Of the 28 cases diagnosed with endometriosis, biopsies were done on just 18 and only 13 of these biopsies histologically confirmed the diagnosis.

Most recently, Vercellini and colleagues[10] looked at 47 adolescent females aged 11–19 who complained of chronic pelvic pain. Their series revealed a 38% incidence of the disease. However, in the first 3 years of the study only 'classic' black lesions of endometriosis were diagnosed, with a 27% rate of diagnosis, while in the last 2 years of the study 'atypical' lesions were also diagnosed, with a 52% rate of diagnosis. Why only the rate in the last 2 years was in line with the rate of diagnosis of endometriosis in the studies of Goldstein and colleagues[8] and Chatman and Ward[9], which did not include atypical lesions, is not clear, but probably is because of the more global definition of chronic pelvic pain in the study of Vercellini and colleagues.

Müllerian malformations and adolescent endometriosis

Endometriosis occurring shortly after menarche is reported frequently, and it is not exclusively associated with Müllerian anomalies, which cause outflow tract obstruction. Müllerian malformations such as bicornuate uterus, rudimentary uterine horn, stenotic hymen or vaginal atresia, enhancing retrograde menstruation, were present in six patients from 15 cases of teenage endometriosis[11]. Sanfilippo and Yussman have also described endometriosis with outflow tract obstruction and have shown that this endometriosis will disappear after the obstruction to the outflow tract has been released[12].

Clinical symptoms and signs

Clinical symptoms of adolescent endometriosis are similar to those in the adult, and the severity of the pain does not correlate with the amount of endometriosis. Approximately half of adolescents complaining of refractory dysmenorrhea or chronic pelvic pain will be diagnosed with endometriosis. The most frequent presenting symptom is pelvic pain, and the most common sign is pelvic tenderness[13].

In teenagers the most common symptom for diagnosis is cyclic or acyclic pain. Adolescents with cyclic pain and those who complain of abdominal pain, nausea, constipation and diarrhea during menses had the largest proportion of red lesions[14]. Pelvic pain is severe enough that the patient has usually missed a lot of school, but she may have scant localizing signs. On the other hand, some tenderness in the uterosacral ligaments or nodularity may be palpated.

Diagnosis

At the present time not enough longitudinal data is available on adolescent endometriosis for us to draw any conclusions as to the benefit of early diagnosis. Therefore most current information is obtained from the extrapolation of endometriosis in adult patients.

When examining the patient, one must be mindful that this may be her first pelvic examination. The mobility of the uterus must be determined, as an important finding in the diagnosis may be a fixed uterus. Pelvic tenderness is the most common sign for endometriosis, and uterosacral ligament nodularity may be better assessed during the patient's menses. The adnexa must also be examined for masses, thickening or tenderness. Recently Davis and colleagues[14] reported that adolescent patients with severe dysmenorrhea may not always have classic signs of endometriosis at laparoscopy. They reported the high incidence of rectal endometriosis (11 patients, 31%).

Menorrhagia and other abnormal findings such as dyspareunia have also been observed in these patients. The abnormal bleeding usually described is not the typical anovulatory bleeding of adolescents, but rather heavy bleeding accompanied by a major component of pain. The patient's cramping and bleeding may be related to prostaglandin formation, and it is well known that the younger implants of endometriosis are usually associated with more symptoms, and the burnt-out old implants do not produce a large amount of prostaglandins. Red endometriosis lesions seem to be the most active producers of prostaglandin F ($PGF_{2\alpha}$) when compared to other lesions[15].

Fedele and colleagues[16], by studying the location of endometriosis implants compared with the localization of pain symptoms in 160 women, evaluated the hypothesis that if endometriosis were a cause of pain, then it should cause pain at its site of implantation. They found no correlation between the location of endometriosis and of pelvic pain[16].

However, Ripps and Martin[17] in a prospective study of 82 women with either pelvic pain or infertility, 59 of whom had endometriosis, found some correlation between location of implants and localization of focal tenderness on pelvic examination. In this study, 76% of the patients found to have endometriosis had localized tenderness that correlated with an area of endometriosis. However, it should be noted that more than half (58%) of these patients also had areas of endometriosis that were not tender. They also attempted to evaluate the types of endometriotic lesion to see if any correlation existed with focal tenderness and found no specific correlation with either typical or atypical lesions. As an aside, in patients with focal tenderness, endometriosis was the most frequent diagnosis (45 of 68 diagnoses, or 66%).

These results comply with our results for push-pull tenderness during the transvaginal detection of endometriotic lesions. Eighty per cent of our adolescent endometriosis patients showed push-pull tenderness at the sites of the typical cartwheel-appearance echoes[18].

Laparoscopic diagnosis

It is important that serosanguinous fluid seen in the cul-de-sac is aspirated with a secondary probe and the back of the uterus, ovarian ligament and other areas in the pelvis are mobilized so that all surfaces are visualized, and early endometriosis is diagnosed and taken care of. We have always used the two- or three-puncture technique and may use a third puncture depending on the extent of the implants. We have been able to use either the monopolar cautery, the endocoagulator, or the CO_2 or Nd:YAG laser in the treatment of these implants. If the implants are deeper, very occasionally they may need excision. Chatman[19] has also described the peritoneal defects that may be suggestive of long-standing endometriosis. Occasionally no obvious implants may be seen, and in this case a biopsy from the cul-de-sac must be obtained to make sure there is no occult endometriosis. Most patients treated surgically are found to have minimal or mild disease, most frequently located in the cul-de-sac. After the diagnosis and treatment of endometriosis has been carried out, the grading and the staging of the patient's condition should be explained to the patient. It is very clear in our own experience that most of these patients usually have minimal or mild endometriosis and a very small percentage have moderate or severe endometriosis.

Age-related appearance

It is becoming increasingly clear in the literature on endometriosis that the implants may vary: they can be clear papules, clear lesions or red, white and black lesions. These earlier lesions may have to be biopsied to make a diagnosis of endometriosis[20]. Color appearance of endometriotic implants is closely related with patient's age, but the number of pelvic areas involved in the disease does not increase with advancing age[5]. No increase of the total pelvic area involved in endometriosis with an advance in age has been reported, although the depth of infiltration of the implants is greater as is the incidence of endometriosis[21].

Limitation of visual diagnosis

Gynecologists could observe the increased frequency of endometriosis with the introduction of the concept of non-pigmented endometriotic lesions[22]. Furthermore, there are controversies on the clinical significance of microscopic endo-metriosis. Redwine and Yocom[23] reported that visually normal peritoneum does not harbor a high prevalence of invisible microscopic endometriosis. A glandular element compatible with possible endometriosis was found in only one patient from 45 patients with biopsy-proven endometriosis and 10 patients without endometriosis.

Laparoscopic diagnosis of endometriosis might be difficult in cases of minimal or micro-scopic endometriosis, atypical non-pigmented endometriosis, subperitoneal endometriosis, adhesions which obscure visualization of endometriotic lesions or differential diagnosis between ovarian endometriomas and corpus lutein cysts. In these situations, imaging diagnosis with pelvic magnetic resonance or trans-rectal sonography might be the choice in terms of non-invasive diagnosis of pelvic endometriosis.

Imaging diagnosis

Wood and Maher[24] reported that conventional magnetic resonance images demonstrated only four lesions among 111 small endometrial implants that measured > 5 mm in diameter. The addition of fat-suppressed magnetic resonance imaging increased the detection rate to 55 of 111 lesions. Fat-suppressed magnetic resonance imaging can, therefore, be useful in detecting small endometrial implants. This result complies with our results that diagnostic accuracy was higher with fat-suppressed imaging (77%) than with conventional imaging (55%) ($p = 0.06$). The overall sensitivity in detecting peritoneal implants was significantly higher with fat-suppressed imaging (61%) than with conventional imaging (27%) ($p = 0.01$)[25].

Magnetic resonance imaging of the pelvis may be preferable to diagnostic laparoscopy in women who wish to preserve their fertility. Obviating surgery or enabling more directed, less invasive surgery has the advantage of eliminating or reducing formation of postoperative pelvic adhesions, which occur after both laparoscopy and laparotomy[26]. The use of pelvic magnetic resonance imaging may alter treatment, decrease the number of invasive surgical procedures and reduce the total health care cost.

Because magnetic resonance imaging is more expensive than other conventional imaging techniques, it might be more convenient to use transvaginal sonography. Unfortunately, sonography is not widely accepted as a non-invasive diagnostic modality to detect tiny endometriotic lesions. Based on our experiences, it might be possible to detect tiny endometriotic lesions, but it needs more studies to confirm our 'cartwheel echoes' with push-pull tenderness at the sites of endometriosis[19].

Management

Estimates of the distribution of endometriosis in the female population might be unreliable due to lack of control of the variables which influence diagnosis of the disease in the initial stages[27]. Early surgical intervention permits accurate staging of endometriosis, debulking of disease and restoration of anatomy. While surgical ablation may prevent progression of endometriosis, the effects remain unknown in adolescents undergoing conservative surgery. In the adolescent presenting with refractory dysmenorrhea or chronic pelvic pain, endometriosis must be high on the list of possible diagnoses. Depending on the symptoms and signs, the physician can choose either medical or surgical management. Because many investigators believe that endometriosis is a progressive disease, these patients should be closely followed and therapy individualized.

Analysis of data from prospective studies on asymptomatic women undergoing tubal sterilization reveals a markedly higher than expected frequency of endometriosis[16]. This raises doubts about the clinical significance of the minimal lesions that are often found. The concept that initial endometriosis should always be treated to avoid worsening of the condition seems to lack a convincing rational basis and is not supported by definitive scientific evidence[27]. Minimal/mild endometriosis could represent a temporary phase in an ongoing process that usually results in cytolysis of recently implanted endometrial cells, whereas in a few immunologically 'tolerant' subjects, nodular, cystic and infiltrating lesions develop, with eventual progression to moderate and severe stages. The results of danazol treatment, diathermy, conservative surgery with postoperative danazol and no treatment were compared at laparoscopy repeated after a mean interval of 12 months: there was no significant worsening in the American Fertility Society classification score in the 11 untreated patients[28].

The individual adolescent endometriotic patients can be divided into two different patient groups based on symptoms and pelvic findings. The first group is presumed adolescent endometriotic patients with minimal symptoms such as dysmenorrhea or pelvic pain and minimal abnormal pelvic findings. In these cases, we can prescribe prostaglandin synthetase inhibitors (PGSIs), cyclic oral contraceptive pills or progestins. The patient should then be re-evaluated at 1–3-month intervals, depending on the nature of her symptoms. At these visits, the treatment can be either continued or a new treatment implemented. If after a reasonable interval (approximately 3–6 months) there is little or no abatement of symptoms despite alternative therapy, a laparoscopy is recommended for definitive diagnosis, with possible surgical treatment and surgical staging.

The second group is symptomatic patients with posterior cul-de-sac nodularities, adnexal mass or fixed uterus. We should perform cytoreductive laparoscopic surgery in these patients, and then we can prescribe oral contraceptive pills, progestins, danazol or gonadotropin-releasing hormone analogs, depending on patients' status, for 3–6 months of medical therapy. Danazol, large doses of progestins (Provera 20 mg or greater daily) and Depo-

Provera (medroxyprogesterone acetate, Pharmacia and Upjohn Inc., USA) have been shown to have significant adverse side-effects and are associated with poor compliance in adolescents[8]. After this, patients can start cyclic premenstrual PGSIs to reduce menstrual regurgitation monthly. Oral contraceptives are the medical treatment most often prescribed for endometriosis. Unfortunately, no data are available to show that these drugs either reduce lesions or alleviate symptoms. Most cases are amenable to modern advanced laparoscopic surgery.

Summary

Endometriosis might not be eradicated from the pelvic cavity with conventional treatments. Therefore more conservative, disease-modifying and non-invasive management of adolescent endometriosis might be acceptable to gynecologists, parents and patients. On the basis of our experiences, adolescent endometriotic patients may not have to receive laparoscopic surgery to confirm the diagnosis of pelvic endometriosis. If this is right, we can make the magnetic resonance images or trans-rectal sonography-guided tentative diagnosis of endometriosis in adolescents with subjective symptoms. Imaging diagnosis using trans-rectal sonography or pelvic magnetic resonance imaging with fat suppression might be helpful in detecting mild or minimal endometriosis in adolescents complaining of severe dysmenorrhea or chronic pelvic pain.

Cycle control with PGSIs to minimize menstrual regurgitation might minimize the recurrences of endometriosis following cytoreductive laparoscopic surgery. Imaging diagnosis can be followed by one of the hormonal drugs such as danazol, progestins, gonadotropin-releasing hormone analogs or oral contraceptive pills. If she is responding to medical therapy, she does not have to receive the invasive diagnostic laparoscopy. If she cannot get the satisfactory clinical response, we can recommend laparoscopic surgery. Invasive laparoscopic diagnosis can be cautiously replaced with non-invasive sonographic or magnetic resonance imaging diagnosis in some selected cases of endometriosis such as in adolescent endometriosis, endometriotic patients without discernible adnexal mass, or recurrent endometriosis. Despite significant development in surgical and medical approaches, the optimal therapy for adolescent endometriosis still needs further innovation.

References

1. Thomas, E.J. (1995). Endometriosis 1995 – confusion or sense? *Int. J. Gynecol. Obstet.*, **48**, 149–55
2. Koninckx, P.R., Oosterlynck, D., D'Hooghe, T. and Meuleman, C. (1994). Deeply infiltrating endometriosis is a disease whereas mild endometriosis could be considered a non-disease. *Ann. N. Y. Acad. Sci.*, **734**, 333–41
3. Hoshiai, H., Ishikawa, M., Saawatari, Y., Noda, K. and Fukaya, T. (1993). Laparoscopic evaluation of the onset and progression of endometriosis. *Am. J. Obstet. Gynecol.*, **169**, 714–19
4. Gidwani, G.P. (1996). Chronic pelvic pain: steps to take before and after operative intervention. In Pokorny, S. (ed.) *Pediatric and Adolescent Gynecology*, pp. 41–54. (New York: Chapman & Hall)
5. Redwine, D. (1987). The distribution of endometriosis in the pelvis by age groups and fertility. *Fertil. Steril.*, **47**, 173–5
6. Houston, D., Noller, K., Melton, L., Selwyn, B.J. and Hardy, R.J. (1987). Incidence of pelvic endometriosis in Rochester, Minnesota, 1970–1979. *Am. J. Epidemiol.*, **125**, 959–69
7. Bullock, J., Massey, F. and Gambrell, R. (1974). Symptomatic endometriosis in teenagers: a reappraisal. *Obstet. Gynecol.*, **43**, 896–900
8. Goldstein, D.P., deCholnoky, C. and Emans, S.J. (1980). Adolescent endometriosis. *J. Adolesc. Health Care*, **1**, 37–41
9. Chatman, D.L. and Ward, A.B. (1982).

Endometriosis in adolescents. *J. Reprod. Med.*, **27**, 156–60

10. Vercellini, P., Fedele, L., Arcaini, L., Bianch, S., Rognoni, M.T. and Candiani, G.B. (1989). Laparoscopy in the diagnosis of chronic pelvic pain in adolescent women. *J. Reprod. Med.*, **34**, 827–30

11. Schifrin, B.S., Erez, S. and Moore, J.G. (1973). Teenage endometriosis. *Am. J. Obstet. Gynecol.*, **116**, 973–80

12. Sanfilippo, J. and Yussman, M. (1985). Gynecologic problems of adolescence. In Lavery, J. and Sanfilippo, J. (eds.) *Pediatric and Adolescent Obstetrics and Gynecology*, pp. 74–83. (New York: Springer-Verlag)

13. Durinzi, K.L. and De Leon, F.D. (1993). Endometriosis in the adolescent and teenage female. *Adolesc. Pediatr. Gynecol.*, **6**, 3–7

14. Davis, G.D., Thillet, E. and Lindemann, J. (1993). Clinical characteristics of adolescent endometriosis. *J. Adolesc. Health*, **14**, 362–8

15. Vernon, M.W., Beard, J.S. Graves, K. and Wilson, E.A. (1986). Classification of endometriotic implants by morphologic appearance and capacity to synthesize prostaglandin F. *Fertil. Steril.*, **46**, 801–6

16. Fedele, L., Parazzini, F., Bianchi, S., Arcaini, L. and Candiani, G.B. (1990). Stage and localization of pelvic endometriosis and pain. *Fertil. Steril.*, **53**, 155–8

17. Ripps, B.A. and Martin, D.C. (1991). Focal pelvic tenderness, pelvic pain, and dysmenorrhea in endometriosis. *J. Reprod. Med.*, **36**, 470–2

18. Cho, S. and Lim, Y.T. (1996). Transvaginal sonographic detection of endometriotic foci with laparoscopic correlation. Presented at the *Vth World Congress on Endometriosis*, October, Yokohama, Japan, 0–96

19. Chatman, D.L. (1981). Pelvic peritoneal defects and endometriosis. Allen-Masters syndrome revisited. *Fertil. Steril.*, **36**, 751–6

20. Redwine, B.D. (1987). Age-related evolution in color appearance of endometriosis. *Fertil. Steril.*, **48**, 1062–3

21. Koninckx, P.R., Meuleman, C., Demeyere, S., Lesaffre, E. and Cornillie, F. (1991). Suggestive evidence that pelvic endometriosis is a progressive disease, whereas deeply infiltrating endometriosis is associated with pelvic pain. *Fertil. Steril.*, **55**, 759–66

22. Jansen, R.P.S. and Russell, G. (1986). Non-pigmented endometriosis: clinical, laparoscopic, and pathologic definition. *Am. J. Obstet. Gynecol.*, **155**, 1154–9

23. Rewine, D.B. and Yocom, L.B. (1990). A serial section study of visually normal pelvic peritoneum in patients with endometriosis. *Fertil. Steril.*, **54**, 648–51

24. Wood, C. and Maher, P. (1996). Peritoneal surgery in the treatment of endometriosis – excision or thermal ablation? *Aust. N. Z. J. Obstet. Gynaecol.*, **36**, 190–7

25. Ha, H.K., Lim, Y.T., Kim, H.S., Seo, J.S., Song, H.H. and Kim, S.J. (1994). Diagnosis of pelvic endometriosis: fat suppressed T_1-weighted vs. conventional MR images. *Am. J. Radiol.*, **163**, 127–31

26. Schwartz, L.B. and Diamond, M.P. (1991). Formation, reduction, and treatment of adhesive disease. *Semin. Reprod. Endocrinol.*, **9**, 89–99

27. Vercellini, P., Bocciolone, L. and Crosignani, P.G. (1992). Is mild endometriosis always a disease? *Hum. Reprod.*, **7**, 627–9

28. Mahmood, T.A. and Templeton, A. (1991). Prevalence and genesis of endometriosis. *Hum. Reprod.*, **6**, 544–9

The onset and progression of endometriosis in humans

T. Fukaya, T. Murakami, J. Sugawara, H. Yoshida, A. Yajima and H. Hoshiai

Introduction

Although several mechanisms have been proposed to explain the pathogenesis of endometriosis, a definitive theory on the overall process has yet to be established. Some studies have suggested that the incidence of endometriosis in teenage girls may be higher than previously anticipated[1,2]. However, the rate of progression of endometriotic lesions is unknown. To define the clinical characteristics of endometriosis better, the clinical records of 690 laparoscopically confirmed cases of endometriosis were analyzed retrospectively with regard to the site of primary lesion, age at onset, rate of progression, and response to drug treatment on the basis of the revised American Fertility Society point system for endometriosis.

In contrast to clinical study, the initiation of endometriosis has not been fully understood. To reveal the process of initiation of endometriosis, the evaluation of the change of pelvic environment in the patient with endometriosis may be important. With regard to these changes, there have been many studies carried out on cytokines, vascularization, etc. In the present study, we focused on the environment of soluble intercellular adhesion molecule-1 (soluble ICAM-1). Soluble ICAM-1 has been implicated in tumor progression by escape from immunosurveillance[3]. Recent studies have disclosed various defects in the cell-mediated immune system and there is a possibility of its relationship to progression of endometriosis. However, little is known about the mechanism of the defect in the cell-mediated immune system in the patient with endometriosis. To determine the mechanism of the defect in the cell-mediated immune system in endometriosis, we assessed the soluble ICAM-1 level in peritoneal fluid and macrophage-conditioned media of women with and without endometriosis.

Materials and methods

Clinical assessment

The subjects were 690 women with laparoscopically confirmed endometriosis at the Department of Obstetrics and Gynecology, Tohoku University School of Medicine, and at the Kinki University School of Medicine, as well as at affiliated hospitals, from 1985 to 1992.

Laparoscopic examination served only as a diagnostic procedure, and the severity of endometriosis was diagnosed according to the revised American Fertility Society (AFS) classification. The revised AFS stage of the 690 subjects was stage I in 250 cases, stage II in 130 cases, stage III in 149 cases, and stage IV in 161 cases. To calculate the frequency of endometriotic lesions by site, each lesion present in a single organ was counted as one occurrence regardless of the lesion size.

Data on the natural course of endometriosis were obtained from seven patients who underwent repeated laparoscopic examinations at varying intervals without receiving any type of treatment. Moreover data from four teenagers were used to estimate the onset of endometriosis.

Evaluation of ICAM-1

Peritoneal fluid samples were obtained at the time of diagnostic or operative laparoscopy for infertility and benign gynecological disease. Among these patients, 18 out of 32 patients were confirmed as having pelvic endometriosis and other patients were normal. All samples were centrifuged at $400\,g$ for 10 min and the supernatant was kept at $-80\,°C$ until ICAM-1 assay. In 13 patients (6 normal and 7 with endometriosis), the cellular pellet obtained after centrifugation was resuspended in 10 ml RPMI–1640 with penicillin, streptomycin and fungisone. Peritoneal macrophages were isolated using selective adherence to plastic plates, and the macrophages were cultured on plastic plates for 1 h at 37 °C with medium. Non-adherent macrophages were then removed by rinsing with warmed RPMI-1640. Adhered macrophages were detached and counted using a hemocytometer and phase-contrast microscopy. Macrophage cells at a concentration of 1×10^6/ml were cultured in 48-well culture plates with γ-interferon and interleukin-6 for 72 h. The supernatant was kept at $-80\,°C$ until assay. Soluble ICAM-1 levels were determined by enzyme-linked immunosorbent assay (ELISA).

Results

Clinical findings

In the 250 patients with stage I disease, lesions were classified according to the primary site into seven categories: right ovary, left ovary, pelvic peritoneum/pouch of Douglas, utero-sacral ligament, vesicouterine pouch, rectum/colon and Fallopian tubes (Table 1). The primary site was the ovary in 16.4% of the cases (right 9.6%, left 6.8%), the pelvic peritoneum/pouch of Douglas in 34.5%, the uterosacral ligament in 38.9%, the vesico-uterine pouch in 6.5%, the rectum/colon in 0.3% and the Fallopian tubes in 0.6% of cases. Other sites (2.8%) where lesions were found included the uterus, round ligament, peritoneum parietale, etc. Lesions on the dorsal side of the uterus, that is those situated on the uterosacral ligament and pelvic peritoneum/pouch of Douglas, accounted for about 73% of the total. However, disease progression was associated with an increasing frequency of ovarian lesions (Figure 1).

In seven patients who had laparoscopically diagnosed endometriosis but were left untreated because they did not visit the hospital for 3 months or more, a second laparoscopic examination was performed when treatment was sought again. The revised AFS point score at the first laparoscopic examination was compared with that given at the second examination to estimate the rate of natural progression of endometriosis. After the second examination, two of these seven patients were untreated again for similar reasons and underwent a third laparoscopic examination. The endometriosis score increased gradually in four of seven patients but was unchanged in one, and distinctly decreased in another. On average, endometriosis in these seven patients progressed at the rate of 0.3 points per month (Figure 2).

ICAM-1

Peritoneal fluid volume and the number of peritoneal macrophages were not different in the patients with and without endometriosis.

Table 1 Incidence of lesions by primary site in patients with stage I endometriosis

Primary site	Incidence (%)
Right ovary	9.6
Left ovary	6.8
Pelvic peritoneum	34.5
Uterosacral ligament	38.9
Vesicouterine pouch	6.5
Rectum/colon	0.3
Fallopian tubes	0.6
Other	2.8

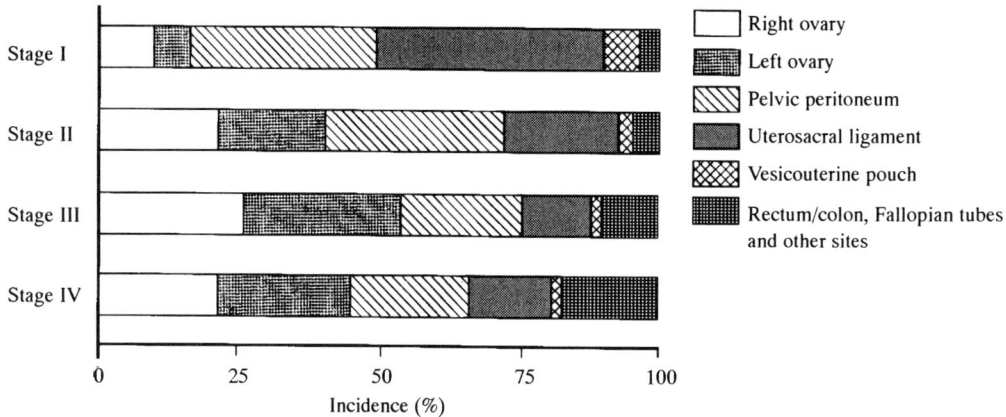

Figure 1 Incidence of lesions at different sites according to stage of endometriosis

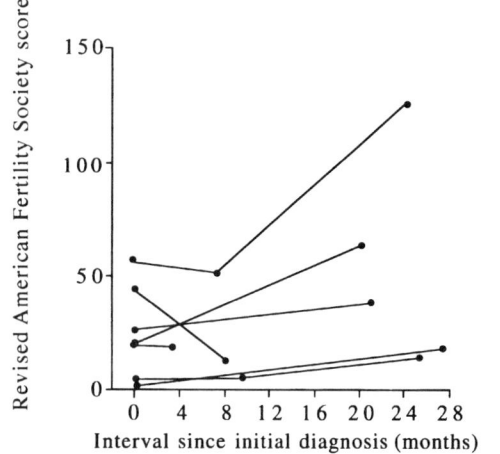

Figure 2 Natural evolution of endometriosis

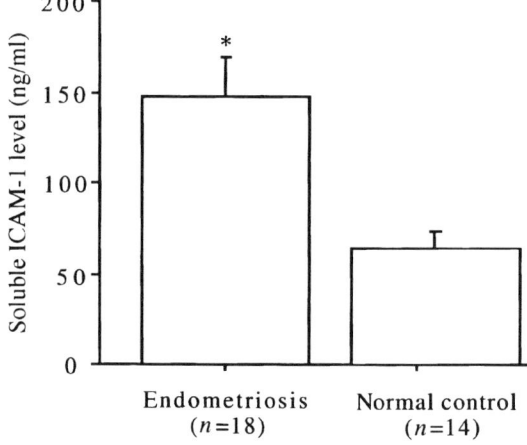

Figure 3 Soluble intercellular adhesion molecule-1 (ICAM-1) levels in peritoneal fluid. Values are expressed as mean ± SD. $*p < 0.01$ compared with controls

The levels of ICAM-1 in the patients with endometriosis were significantly higher than in the patients with endometriosis ($p < 0.01$) (Figure 3). When macrophages were cultured with γ-interferon and interleukin-6, the levels of soluble ICAM-1 were significantly elevated in the patients with endometriosis compared to the normal subjects. Moreover, soluble ICAM-1 levels in culture media were significantly increased in a dose-dependent manner in the patients with endometriosis ($p < 0.05$) (Figures 4 and 5).

Discussion

Several hypotheses have been proposed for the pathogenesis of endometriosis; of them the implantation theory, including the mechanisms of benign metastasis and mechanical transplantation, and the celomic metaplasia theory, are currently the most plausible. The fact that in revised AFS stage I endometriosis primary lesions on the dorsal wall of the uterus, including the uterosacral ligament and the pelvic peritoneum/pouch of Douglas,

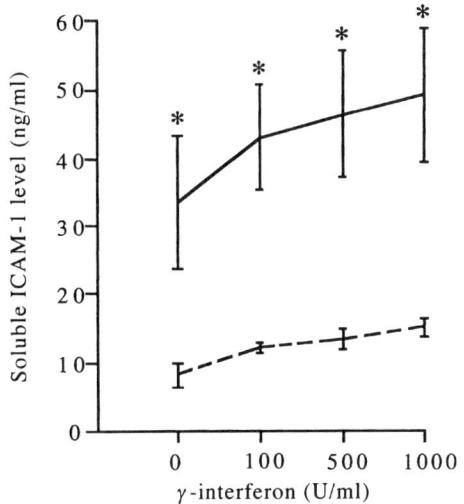

Figure 4 Production of soluble intercellular adhesion molecule-1 (ICAM-1) from peritoneal macrophages cultured with γ-interferon. Values are expressed as mean ± SD. Closed line and dotted line represent the levels of soluble ICAM-1 production in macrophages obtained from patients with endometriosis ($n = 6$) and without endometriosis ($n = 7$), respectively. *$p < 0.01$ compared with controls

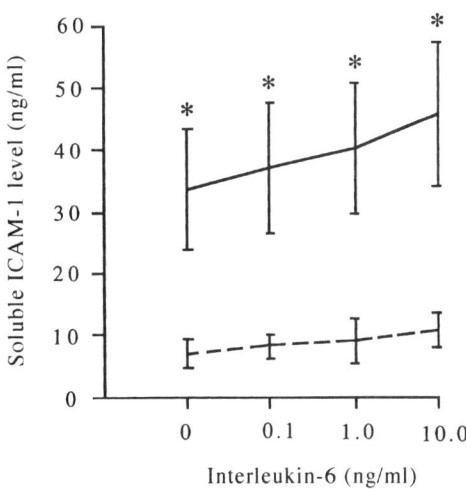

Figure 5 Production of soluble intercellular adhesion molecule-1 (ICAM-1) from peritoneal macrophages cultured with interleukin-6. Values are expressed as mean ± SD. Closed line and dotted line represent the levels of soluble ICAM-1 production in macrophages obtained from patients with endometriosis ($n = 6$) and without endometriosis ($n = 7$), respectively. *$p < 0.05$ compared with controls

made up 73% of all lesions observed in the present study indicates that endometriosis occurred preferentially at sites that are anatomically receptive to implants of aberrant endometrium. Likewise, the fact that the frequency of lesions was 6.5% or lower in regions such as the vesicouterine pouch in which access is poor, supports the implantation theory. In revised AFS stage II endometriosis, the frequency of ovarian lesions increased dramatically compared with the 16% incidence observed in patients with stage I disease. In revised AFS stage II endometriosis, lesions on the uterosacral ligament and pouch of Douglas were often not in contact with ovarian lesions. Thus it was difficult to judge from the present data whether lesions originating in the uterosacral ligament and pouch of Douglas had spread to the ovaries or if newly migrant endometrium had implanted in the ovaries.

Once initiated, endometriosis occasionally regressed, but in most cases it progressed gradually by about 0.3 revised AFS points per month. The natural course of endometriosis has been described by Telimaa[4], Thomas and Cooke[5], and Mahmood and Templeton[6] in comparison with a drug-treated control group. However, because these studies did not use the revised AFS scoring system to evaluate disease status, a direct comparison with the results of the present investigation is not feasible.

Adhesion molecules have been implicated in tumor progression and metastasis by escape from immunosurveillance[3]. Among the adhesion molecules, the elevated level of circulating soluble ICAM-1 is demonstrated in several diseases[7]. Accordingly, in endometriosis, various defects in the cell-mediated immune system in the pelvic cavity have been speculated as one of the causes of the pathogenesis of endometriosis. We therefore focused on the role that soluble ICAM-1 may contribute to the pathogenesis and implantation of endometriosis by measuring the levels of soluble ICAM-1 in peritoneal fluid and evaluating the production of soluble ICAM-1 from peritoneal macrophages cultured with γ-interferon and interleukin-6.

In the present study, the levels of soluble ICAM-1 in the pelvic fluid of patients with endometriosis were significantly higher than in normal subjects. Nevertheless, the population of macrophages was not different in patients with and without endometriosis. Moreover, the production of soluble ICAM-1 from cultured macrophages was significantly higher in patients with endometriosis than in normal subjects. These results indicate that there is a relationship between adhesion molecules and progression of endometriosis. Although the major source of soluble ICAM-1 is considered to be endometrial stromal cells[8], our results indicated that some p ortion of peritoneal soluble ICAM-1 is produced by peritoneal macrophages. Elevated soluble ICAM-1 may also contribute to the pathogenesis and/or progression by the cell-mediated immune system, especially by escape from immunosurveillance through the reduction of natural killer cell activity[9]. It is difficult to determine whether soluble ICAM-1 is responsible for the initiation of endometriosis. However, our results indicate that cytokine(s) from the uterus may stimulate soluble ICAM-1 production and consequently reduce the natural killer cell activity, and these changes of pelvic environment may be important for the pathogenesis of this disease.

References

1. Ranney, B. (1980). Etiology prevention and inhibition of endometriosis. *Clin. Obstet. Gynecol.*, **23**, 875–82
2. Chatman, D.L. (1976). Endometriosis in black women. *Am. J. Obstet. Gynecol.*, **125**, 987–9
3. McCarthy, J.B., Skubitz, A.P.N., Iida, J., Mooradian, D.L., Wilke, M.S. and Furcht, L.T. (1991). Tumor cell adhesive mechanism and their relationship to metastasis. *Semin. Cancer Biol.*, **2**, 155–67
4. Telimaa, S. (1988). Danazol and medroxyprogesterone acetate are inefficacious in the treatment of infertility in endometriosis. *Fertil. Steril.*, **50**, 872–5
5. Thomas, E.J. and Cooke, I.D. (1987). Impact of Gestrinone on the course of asymptomatic endo-metriosis. *Br. Med. J.*, **294**, 272–4
6. Mahmood, T.A. and Templeton, A. (1990). The impact of treatment on the natural history of endometriosis. *Hum. Reprod.*, **5**, 965–70
7. Banks, R.E., Gearing, A.J.H., Hemingway, I.K., Norfork, D.R., Perren, T.J. and Selby, P.J. (1993). Circulating intercellular adhesion molecule-1 (ICAM-1), E-selectin and vascular cell adhesion molecule-1 (VCAM-1) in human malignancies. *Br. J. Cancer*, **68**, 122–4
8. Somigliana, E., Vigano, P., Gaffuri, B., Guarneri, D., Busacca, M. and Vignali, M. (1996). Human endometrial stroma cell as a source of soluble intercellular adhesion molecule (ICAM)-1 molecules. *Hum. Reprod.*, **11**, 1190–4
9. Vigano, P., Pardi, R., Magri, B., Busacca, M., DiBlasio, A.M. and Vignali, M. (1994). Expression of intercellular adhesion molecule-1 (ICAM-1) on cultured human endometrial stromal cells and its role in the interaction with natural killers. *Am. J. Reprod. Immunol.*, **32**, 139–45

The ovarian endometrioma

I.A. Brosens

Although the features of ovarian endometrioma were fully described by Russell in 1899 it took more than 20 years before the hemorrhagic cyst was recognized as an endometrial cyst by Sampson in 1921[1]. The discovery of the endometrial origin by Sampson was based on the presence of endometrial-like tissue and the functional evidence of menstrual bleeding at the time of menstruation. Two types of endometrial implants were described by Sampson in association with large ovarian endometriomas: first, the lining of the cyst by surface epithelium with or without stroma and usually without glandular structures, and second, implants of glands and stroma enclosed at the site where the cyst was adherent to pelvic structures such as the posterior side of the uterus. Menstrual bleeding was observed in the free implants lining the cavity of the cyst, while proliferation of the smooth muscle cells was described in the enclosed implants at the sites of the adhesions with other pelvic structures. Sampson made these observations on hysterectomy and bilateral salpingoophorectomy with endometriomas *in situ*, and as four specimens obtained at the time of menstruation showed the menstrual changes which are specific for endometrial tissue, the endometrial origin of the cyst was firmly established.

In 1957 Hughesdon[2] could also demonstrate on ovaries with the endometrioma *in situ* that in 93% of cases the wall of the cyst was formed by the invagination of the ovarian cortex and that there was no evidence of invasion of the ovary by endometrial tissue. He concluded therefore that the majority of endometriomas are extra-ovarian pseudocysts. Both Sampson and Hughesdon found in 9% and 3% of cases, respectively, an ovarian endometrioma communicating with a luteal cyst, which is of no surprise when it is realized that the pseudocyst

Table 1 Gross features of ovarian endometrial cysts

Size 2–10 cm (Sampson[1])
Bilateral 1/3 (Sampson[1])
Caudal pole
Adhesions
Spilling at adhesiolysis
Chocolate content

is lined by cortex. This observation, however, is usually used as an argument for the theory that endometriomas originate from invasion and colonization of ruptured follicles by endometriotic cells.

The exploration of the endometrioma *in situ* by ovarian cystoscopy[3] has allowed investigations in young women and has confirmed the previous observations. In addition, it has been observed that in young women the wall has the pearl-white or slightly pigmented appearance of ovarian cortex. The endometrial lining is a highly vascularized and loosely attached, very thin layer which can easily be detached from the wall. The macroscopic, histological and endoscopic features of the ovarian endometrioma are summarized in Tables 1, 2 and 3, respectively.

At the site of adhesions the wall of the cyst shows retraction or a niche suggesting extension of the initially small pseudocyst from this area. The pattern of neoangiogenesis is also suggestive of colonization of the wall by the endometrial epithelium from the site of inversion. In summary, the typical ovarian endometrioma has the structure of a pseudo-uterine cavity which is created by adhesions and inclusion of endometriotic implants and developing into a pseudo-hematometra.

Endometriomas larger than 2 cm show in 83–100% of adhesions with the opposing

Table 2 Histological features of ovarian endometrial cysts

Lining	endometrial epithelium with/without stroma
	cortex
	fibro-reactive tissue
	non-specific lining
Wall	hemosiderin-laden macrophages
	fibrosis
	smooth muscle cell hyperplasia
Adhesion site	glands and stroma
	adenomyosis

Table 3 Ovarioscopic features of ovarian endometrial cysts

Non-fibrotic (red) cysts
  red implants
  highly vascularized
  superficial and loosely adherent to wall
  white, yellow wall
  retraction, niche at site of adhesions
Fibrotic (black) cysts
  brown dark wall
  focal vascularization

Table 4 Technique of extra-ovarian reconstruction of the ovarian endometrioma

Adhesiolysis and identification of invagination site
Opening and resection of invagination site
Coagulation of red implants
Full hemostasis

pelvic structures[1,4]. At this site enclosed adenomyotic implants are frequently found. It is therefore recommended that this site is explored for deep or nodular endometriosis which could explain the correlation between endometriomas and pelvic pain[5].

Reconstructive surgery of the ovaries with endometriomas in young women can be achieved by an extra-ovarian technique (Table 4)[6]. In addition, at the site of adhesions nodular or adenomyotic lesions should be carefully coagulated or excised. In the presence of adhesions a second-look laparoscopy is recommended to evaluate and treat postsurgical recurrent adhesions. Treatment with gonadotropin-releasing hormone agonist during the 2 months before the second-look laparoscopy has been proposed to reduce the risk of recurrent adhesion formation[7]. Excision of the ovarian cortex which forms the wall of the pseudocyst should be avoided in young women. In addition to the increased risk of adhesion formation, recent data suggest that cystectomy results in a poor response during ovarian stimulation in IVF treatment.

References

1. Sampson, J.A. (1921). Perforating hemorrhagic (chocolate) cysts of the ovary. *Arch. Surg.*, **3**, 245–323
2. Hughesdon, P.E. (1957). The structure of endometrial cysts of the ovary. *J. Obstet. Gynaecol. Br. Emp.*, **44**, 481–7
3. Brosens, I.A., Puttemans, P.J. and Deprest, J. (1994). The endoscopic localization of endometrial implants in the ovarian chocolate cyst. *Fertil. Steril.*, **61**, 1034–8
4. Nezhat, F., Nezhat, C., Allan, C.J., Metzger, D.A. and Sears, D.L. (1992). A clinical and histologic classification of endometriomas: implications for a mechanism of pathogenesis. *J. Reprod. Med.*, **37**, 771–6
5. Fedele, L., Bianchi, S., Bocciolone, L., Di Nola, G. and Parazzini, F. (1992). Pain symptoms associated with endometriosis. *Obstet. Gynecol.*, **79**, 767–9
6. Brosens, I.A., Van Ballaer, P., Puttemans, P. and Deprest, J. (1996). Reconstruction of the ovary containing large endometriomas by an extra-ovarian endosurgical technique. *Fertil. Steril.*, **66**, 517–21
7. Donnez, J., Nisolle, M., Gillerot, S., Anaf, V., Clerckx-Braun, F. and Casanas-Roux, F. (1994). Ovarian endometrial cysts: the role of gonadotropin-releasing hormone agonist and/or drainage. *Fertil. Steril.*, **62**, 63–6

Rectovaginal septum adenomyotic nodule: a distinct entity

J. Donnez, M. Nisolle and F. Casanas-Roux

Introduction

In the pelvis, three different forms of endometriosis must be considered[1]: peritoneal endometriosis, ovarian endometriosis and rectovaginal endometriosis. Recently, Nisolle[2] demonstrated that the three entities are distinct and have a different histopathogenesis.

Red lesions (red vesicles, polypoid lesions, red flame-like lesions, hypervascularized areas or even petechial peritoneum)[1,3,4] have recently been proved to be a very active form of the disease[5]. In women, our hypothesis is that red lesions are more aggressive and progress to the so-called typical or black lesions which must be considered as an enclosed implant surrounded by fibrosis. Ovarian chocolate-colored fluid cysts are, according to the hypothesis of Hughesdon[6], the consequence of the invagination of superficial implants into the ovary. Our hypothesis[2,7] claims that the endometrioma is the consequence of the metaplasia of invaginated mesothelium. Endometrioma can also develop in the ovaries and this type of cystic ovarian endometriosis must be considered as another severe form of endometriosis, often related to infertility.

A third form of the disease is deep-infiltrating endometriosis of the rectovaginal septum. Sampson[8] defined cul-de-sac obliteration as 'extensive adhesions in the cul-de-sac, obliterating its lower portion and uniting the cervix or the lower portion of the uterus to the rectum, with adenoma of the endometrial type invading the cervical and the uterine tissue and probably also (but to a lesser degree) the anterior wall of the rectum'. For us, rectovaginal septum endometriosis is, in fact, an 'adenomyotic nodule'.

Treatment options for pain or infertility secondary to cul-de-sac obliteration include ovarian suppression therapy with danazol or gonadotropin-releasing hormone agonists, or surgery[9–11]. Recently, some gynecologists[10,12–14] have developed the endoscopic technique.

Methods and results

Our series of 500 cases of rectovaginal septum endometriosis is presented here. In the majority of cases, the main symptom was severe pelvic pain. Twenty-five per cent of patients suffered pelvic pain and infertility. In cases of infertility, all patients underwent an evaluation of ovulation, cervical mucus–sperm interaction (post-coital test) and male factor infertility (defined as < 15 million sperm per ml using a Makler counting chamber). Preoperative radiography of the colon was carried out in order to evaluate the involvement of the rectal surface. Profile radiography of an air-contrast barium enema offers the best evaluation of the infiltration of the rectal anterior wall (Figure 1).

The surgical techniques have evolved gradually but all of them involve the separation of the anterior rectum from the posterior vagina and the excision or ablation of the endometriosis in that area. Aquadissection, scissor dissection and electrosurgery with an unmodulated (cutting) current are used by some authors[10], while others[12,15] prefer the use of the CO_2 laser. A mechanical bowel preparation was administered orally on the afternoon before surgery to induce brisk, self-

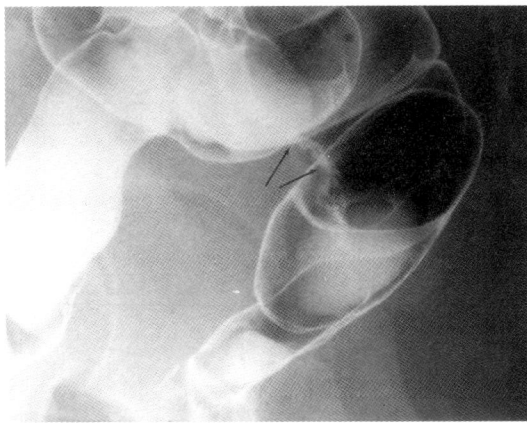

Figure 1 Profile radiography of an air-contrast barium enema offers the best evaluation of the infiltration of the anterior rectal wall. Typical 'endometriotic' infiltration of the anterior rectal wall (arrows)

Table 1 Rectovaginal endometriosis: technical aspects ($n = 500$)

Technical aspects	Mean (range)
Duration of surgery	69 (40–132) mins
Hospitalization time	2.8 (2–5) days
Laparoscopic bowel resections	0

limiting diarrhea that rapidly cleanses the bowel without disrupting the electrolyte balance. All the laparoscopic procedures were performed using general anesthesia. A 12-mm operative laparoscope was inserted through a vertical intraumbilical incision. Three other puncture sites were made 2–3 cm above the pubis, on the midline and in the areas adjacent to the deep inferior epigastric vessels, which were visualized directly.

Clinical and laparoscopic aspects (Table 1)

Examination with a speculum reveals either a normal vaginal mucosa or a protruded endometriotic nodule in the posterior fornix. By palpation, the diameter of the lesion can be evaluated. Palpation is very often painful and the presence of the nodule accounts for symptoms like deep dyspareunia and dysmenorrhea. To determine the cul-de-sac obliteration, a sponge on a ring forceps was inserted into the posterior vaginal fornix. A dilator (Hegar 25) was systematically inserted into the rectum. Complete obliteration was diagnosed when the outline of the posterior fornix could not be seen through the laparoscope. Cul-de-sac obliteration was partial when rectal tenting was visible but a protrusion of the sponge in the posterior vaginal fornix was identified between the rectum and the inverted U of the utero-sacral ligaments. Sometimes, however, a deep-infiltrating lesion of the rectovaginal septum is only barely visible by laparoscopy.

Surgical technique

Deep fibrotic nodular endometriosis involving the cul-de-sac requires an excision of the nodular fibrotic tissue from the posterior vagina, rectum, posterior cervix and uterosacral ligaments. As described by Reich and associates[10], attention was first directed toward a complete dissection of the anterior rectum throughout its area of involvement until the loose tissue of the rectovaginal space was reached. A sponge on a ring forceps was inserted into the posterior vaginal fornix and a dilator (Hegar 25) was placed in the rectum. In addition, a cannula was inserted into the endometrial cavity to antevert the uterus markedly. The peritoneum covering the cul-de-sac of Douglas was opened between the 'adenomyotic' lesion and the rectum.

We used a technique of first freeing the anterior rectum from the loose areolar tissue of the rectovaginal septum, prior to excising and/or vaporizing visible and palpable deep fibrotic endometriosis. This approach is possible even when anterior rectal muscularis infiltration is present. Careful dissection was then carried out using the aquadissector for aquadissection and the CO_2 laser for sharp dissection until the rectum was completely freed

Table 2 Rectovaginal endometriosis: complications ($n = 500$)

Complications	n (%)
Rectal perforation*	4 (0.9)
Delayed hemorrhage (< 24 h post-operative)	2 (0.4)
Urinary retention	4 (0.6)
Ureteral injury	0
Bladder injury	0

*Rectal perforation: the perforation was recognized during the procedure. The defect was repaired either by colpotomy ($n = 2$) or by minilaparotomy ($n = 2$).

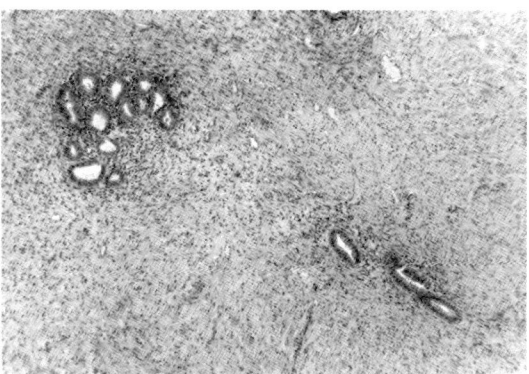

Figure 2 Rectovaginal adenomyosis (Gomori's trichrome ×66). Scanty endometrial type stroma and glandular epithelium are disseminated in muscular tissue

and identifiable below the lesion. Excision of the fibrotic tissue on the side of the rectum was attempted only after the rectal dissection was complete. A partial rectal resection was never performed in our series. In cases of deep-infiltrating lesions, the vaginal wall is more or less penetrated by the adenomyosis, and excision of a part of the vagina is essential.

Dissection was performed accordingly, not only with the removal of all visible endometriotic lesions, but also of the vaginal mucosa with at least a 0.5-cm disease-free margin. Lesions extending totally through the vagina were treated by *en bloc* laparoscopic resection from the cul-de-sac to the posterior vaginal wall; the pneumoperitoneum was maintained and the posterior vaginal wall was closed vaginally. The anterior rectum can be reperitonealized by plicating the uterosacral ligaments and lateral rectal peritoneum across the midline using 4–0 Polydioxanone[10] or Tissucol or Interceed (Johnson and Johnson, Ascot, UK)[16]. In our series of 500 cases, laparoscopic rectal perforation occurred in four cases (Table 2). Perforation was diagnosed at the time of the laparoscopy. In two cases, the rectum was repaired by laparotomy and in the other two cases by colpotomy. Laparoscopic dissection was successfully performed in all cases, even when the radiography of the colon showed bowel involvement. During the same period, five cases of rectal endometriosis and eight cases of sigmoid colon endometriosis were diagnosed. None of the 13 patients had nodules of the septum, but bowel wall endometriosis which provoked menstrual rectorrhagia. In the 13 cases, laparotomy and bowel resection were performed. In all cases, histology proved the invasion of the mucosa by endometriotic tissue.

Histology

Deep vaginal endometriosis associated with pelvic endometriosis can take the form of nodular or polypoid masses involving the posterior vaginal fornix. It has been called an 'adenomyotic nodule of the rectovaginal septum'[17,18]. An adenomyoma is a circumscribed, nodular aggregate of smooth muscle, endometrial glands and usually, endometrial stroma (Figure 2). This type of lesion is not actually endometriosis, but a specific disease called adenomyosis characterized by the presence of abundant muscular tissue invaded by glandular epithelium covered with a scanty stroma. Adenomyosis exhibits a varied functional response to ovarian hormones. It may not respond to physiological levels of progesterone, and secretory changes are frequently absent or incomplete during the second half of the cycle[17]. Proliferative glands and stroma

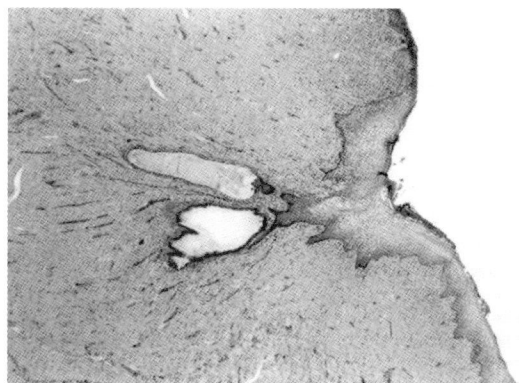

Figure 3 Endometrial glands and stroma are found up to the vaginal mucosa (Gomori's trichrome × 50)

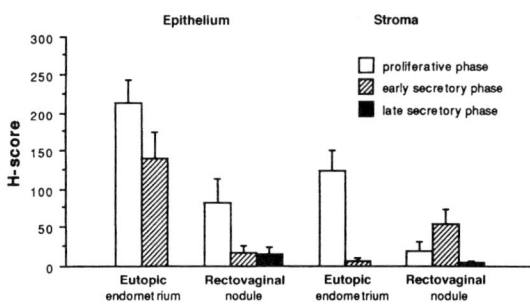

Figure 4 Estrogen receptors. Mean ± SEM quantitative H-score in nuclei of glandular epithelium and stroma of eutopic endometrium and rectovaginal nodule adenomyosis during the proliferative phase and the secretory phase

are generally observed in the first half of the menstrual cycle. Very often, endometriotic glands and stroma were found by serial section up to the vaginal mucosa (Figure 3) which was sometimes replaced by endometrial epithelium.

Sometimes, the 'invasion' of the muscle by a very active glandular epithelium proved that the stroma is not necessary for the invasion in this particular type of pathology called adenomyosis.

Cytokeratin and vimentin staining

The evaluation of intermediate filaments by cytokeratin staining[19] showed a similar pattern throughout the menstrual cycle when compared to eutopic endometrium, the cytokeratin H-score in glandular epithelium during the luteal phase being significantly lower in the nodules than in the other tissue. Vimentin was never expressed during the follicular phase in the glandular epithelium and stroma of nodules. During the luteal phase, the vimentin H-score in the stroma was similar to that of eutopic endometrium, but significantly lower in the glandular epithelium. The presence of a lower expression of cytokeratin in glandular epithelium could be interpreted as a lower degree of differentiation or as a delay in the differentiation. The very low vimentin reactivity and the absence of any decrease throughout the cycle in the glandular epithelium of nodules account for the low degree of differentiation and their unresponsiveness to endogenic hormonal variations.

Estrogen receptor and progesterone receptor content

The pattern of the estrogen receptor content (Figure 4) of the glandular epithelium of nodules was similar to that observed in eutopic endometrium throughout the cycle, a significant decrease occurring during the luteal phase in both tissues. But at the stroma level, a significant increase in estrogen receptor was observed in the nodules throughout the cycle whereas a significant decrease occurred in eutopic endometrium. The progesterone receptor content pattern throughout the menstrual cycle was different in the two tissues (Figure 5). Indeed, although a significant decrease was observed in eutopic endometrium, a significant increase was noted in the nodules throughout the cycle, in the glandular epithelium as well as the stroma.

The variations in the estrogen receptor and progesterone receptor content of the nodules

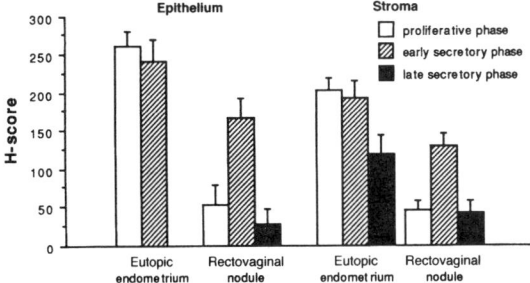

Figure 5 Progesterone receptors. Mean ± SEM quantitative H-score in nuclei of glandular epithelium and stroma of eutopic endometrium and rectovaginal nodule adenomyosis during the proliferative phase and the secretory phase

throughout the cycle suggest that they are probably not regulated by steroids. The absence of response to progesterone levels also suggest different regulatory mechanisms of endometriotic steroid receptors.

Discussion

In the pelvis, three different forms of endometriosis must be considered[18]: peritoneal, ovarian and rectovaginal septum. By evaluation of the mitotic activity and the stromal vascularization, we recently proved[5] that red peritoneal lesions were the most aggressive form of the disease and progress to the so-called typical or black lesion which must be considered as an enclosed implant surrounded by fibrosis. This type of infiltration must be clearly differentiated from the rectovaginal endometriotic nodule. Koninckx[11] recently described three types of deep-infiltrating endometriosis. Deep-infiltrating endometriosis of Type I is a rather large lesion in the peritoneal cavity, infiltrating conically with the deeper parts becoming progressively smaller. It has been suggested that this type of endometriosis is caused by infiltration. In Type II lesions, the main feature is the bowel retracted over the lesion which thus becomes deeply situated in the rectovaginal septum although not really infiltrating it. Type III lesions are the deepest and most severe. They are sphere-shaped, situated deep in the rectovaginal septum, and often only visible as a small typical lesion at laparoscopy. This lesion is often more palpable than visible, originates from the rectovaginal septum tissue and consists essentially of smooth muscle with active glandular epithelium and scanty stroma. In our study, the rectovaginal nodule was histologically similar to an adenomyoma[20]. It was a circumscribed, nodular aggregate of smooth muscle, endometrial glands and endometrial stroma. As in the 'adenomyoma', secretory changes were frequently absent in 'endometriotic' rectovaginal nodules, and this can be explained by the very low epithelial and stromal estrogen receptor content during the follicular phase, which could be the key factor of the out-of-phase endometrium despite normal progesterone levels[21]. Sometimes, the invasion of the muscle by a very active glandular epithelium without stroma proved that the stroma is not mandatory for invasion in this particular type of pathology called adenomyosis. In some instances, it could be seen that the vaginal pluristratified epithelium was replaced by glandular epithelium. The presence of ciliated cells and the coexpression of both vimentin and cytokeratin proved the Müllerian origin of the nodule, of which certain histological characteristics are completely different from those observed in peritoneal lesions[4].

In our series, deep fibrotic tissue assumed to contain endometriosis was excised or vaporized from the anterior rectum with the aid of multiple rectovaginal examinations. Cul-de-sac dissection was followed by excision of deep fibrotic endometriosis, without cul-de-sac reconstruction. In four cases, the bowel lumen was entered. A comprehensive laparoscopic procedure, while not eradicating all the endometriosis, may result in considerable pain relief or a desired pregnancy. While we recognize that bowel resection may be necessary in rare cases, it seems prudent to curtail, rather than encourage, the widespread use of an aggressive, potentially morbid procedure.

In conclusion, deep-infiltrating endometriosis should be considered as a specific disease, different from mild or minimal endometriosis and ovarian cystic endometriosis. We suggest calling this disease 'rectovaginal adenmyosis'.

Acknowledgements

This study was supported by Fonds de la Recherche Scientifique, grant number 3.4587.90, Brussels, Belgium, and by a grant from Ipsen Biotech, Paris, France.

References

1. Donnez, J., Nisolle, M. and Casanas-Roux, F. (1992). Three dimensional architectures of peritoneal endometriosis. *Fertil. Steril.*, **57**, 980–3
2. Nisolle, M. (1996). Peritoneal, ovarian and rectovaginal endometriosis are three distinct entities. *Thèse d'Agrégation de l'Enseignement Supérieur Université Catholique de Louvain*
3. Donnez, J. and Nisolle, M. (1988). Appear-ances of peritoneal endometriosis. In *Proceedings of the 3rd International Laser Surgery Symposium*, Brussels
4. Nisolle, M., Paindaveine, B., Bourdon, A., Berliere, M., Casanas-Roux, F. and Donnez, J. (1990). Histologic study of peritoneal endometriosis in infertile women. *Fertil. Steril.*, **53**, 984–8
5. Nisolle, M., Casanas-Roux, F., Anaf, V., Mine, J.M. and Donnez, J. (1993). Morphometric study of the stromal vascularization in peritoneal endometriosis. *Fertil. Steril.*, **59**, 681–4
6. Hughesdon, P.E. (1957). The structure of endometrial cysts of the ovary. *J. Obstet. Gynaecol. Br. Emp.*, **64**, 481–7
7. Donnez, J., Nisolle, M., Gillet, N., Smets, M., Bassil, S. and Casanas-Roux, F. (1996). Large ovarian endometriomas. *Hum. Reprod.*, **11**, 641–6
8. Sampson, J.A. (1922). Intestinal adenomas of endometrial type. *Arch. Surg.*, **5**, 217
9. Donnez, J., Nisolle, M. and Casanas-Roux, F. (1990). Endometriosis-associated infertility: evaluation of preoperative use of danazol, gestrinone and buserelin. *Int. J. Fertil.*, **35**, 297–301
10. Reich, H., McGlynn, F. and Salvat, J. (1991). Laparoscopic treatment of cul-de-sac obliteration secondary to retrocervical deep fibrotic endometriosis. *Reprod. Med.*, **36**, 516
11. Koninckx, P.D. (1993). Deeply infiltrating endometriosis. In Brosens, I. and Donnez, J. (eds.) *Endometriosis: Research and Management*, pp. 437–46. (Carnforth, UK: Parthenon Publishing)
12. Nezhat, C., Nezhat, F. and Pennington, E. (1992). Laparoscopic treatment of lower colorectal and infiltrative rectovaginal septum endometriosis by the technique of video laparoscopy. *Br. J. Obstet. Gynaecol.*, **99**, 664–7
13. Canis, M., Wattiez, A., Pouly, J.L., Bassil, S., Bouquet de Joliniere, J., Chapron, C., Manhes, H., Mage, G. and Bruhat, M.A. (1993). Laparoscopic treatment of endometriosis. In Brosens, I. and Donnez, J. (eds.) *Endometriosis: Research and Management*, pp. 407–17. (Carnforth, UK: Parthenon Publishing)
14. Donnez, J., Nisolle, M., Casanas-Roux, F. and Clerckx, F. (1993). Endometriosis: rationale for surgery. In Brosens, I. and Donnez, J. (eds.) *Endometriosis: Research and Management*, pp. 385–93. (Carnforth, UK: Parthenon Publishing)
15. Donnez, J., Nisolle, M., Casanas-Roux, F., Anaf, V. and Smets, M. (1994). Laparoscopic treatment of rectovaginal septum endometriosis. In Donnez, J. and Nisolle, M. (eds.) *An Atlas of Laser Operative Laparoscopy and Hysteroscopy*, pp. 75–86. (Carnforth, UK: Parthenon Publishing)
16. Donnez, J. and Nisolle, M. (1995). Advanced laparoscopic surgery for the removal of rectovaginal septum endometriotic or adenomyotic nodules. *Baill. Clin. Obstet. Gynecol.*, **9**, 769–74
17. Donnez, J., Nisolle, M., Casanas-Roux, F., Bassil, S. and Anaf, V. (1995). Rectovaginal septum endometriosis or adenomyosis: laparoscopic management in a series of 231 patients. *Hum. Reprod.*, **10**, 630–5
18. Donnez, J. and Nisolle. M. (1995). Peritoneal endometriosis, ovarian endometrioma and 'endometriotic' nodules of the rectovaginal septum are three distinct entities. *Réf. en*

Gynécol. Obstét., **3**, 121–3
19. Donnez, J., Nisolle, M., Smoes, P., Gillet, N., Beguin, S. and Casanas-Roux, F. (1996). Peritoneal endometriosis and 'endometriotic' nodules of the rectovaginal septum are two different entities. *Fertil. Steril.*, **66**, 362–8
20. Zaloudek, C. and Norris, H.J. (1987). Mesenchymal tumors of the uterus. In Kurman, R. (ed.) *Blaustein's Pathology of the Female Genital Tract*, p. 373. (New York: Springer-Verlag)
21. Hirama, Y and Ochiai K (1995). Estrogen and progesterone receptors of the out-of-phase endometrium in female infertile patients. *Fertil. Steril.*, **63**, 984–8

Large ovarian endometriomas: new perspectives on histogenesis

M. Nisolle, F. Casanas-Roux and J. Donnez

The pathogenesis of typical ovarian endometriosis is a source of controversy. The original paper by Sampson on this condition reported that perforation of the so-called chocolate cyst led to spillage of adhesions and the spread of peritoneal endometriosis[1]. The findings of Hughesdon[2] contradicted Sampson's hypothesis and suggested that adhesions are not the consequence but the cause of endometriomas. In 93% of typical endometriomas, the pseudocyst is formed by an accumulation of menstrual debris from the shedding and bleeding of active implants located by ovarioscopy at the site of inversion, resulting in a progressive invagination of the ovarian cortex[3-5]. Other authors[6-8] have suggested that large endometriomas may develop as a result of the secondary involvement of functional ovarian cysts in the endometriotic process. According to our classification[9], there are three different types of ovarian endometriosis: superficial hemorrhagic lesions, hemorrhagic cysts (endometriomas), and deep-infiltrating ovarian endometriosis. The presence of active foci deeply infiltrating the ovarian cortex led us to suggest that different pathogeneses must be considered as such a development from epithelial inclusions in the ovary[10,11]. The aim of this manuscript is to describe the management and the histological data from a series of 814 patients with endometriomas of more than 3 cm in size.

Patients and methods

From January 1982 to March 1994, 3980 patients underwent laparoscopy for endometriosis. Of these, 814 had ovarian cysts larger than 3 cm in size. Bilateral endometriomas were found in 639 cases (79%). The largest endometriomas were > 15 cm ($n = 8$). All peritoneal lesions were noted and the ovarian endometriomas often adherent to the ovarian fossa were mobilized. During laparoscopy, the degree of endometriosis was assessed according to the revised American Fertility Society (AFS) classification system[12] and the ovarian cyst diameter was measured with a probe introduced through a second-puncture incision. After careful examination of the pelvic cavity, the ovarian cyst was incised to a length of 2–3 cm, rinsed and flushed out. All the chocolate-colored fluid was aspirated and the internal wall of the cyst was inspected to ensure the absence of any intracystic polypoid projections. The ovarian endometrial cyst wall was biopsied with a biopsy punch forceps (26–175 DH; Storz, Tuttlingen, Germany) to ascertain the diagnosis of endometriosis. Patients received a subcutaneous injection of goserelin (Zoladex, Zenaca) implant at weeks 0, 4, 8 and 12. The initial pituitary stimulation phase, associated with a rise in estrogens, was curtailed in our study by injecting the implant during the luteal phase.

Twelve weeks after the first-look laparoscopy, another laparoscopy was performed. The degree of endometriosis was assessed by the same two observers (JD and MN) according to the revised AFS classification system. The size of the ovarian cyst was measured.

After biopsy, the internal wall of the ovarian cyst was vaporized with the help of the CO_2 laser[13,14], equipped since 1990 with the Swiftlase® (Sharplan, Laser Industries, Tel Aviv, Israel). Patients were followed up for a maximum of 13 years.

In 93 cases, large biopsies of more than 1 cm in size were taken in order to allow the evaluation of different parameters, including the three-dimensional architecture. Biopsies from eutopic endometrium were taken simultaneously. Six-μm serial sections were stained with Gomori's trichrome and then examined on a blind basis. In all cases, the mitotic index and the epithelial height were calculated, as previously described[15]. Ovarian biopsy specimens were taken from the endometrial cyst wall in 48 cases in order to compare histological data before and after therapy. The three-dimensional architecture evaluation was made whenever reconstruction was possible in order to evaluate histologically the underlying ovarian cortex[16].

The χ^2 test, the median test and the Student's test were used for statistical analysis.

Table 1 Scores (revised AFS classification[12]) and ovarian cyst diameter after drainage and GnRH agonist therapy. Incidence of 'active' endometriosis and tubal meta-plasia. Mitotic index and epithelial height in active ovarian endometriotic foci

	First look	Second look
Laparoscopic findings ($n = 814$)		
Revised AFS scores		
Total	43.4 ± 2.1	33.2 ± 2.1*
Implants	27.1 ± 1.8	16.9 ± 1.7*
Adhesions	16.3 ± 1.7	16.3 ± 1.7
Cyst diameter (mm)	47.3 ± 4.2	21.7 ± 3.8*
Histological findings ($n = 48$)		
Active endometriosis (%)	84	41*
Tubal metaplasia (%)	62	51
Mitotic index (%)	0.2	0.06*
Epithelial height (μm)	16.0 ± 4.9	17.2 ± 4.8

*Significantly different ($p < 0.001$) from initial values

Results

Modifications of AFS scores

The mean laparoscopic scores found before and at the end of treatment are compared in Table 1. The mean score decreased from 43.4 ± 2.1 to 33.2 ± 2.1. The difference was statistically significant ($p < 0.001$). Laparoscopic scoring was carried out separately for implants and adhesions. In the case of implants, the score decreased from 27.1 ± 1.8 to 16.9 ± 1.7. The difference was statistically significant ($p < 0.005$). The initial adhesion score did not decrease.

Modifications of cyst diameter

In all cases, a residual cyst was present. A complete disappearance of the cyst was never observed. The response of the ovarian disease was evaluated by measuring the modifications of the ovarian cyst diameter (Table 1). After drainage and a 12-week gonadotropin-releasing hormone (GnRH) agonist therapy, a significant ($p < 0.001$) decrease was observed from 47.3 ± 4.2 mm to 21.7 ± 3.8 mm. In eight cases, the endometrioma was larger than 15 cm (mean 17.5 ± 2.8). The ovarian cortex was evaluated by echography as being less than 2 mm in thickness. Eight weeks after drainage and GnRH agonist therapy, the size was 8.8 ± 4.2 cm. Aspiration of the remaining chocolate-colored fluid and flushing out were then performed by vaginal puncture under echography. Four weeks later, the diameter was 4.6 ± 2.4 cm. It was obvious that the remaining ovarian cortex surrounding the endometrioma became significantly ($p < 0.001$) thicker (between 8 mm and 1 cm) when compared to the values obtained before drainage. In all cases, vaporization of the internal lining of the cyst was easily performed at week 12.

Pregnancy rate and recurrence rate

The cumulative pregnancy rate was evaluated from the first postoperative menstruation. Forty-two patients who did not menstruate (because they became pregnant from the first ovulation) were included in the 'first cycle'.

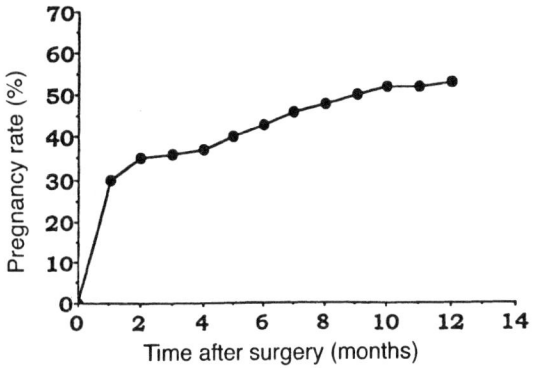

Figure 1 Cumulative pregnancy rate during the first year after surgery

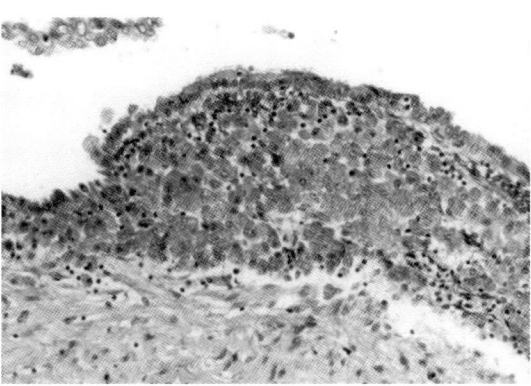

Figure 2 Ovarian endometrioma wall biopsy: glandular epithelium and stroma with numerous hemosiderin-laden macrophages

A pregnancy rate of more than 51% was achieved (Figure 1). The majority of pregnancies occurred during the first 10 months following surgery. In our series of 814 patients with ovarian endometriomas treated with the combined therapy (GnRH agonist and laser surgery), 607 patients were followed up for 2–13 years. A recurrence of ovarian endometriomas was suspected by vaginal echography and then confirmed by laparoscopy in 51 cases (8%). Among the 51 cases, previous laparoscopy had revealed a unilateral endometrioma in 15 cases (30%). A recurrence was observed in eight cases in the heterolateral ovary, and in seven cases in the previously treated ovary.

Ovarian cyst histology

The diagnosis of ovarian endometriosis was confirmed morphologically in all cases except two, in which glandular epithelium and stroma were absent and replaced by fibrous tissue.

Serial sections were carried out in a series of 93 large biopsies in order to observe endometrial epithelium which is often very thin and flattened. Biopsies of the endometrioma wall frequently reveal flattened columnar epithelium with stroma of an endometrial type, often surrounded by fibroreactive tissue with hemosiderin-like macrophages. There is no real plane of 'cleavage' between the endometrial-type stroma and the ovarian cortex and it is not unusual to find ovocytes in the vicinity of the endometrial stroma (Figure 2). In some areas, mucosal endometrium can be seen. In other areas, the epithelium is very thin, often detached from the subepithelial layers. The epithelial and stromal lining of an endometriotic cyst frequently becomes attenuated and the former may be reduced to a single layer of cuboidal cells which is frequently devoid of specific features. In such circumstances, recognition of the cyst as endometriotic may only be possible if a rim of subjacent endometrial stroma persists. Commonly, the cyst lining of endometrial epithelium and stroma is totally lost and replaced by granulation tissue, dense, fibrous and numerous pigmented macrophages. In this case, diagnosis of endometriosis can be difficult because similar findings can be seen in an old corpus luteum cyst. In our series, serial sections enabled us to diagnose endometriosis in all cases ($n = 93$). Nuclear atypia (Figure 3) were seen in 12% of cases. Metaplastic changes similar to those occurring in eutopic endometrial glands were observed. These included tubal (ciliated cell) metaplasia and hobnail metaplasia. Ciliated cells were demonstrated in more than 62% of cases.

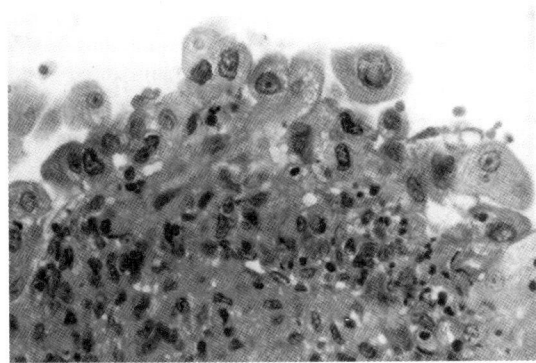

Figure 3 Ovarian endometrioma: glandular epithelium with nuclear atypia

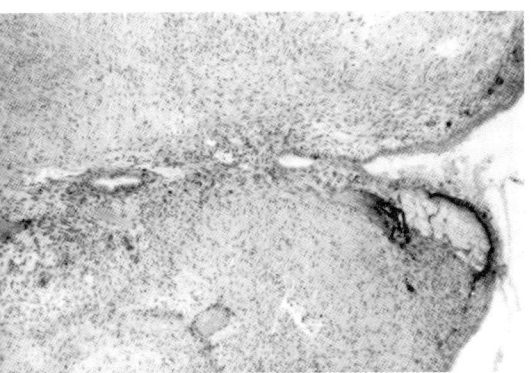

Figure 4 'Extracystic' endometriotic lesions. Serial sections demonstrated that these lesions must be considered as invagination of the endometrial glands

When biopsies were obtained from the site of adhesions (inversion stigma according to Hughesdon's hypothesis[2]) and from the deepest area of the endometrioma, histology revealed the same data in both areas: areas of fibrosis covered with flattened epithelium surrounded by stroma with hemosiderin-laden macrophages were observed and small foci of full-thickness endometrial tissue were found with the same incidence close to the inversion stigma as well as in the other parts. Flattened epithelium was in continuum with active glandular epithelium. During the luteal phase, in areas both with non-flattened glandular epithelium and with the flattened epithelium, the endometrium was never found to be in phase with the eutopic endometrium.

Extracystic endometriotic lesions (Figure 4) were observed in the endometriotic stroma or deeper in the ovarian cortex in 33% of cases. These endometriotic lesions were considered as invaginations of the ovarian cortex by epithelium surrounded by endometrial-type stroma. The three-dimensional architecture revealed this process of invagination. The multifocal appearance of these lesions in two dimensions was not confirmed by the three-dimensional reconstruction. Indeed, these 'extracystic' endometriotic inclusions were clearly defined as ramified invaginations by the glandular epithelium and stroma. In

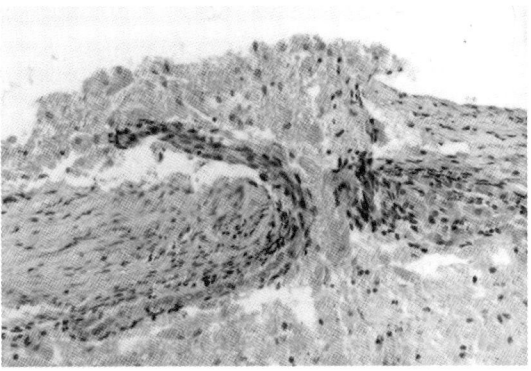

Figure 5 Clear continuum between the invaginated mesothelium and endometriotic tissue at the site of invagination (endometrioma ostium). The endometrioma ostium is clearly visible as well as the cyst with the chocolate-colored fluid

some cases, invagination of the mesothelial cells covering the ovary was clearly demonstrated and metaplasia into endometrial tissue could be observed. A continuum between the invaginated mesothelium and the endometriotic tissue was observed in some serial sections (Figure 5).

In 48 cases, biopsies before and after therapy were available and a comparison was then possible in order to evaluate the influence of GnRH agonist therapy. An endometriotic lesion was considered 'active' when typical glandular epithelium that appeared either proliferative or completely unresponsive to hormones was found with typical stroma. 'Active' endometriosis was found in, respectively, 84% and 41% of cases before and after GnRH agonist therapy, which is significantly different ($p < 0.001$). The mitotic index was calculated in typical glandular epithelium. Its value was, respectively, 0.2% and 0.06% before and after GnRH agonist therapy. The value observed after GnRH agonist therapy was significantly lower than that observed before therapy ($p < 0.001$). No difference in the epithelial height was observed after therapy. After GnRH agonist therapy, no decrease in nuclear atypia and hyperplasia was observed. Some areas revealed the presence of cells showing no signs of degeneration.

Discussion

Since 1992, different suggestions have been put forward in order to improve our knowledge of the physiopathology of endometriomas (chocolate cysts)[4-6,9]. The term 'chocolate cyst' was applied by Sampson to describe the endometrial cyst of the ovary[1]. According to Hughesdon, the internal surface of a chocolate cyst is really the external surface of the ovary[2]; the ovarian cortex is identifiable by the presence of primordial follicles. The endometrial cyst may be lined with free endometrial tissue, similar histologically and functionally to eutopic endometrium[3]. It was thus suggested that the endometrioma is a pseudocyst formed by an accumulation of menstrual debris from endometrial implants adherent to the peritoneal layer[2,4,5]. The adhesions are the cause of the endometrioma by the shedding of active superficial implants.

We have focused our study on the evaluation of 'endometriomas' (larger than 3 cm) in order to analyze the histological data and the clinical implications. Ovarian endometriomas do not respond very well to medical therapy[15-19]. After drainage alone, a quick recurrence of the cyst size proved that drainage, by itself, is completely ineffective in the management of large endometriomas[18], although some authors have suggested its efficacy[20]. However, 3 months after drainage of the endometrioma and GnRH agonist therapy (which provokes amenorrhea), a significant reduction (from $47.3 \pm 4.2\,\mu m$ to 21.7 ± 3.8) was observed. The reformation of chocolate-colored fluid during an amenorrheic period suggests, however, that endometrial shedding is not responsible, by itself, for chocolate-colored fluid formation. In our opinion, its origin could be: cyst wall exudation, congested blood vessels of the cyst wall or inflammation around persistent intracystic endometrial foci which are resistant to medical therapy.

The persistence of a chocolate cyst at laparoscopy after GnRH agonist therapy was confirmed by the histological study. Indeed, in all cases, histological examination of residual ovarian endometriotic lesions after hormonal therapy revealed glandular epithelium and stroma. In more than 40% of cases, areas with persistent active endometriosis were observed after GnRH agonist therapy. The precise reason why a number of endometrial cells of endometriotic cysts do not respond to hormonal therapy is unknown but five hypotheses can be proposed:

(1) The drug does not gain access to the ovarian endometriotic foci because fibrosis surrounding the foci prevents access locally.

(2) Endometriotic cells may have their own genetic programming, while an endocrine influence appears to be only secondary and dependent on the degree of differentiation of the individual cell.

(3) The low number of endometriotic steroid receptors and their different regulatory mechanisms in ectopic and eutopic endometrium may result in deficient endocrine dependency[21].

(4) There may be an absence of control by the steroid receptors which are

biologically inactive (unable to induce typical secretory changes).

(5) It could be due to the intraovarian environment with paracrine-stimulating growth factors.

The persistence of active endometriotic tissue after GnRH agonist therapy suggests the need for the surgical removal of invasive endometriosis[4–9,13,16,17,22]. The cumulative pregnancy rate achieved after combined therapy (GnRH agonist and endoscopy) was similar to that obtained after microsurgery[23], and allows us to propose this form of therapy in the management of large endometriomas. Indeed, the reduction in both cyst size and internal wall thickness observed in our study after GnRH agonist therapy facilitates the laparoscopic management of large endometrial cysts. In our series of large cysts (more than 15 cm), an echoguided puncture was performed after an 8-week GnRH agonist therapy and the size of the cyst decreased to a diameter of 4.6 ± 2.4 cm. The recurrence rate of ovarian endometriomas was low (8%), similar to the rate observed after microsurgery[23] or after a laparoscopic procedure (cystectomy)[24,25].

We recommend the vaporization of the internal wall of the endometrioma because the active implants are located on the internal surface of the cyst. The incidence of endometriotic lesions found deep in the stroma in our study (33%) cannot be considered as an argument in favor of cystectomy because deep-infiltrating intraovarian endometriosis was found with the same incidence. Another argument in favor of vaporization is the frequent absence of a thickened capsule around the endometrial cyst, which makes capsule removal difficult and is responsible for the simultaneous removal of numerous ovocytes. In large cysts, the remaining ovarian cortex surrounding the endometrioma is often thinner than 5 mm. There is a risk of removing the normal ovarian cortex containing ovocytes during the attempt at endometrioma wall removal.

We do not agree with a recent paper by Dubuisson and Chapron[26] which recommended cystectomy in every case because histological analysis of endometriotic lesions of the ovary showed that 4% of cases were atypical as described in 1979 by Czernobilsky and Morris[27]. This incidence was interpreted by Dubuisson and Chapron[26] as a risk factor for the development of cancer. It has never been proved that atypical cells can lead to ovarian cancer. We encountered no cases of ovarian cancer in our series of 814 patients, although we observed atypical areas in 12% of cases. As reported by Czernobilsky and Morris[27] and by our group[15], hyperplasia and atypia have to be considered as endometriotic tissue completely unresponsive to hormones and not as a potential for ovarian cancer.

Although two recent papers and debates[4,5,8] have tried to classify endometriomas, considerable uncertainty still exists about their histogenesis. Our arguments in favor of metaplasia of the invaginated mesothelium covering the ovary are the following:

(1) In our series, we found 12% of endometriomas not fixed to the broad ligament. The theory of Hughesdon[2] cannot explain the formation of the endometrioma in these cases.

(2) It was not unusual to find multilocular endometriomas, as shown by the computed tomography scan (Figure 6), which cannot be explained by the theory of adhesions and bleeding of active superficial implants adherent to the peritoneum.

(3) The epithelium covering the ovary, which is the mesothelium able to form any type of tissue, can invaginate into the ovarian cortex. Indeed, invaginations of the mesothelial layer covering the ovarian tissue were described by Motta and colleagues in animal and fetal ovaries[28], and this was also visualized in our study in human adult ovaries. Moreover, in our serial sections of the ovary,

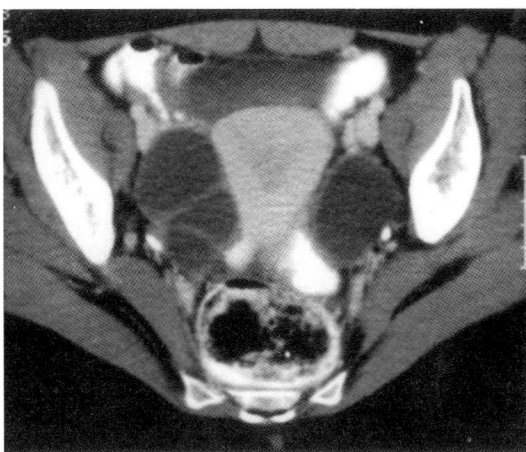

Figure 6 Computed tomography: multilocular endometriomas

mesothelial inclusions were frequently seen. Under the influence of so far unknown growth factors, these inclusions could be transformed into intraovarian endometriosis by metaplasia.

(4) The fact that primordial follicles were found surrounding the endometriotic cyst is also in agreement with our hypothesis. When the mesothelium invaginates deep in the ovary, the follicles located at the invagination site are pushed concomitantly with the mesothelium.

(5) Our main argument is the presence of epithelial invaginations in continuum with endometrial tissue, proving the metaplasia theory (Figure 5).

(6) Another major argument is the demonstration in our study of the capacity of the tissue to invaginate secondarily from the endometrial wall itself.

(7) Arguments can also be found in the literature. Endometriomas have been described in patients suffering from the Rokitansky–Kuster–Hauser syndrome characterized by the absence of a uterus and, therefore, without retrograde menstruation[29].

Common epithelial tumors of the ovary are considered to be derived from the surface epithelium covering the ovary and from the underlying stroma[30]. Our theory is thus different from the theories of Hughesdon[2], Brosens et al.[3] and Brosens[4,5], who consider that the pathogenesis of the typical ovarian endometrioma has now been clarified as a process originating from a free superficial implant which is in contact with the ovarian surface and is sealed off by adhesions, the menstrual shedding and bleeding of this small implant resulting in a progressive invagination of the ovarian cortex and the formation of the pseudocyst.

In our opinion, the endometrioma must be considered as an invagination and not as the result of the bleeding of a superficial implant. Indeed, metaplasia of the celomic epithelium invaginated in the ovarian cortex was proved in our study and explains the endometrioma formation. The 'deep-infiltrating ovarian endometriosis' described by Donnez in 1993[9] is, in fact, invagination of the ovary by the endometriotic tissue and is probably responsible for the recurrence of ovarian endometriosis after cyst excision or vaporization.

References

1. Sampson, J.A. (1921). Perforating haemorrhagic (chocolate) cysts of the ovary. *Arch. Surg.*, **3**, 245–323
2. Hughesdon, P.E. (1957). The structure of endometrial cysts of the ovary. *J. Obstet. Gynaecol. Br. Emp.*, **44**, 481–7
3. Brosens, I., Puttemans, P. and Deprest, J. (1994). The endoscopic localization of endometrial implants in the ovarian chocolate cyst. *Fertil. Steril.*, **61**, 1034–8
4. Brosens, I. (1995). Endoscopic exploration and classification of the chocolate cyst. *Hum. Reprod.*, **9**, 2213–14
5. Brosens, I. (1995). Ovarian endometriosis. In Shaw, R. (ed.) *Endometriosis*, p. 97. (London,

Carnforth, UK: Parthenon Publishing)
6. Nezhat, F., Nezhat, C., Allan, C.J., Metzger, D.A. and Sears, D.L. (1992). A clinical and histologic classification of endometriomas: implications for a mechanism of pathogenesis. *J. Reprod. Med.*, **37**, 771–6
7. Nezhat, F., Nezhat, C., Nezhat, C. and Admon, D. (1994). A fresh look at ovarian endometriomas. *Contemp. Obstet. Gynecol.*, 81–94
8. Nezhat, C., Nezhat, F., Nezhat, C. and Siedman, D. (1995). Classification of endometriosis. Improving the classification of endometriotic ovarian cysts. *Hum. Reprod.*, **9**, 2212–13
9. Donnez, J. (1993). Rationale for surgery. In Brosens, I. and Donnez, J. (eds.) *Current Status of Endometriosis*, pp. 385–95. (Carnforth, UK: Parthenon Publishing)
10. Donnez, J., Nisolle, M., Gillet, N., Smets, M., Bassil, S. and Casanas-Roux, F. (1996). Large ovarian endometriomas. *Hum. Reprod.*, **11**, 641–6
11. Nisolle, M. and Donnez, J. (1996). *The Peritoneal, Ovarian and Rectovaginal Endometriosis. The Identification of Three Separate Diseases.* (Carnforth, UK: Parthenon Publishing)
12. American Fertility Society (1985). Revised American Fertility Society classification of endometriosis. *Fertil. Steril.*, **58**, 351–62
13. Donnez, J. (1987). CO_2 laser laparoscopy in infertile women with adhesions or endometriosis. *Fertil. Steril.*, **48**, 390–4
14. Donnez, J. and Nisolle, M. (1991). Laparoscopic management of large ovarian endometrial cyst: use of fibrin sealant. *J. Gynecol. Surg.*, **7**, 163–7
15. Nisolle, M., Casanas-Roux, F. and Donnez, J. (1988). Histologic study of ovarian endometriosis after hormonal therapy. *Fertil. Steril.*, **49**, 423–6
16. Donnez, J., Nisolle, M. and Casanas-Roux, F. (1992). Three-dimensional architectures of peritoneal endometriosis. *Fertil. Steril.*, **57**, 980–3
17. Donnez, J., Nisolle, M. and Casanas-Roux, F. (1990). Endometriosis-associated infertility: evaluation of preoperative use of danazol, gestrinone and buserelin. *Int. J. Fertil.*, **42**, 128
18. Donnez, J., Nisolle, M., Gillerot, S., Anaf, V., Clerck, F. and Casanas-Roux, F. (1994). Ovarian endometrial cysts: the role of gonadotropin-releasing hormone agonist and/or drainage. *Fertil. Steril.*, **62**, 63–6
19. Shaw, R.W. (1992). The role of GnRH analogues in the treatment of endometriosis. *Br. J. Obstet. Gynecol.*, **99**, 7, 9–12
20. Fayez, J.A. and Vogel, M.S. (1991). Comparison of different treatment methods of endometriosis by laparoscopy. *Obstet. Gynecol.*, **78**, 660–5
21. Nisolle, M., Casanas-Roux, F., Wyns, C., de Menten, Y., Mathieu, P.E. and Donnez, J. (1994). Immunohistochemical analysis of estrogen and progesterone receptors in endometrium and peritoneal endometriosis: a new quantitative method. *Fertil. Steril.*, **62**, 751–9
22. Donnez, J., Nisolle, M. and Casanas-Roux, F. (1989). Administration of nasal buserelin as compared with subcutaneous buserelin implant for endometriosis. *Fertil. Steril.*, **52**, 27–30
23. Gordts, S., Boeckx, W. and Brosens, I. (1994). Microsurgery of endometriosis in infertile patients. *Fertil. Steril.*, **42**, 520–5
24. Canis, M., Mage, G., Wattiez, A., Chapron, C., Pouly, J.L. and Bassil, S. (1992). Second-look laparoscopy after laparoscopic cystectomy of large endometriomas. *Fertil. Steril.*, **58**, 617–19
25. Canis, M., Wattiez, A., Pouly, J.L., Bassil, S., Bouquet, J., Chapron, C., Manhes, H., Mage, G. and Bruhat, M.A. (1993). Laparoscopic treatment of endometriosis. In Brosens, I. and Donnez, J. (eds.) *The Current Status of Endometriosis. Research and Management*, p. 407. (Carnforth, UK: Parthenon Publishing)
26. Dubuisson, J.B. and Chapron, C. (1995). The need for modification. *Hum. Reprod.*, **9**, 2214–15
27. Czernobilsky, O. and Morris, W.J. (1979). A histologic study of ovarian endometriosis with emphasis on hyperplastic and atypical changes. *Obstet. Gynecol.*, **53**, 318
28. Motta, P.M., Van Blerkom, J. and Makabe, S. (1980). Changes to the surface morphology of ovarian germinal epithelium during the reproductive life and in some pathological conditions. *J. Sub. Cytol.*, **12**, 407–25
29. Rosenfeld, D.L. and Lecher, D.B. (1981). Endometriosis in a patient with Rokitansky–Kuster–Hauser syndrome. *Am. J. Obstet. Gynecol.*, **124**, 722–3
30. Serov, S.F., Scully, R.E. and Sobin, L.H. (1973). Histological typing of ovarian tumors. In *International Histological Classification of Tumors*, pp. 17–21. (Geneva: World Health Organization)

Deep endometriosis 8

D.C. Martin, P.R. Koninckx, R.E. Batt and R. Smith

Introduction

Deep endometriosis occurs in a small group of patients diagnosed with endometriosis. Almost all of these patients have significant pain. In this small group, diagnosis and surgery can be difficult. Preoperative and intraoperative care requires significant attention[1]. Complete resection might require removal of parts of the bowel, bladder, uterus, diaphragm or other organs.

Diagnosis

The unpredictable progression and regression of endometriosis suggest that many women have endometriosis as a self-limited disease[2-10]. Furthermore, 100% of women may have endometriosis at sometime in their lives[11-15]. However, the diagnosis is made in only 1–8%[16,17]. The expression of symptoms appears to be related to genetics, but an alternate interpretation is that there is increased surveillance in a family when endometriosis is known. Diagnosis increases with increased surveillance[11,18].

Both visualization and lack of visualization can be a problem. Visualization of endometriosis has occurred in up to 87% of patients as an incidental finding. This was asymptomatic in 93%; the other 7% had disease without pain[19]. But a larger concern is lesions that are not seen. Lesions that may not be seen include deep intra-ovarian endometriosis, retroperitoneal disease, endometriosis in adhesions and microscopic lesions[1,20-25].

Deep endometriosis can be common in a referral practice. In two different series, the depth of endometriosis was greater than 3 mm in 43% and 53% of patients and greater than 5 mm in 25% and 29% of patients[26,27]. These projections are based on the expected incidence in populations of 0.8% to 8.1%[16]. Of patients who are diagnosed with endometriosis, those with deep endometriosis were found in a subset of the population which was 13.8% of that study[28]. The minimal projection is based on 0.8% of 13.8% multiplied by the lowest figure for deep penetration of 25%[26]. The maximum uses the same calculations and the highest percent for deep infiltration of 53%[28]. However, deep endometriosis may be found in only 1/170 to 1/3800 women in a primary care practice[16,26-28] (Table 1).

The diagnosis of endometriosis at the time of pelvic surgery is higher than in a random population. At gynecological surgery, 5–28% of patients have endometriosis[29]. At reproductive surgery, this is 20–71%[18,30]. Deep hidden endometriosis was found in 4.5% of patients with pain and infertility[31]. Using the combined data from several studies, as in Table 1, deep endometriosis is anticipated in 0.17–2.0% of patients having pelvic surgery[26-29] (Table 2). The prevalence of deep endometriosis as shown in Tables 1 and 2 may be high because these include referral patients, from outside of the area or they may

Table 1 Expected prevalence of endometriosis in a general population

	All patients[16]	Deep endometriosis[26-28]
Minimum projection	0.008	0.00028
Maximum projection	0.081	0.0059

See text for explanation

Table 2 Expected prevalence of endometriosis in pelvic surgery populations

	All pelvic surgery[29]	Deep endometriosis population[26,27]	Deep endometriosis all patients[28]
Minimum projection	0.05	0.25	0.0017
Maximum projection	0.28	0.53	0.020

See text for explanation

be low due to missed lesions in some patients. In either situation, they are a starting point for ongoing study.

Progression does not occur in all patients[2-10]. When progression occurs, changes in appearance take time. Water blister lesions progress to scarred blue dome cysts over 4–10 years[32]. The occurrence of scarred black lesions increases from 23 to 63% over 20 years. This is accompanied by a progressive decrease in red and clear early type lesions[33]. Although the time progression of appearance is important, young patients may have dark scarred lesions while older patients may have red lesions.

Identification

Ripps and Martin[34] studied the predictive positivity and specificity of pelvic examination for focal tenderness. This study revealed that 45 of 70 patients with focal tenderness had endometriosis while 25 had non-endometriotic lesions. Tenderness did predict disease, but not specifically endometriosis[34]. In a follow-up study, these authors noted that tender endometriotic lesions are associated with an increased depth and increased volume. Tender lesions had an average depth of 5.3 mm while non-tender lesions averaged 3.3 mm in depth. The volume averaged 1213 mm^3 in tender lesions and 194 mm^3 in non-tender lesions[35].

Deep endometriosis can be difficult to identify. This is particularly true when it is retroperitoneal[1]. Hidden retroperitoneal endometriosis was found in 3.2% of patients with pain and 4.5% with both infertility and pain[31].

Clinical diagnosis is aided by pain mapping, single finger examinations and a rectovaginal examination[36,37]. Examination is timed during menses to increase the findings. In 61 patients, random examination demonstrated nodular infiltrating endometriosis in four women. Examination during menses increased this by 450% to 22 patients. With deep endometriosis, bowel is routinely prepared for repair as the possibility of entering bowel in these patients is increased[25].

Clinical and histological findings

Classical endometriosis is infiltrating adenomyomata[38-41]. Adenomyomata is a combination of a fibromuscular matrix, characteristic glands and/or epithelium in addition to endometrial stroma[40]. A fibromuscular component can be noted in superficial endometriosis[42-44], and is a dominant feature in rectovaginal and bowel endometriosis. The peritoneal component may be related to the development of leiomyomatosis peritonealis disseminata[45-47].

Donnez and colleagues have added to the description of retroperitoneal disease and reconfirmed the fibromuscular component[48]. In their studies, the glands and stroma are in contiguous tongues infiltrating through these areas[48]. Deep rectovaginal endometriosis and peritoneal endometriosis differ in several factors. The location, three-dimensional architecture, mitotic activity, existence of tubal metaplasia, synchronicity, expression of cytokeratin, amount of vimetin and degree of estrogen and progesterone receptors vary in these two areas. This leads to the conclusion that deep and peritoneal endometriosis are different entities with different sources. The histological similarities with uterine adenomyomata lead to the conclusion that both are

Müllerian. The authors concluded that peritoneal lesions are related to retrograde menstruation whereas retroperitoneal lesions are from Müllerian remnants[49,50].

The carefully documented findings of Donnez and colleagues[48,49] demonstrate different biochemistries of deep and superficial endometriosis. However, these do not explain why two Müllerian derivatives (transplanted endometrium and Müllerian remnant) have different expressions. There is not an explanation for similar fibromuscular findings in superficial lesions and lesions of the ovaries, peritoneum, omentum, lymph nodes and bowel[42–46]. Clarification of recent (type 3 collagen) or past (type 1 collagen) differentiation may be useful[44]. Since the Müllerian system is the original source of both endometrium and Müllerian remnant, the biochemical and histological expression may be related to the peritoneal fluid microenvironment[51], vascularization[52,53], local immunology, tissue resistance, loose connective tissue characteristics, genetics or other factors.

Donnez and colleagues found no in-phase cellular differentiation between deep and eutopic endometrium[49]. On the other hand, Cornillie and associates noted good correlation between eutopic and ectopic endometrium[27]. The reason for this difference needs clarification. Also, it is not clear if adenomyomata is metaplasia or is growth and hypertrophy.

The distribution near or in the rectovaginal septum[54,55] in the area of the obliterated fetal peritoneum supports a Müllerian remnant origin[52,53,56,57]. However, the distribution is also similar to that of other peritoneal endometriosis and supports implantation, growth, and infiltration of the peritoneum. Furthermore, the finding that most if not all deep paravaginal lesions extend from or to the peritoneum[58] argues for infiltration or implantation into pockets with subsequent growth. The observation that most pockets are in and around the septum[52,53,59] and isolated midvaginal lesions are rare, if at all existent, argues for infiltration, implantation into pockets or metaplasia in pockets.

Other paravaginal possibilities are implantation into the rectovaginal septum as a Müllerian derived body of increased susceptibility or into a persistence of the fetal peritoneum presenting as a peritoneal pocket. If the septum is perirectal[60] rather than paravaginal, there is a possibility that this mature Müllerian structure might protect the rectum from infiltrating retrocervical endometriosis.

As an alternative, Koninckx and Martin have postulated three types of infiltrating implants[31]. Type I lesions are infiltrating lesions starting at the surface and have a conical distribution. Type II lesions involve peritoneal retraction and adhesions. Type II lesions appear to be an extension of the observations of Sampson[41] and Chatman and Zbella[61] that lesions can hide in or at the rim of peritoneal pockets. As such, type II lesions are not true infiltration but are deep hidden endometriosis. This can often be grasped and everted for excision. Immediate hemostasis is important. If vessels are cut in the everted tissue, these will retract deep into the pelvis. In addition, type II lesions may be precursors to type III deep infiltration, but these are not Allen-Masters syndrome[62].

Type III lesions are deep spherical lesions. These may be the result of ballooning after infiltration into deep loose connective tissue, expansion of type II lesions, metaplasia of Müllerian remnants or growth from Müllerian remnants[31]. A combination of these origins may be needed to account for all findings.

A staging system has been proposed by Adamyan[63]. Retrocervical endometriosis is stage I. Stage II involves the vagina. Stage III involves the vagina and rectum while stage IV includes cul-de-sac obliteration. Stages I and II in this classification have no cul-de-sac distortion and are compatible with deep Müllerian[49,50] or type III endometriosis[31]. Stages III and IV have significant cul-de-sac distortion and/or obliteration. These appear to be type I or a combination of types I and III[31].

Deep rectovaginal nodules tend to invade the vagina and not the rectum[50,58,63,64]. This finding may be related to infiltration to the loose connective tissue of the paravaginal tissue above the rectovaginal septum or pararectal fascia. This conjecture that these lesions are on the vaginal side of the septum or of the perirectal fascia suggests the fascia can protect the bowel. If so, these lesions may be better represented by a concept of retrocervical endometriosis[63,65] or paravaginal endometriosis rather than rectovaginal involvement. Ongoing study may reveal new anatomical associations.

Treatment

Most patients will require excision of deep lesions for pain relief[26,50,51,64,66,67]. Using coagulation rather than excision will increase persistence in certain patients[59,66,68]. However, the routine use of excisional techniques can result in increased expense and complications[67,69].

Preparation for any lesion in the rectovaginal septum or near the colon generally utilizes sigmoidoscopy and bowel preparation. If there is cul-de-sac obliteration, blood banking is also considered. Bowel is usually spared with retrocervical or retrovaginal endometriosis when the cul-de-sac is intact. These patients appear to be the best candidates for a laparoscopic or combined laparoscopic and vaginal approach[58,63,70]. On the other hand, those who have cul-de-sac obliteration often have bowel involvement and require laparotomy[51,71].

Medical suppression may be useful in certain patients. Preoperatively, medical suppression may avoid surgery in some patients and decrease complications in others. Medical suppression has been useful in providing long-term relief of pain in 26% of patients with severe endometriosis[72]. Furthermore, natural or surgical menopause has been used in the treatment of deep bowel disease[19,71]. Although deep endometriosis is poorly represented by the American Fertility Society classification[1], the combination of clinical findings leads to the conclusion that certain patients may avoid surgery and its risks by using medical menopause.

A second preoperative concern is in decreasing complications. Bowel and ureteral complications have accompanied resection of endometriosis[67,69,73,74]. In a study by Koninckx, complications occurred more often in patients with no pretreatment, and it was concluded that pretreatment makes dissection easier and limits complications[67].

Postoperative medical suppression following laser ablation decreases residual scores[75]. This appears to be important for those physicians using laser vaporization and/or electrosurgical coagulation. However, this may be less important if complete excision is used[36].

Summary

In summary, the natural course of endometriosis is occurrence in 100% of women, diagnosis in 1–8%, and deep endometriosis in 0.03–53%, in different populations. Deep endometriosis may represent infiltration, metaplasia or other pathophysiology. The potential is more pronounced in the cul-de-sac, but it is not known whether this is related to peritoneal fluid micro-environment, local vascularity, immunology, embryonal rests or other factors.

In order to identify these women, examination during menses is needed. When deep nodules are found, bowel preparation is used prior to surgery. Deep retrocervical or paravaginal lesions may occur due to metaplasia in Müllerian rests, metaplasia in peritoneal pockets, infiltration into peritoneal pockets or infiltration into the area of the rectovaginal septum (embryonic peritoneum). These tend to spare the bowel and cul-de-sac. These can be resected using a laparoscopic or combined laparoscopic and vaginal approach. On the other hand, lesions with cul-de-sac distortion or obliteration are more likely to be infiltration and to involve bowel. Bowel surgery is more likely in this group. Deep pockets are a variant which can often be everted and resected at laparoscopy. Preoperative medical treatment may avoid surgical treatment in some patients and complications in others. Furthermore, postoperative suppression may decrease residual disease in those patients who have laser ablation or electrosurgical coagulation.

Acknowledgements

Appreciation is expressed to Dr David Nichols for discussing embryogenesis and the recto-vaginal septum and to Parthenon Publishing and Mrs Melanie Savage for the ongoing revisions of this manuscript.

References

1. Moore, J.G., Binstock, M.A. and Growdon, W.A. (1988). The clinical implications of retroperitoneal endometriosis. *Am. J. Obstet. Gynecol.*, **158**, 1291–8
2. Telimaa, S., Puolakka, J., Rönnberg, L. and Kauppila, A. (1987). Placebo-controlled comparison of danazol and high-dose medroxyprogesterone acetate in the treatment of endometriosis. *Gynecol. Endocrinol.*, **1**, 13–23
3. Telimaa, S., Rönnberg, L. and Kauppila, A. (1987). Placebo-controlled comparison of danazol and high-dose medroxyprogesterone acetate in the treatment of endometriosis after conservative surgery. *Gynecol. Endocrinol.*, **1**, 363–71
4. Thomas, E.J. and Cooke, I.D. (1987). Impact of gestrinone on the course of asymptomatic endometriosis. *Br. Med. J.*, **294**, 272–4
5. Mahmood, T.A. and Templeton, A. (1990). The impact of treatment on the natural history of endometriosis. *Hum. Reprod.*, **5**, 965–70
6. D'Hooghe, T.M., Bambra, C.S., Isahakia, M. and Koninckx, P.R. (1992). Evolution of spontaneous endometriosis in the baboon (*Papio anubis*, *Papio cynocephalus*) over a 12-month period. *Fertil. Steril.*, **58**, 409–41
7. Hoshiai, H., Ishikawa, M., Sawatari, Y., Noda, K. and Fukaya, T. (1993). Laparoscopic evaluation of the onset and progression of endometriosis. *Am. J. Obstet. Gynecol.*, **169**, 714–19
8. Wiegerinck, M.A.H.M., Van Dop, P.A. and Brosens, I.A. (1993). The staging of peritoneal endometriosis by the type of active lesion in addition to the revised American Fertility Society classification. *Fertil. Steril.*, **60** (3), 461–4
9. Vercellini, P., Vendola, N., Presti, M. and Bolis, G. (1993). Multifocal endometriosis: a case report. *J. Reprod. Med.*, **38**, 815–19
10. Brosens, I.A. (1994). Is mild endometriosis a progressive disease? *Hum. Reprod.*, **9** (12), 2209–11
11. Scott, R.B., Te Linde, R.W. and Wharton, L.R.J. (1953). Further studies on experimental endometriosis. *Am. J. Obstet. Gynecol.*, **63**, 1082–103
12. Rawson, J.M.R. (1991). Prevalence of endometriosis in asymptomatic women. *J. Reprod. Med.*, **36**, 513–15
13. Evers, J.L.H. (1994). Endometriosis does not exist; all women have endometriosis. *Hum. Reprod.*, **9**, 2206–9
14. Koninckx, P.R. (1994). Is mild endometriosis a condition occurring intermittently in all women? *Hum. Reprod.*, **9**, 2202–5
15. Moen, M.H. (1995). Is mild endometriosis a disease? Why do women develop endometriosis and why is it diagnosed? *Hum. Reprod.*, **10**, 8–11
16. Simpson, J., Elias, S., Malinak, L. and Buttram, V.J. (1980). Heritable aspects of endometriosis. I. Genetic studies. *Am. J. Obstet. Gynecol.*, **137**, 327
17. Strathy, J.H., Molgaard, C.A., Coulam, C.B. and Melton, L.J. (1982). Endometriosis and infertility: a laparoscopic study of endometriosis among fertile and infertile women. *Fertil. Steril.*, **38**, 667–72
18. Martin, D.C., Hubert, G.D., Vander Zwaag, R. and El-Zeky, F.A. (1989). Laparoscopic appearances of peritoneal endometriosis. *Fertil. Steril.*, **51**, 63–7
19. Kempers, R.D., Dockerty, M.B., Hunt, A.B. and Symmonds, R.E. (1960). Significant postmenopausal endometriosis. *Surg. Gynecol. Obstet.*, **111**, 348–56

20. Russell, W.W. (1899). Aberrant portions of the Mullerian duct found in an ovary. *Johns Hopkins Hosp. Bull.*, **94–96**, 8–10
21. Vasquez, G., Cornillie, F. and Brosens, I.A. (1983). Peritoneal endometriosis: scanning electron microscopy and histology of minimal pelvic endometriotic lesions. *Fertil. Steril.*, **42**, 696–703
22. Murphy, A.A., Green, W.R., Bobbie, D., Dela Cruz, Z.C. and Rock, J.A. (1986). Unsuspected endometriosis documented by scanning electron microscopy in visually normal peritoneum. *Fertil. Steril.*, **46**, 522–4
23. Jansen, R.P.S. and Russell, P. (1986). Non-pigmented endometriosis: clinical laparoscopic, and pathologic definition. *Am. J. Obstet. Gynecol.*, **155**, 1154–9
24. Nisolle, M., Paindaveine, B., Bourdon, A., Berlière, M., Casanas-Roux, F. and Donnez, J. (1990). Histologic study of peritoneal endometriosis in infertile women. *Fertil. Steril.*, **53**, 984–8
25. Koninckx, P.R., Meuleman, C., Oosterlynck, D. and Cornillie, F.J. (1996). Diagnosis of deep endometriosis by clinical examination during menstruation and plasma CA-125 concentrations. *Fertil. Steril.*, **65**, 280–7
26. Martin, D.C., Hubert, G.D. and Levy, B.S. (1989). Depth of infiltration of endometriosis. *J. Gynecol. Surg.*, **5**, 55–60
27. Cornillie, F.J., Oosterlynck, D., Lauweryns, J.M. and Koninckx, P.R. (1990). Deeply infiltrating pelvic endometriosis: histology and clinical significance. *Fertil. Steril.*, **53**, 978–83
28. Martin, D.C., Ahmic, R., El-Zeky, F.A., Vander Zwaag, R., Pickens, M.T. and Cherry, K. (1990). Increased histologic confirmation of endometriosis. *J. Gynecol. Surg.*, **6**, 275–9
29. Ramzy, I. (1989). Pathology. In Schenken, R.S. (ed.) *Endometriosis. Contemporary Concepts in Clinical Management*, pp. 49–81. (Philadelphia: J.P. Lippincott Co.)
30. Klein, N.A. and Olive, D.L. (1993). Management of endometriosis-associated infertility. In Schlaff, W.D. and Rock, J.A. (eds.) *Decision Making in Reproductive Endocrinology*, pp. 488–94. (Oxford: Blackwell Scientific)
31. Koninckx, P.R. and Martin, D.C. (1992). Deep endometriosis: a consequence of infiltration or retraction or possibly adenomyosis externa? *Fertil. Steril.*, **58**, 924–8
32. Karnaky, K.J. (1969). Theories and known observations about hormonal treatment of endometriosis *in situ*, and endometriosis at the enzyme level. *Arizona Med.*, January, 37–41
33. Koninckx, P.R., Meuleman, C., Demeyere, S., Lesaffre, E. and Cornillie, F.J. (1991). Suggestive evidence that pelvic endometriosis is a progressive disease, whereas deeply infiltrating endometriosis is associated with pelvic pain. *Fertil. Steril.*, **55**, 759–65
34. Ripps, B.A. and Martin, D.C. (1991). Focal pelvic tenderness, pelvic pain and dysmenorrhea in endometriosis. *J. Reprod. Med.*, **36**, 470–2
35. Ripps, B.A. and Martin, D.C. (1992). Correlation of focal pelvic tenderness with implant dimension and stage of endometriosis. *J. Reprod. Med.*, **37**, 620–4
36. Redwine, D.B. (1991). Conservative laparoscopic excision of endometriosis by sharp dissection: life table analysis of reoperation and persistent or recurrent disease. *Fertil. Steril.*, **56**, 628–34
37. Kresch, A.J. (1993). Clinical assessment. In Martin, D.C. (ed.) *Atlas of Endometriosis*, pp. 3.1–3.8. (London: Gower Medical Publishing)
38. Cullen, T.S. (1896). Adenomyoma of the round ligament. *Johns Hopkins Hosp. Bull.*, **896**, 62–3
39. Lockyer, C. (1913). Adenomyoma in the recto-uterine and recto-vaginal septa. *Proc. R. Soc. Med. (Obstet.)*, **6**, 112–20
40. Cullen, T.S. (1919). The distribution of adenomyomata containing uterine mucosa. *Am. J. Obstet. Gynecol.*, **80**, 130–8
41. Sampson, J.A. (1921). Perforating hemorrhagic (chocolate) cysts of the ovary. Their importance and especially their relation to pelvic adenomas of the endometrial type ('adenomyoma' of the uterus, rectovaginal septum, sigmoid, etc.). *Arch. Surg.*, **3**, 245–323
42. Stripling, M.C., Martin, D.C., Chatman, D.L., Vander Zwaag, R. and Poston, W.M. (1988). Subtle appearance of pelvic endometriosis. *Fertil. Steril.*, **49**, 427–31
43. Clement, P.B. (1990). Pathology of endometriosis. *Pathol. Ann.*, **25**, (Part 1), 245–95
44. Khare, V.K., Martin, D.C. and Eltorky, M. (1996). A comparative study of ovarian and pelvic wall-infiltrating endometriosis. *J. Am. Assoc. Gynecol. Laparoscop.*, **3**, 235–9
45. Parmley, T.H., Woodruff, J.D., Winn, K., Johnson, J.W.C. and Douglas, P.H. (1975). Histogenesis of leiomyomatosis peritonealis

45. ... disseminata (disseminating fibrosing deciduosis). *Obstet. Gynecol.*, **46**, 511–16
46. Fujii, S., Okamura, H., Nakashima, N., Bann, C., Aso, T. and Nishimura, T. (1980). Leiomyomatosis peritonealis disseminata. *Obstet. Gynecol.*, **55**, 79–83
47. Woodruff, J.D. and Parmley, T.H. (1988). *Atlas of Gynecologic Pathology.* (New York: Gower Medical Publishing)
48. Donnez, J., Nisolle, M. and Casanas-Roux, F. (1992). Three-dimensional architectures of peritoneal endometriosis. *Fertil. Steril.*, **57**, 980–3
49. Donnez, J., Nisolle, M., Smoes, P., Gillet, N., Beguin, S. and Casanas-Roux, F. (1996). Peritoneal endometriosis and endometriotic nodules of the rectovaginal septum are two different entities. *Fertil. Steril.*, **66**, 362–8
50. Nisolle, M. and Donnez, J. (1997). *Peritoneal Ovarian and Rectovaginal Endometriosis.* (Carnforth, UK: Parthenon Publishing)
51. Koninckx, P.R. and Martin, D.C. (1994). Treatment of deeply infiltrating endometriosis. *Curr. Opin. Obstet. Gynecol.*, **6**, 231–41
52. Batt, R., Smith, R., Buck, G., Naples, J. and Severino, M. (1989). A case series – peritoneal pockets and endometriosis: rudimentary duplications of the Mullerian system. *Adolesc. Pediatr. Gynecol.*, **2**, 47–56
53. Batt, R.E. and Smith, R.A. (1989). Embryologic theory of histogenesis of endometriosis in peritoneal pockets. *Obstet. Gynecol. Clin. North. Am.*, **16**, 15–28
54. Milley, P.S. and Nichols, D.H. (1969). A correlative investigation of the human rectovaginal septum. *Anat. Rec.*, **163**, 443–52
55. Nichols, D. and Randall, C.L. (1996). *Vaginal Surgery.* (Baltimore: Williams and Wilkins)
56. Redwine, D.B. (1988). Mulleriosis. The single best-fit model of the origin of endometriosis. *J. Reprod. Med.*, **11**, 915–20
57. Redwine, D.B. (1989). Peritoneal pockets of endometriosis. Confirmation of an important relationship, with further observations. *J. Reprod. Med.*, **34**, 270–2
58. Martin, D.C. (1988). Laparoscopic and vaginal colpotomy for the excision of infiltrating cul-de-sac endometriosis. *J. Reprod. Med.*, **33**, 806–8
59. Davis, G.D. and Brooks, R.A. (1988). Excision of pelvic endometriosis with the carbon dioxide laser laparoscope. *Obstet. Gynecol.*, **72**, 816–19
60. Thompson, J.D. (1992). Malpositions of the uterus. In Thompson, J.D. and Rock, J.A. (eds.) *Te Linde's Operative Gynecology*, p. 832. (Philadelphia: J.B. Lippincott Co.)
61. Chatman, D.L. and Zbella, E.A. (1986). Pelvic peritoneal defects and endometriosis: further observation. *Fertil. Steril.*, **46**, 711–14
62. Batt, R.E. (1995). Allen-Masters syndrome is caused by trauma, not by endometriosis. *J. Am. Assoc. Gynecol. Laparoscopists*, **2**, 245–7
63. Adamyan, L. (1993). Additional international perspectives. In Nichols, D.H. (ed.) *Gynecologic and Obstetric Surgery*, pp. 1167–82. (St. Louis: Mosby Year Book)
64. Donnez, J., Nisolle, M., Casanas-Roux, F., Bassil, S. and Anaf, V. (1995). Rectovaginal septum, endometriosis or adenomyosis: laparoscopic management in a series of 231 patients. *Hum. Reprod.*, **10**, 630–5
65. Perry, C.P. and Victoria, M.M. (1995). Occult retrocervical endometriosis. *J. Reprod. Med.*, **40**, 652–4
66. Martin, D. (1995). Rationale for surgical treatment of endometriosis. In Nezhat, C.R., Berger, G.S., Nezhat, F.R., Buttram, V.C. and Nezhat, C. (eds.) *Endometriosis: Advanced Management and Surgical Techniques*, pp. 69–76. (New York: Springer-Verlag)
67. Koninckx, P.R. (1996). Complications of CO_2 laser endoscopic excision of deep endometriosis. *Hum. Reprod.*, **11**, 2263–8
68. Martin, D.C. (1995). Pain and infertility – a rationale for different treatment approaches. *Br. J. Obstet. Gynaecol.*, **102** (Suppl. 12), 2–3
69. Maxson, W.S., Hoffman, D.I., Nezhat, F. and Adamson, G.D. (1996). Complications of operative laparoscopy. In Adamson, G.D. and Martin, D.C. (eds.) *Endoscopic Management of Gynecologic Disease*, pp. 361–83. (Philadelphia: Lippincott-Raven Publishers)
70. Davis, G.D., Wolgamott, G. and Moon, J. (1993). Laparoscopically assisted vaginal hysterectomy as definitive therapy for stage III and IV endometriosis. *J. Reprod. Med.*, **38**, 577–81
71. Weed, J.C. and Ray, J.E. (1987). Endometriosis of the bowel. *Obstet. Gynecol.*, **69**, 727–30
72. Waller, K.G. and Shaw, R.W. (1993). Gonadotropin-releasing hormone analogues for the treatment of endometriosis: long-term follow-up. *Fertil. Steril.*, **59** (3), 511–15
73. Nezhat, C. and Nezhat, F. (1992). Laparoscopic repair of ureter resected during operative laparoscopy. *Obstet. Gynecol.*, **80**, 543–4

74. Khare, V.K., Martin, D.C. and Kaigh, J. (1993). Buttonhole ulceration and perforation of the rectum. *J. Am. Assoc. Gynecol. Laparoscopists*, **1**, 12–15
75. Shaw, R.W. (1996). A prospective randomized open study comparing laser ablation plus gosereline therapy and laser ablation alone in the treatment of endometriosis. Presented at the *Vth World Congress on Endometriosis*, Yokohama, October, Abstract 0–116, p60

Natural history of endometriosis in baboons

T.M. D'Hooghe

Introduction

Endometriosis has been well described and known for over 50 years. However, our current knowledge of pathogenesis, pathophysiology of related infertility and spontaneous evolution remains unclear. This may be explained by several factors. Firstly, at the time of diagnosis most patients with endometriosis have had the disease for some period of time. Therefore, it is difficult to initiate any clinical experiments that would definitely determine the etiology or progression of the disease[1]. Secondly, it is hard to carry out studies as mentioned above with sufficient numbers of patients and meaningful controls, which obviates the need for multicenter orientated research[2]. Thirdly, endometriosis occurs naturally in humans and non-human primates only. Due to ethical considerations, properly controlled studies are very difficult and invasive experiments cannot be performed in humans. Therefore, there is an obvious need for the development of a good animal model with spontaneous endometriosis.

Animal models for the study of endometriosis

Both rodents and primates have been studied as models for the study of endometriosis. The main advantage of rodent (rat and rabbit) models is the low cost relative to the monkey, but the disadvantages are numerous. Rodents lack a menstrual cycle and do not have spontaneous endometriosis. While the rat is a spontaneous ovulator, it has a shorter luteal phase than the human. The reproductive pattern of the rabbit lacks even a luteal phase. In addition to this, there is a wide phylogenetic gap between these two species and the human. In both rodent models, induction is performed through the autotransplantation of endometrial fragments or uterine squares[3], which is not physiological, damages the uterus and causes adhesions interfering with fertility. The resulting 'endometriotic lesions' consist of cysts containing clear serous fluid in the rat, while vascularized hemorrhagic solid masses can also be found in the rabbit. These types of lesions in both species seem to be quite different from the variety of pigmented and non-pigmented lesions found in the human[4–6].

Monkeys, although difficult and expensive to maintain in captivity, offer unique advantages in endometriosis research when compared to rodents. Firstly, they are phylogenetically much closer to the human and have a comparable menstrual cycle. Secondly, non-human primates are known to be afflicted with spontaneous endometriosis: the rhesus monkey[7], the pigtailed macaque[8], the cynomolgus monkey, the De Brazza monkey[9] and the baboon[10,11]. It has been reported that irradiation is associated with an increased incidence of spontaneous endometriosis in rhesus monkeys, but only after at least 6 years[12]. In the same species, a positive correlation was found between dioxin dose and severity of endometriosis[13]. Thirdly, induced endometriosis results in macroscopic lesions which show similarity to the human disease[14–19].

The great apes (chimpanzee, gorilla, orangutan) are closest to man in many anatomical and physiological aspects of reproduction. However, since all of them are protected, endangered species in the wild, they are not practical models for most studies. So far, most endometriosis research has been done in rhesus monkeys and cynomolgus monkeys. However, the baboon may offer clear advantages compared to the rhesus and cynomolgus monkeys. It is phylogenetically very close, since human (46 chromosomes) and baboon (42 chromosomes) karyotypes, evolving slowly, share many ancestral characteristics[20]. Baboons are very intelligent animals with a well-studied and interesting social life. Hypotheses about the early evolution of human social behavior have been developed by carefully studying the behavior of baboon troops living on the grassy plains of Africa[21]. Detailed accounts of baboon reproductive anatomy and physiology, similar to the human, are available including menstrual cycle characteristics, embryo implantation and fetal development[22]. Perineal skin inflation and deflation correspond with relative precision to follicular and luteal phase, offering external follow-up of the menstrual cycle without the need for serial blood samples for determination of estradiol and progesterone levels. The baboon is a proven model for research in cardiovascular and endoscopic surgery[23], endocrinology, teratology, toxicology, testing of contraceptive agents[24] and placental development[25]. The baboon is also a continuous breeder with menstrual cycles throughout the year, also in captivity. It is a larger and stronger primate than rhesus or cynomolgus monkeys, allowing repetitive blood sampling and complex experimental surgery[24]. Specific advantages of the baboon model in gynecological research include the spontaneous presence of peritoneal fluid and the accessibility of the uterine cavity via the cervix, allowing endometrial sampling without hysterotomy[26]. For all these reasons, the baboon is considered to be a good model for research in reproduction[24]. Spontaneous endometriosis in the baboon has been found to be both minimal[11] and disseminated[10], similar to the different disease stages in women. In summary, the baboon seems to offer interesting advantages and merits to be studied as a possible model for the study of endometriosis.

Natural history of endometriosis in baboons

The natural history of endometriosis in women is poorly understood, due to the lack of follow-up beyond 6–12 months after diagnosis[27,28]. During serial observations, progression of endometriosis was reported in 47% after 6 months[27] and 64% after 12 months[28], whereas *status quo* was found in 9% after 12 months[28]. In these studies, improvement was seen in 29% after 6 months[27] and 27% after 12 months[28], and elimination was observed in 23% after 6 months[27]. Repetitive laparoscopies over more than 12 months cannot be done in women for ethical reasons. Recently, minimal endometriosis has been reported to occur in 25% of healthy female baboons of proven fertility[29,30].

The aim of this review is to summarize the clinical value of the baboon as a model for the study of spontaneous evolution of endometriosis. The studies reviewed were carried out at the Institute of Primate Research, Nairobi, Kenya, from 1990 until 1994.

The prevalence of spontaneous endometriosis in the baboon increases with the duration of captivity[31]

This study[31] was done to compare the prevalence of endometriosis between baboons recently captured in the wild and those living in captivity for several years. A diagnostic laparoscopy was performed for endometriosis screening and obtaining biopsies in 104 female baboons including animals that had been recently captured in the wild ($n = 52$,

Group I), primates that had been living in captivity for 1–2 years ($n = 30$, Group II) and animals that had been captured for more than 2 years ($n = 22$, Group III). The prevalence of clinical and biopsy-proven endometriosis in all baboons was 17% and 12%, respectively.

Clinical endometriosis was found more frequently in Group III (27%) than in Group II (17%) or Group I (11%). The prevalence of biopsy-proven endometriosis was also significantly higher in Group III (27%) than in Groups I and II combined (10%, $p = 0.03$). The results of this study indicate that the prevalence of endometriosis increases with the time spent in captivity. This trend may be explained by more menstrual cycles uninterrupted by pregnancy in captive than in wild baboons, and/or by captivity-associated stress[31].

Spontaneous evolution over 12 months[32]

In an initial study[32] repeat laparoscopy of 11 baboons with initial endometriosis showed a significant increase in the lesion number after 10 months. Moreover, endometriosis was present after 10–12 months in seven of ten animals with a previously normal pelvis[32]. All endometriosis observed was minimal or American Fertility Society (AFS) stage I[33]. This observation, together with the high incidence of endometriosis (70%) in control animals, suggests that there was no fundamental difference between both groups and that endometriosis in baboons is either a moderately progressive disease or a stable condition that may have transitory surges of development followed by regression[32]. We speculated that peritoneal trauma and/or irritation during repeated laparoscopies could favor the development of endometriosis, eventually through local or systemic immunological factors[34]. Remodeling of the lesions was apparent when data at 10 and 12 months were compared[32]. These results suggest that there is transition between subtle and typical lesions. White plaques should not be considered as burnt-out lesions, because they can become white vesicles at a later stage[32]. This concept of remodeling which was first demonstrated in baboons[32] has recently been confirmed in studies in women with endometriosis[35].

Cumulative incidence rate of endometriosis over 30 months[36]

The aim of this study[36] was to document the incidence of endometriosis over 30 months in baboons with an initially normal pelvis. In 24 baboons with a laparoscopically confirmed normal pelvis, 67 serial laparoscopies (2.8 ± 1.9 per animal, range 1–6) were performed after 1–3 months ($n = 8$), 4–6 months ($n = 11$), 7–9 months ($n = 9$), 10–12 months ($n = 17$), 13–15 months ($n = 6$), 16–18 months ($n = 4$), 19–21 months ($n = 3$), 22–24 months ($n = 4$), 25–27 months ($n = 1$) and 30–32 months ($n = 4$). During each laparoscopy the pelvis was examined for the presence of endometriosis; the number, size and type of endometriotic implants were noted on a pelvic map; the endometriosis score and stage was calculated according to the revised classification of the American Fertility Society[33]. The cumulative incidence of minimal endometriosis was 70% after 30–32 months of follow-up. The ten baboons that developed endometriosis were followed during a longer period of time and had undergone more serial laparoscopies than the animals that did not get the disease[36]. The increase in number and surface of lesions was caused largely by subtle implants. Although fluctuations were observed in both number and surface of implants, regression of endometriosis was not observed in any animal. Progression beyond AFS stage I or minimal endometriosis was not found[36]. The results of this study show a high incidence of minimal endometriosis in baboons increasing with the time of follow-up and with the number of repeat laparoscopies[36].

Spontaneous evolution over 30 months[37]

In 12 baboons with histologically proven spontaneous endometriosis, 54 serial laparoscopies (4.2 ± 1.9 per animal, range 1–7) were performed after 1–3 months ($n = 2$), 4–6 months ($n = 1$), 7–9 months ($n = 6$), 10–12 months ($n = 17$), 13–15 months ($n = 7$), 16–18 months ($n = 1$), 19–21 months ($n = 8$), 22–24 months ($n = 8$), 25–27 months ($n = 2$) and 30–32 months ($n = 2$). During each laparoscopy the pelvis was examined for the presence of endometriosis. The number, size and type of endometriotic implants were noted on a pelvic map and both endometriosis score and stage were calculated. Remodeling was defined as a change in laparoscopic appearance (typical, subtle, suspicious) of an individual endometriotic lesion. Endometriosis was progressive as shown by the significant increase in the number and surface of lesions and in endometriosis scores after 24 months. The total number of endometriotic lesions after 24 months consisted of 69% new (and mostly subtle) implants, 10% remodeled lesions and 21% unchanged implants. This study demonstrated that endometriosis in captive baboons undergoing repeated laparoscopies is a dynamic and moderately progressive disease with periods of development and regression and active remodeling between different types of lesions.

Spontaneous evolution during pregnancy[38]

This study[38] was performed on 11 baboons with histologically proven endometriosis to test the hypothesis that endometriosis undergoes regression during pregnancy. In each individual baboon paired laparoscopies were performed prior to and during pregnancy (six during first and five during second trimester of gestation) with an interval of 5 ± 3 months (range 2–11) and the observations prior to and during pregnancy were compared. No significant change in the AFS score or stage of endometriosis, or in the number, size and type of endometriotic lesions was observed in pregnant baboons when compared to the non-pregnant state[38]. Although in baboons pregnancy had no significant effect on endometriosis during the first or second trimester of gestation, a beneficial effect of the third trimester of gestation and of the postpartum period on endometriosis cannot be excluded in baboons. These results may also offer a partial explanation as to why hormonal 'pseudopregnancy' regimens apparently do not result in a cure with complete fibrosis of endometriotic implants.

Intrapelvic injection of menstrual endometrium causes endometriosis in baboons[26]

The goal of this study[26] was to test the Sampson hypothesis of retrograde menstruation as a cause of endometriosis[39], by determining the effect of intrapelvic injection of menstrual versus luteal endometrium on the incidence, peritoneal involvement and stage of endometriosis. Seventeen baboons were injected retroperitoneally with luteal ($n = 6$) or menstrual ($n = 7$) endometrium and intraperitoneally with menstrual endometrium ($n = 4$). Laparoscopies were performed after 2 months in all animals, and after 5 and 12 months in six and five primates injected with luteal and menstrual endometrium, respectively. The peritoneal endometriosis surface area, number of implants and incidence of typical and red subtle lesions were significantly higher after retroperitoneal injection of menstrual than of luteal endometrium. Using menstrual endometrium, intraperitoneal seeding was more successful in causing endometriosis than retroperitoneal injection.

The spontaneous evolution of endometriosis in this study[26] revealed that endometriosis remained unchanged in all primates induced with luteal endometrium after 5 months and increased in three of four regularly cycling baboons induced with menstrual endometrium after 12 months. These findings support the observation that injection of menstrual endometrium is more successful than luteal endometrium in inducing endometriosis. The incidence of red lesions decreased and typical lesions increased during the follow-up period in all animals. This finding supports the hypothesis that red lesions represent early while typical implants represent late manifestations of pelvic endometriosis[40] and confirms our observation that remodeling and transformation of typical and subtle lesions occur[32,36,37].

Immunosuppression can increase progression of spontaneous endometriosis in baboons[41]

The goal of this study[41] was to test the hypothesis that immunosuppression increases the development and progression of endometriosis in baboons. Thirty-two baboons (eight with normal pelvis, ten with spontaneous endometriosis and fourteen with endometriosis induced by intraperitoneal seeding of menstrual endometrium) were studied. Immunosuppression was obtained by daily intramuscular injection of methylprednisolone 0.8 mg/kg and azathioprine 2 mg/kg for 3 months in 16 baboons (four with normal pelvis, five with spontaneous and seven with induced endometriosis). No treatment was given to the remaining 16 primates. Immunosuppressed baboons with spontaneous endometriosis had a significantly higher number ($p < 0.02$) and larger surface area ($p = 0.03$) of endometriotic lesions than non-treated animals[41]. However, immunosuppressed and non-treated primates with induced endometriosis were comparable with respect to both number and surface area of implants. In immunosuppressed baboons with either spontaneous or induced disease, a temporary increase in subtle and decrease in typical endometriotic lesions was noted[41]. This suggests that immunosuppression may favor the development of subtle implants and retard the physiological transition from subtle lesions to more typical implants[41].

The spontaneous evolution of endometriosis after immunosuppression was different in animals with spontaneous disease and those with the induced condition[41]. In baboons with spontaneous endometriosis, significant progression of disease was observed in immunosuppressed primates as compared to animals that had not been immunosuppressed, as evidenced by a significantly higher ($p < 0.01$) difference in number of endometriotic lesions between the first laparoscopy and follow-up laparoscopy 9 months later[41]. In contrast, in baboons with induced endometriosis both mean number and surface area of lesions were comparable in immunosuppressed and non-immunosuppressed animals, and were similar to the findings at the first laparoscopy[41]. During spontaneous evolution, the surface area covered by subtle lesions decreased in both immunosuppressed and control animals with induced or spontaneous endometriosis[41].

Immunosuppression did not cause the development of endometriosis in baboons with previously documented normal pelvis[41]. It is possible that in baboons with a normal pelvis the immunosuppression period was too short to significantly favor the implantation of retrogradally-shed endometrium. In a previous study in rhesus monkeys, 7 years of exposure to proton irradiation were required for the development of endometriosis[12].

Conclusions

The data on spontaneous evolution of endometriosis in baboons[26,31,32,36–38,41] show that endometriosis is a moderately progressive disease, that minimal endometriosis can be found with a high incidence in baboons with a previously normal pelvis, and that immunosuppression may favor the progression of spontaneous endometriosis in baboons.

Minimal endometriosis can be considered as a risk factor for the development of more advanced (mild–severe) disease. This is clinically important because a reduced cycle fecundity rate has been reported in baboons with mild to severe disease[42], whereas the normal cycle fecundity rate was observed in baboons with minimal disease in two different prospective controlled studies[42,43].

Acknowledgments

We thank the mentors of this project: C.S. Bambra, Nairobi, Kenya; P.R. Koninckx, Leuven, Belgium and J.A. Hill, Harvard Medical School, Boston, MA, USA. We are grateful for critical comments from the collaborating European centers: M. Bruhat, Clermont-Ferrand, France; J. Calaf, Barcelona, Spain; H. Evers, Maastricht, The Netherlands; J. Raus, Diepenbeek, Belgium and M. Dhont, Gent, Belgium. The help of advisers, A.F. Haney, Duke University, Durham, NC, USA; D.C. Martin, Memphis, TN, USA; R.S. Schenken, San Antonio, TX, USA and E.R. te Velde, University of Utrecht, The Netherlands, is greatly appreciated. The laparoscopy equipment was kindly donated by Mrs Storz-Rehling (Storz Company, D-7200 Tuttlingen, Germany). The authors also thank Mr Z. Maheli Karanja, Mr S. Kago and Mr S. Kisara for their clinical assistance and for logistic and administrative support provided by the VVOB (Flemish Organization for Development Programs Abroad, Belgium).

References

1. Haney, A.F. (1987). Endometriosis: pathogenesis and pathophysiology. In Wilson, E.A. (ed.) *Endometriosis*, pp. 23–51. (New York: A.R. Liss Inc.)
2. Hill, J.A. (1992). Immunological factors in endometriosis and endometriosis-associated reproductive failure. *Infertil. Reprod. Med. Clin. North Am.*, **3**, 583–96
3. Vernon, M.W. and Wilson, E.A. (1985). Studies on the surgical induction of endometriosis in the rat. *Fertil. Steril.*, **44**, 684–94
4. Jansen, R.P.S. and Russell, P. (1986). Nonpigmented endometriosis: clinical, laparoscopic and pathologic definition. *Am. J. Obstet. Gynecol.*, **155**, 1160–3
5. Martin, D.C., Hubert, G.D., Vander Zwaag, R. and El-Zeky, F.A. (1989). Laparoscopic appearances of peritoneal endometriosis. *Fertil. Steril.*, **51**, 63–7
6. Nisolle, M., Casanas-Roux, F., Anaf, V., Mine, J. and Donnez, J. (1993). Morphometric study of the stromal vascularization in peritoneal endometriosis. *Fertil. Steril.*, **59**, 681–4
7. McCann, T.O. and Myers, R.E. (1970). Endometriosis in rhesus monkeys. *Am. J. Obstet. Gynecol.*, **106**, 516–23
8. Digiacomo, R.F. (1977). Gynecologic pathology in the rhesus monkey (*Macaca mulatta*). *Vet. Pathol.*, **14**, 539–46
9. Binhazim, A.A., Tarara, R.P. and Suleman, M.A. (1989). Spontaneous external endometriosis in a DeBrazza's monkey. *J. Comp. Pathol.*, **101**, 471–4
10. Folse, D.S. and Stout, L.C. (1978). Endometriosis in a baboon. *Lab. Anim. Sci.*, **28**, 217–19
11. Merrill, J.A. (1968). Spontaneous endometriosis in the Kenya baboon. *Am. J. Obstet. Gynecol.*, **101**, 569–70
12. Wood, D.H. (1991). Long-term mortality and cancer-risk in irradiated rhesus monkeys. *Radiat. Res.*, **126**, 132–40
13. Rier, S.E., Martin, D.C., Bowman, R.E., Dmowski, W.P. and Becker, J.L. (1993). Endometriosis in rhesus monkeys (*Macaca mulatta*) following chronic exposure to 2,3,7,8-tetrachlorodibenzo-p-dioxin. *Fundam. Appl. Toxicol.*, **21**, 433–41
14. Jacobson, V.C. (1926). The intraperitoneal transplantation of endometrial tissue in the rabbit. *Arch. Pathol. Lab. Med.*, **1**, 169–74
15. Te Linde, R.W. and Scott, R.B. (1950). Experimental endometriosis. *Am. J. Obstet. Gynecol.*, **60**, 1147–73
16. Allen, E., Peterson, L.F. and Campbell, Z.B. (1954). Clinical and experimental endometriosis. *Am. J. Obstet. Gynecol.*, **68**, 356–75

17. Dizerega, G.S., Barber, D.L. and Hodgen, G.D. (1980). Endometriosis: role of ovarian steroids in initiation, maintenance and suppression. *Fertil. Steril.*, **33**, 649–53
18. Schenken, R.S., Asch, R.H., Williams, R.F. and Hodgen, G.D. (1984). Etiology of infertility in monkeys with endometriosis: luteinized unruptured follicles, luteal phase defects, pelvic adhesions, and spontaneous abortions. *Fertil. Steril.*, **41**, 122–30
19. Mann, D.R., Collins, D.C., Smith, M.M., Kessler, M.J. and Gould, K.G. (1986). Treatment of endometriosis in rhesus monkeys: effectiveness of a gonadotropin-releasing hormone agonist compared to treatment with a progestational steroid. *J. Clin. Endocrinol. Metab.*, **63**, 1277–83
20. Marks, J. (1982). Evolutionary tempo and phylogenetic inference based on primate karyotypes. *Gytogenet. Cell. Genet.*, **34**, 261–4
21. Strum, S.C. (1987). Almost human: a journey into the world of baboons. (London: Elm Tree Books)
22. Hendrickx, A.G. (1971). Reproduction: methods. In Hendrickx, A.G. (ed.) *Embryology of the Baboon*, pp. 1–44. (Chicago and London: University of Chicago Press)
23. D'Hooghe, T.M., Bambra, C.S., Farah, I.O., Raeymaekers, B. and Koninckx, P.R. (1993). High intra-abdominal pressure during laparoscopy: effects on clinical parameters and lung pathology in baboons (*Papio anubis, Papio cynocephalus*). *Am. J. Obstet. Gynecol.*, **169**, 1352–6
24. Isahakia, M.A. and Bambra, C.S. (1990). Primate models for research in reproduction. In *Gamete Interaction: Prospects for Immunocontraception*, pp. 487–500. (New York: Wiley-Liss, Inc.)
25. Pijnenborg, R., D'Hooghe, T., Vercruysse, L. and Bambra, C. (1996). Evaluation of trophoblast invasion in placental bed biopsies of the baboon, with immunohistochemical localization of cytokeratin, fibronectin and laminin. *J. Med. Primatol.*, **25**, 272–81
26. D'Hooghe, T.M., Bambra, C.S., Raeymaekers, B.M., De Jonge, I., Lauweryns, J.M. and Koninckx, P.R. (1995). Intrapelvic injection of menstrual endometrium causes endometriosis in baboons (*Papio cynocephalus, Papio anubis*). *Am. J. Obstet. Gynecol.*, **173**, 125–34
27. Thomas, E.J. and Cooke, I.D. (1987). Impact of gestrinone on the course of asymptomatic endometriosis. *Br. Med. J.*, **294**, 272–4
28. Mahmood, T.A. (1990). The impact of treatment on the natural history of endometriosis. *Hum. Reprod.*, **5**, 965–70
29. D'Hooghe, T.M., Bambra, C.S., Cornillie, F.J., Isahakia, M. and Koninckx, P.R. (1991). Prevalence and laparoscopic appearance of spontaneous endometriosis in the baboon (*Papio anubis, Papio cynocephalus*). *Biol. Reprod.*, **45**, 411–16
30. Cornillie, F.J., D'Hooghe, T.M., Bambra, C.S., Lauweryns, J.M., Isahakia, M. and Koninckx, P.R. (1992). Morphological characteristics of spontaneous endometriosis in the baboon (*Papio anubis, Papio cynocephalus*). *Gynecol. Obstet. Invest.*, **34**, 225–8
31. D'Hooghe, T.M., Bambra, C.S., De Jonge, I., Lauweryns, J.M. and Koninckx, P.R. (1996). The prevalence of spontaneous endometriosis in the baboon increases with the time spent in captivity. *Acta Obstet. Gynecol. Scand.*, **75**, 98–101
32. D'Hooghe, T.M., Bambra, C.S., Isahakia, M. and Koninckx, P.R. (1992). Evolution of minimal endometriosis in the baboon (*Papio anubis, Papio cynocephalus*) over a 12-month period. *Fertil. Steril.*, **58**, 409–12
33. American Fertility Society (1985). Revised American Fertility Society classification of endometriosis. *Fertil. Steril.*, **43**, 351–2
34. D'Hooghe, T.M. and Hill, J.A. (1996). Immunobiology of endometriosis. In Bronson, R.A., Alexander, N.J., Anderson, D.J., Branch, D.W. and Kutteh, W.H. (eds.) *Immunology of Reproduction*, pp. 322–58. (Cambridge, MA: Blackwell Science)
35. Wiegerinck, M.A.H.M., Van Dop, P.A. and Brosens, I.A. (1993). The staging of peritoneal endometriosis by the type of active lesion in addition to the revised American Fertility Society classification. *Fertil. Steril.*, **60**, 461–4
36. D'Hooghe, T.M., Bambra, C.S., Raeymaekers, B.M. and Koninckx, P.R. (1996). The cumulative incidence rate of endometriosis in baboons (*Papio anubis, Papio cynocephalus*) with an initially normal pelvis is 70% after 30 months. *Obstet. Gynecol.*, **88**, 462–6
37. D'Hooghe, T.M., Bambra, C.S., Raeymaekers, B.M. and Koninckx, P.R. (1996). Serial laparoscopies over 30 months show that endometriosis is a progressive disease in captive baboons (*Papio anubis, Papio cynocephalus*). *Fertil. Steril.*, **65**, 645–9

38. D'Hooghe, T.M., Bambra, C.S., De Jonge, I., Lauweryns, J.M., Raeymaekers, B.M. and Koninckx, P.R. (1995). Pregnancy does not affect endometriosis in baboons (*Papio anubis, Papio cynocephalus*). Presented at the *15th World Congress on Fertility and Sterility*, Montpellier, France, September
39. Sampson, J.A. (1927). Peritoneal endometriosis due to menstrual dissemination of endometrial tissue into the pelvic cavity. *Am. J. Obstet. Gynecol.*, **14**, 422–69
40. Redwine, D.B. (1987). Age-related evolution in color appearance of endometriosis. *Fertil. Steril.*, **48**, 1062–3
41. D'Hooghe, T.M., Bambra, C.S., Raeymaekers, B.M., Hill, J.A. and Koninckx, P.R. (1995). Immunosuppression can increase progression of spontaneous endometriosis in baboons. *Fertil. Steril.*, **64**, 172–8
42. D'Hooghe, T.M., Bambra, C.S., Raeymaekers, B.M., Riday, A.M., Suleman, M.A. and Koninckx, P.R. (1996). A prospective controlled study over 2 years shows a normal monthly fertility rate (MFR) in baboons with stage I endometriosis and a decreased MFR in primates with stage II and stage III–IV disease. *Fertil. Steril.*, **66**, 809–13
43. D'Hooghe, T.M., Bambra, C.S. and Koninckx, P.R. (1994). Cycle fecundity in baboons of proven fertility with minimal endometriosis. *Gynecol. Obstet. Invest.*, **37**, 63–5

Section 2

The physiology of the endometrium, uterus and endometriosis

Endometrium in endometriosis

M. Wingfield, A. Macpherson, P.A.W. Rogers and D.L. Healy

Introduction

The most widely accepted hypothesis for the development of endometriosis is retrograde menstruation[1]. However, this phenomenon has been demonstrated in 90% of all women undergoing laparoscopy during menses[2], suggesting that retrograde menstruation facilitates transport of endometrial tissue to the peritoneal cavity but that some other factor renders certain women susceptible to the implantation and growth of this ectopic endometrium. Theories proposed to account for this susceptibility include genetic predisposition[3], a greater amount of retrograde menstruation[4], an altered peritoneal environment[5] or an immunological susceptibility[6].

Surprisingly little attention has focused on the possible role of the intrauterine endometrium in the pathogenesis of endometriosis. We propose that women develop endometriosis because of abnormalities inherent in their ectopic or intrauterine endometrium. Endometrium is unique among adult tissues because it undergoes intense proliferation, secretion, regression, and regeneration during each menstrual cycle. It is plausible that subtle alterations in this complex series of events could lead to pathological proliferation of endometrial tissue. Our hypothesis is that the endometrium of women with endometriosis has an increased capacity to proliferate and therefore implant and grow in the peritoneal cavity.

Central to the complex changes occurring in the endometrium throughout the menstrual cycle is angiogenesis or new blood vessel growth. Three separate episodes of angiogenesis have been described in primate endometrium[7]. These comprise postmenstrual repair during the early proliferative phase, midproliferative vessel growth under the influence of estrogen, and finally growth of coiled arterioles under the influence of progesterone in the secretory phase.

There is evidence that angiogenesis may be important in the pathophysiology of endometriosis. It is obvious at laparoscopy that most endometriotic lesions are surrounded by peritoneal blood vessels. The peritoneal fluid of women with endometriosis contains more angiogenic factors than that of women without the disease[8]. Histological studies and animal experiments have shown that endometriotic deposits derive their blood supply from the surrounding microvasculature[9], that larger deposits grow in areas with a rich blood supply[10], and that the more vascular endometriotic deposits are more active[10].

Angiogenesis is a complex process involving local degradation of the basement membrane of the native blood vessel followed by the migration and proliferation of endothelial cells to form a new vessel[11]. The primary aim of our study was to compare endothelial cell proliferation (one of the stages of angiogenesis) in the endometrium of women with and without endometriosis[12]. The immunohistochemistry technique used also enabled evaluation of endometrial epithelial and stromal cell proliferation.

Cell proliferation in the endometrium of women with endometriosis

To study endothelial cell proliferation in the endometrium of women with and without endometriosis, endometrium was sampled at dilatation and curettage in 30 women with endometriosis and 27 normal controls. Endo-

Table 1 Proliferation indices for endothelial cells and proliferation scores for glandular and luminal epithelium and stroma in endometrium of endometriosis patients and controls. Values are given as means ± SEM, with the number of patients in parentheses

	Cycle stage	Endometriosis patients	Controls	p-value
Endothelial cells	all stages	12.9 ± 2.6 (30)	4.0 ± 3.2 (27)	0.0014
	menstrual	16.6 ± 16.4 (2)	3.0 ± 2.2 (2)	NS
	proliferative	15.1 ± 3.7 (18)	3.8 ± 1.0 (12)	0.0019
	secretory	8.1 ± 3.0 (10)	4.3 ± 1.2 (13)	NS
Glandular epithelium	all stages	6.9 ± 0.7 (30)	2.7 ± 0.5 (27)	0.0002
	menstrual	7.0 ± 5.0 (2)	1.0 ± 0.0 (2)	NS
	proliferative	8.7 ± 0.8 (18)	4.0 ± 0.8 (12)	0.0014
	secretory	3.6 ± 1.0 (10)	1.9 ± 0.4 (13)	NS
Luminal epithelium	all stages	4.0 ± 0.8 (22)	1.1 ± 0.5 (12)	0.0100
	menstrual	0.0 ± 0.0 (1)	—	—
	proliferative	6.7 ± 1.0 (12)	2.0 ± 1.0 (5)	0.0177
	secretory	0.9 ± 0.2 (9)	0.4 ± 0.4 (7)	NS
Stroma	all stages	3.5 ± 0.4 (30)	2.1 ± 0.3 (27)	0.0006
	menstrual	2.0 ± 0.0 (2)	1.0 ± 0.0 (2)	NS
	proliferative	4.2 ± 0.6 (18)	2.5 ± 0.8 (12)	0.0141
	secretory	2.5 ± 0.4 (10)	1.9 ± 0.2 (13)	NS

p-values derived using the Mann–Whitney U-test; NS, not significant

metriosis was diagnosed at concurrent laparoscopy and staged according to the revised American Fertility Society (AFS) score[13]. Ten women had stage I disease, 12 had stage II, six had stage III, and two had stage IV. The overall laparoscopic appearance of endometriosis was also described as predominantly red lesions (n = 8), predominantly black lesions (n = 10), combined red and black lesions (n = 8) or deep lesions (infiltrating deeply into the vagina or rectovaginal septum, n = 4). Controls were women with a normal pelvis at laparoscopy performed for tubal sterilization or for infertility where the sole cause of infertility was a male factor. All women had normal menstrual cycles and had not received any hormonal therapy, used an intrauterine device, been pregnant or lactated during the previous 2 months. Institutional ethical approval was obtained and all subjects gave informed consent.

Endometrial biopsies were fixed in 10% buffered formalin for 4–6 h, washed in phosphate buffered saline, and processed through increasing concentrations of ethanol to Safsolvent (Ajax Chemicals, Auburn, New South Wales, Australia) and finally to wax (Paraplast X-TRA; Oxford Labware, St. Louis, MO, USA). Serial 5-µm sections were cut for immunohistochemistry and hematoxylin and eosin staining. Sections were dated by a gynecological pathologist according to the histological criteria of Noyes and colleagues[14] and classified as menstrual, proliferative or secretory. The number of samples for each cycle stage is shown in Table 1. Samples incorporating the basalis layer of endometrium were excluded from the analyses because of known differences in cell proliferation between the functionalis and basalis layers of the endometrium[15].

Immunohistochemistry involved a double staining technique. Endothelial cells were stained using a mouse monoclonal antibody against CD34 antigen, a glycoprotein expressed on the luminal surface of endothelial cells[16] (clone QBED/10; Serotex, Oxford, UK). All proliferating nuclei in the section (i.e. stromal and epithelial cells in addition to endothelial cells) were stained with a mouse monoclonal antibody against proliferating cell nuclear antigen (PCNA) (Clone PC10; Novocastra Laboratories, Newcastle upon Tyne, UK). Proliferating cell nuclear antigen is a nuclear protein whose expression peaks during the S phase of the cell cycle and which has been used previously to identify proliferating cells[17]. The staining protocol has been described in detail elsewhere[17]. Briefly, a Histostain-DS Kit (Zymed Laboratories Inc., San Francisco, CA, USA) was used. This involves a peroxidase and biotin-streptavidin detection system. Proliferating cell nuclear antigen is stained red with aminoethylcarbazole chromogen and CD34 blue with alkaline phosphatase-blue. A separate section was stained with CD34 (in this case stained red) and hematoxylin and eosin to identify the total number of endothelial cell nuclei. In each run, a control section (early proliferative to midproliferative phase endometrium) of known immunostaining intensity was included as a positive interassay control. Negative controls of mouse immunoglobulin of the same immunoglobulin class and concentration as the primary antibody were used instead of the primary antibody.

Endothelial cell proliferation was quantified by calculating an endothelial cell proliferation index for each section, i.e. the number of proliferating endothelial cells per mm^2 divided by the total number of endothelial cells per mm^2, expressed as a percentage. Cells were counted with the aid of a microscope at ×400 linked via a color CCD video camera (MW-F15e; Panasonic, Matsushita Electrical Industrial Co. Ltd, Osaka, Japan) to a personal computer (Amiga model 2000; Commodore, Lane Cove, New South Wales, Australia) with stereology software (Grid version 2.1; Graffiti Data, Silkeborg, Denmark).

Nuclear proliferation in glandular and luminal epithelial cells and in stromal cells (excluding endothelial cells) was scored semi-quantitatively. For each tissue compartment, the fraction of positively stained cells was expressed as either 0 (no staining), 1 (≤ 1/250 cells stained), 2 (≤ 1/50), 3 (≤ 1/10) or 4 (> 1/10 cells stained), and the intensity of staining was graded as either 0 (none), 1 (mild), 2 (moderate) or 3 (intense). These two scores were then multiplied to derive a total immunostaining score[18]. The author who scored these sections and who counted the endothelial cells as described above was blinded as to which sections were from women with endometriosis and which were from control women.

Data were analyzed using Excel (version 5.0; Microsoft Corporation, Redmond, WS, USA) and Minitab (Minitab Inc., University Park, PA, USA) software. Comparisons were performed using the Mann–Whitney U-test for nonparametric data. Correlations were performed using regression analysis. Results with $p \leq 0.05$ were considered significant.

The mean endothelial cell proliferative index was significantly greater in those with endometriosis compared with controls (mean ± SEM, 12.9 ± 2.6 vs. 4.0 ± 3.2, $p = 0.0014$; Table 1). However, there was wide interpatient variability particularly among women with endometriosis. In this group, 11/30 women had proliferative indices exceeding the mean value for the group (12.9). Only one control endometrium had a proliferative index exceeding this value. If a proliferative index of ≥ 12 were used as a cut-off point to predict endometriosis, it would have a specificity of 96% and a sensitivity of 40%.

When endothelial cell proliferative indices were analyzed according to menstrual cycle stage, proliferative phase values showed a significant different between endometriosis patients and controls. Secretory phase proliferation indices were similar in each group and there were insufficient samples in the menstrual phase to achieve statistically meaningful results.

Epithelial (glandular and luminal) and stromal cells demonstrated significantly higher immunostaining scores in endometriosis patients compared with controls (Table 1). As with endothelial cells the difference was statistically significant in the proliferative phase of the cycle. Using regression analysis, endothelial cell proliferation correlated with glandular proliferation in the endometriosis group (Pearson $r = 0.51$, $p = 0.004$) but not in control endometrium (Pearson $r = 0.01$, $p = 0.98$). There was no correlation between endothelial cell proliferation and either stromal or luminal proliferation.

Endothelial cell proliferation showed no significant variation throughout the menstrual cycle in either endometriosis or control endometrium. In endometrium from endometriosis patients, however, mean proliferation scores were significantly higher in the proliferative phase compared with the secretory phase in glandular epithelial cells (mean ± SEM, 8.7 ± 0.8 vs. 3.6 ± 1.0, $p = 0.002$), luminal epithelial cells (6.7 ± 1.0 vs. 0.9 ± 0.2, $p = 0.0002$), and stromal cells (4.2 ± 0.6 vs. 2.5 ± 0.4, $p = 0.04$).

Proliferation scores in the endometriosis group were analyzed according to various clinical characteristics. None of the endometrial parameters studied (endothelial cell proliferative indices and immunostaining scores for glandular and luminal epithelial and stromal cells) showed any significant difference between women with endometriosis who presented with pain or asymptomatic infertility or between those with revised AFS stages I to IV of endometriosis. When endometrial data were analyzed according to general laparoscopic appearance of endometriosis (i.e. red, black, mixed or deep), three of four women with deeply infiltrating disease had very high endothelial cell proliferative indices (> 32) in their uterine endometrium, but this was not significantly different from the other groups, possibly because of small numbers.

These results support the hypothesis that the endometrium of some women with endometriosis is significantly different from that of women without the disease. Using immunohistochemistry, we have demonstrated increased numbers of proliferating endothelial cells as well as glandular and luminal epithelial and stromal cells in the endometrium of these women. These findings suggest that the intrauterine endometrium may be central to the pathogenesis of endometriosis.

Future directions

There is growing evidence that the endometrium of women with endometriosis is not 'normal'. Endometrium from patients with minimal endometriosis has been shown to secrete more complement-3 than that of patients without endometriosis or those with severe disease[19]. Others have demonstrated an increased presence of complement receptor type 3 positive macrophages infiltrating the proliferative endometrial stroma of patients with mild-to-moderate endometriosis[19]. These authors also showed that endometrial extracts from patients with endometriosis have enhanced chemotactic activity for neutrophils and macrophages in the proliferative phase of the cycle compared with controls. Oosterlynck and colleagues[6] demonstrated that the endometrium of women with endometriosis is more resistant to the cytotoxic effect of heterologous lymphocytes than that of control women. Another study has shown significant reduction in glycogen content and glycogen synthetase in the endometrium of women with endometriosis[20]. Menstrual fluid cancer antigen-125 (CA-125) levels are almost three times greater in women with endometriosis compared with controls[21], while a recent study employing endometrial cell culture has demonstrated two to four times more *in vitro* CA-125 production by endometrium from women with endometriosis compared with that from control women[22].

Our data suggests that the endometrium in women with endometriosis has enhanced proliferation and increased ability to implant and survive in ectopic locations. The concept of enhanced endothelial cell proliferation is attractive since angiogenesis is essential if endometrium is to survive outside the uterus.

If, as is widely accepted, endometriosis occurs via retrograde menstruation, an enhanced ability of the endometrium to induce angiogenesis and proliferate would make it more likely to acquire an adequate blood supply and survive in ectopic locations. Moreover, enhanced proliferation in eutopic endometrium might also interfere with normal implantation, and so contribute to infertility and increase the risk of miscarriage associated with endometriosis.

Acknowledgements

We thank Beatrice Susil from the Department of Anatomical Pathology, Monash Medical Center, Clayton, Victoria, Australia, for dating the endometrial biopsies, and Dr Nigel Wreford from the Institute of Reproduction and Development, Monash University, Melbourne, Victoria, Australia, for advice and use of his equipment for endothelial cell quantification.

References

1. Sampson, J.A. (1927). Peritoneal endometriosis due to the menstrual dissemination of endometrial tissue into the peritoneal cavity. *Am. J. Obstet. Gynecol.*, **14**, 422–69
2. Halme, J., Hammond, M.G., Hulka, J.F., Raj, S.G. and Talbert, L.M. (1984). Retrograde menstruation in healthy women and in patients with endometriosis. *Obstet. Gynecol.*, **64**, 151–4
3. Lamb, K., Hoffman, R.G. and Nichols, T.R. (1986). Family trait analysis: a case–control study of 43 women with endometriosis and their best friends. *Am. J. Obstet. Gynecol.*, **154**, 596–601
4. Cramer, D.W., Wilson, E., Stillman, R.J., Berger, M.J., Belisle, S. and Schiff, I. (1986). The relation of endometriosis to menstrual characteristics, smoking and exercise. *J. Am. Med. Assoc.*, **255**, 1904–8
5. Ramey, J.W. and Archer, D.F. (1993). Peritoneal fluid: its relevance to the development of endometriosis. *Fertil. Steril.*, **60**, 1–14
6. Oosterlynck, D.J., Cornillie, F.J., Waer, M., Vandeputte, M. and Koninckx, P.R. (1991). Women with endometriosis show a defect in natural killer activity resulting in a decreased cytotoxicity to autologous endometrium. *Fertil. Steril.*, **56**, 45–51
7. Rogers, P.A.W., Abberton, K.M. and Susil, B. (1992). Endothelial cell migratory signal produced by human endometrium during the menstrual cycle. *Hum. Reprod.*, **7**, 1061–6
8. Oosterlynck, D.J., Meuleman, C., Sobis, H., Vandeputte, M. and Koninckx, P.R. (1993). Angiogenic activity of peritoneal fluid from women with endometriosis. *Fertil. Steril.*, **59**, 778–82
9. Nieminen, U. (1962). Studies on the vascular pattern of ectopic endometrium with special reference to cyclic changes. *Acta Obstet. Gynecol. Scand.*, **41**(Suppl. 3), 9–81
10. Vernon, M.W. and Wilson, E.A. (1985). Studies on the surgical induction of endometriosis in the rat. *Fertil. Steril.*, **44**, 684–94
11. Findlay, J.K. (1986). Angiogenesis in reproductive tissues. *J. Endocrinol.*, **111**, 357–66
12. Wingfield, M., Macpherson, A., Healy, D.L. and Rogers, P.A.W. (1995). Cell proliferation is increased in the endometrium of women with endometriosis. *Fertil. Steril.*, **64**, 340–6
13. The American Fertility Society (1985). Revised American Fertility Society classification of endometriosis. *Fertil. Steril.*, **43**, 351–2
14. Noyes, R.W., Hertig, A.T. and Rock, J. (1950). Dating the endometrial biopsy. *Fertil. Steril.*, **1**, 3–25
15. Ferenczy, A., Bertrand, G. and Gelfand, M.M. (1979). Proliferation kinetics of human endometrium during the normal menstrual cycle. *Am. J. Obstet. Gynecol.*, **133**, 859–67
16. Traweek, S.T., Kandalaft, P.L., Mehta, P. and Battifora, H. (1991). The human haematopoietic progenitor cell antigen (CD34) in vascular neoplasia. *Am. J. Clin. Pathol.*, **96**, 25–31
17. Goodger, A.M. and Rogers, P.A.W. (1994). Endometrial endothelial cell proliferation during the menstrual cycle. *Hum. Reprod.*, **9**, 399–405
18. Bergqvist, A., Ljungberg, O. and Skoog, L. (1993). Immunohistochemical analysis of estrogen and progesterone receptors in

endometriotic tissue and endometrium. *Hum. Reprod.*, **8**, 1915–22
19. Isaacson, K. B., Galman, M., Coutifaris, C. and Lyttle, C.R. (1990). Endometrial synthesis and secretion of complement component-3 by patients with and without endometriosis. *Fertil. Steril.*, **53**, 836–41
20. Ishihara, S., Taketani, Y. and Mizuno, M. (1991). Endometriosis impairs glycogen synthesis in human endometrium. *Int. J. Fertil.*, **36**, 287–90
21. Takahashi, K., Nagata, H., Abu Musa, A., Shibukawa, T., Yamasaki, H. and Kitao, M. (1990). Clinical usefulness of CA125 levels in the menstrual discharge in patients with endometriosis. *Fertil. Steril.*, **54**, 360–2
22. McBean, J.H. and Brunsted, J.R. (1993). *In vitro* CA-125 secretion by endometrium from women with advanced endometriosis. *Fertil. Steril.*, **59**, 89–92

Endometriosis and pain: the role of prostaglandins

K. Satoh, M. Tochigi and J.M. Teng

There has been a recent increase in numbers of patients with endometriosis. The most frequent symptoms and signs in endometriosis are usually pain such as menstrual pain (dysmenorrhea), dyspareunia, lumbago, lower abdominal pain, defecation pain, etc. Since it was reported that the concentration of prostaglandin $F_{2\alpha}$ ($PGF_{2\alpha}$) is increased in the menstrual fluid of the dysmenorrheic woman[1], prostaglandins have been focused on as the cause of the pains. Furthermore, increased levels of prostaglandins have been found in the endometrial tissue of dysmenorrheic women[2,3], and in the menstrual fluid of endometriotic patients[4].

After these phenomena were observed, non-steroidal anti-inflammatory drugs which inhibited the synthesis of prostaglandins were applied for the clinical treatment of menstrual disorders such as dysmenorrhea and menorrhagia[5,6]. From these findings, the involvement of prostaglandins in the pain caused by endometriosis is now generally recognized, but it still remains unclear how prostaglandins act in such pain. In order to clarify the role of prostaglandins in endometriotic pain, the characteristics of the pain, the mechanism of prostaglandin action in the algesic process and the relief of the pain will be discussed in this paper.

Endometriotic pain in reproductive women

By laparoscopic examination, 127 out of the 367 sterile patients were found to have endometriosis and the incidence of endometriosis was 35% in our department during 1982–89. In these 127 patients, the characteristics of the complaints and the findings by internal examination are shown in Table 1. About 60% of endometriotic patients complained of some concomitant pains, among which menstrual pain was complained of most frequently, and by internal examination, cul-de-sac tenderness was the most obvious sign.

Since pain is the most typical symptom in endometriosis, whether the severity of the pain is parallel to the stage of endometriosis is one of the interesting questions in the pathogenesis. As shown in Table 2, 13/17 patients with stage I disease complained of mild menstrual pain and 2/6 patients with stage IV disease complained of moderate pain, but little correspondence was found between the stage and the severity of the pain.

Table 1 Concomitant symptoms in 127 patients with endometriosis

Concomitant symptoms	n	%
Complaints		
menstrual pain	41	32.3
dyspareunia	16	12.6
lower abdominal pain	12	9.4
lumbago	8	6.3
defecation pain	4	3.1
Internal examination		
cul-de-sac tenderness	48	37.8
uterine tenderness	16	12.6
immobilization of the uterus	8	6.3
ovary enlargement	17	13.4

Local concentration of prostaglandins

Prostaglandins might play an important role in endometriotic pain, because prostaglandin

Table 2 The revised American Fertility Society stage of endometriosis and severity of menstrual pain

Stage	n	Menstrual pain		
		Mild	Moderate	Severe
I	17	13	4	0
II	12	9	2	1
III	6	4	2	0
IV	6	2	2	2
Total	41	28	10	3

Table 3 Concentration of prostaglandins (ng/ml, mean ± SD) in the peritoneal fluid, measured by radioimmunoassay

	Endometriosis ($n = 8$)	Non-endometriosis ($n = 7$)	p
PGE_2	0.568 ± 0.397	0.396 ± 0.330	NS
$PGF_{2\alpha}$	0.936 ± 0.495	0.802 ± 0.486	NS
6-keto-$PGF_{1\alpha}$	0.651 ± 0.473	0.511 ± 0.398	NS

NS, not significant

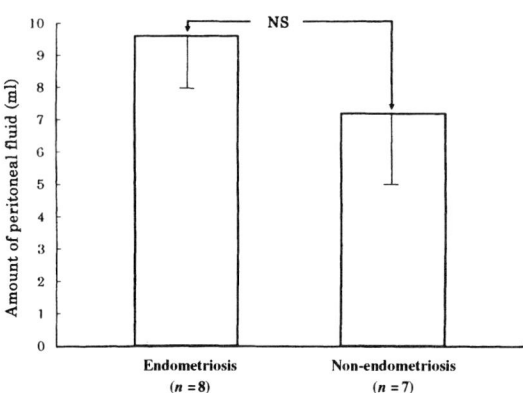

Figure 1 Comparison of the amount of peritoneal fluid in patients with or without endometriosis

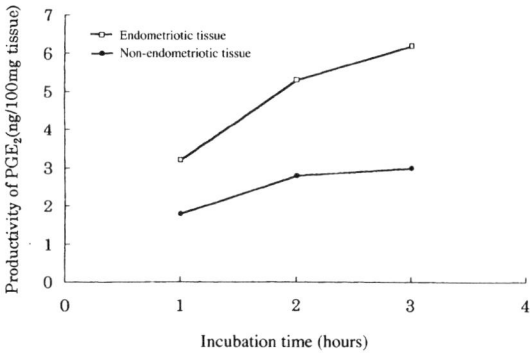

Figure 2 Prostaglandin E_2 (PGE_2) production of the peritoneal endometriotic and non-endometriotic tissue

levels increase in the menstrual fluid and the endometrial tissue of endometriotic patients. As endometriosis occurs outside of the uterus and the symptoms such as cul-de-sac tenderness are also caused by the extrauterine pathological changes, it is necessary to investigate the extrauterine condition, such as the peritoneal fluid.

As shown in Figure 1, when the volume of the peritoneal fluid in the cul-de-sac was measured in patients with or without endometriosis, the volume was slightly increased in endometriotic patients. Then in order to analyze the relationship between the local concentrations of prostaglandins and the endometriosis, the concentrations of prostaglandin E_2 (PGE_2), $PGF_{2\alpha}$ and 6-keto-$PGF_{1\alpha}$ in the peritoneal fluid were measured by radioimmunoassay (Table 3). The concentrations of these prostaglandins were slightly increased in the patients with endometriosis but the difference was not statistically significant.

In Figure 2, productivity of PGE_2 by the peritoneal tissue with or without endometriosis was investigated. After incubation, productivity of PGE_2 by the tissue with endometriosis was almost twice as high as that without endometriosis. These results may show that the total amount of prostaglandins in the peritoneal fluid was elevated by the high productivity of prostaglandins by endometriotic tissue.

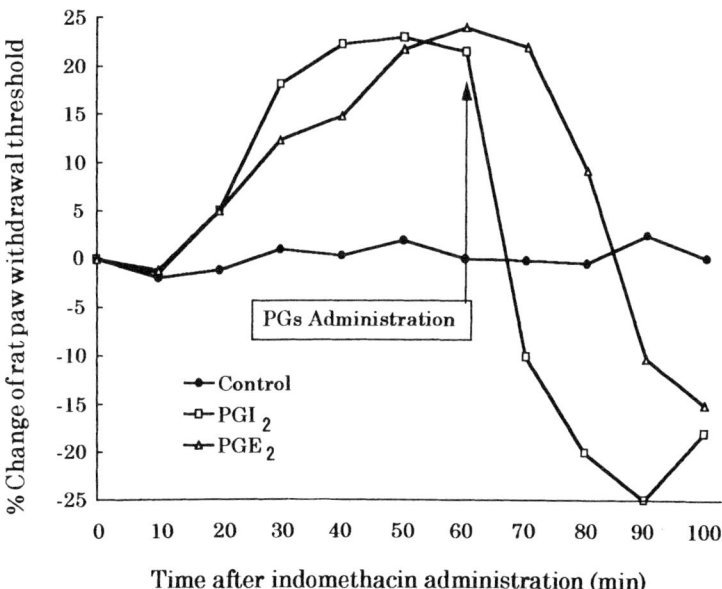

Figure 4 Change of rat paw withdrawal threshold by prostaglandins in the indomethacin-treated rat (200 ng in 50 μl was injected into the rat paw. The rate of nociceptive stimulus was 48 g/s and the data are the mean value of the two experiments)

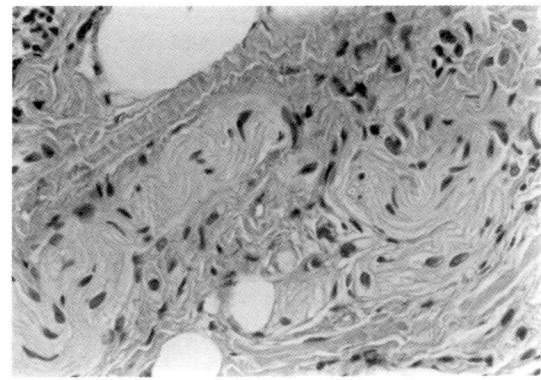

Figure 3 Microscopic finding of nerve fibers in the peritoneal tissue. Nerve fibers were detected as a wave-shaped structure in the specimen of peritoneal tissue taken from the cul-de-sac

Distribution of nerve fibers in peritoneal tissue

The clinical data showed that pain is the most common complaint and that cul-de-sac tenderness is the characteristic sign of endometriosis, thus it is important whether there is any histological difference in the peritoneal tissue taken from the cul-de-sac and other portions. Detection of nerve fibers in the peritoneal tissues (size 5×5 mm) excised from several parts of the abdominal cavity was carried out by hematoxylin-eosin (H-E) staining, and the nerve fibers were detected in 4/5 samples taken from the cul-de-sac (see Figure 3) and in 0/5 from locations other than the cul-de-sac. The densely located nerve fibers in the cul-de-sac and the high concentration of prostaglandins may be two corresponding factors causing endometriotic pain.

Enhancing effect of prostaglandins on nociceptive stimulus

In order to examine the effect of prostaglandins on algesia, the change of the rat paw withdrawal threshold by prostaglandins was investigated using a Randoll-Selitto method.

As shown in Figure 4, the threshold was increased by the intraperitoneal administration of indomethacin and, on the contrary, the threshold was decreased by the local injection of PGE_2 after the latent period of about 20 min. Furthermore, we investigated the effects of several other prostaglandins (PGI_2, $PGF_{2\alpha}$ and PGE_1) on the rat paw withdrawal threshold under the condition of no treatment. Among them, PGI_2 was the most rapidly acting agent on the change of the threshold, and the decrease of the threshold was observed within 5 min after the administration. These animal data clearly show that the nociceptive stimulus will be easily recognized as pain through the decrease of the threshold by prostaglandins.

Discussion

The present clinical and experimental data confirm that prostaglandins play some role in inducing endometriotic pains. In the endometriotic patients, prostaglandin levels increased in the endometrial tissue[3] and menstrual fluid[4]. The macrophages in the peritoneal fluid of endometriotic patients were reported to have a much higher concentration[7], and so produce a significantly higher amount of prostaglandins[8] and cytokines such as interleukin-1. Our data showed that the concentration of prostaglandins in the peritoneal fluid of the endometriotic patients was slightly increased, but *in vitro* production of PGE_2 by the peritoneum of the endometriotic lesions was twice as high as that of non-endometriotic lesions. A line of evidence indicates that there is no relationship between the stages and pain[7], and severity of the pain may rather correspond to the local production of prostaglandins in the endometriotic tissue.

Bradykinin is one of the main substances to induce the pain in tissue injuries (nociceptive stimuli) and to stimulate the permeability of small vessels and PGE_2 enhances the permeability caused by bradykinin tenfold[9]. In our experiment, prostaglandins decreased the rat paw withdrawal threshold. Thus it is reasonable to deduce that prostaglandins play a role in endometriotic pain as a pain enhancer.

In endometriosis, nociceptive stimuli to endometriotic lesions, such as compression, sexual intercourse and menstruation, may cause local release of bradykinin which acts not only as a pain inducer by stimulating the nerve fiber endings but also as a key substance to activate phospholipase A_2, which in turn triggers the cascade of arachidonic acid. The algesic effect of bradykinin is therefore highly amplified by the prostaglandins locally produced. Consequently, it is reasoned that in endometriosis the decrease of the pain threshold by the high local concentration of prostaglandins induces hyperalgesthesia such as tenderness, dysmenorrhea and so on. Free nerve endings as nociceptors are distributed in the peritoneum and our data showed that the nerve fibers which may be terminated to free nerve endings existed very densely in the cul-de-sac, and this may contribute to the tenderness of this portion as the most characteristic sign of this disease.

It is now clear that treatment using prostaglandin synthetase inhibitors (non-steroidal anti-inflammatory drugs, NSAIDs) will produce significant relief from pain such as dysmenorrhea. The mechanism of pain relief by NSAIDs is the inhibition of prostaglandin production and, furthermore, the competitive effects on receptors of prostaglandins. The competitive effects on prostaglandin receptors may be a good explanation of the rapid pain relief by NSAIDs.

References

1. Pickles, V.R., Hall, W.J., Best, F.A. and Smith, G.N. (1965). Prostaglandins in endometrium and menstrual fluid from normal and dysmenorrheic subjects. *J. Obstet. Gynecol. Br. Commonw.*, **72**, 185–92
2. Willaman, E.A., Collins, W.P. and Clayton, S.G. (1976). Studies in the involvement of prostaglandins in uterine symptomatology and pathology. *Br. J. Obstet. Gynaecol.*, **83** (5), 337–41
3. Koike, H., Egawa, H., Ohtsuka, T., Yamagushi, M., Ikenoue, T. and Mori, N. (1992). Correlation between dysmenorrheic severity and prostaglandin production in women with endometriosis. *Prostaglandins Leukot. Essent. Fatty Acids*, **46** (2), 133–7
4. Lumsden, M.A., Kelly, R.W. and Baird, D.T. (1983). Primary dysmenorrhea: the importance of both prostaglandin E_2 and $F_{2\alpha}$. *Br. J. Obstet. Gynaecol.*, **90**, 1135–40
5. Schwartz, A., Zor, U., Lindner, H.R. and Naor, S. (1974). Primary dysmenorrhea. Alleviation by an inhibitor of prostaglandin synthesis and action. *Obstet. Gynecol.*, **44**, 709–12
6. Satoh, K. and Sakamoto, H. (1990). Arachidonic acid cascade products in obstetric and gynecologic diseases. *Nippon Rinsho*, **48**, 1282–8
7. Vernon, M.W., Beard, J:S., Graves, K. and Wilson, E.A. (1986). Classification of endometriotic implants by morphologic appearance and capacity to synthesize prostaglandin F. *Fertil. Steril.*, **46**, 801–6
8. Karck, U., Reister, F., Schäfer, W., Zahradnik, H.P. and Breckwoldt, M. (1996). PGE_2 and $PGF_{2\alpha}$ release by human peritoneal macrophages in endometriosis. *Prostaglandins*, **51**, 49–60
9. Ikeda, K., Tanaka, K. and Katori, M. (1975). Potentiation of bradykinin-induced vascular permeability increase by prostaglandin E_2 and arachidonic acid in rabbit skin. *Prostaglandins*, **18** (4), 655–61

Uterine contractility in patients with endometriosis

C. Bulletti, S. Rossi, A. Albonetti, V. Negrini, V. Polli, E. Giacomucci, D. De Ziegler and C. Flamigni

Introduction

Endometriosis is a very common debilitating disease occurring in 1–50% of premenopausal women[1], and which prevails in infertile women (38.5%)[2]. A variety of symptoms have been attributed to endometriosis; the most common symptoms are pelvic pain, dysmenorrhea and dyspareunia[3]. However, it seems that there is not any correlation between seriousness of symptoms and severity of disease[4]. Many theories have been proposed about the pathogenesis of endometriosis, but none is effective.

The principal mechanism of histogenesis of the disease was postulated by Sampson in 1927. It concerns the retrograde efflux of blood and endometrial debris during menstruation, through the Fallopian tubes, and their implantation upon peritoneal surfaces or abdominopelvic organs[5]. Among the other important theories are: the lymphatic and vascular dissemination of endometrial cells, which can explain unusual sites of endometriosis; the direct extension which results in adenomyosis; and activation of embryonic cell rests. In addition, all these theories can be combined[6].

Recently, the evaluation of electromechanical activities of the uterus *in vitro*[7] and *in vivo* has opened the field of uterine contractility and possible related pathologies, such as endometriosis deriving from abnormal patterns of contractility. Uterine contractility may in fact influence gamete transportation, failure of embryo implantation, spontaneous abortion, retrograde efflux of eutopic endometrium to ectopic implants and ectopic pregnancies.

The present study attempts to establish a correlation between abnormal uterine contractility and endometriosis, including this factor among the possible causes of the disease. The hypercontractility of the uterus is the main cause of dysmenorrhea[8]. There is an increase in cytokines, with an activation of prostaglandins followed by a secondary increase of spontaneous contractility[9]. In recent years the electromechanical activity of myometrium has been investigated *in vitro* in muscle strip, cell cultures and animal organs, but there is not a true correspondence with human responses. Recently a new experimental system was designed to study human uterine activities based on extracorporeal perfusion of isolated human uteri, which reproduces the physiological conditions of the organ[10,11]. The mechanical activation of uterus results in electromechanical coupling, which means that electrical activity is associated with uterine contractions. There is isolated electrical activity, or spikes and a rhythmic activity; only the rhythmic activity is correlated with mechanical events[7]. There is also a pharmacological activation which explains the action of many drugs[12].

The present study was undertaken to estimate the mechanical activity of human uterus *in vivo* by recording the intraluminal pressures in women with endometriosis compared with controls.

Material and methods

Patients

Twenty-two women were recruited for this study and divided in two groups. Group 1 consisted of 12 women (mean age ± SD, 36.40 ± 9.26 years) with a laparoscopic diagnosis of endometriosis. The diagnosis of endometriosis was made by histological evaluation of specimens collected during laparoscopy. Clinical symptoms (pelvic pain, dysmenorrhea and dyspareunia), sonography and biochemical data (cancer antigen-125, CA-125) were also used to properly identify the patients. Group 2 consisted of 10 normal menstruating women (age 34.88 ± 7.21 years) who had never had symptoms suggesting endometriosis, and these were used as controls.

Instrumentation and procedure for mechanical signal acquisition

The intraluminal pressure of the uterus was examined using two ureteral probes, graduated in centimeters, with a 1.2-mm side opening (Neoplex AC 5907 ureteral catheters, Sarlat, France), continuously perfused with 0.45 ml/min distilled water by a constant-perfusion syringe pump (LEM P8). They were introduced at different levels of the lumen cavity, near the fundus (2 cm) and near to the internal os of the cervix. The probes were connected to a transducer (Bakster R611), properly calibrated to convert mechanical signals to electrical signals, which were transferred to an amplifier and an analog–digital converter and stored in a personal computer. The computer was provided with software specifically designed to graphically visualize the mechanical events in real time during the recording period (Reddy-gipc) (Figure 1). The length of each examination was about 20 min. In the first 3 min the intraluminal pressure of the lumen cavity was progressively evaluated from the fundus to the cervix, moving down with one pressure transducer by 1 cm every 30 s. The recording of contractility was then carried out for 15 min by two probes positioned as previously reported. Recording was then carried out for a further 3 min by moving down progressively with the two probes, by 1 cm every 30 s, until the probes were out of the organ.

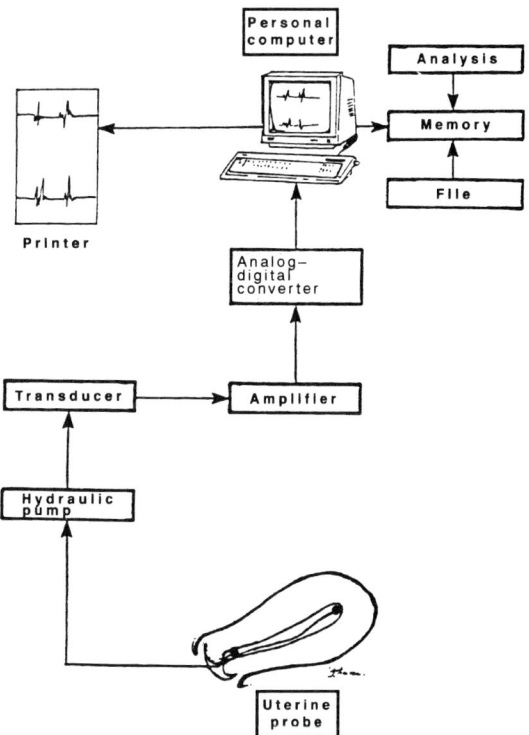

Figure 1 Instrumentation and procedure for mechanical signal acquisition

Analysis

Analysis of data was performed by considering the frequency and amplitude of each oscillation, as well as the basal pressure tone of the organ, during 10 min of the entire 20 min record. Statistical analysis was performed by using the unpaired Student's t-test and the MacNemar test.

Results

Uterine fundus

The number of oscillations in a 10-min period (mean ± SD) in patients with endometriosis was 21.86 ± 9.75, compared with 10.20 ± 5.26 in the controls ($p < 0.05$). The amplitude of the oscillations was 20.04 ± 27.56 mmHg in

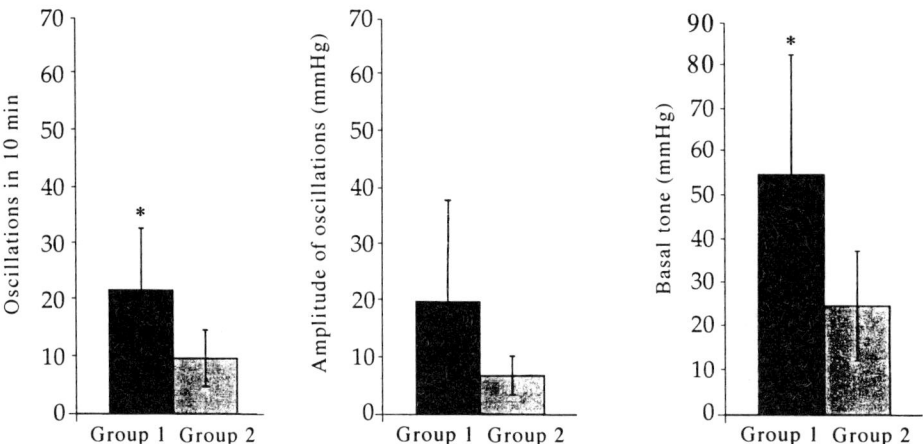

Figure 2 Results of mechanical evaluation of uterine pressure on the fundus. Values are given as means ± SD. Group 1 consists of patients with endometriosis, Group 2 is the control. *$p < 0.05$ compared with the control group

patients with endometriosis, compared with 6.95 ± 5.86 mmHg in the controls (not significant). The basal pressure uterine tone of patients with endometriosis was 55.54 ± 21.04 mmHg compared with 25.28 ± 19.94 mmHg relieved in the controls ($p < 0.05$) (Figure 2).

Uterine cervix

The number of oscillations in a 10-min period in patients with endometriosis was 25.17 ± 14.03 compared with 15.00 ± 11.47 in the controls (not significant), while the amplitude of the oscillations was 10.94 ± 8.39 mmHg in patients with endometriosis, compared with 7.06 ± 5.94 mmHg in the controls (not significant). The basal pressure uterine tone of patients with endometriosis was 55.53 ± 19.90 mmHg compared with 45.86 ± 21.91 mmHg relieved in the controls (not significant) (Figure 3).

Discussion

The present study introduces the role of myometrial contractility in the development of endometriosis. The data show that patients with endometriosis have both a higher frequency of oscillations of the uterine fundus, and higher basal tone, compared with controls. The abnormal contractility pattern demonstrated in patients with endometriosis may be a cause of the disease, inducing expulsion of endometrial debris at the time of menstruation. The hypercontractility is also important in explaining some of the symptoms of endometriosis, such as dysmenorrhea and pelvic pain. This observation may be completed by the acquisition of patterns of different propagation of endometrial contractions, which may further support the hypothesis that contractility is the crucial event in the etiology of endometriosis as well as in its recurrence after therapy. Recently, a relation between subendometrial uterine activity, ultrasonographically observed, and the phase of the menstrual cycle, has been reported[13]. The propagation of contractile waves is anterograde (from fundus to cervix) during menstruation in normal women. In patients with endometriosis there is also a predominant retrograde pattern (from cervix to fundus) during menstruation[14].

The cause of this inversion of the contractile waves in the patients with endometriosis may

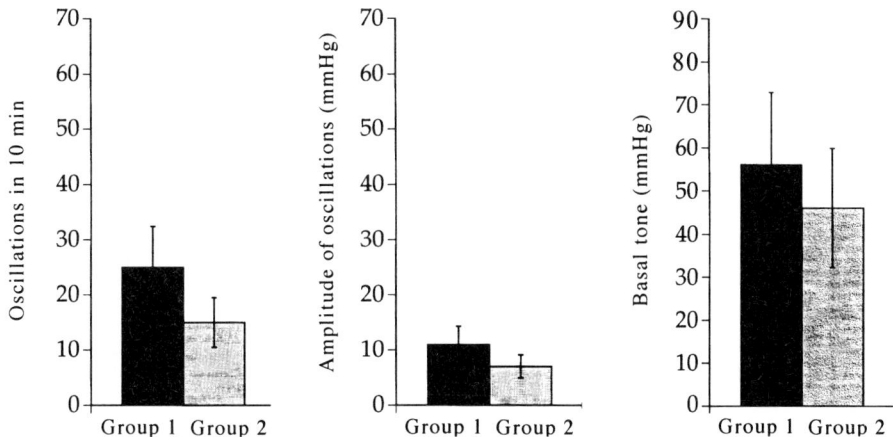

Figure 3 Results of mechanical evaluation of uterine pressure on the cervix. Values are given as means ± SD. Group 1 consists of patients with endometriosis, Group 2 is the control. None of the differences were significant

be related to an alteration of the endometrial prostaglandin activity[15]. In fact, the release of prostaglandins increases the uterine contractility in women with dysmenorrhea, producing an increase of intrauterine pressure and of myometrial tone. This could be a factor favoring the retrograde spillage of menstrual blood, which is one of the causes of endometriosis.

We should also remark that there is an increased incidence of spontaneous abortion in patients with endometriosis[16], and we have already demonstrated an abnormal uterine contractility in patients with spontaneous abortions.

Recent studies are introducing new agents to control contractions, which may serve to prevent the pathologies related to an abnormal uterine contractile pattern, such as abortion, through their uterorelaxant properties[17]. We can also apply this information to endometriosis, for the prevention of new foci of ectopic endometrial implants, and the reduction of symptoms. The medical therapy now utilized is based on the use of progestogens, antisteroids (such as danazol and gestrinone) and gonadotropin-releasing hormone agonists[18]. Progesterone is a potent uterorelaxant hormone; the inhibition of uterine contractility is regulated by progesterone receptors which are present in the uterus[19].

It is possible that the myometrial quiescence induced by progesterone does not affect the uteri of patients with endometriosis because of an intrinsic 'lowered steroid response' characteristic of these myometria. A direct vagina-to-uterus administration of progesterone would aim at increasing the tissue concentrations of progesterone, reducing the systemic adversal effect.

Further *in vivo* and *in vitro* studies will be able to include the evaluation of this hypothesis, by vaginal administration of progesterone and investigation of its effect on contractility.

Acknowledgement

This work was supported by the Italian National Council of Research grant 940840.

References

1. Weeler, J.M. (1989). Epidemiology of endometriosis-associated infertility. *J. Reprod. Med.*, **34**, 41–6
2. Verkauf, B.S. (1987). The incidence, symptoms, and signs of endometriosis in fertile and infertile women. *J. Fla. Med. Assoc.*, **74**, 671–5
3. Rock, J.A. and Markham, S.M. (1992). Pathogenesis of endometriosis. *Lancet*, **340**, 1264–7
4. Schenken, R.S. (1989). *Endometriosis. Contemporary Concepts in Clinical Management*, pp. 83–93. (Philadelphia: J.B. Lippincott Company)
5. Sampson, J.A. (1927). Peritoneal endometriosis, due to menstrual dissemination of endometrial tissue into venous circulation. *Am. J. Pathol.*, **3**, 93
6. Schenken, R.S. (1989). *Endometriosis. Contemporary Concepts in Clinical Management*, pp. 3–20. (Philadelphia: J.B. Lippincott Company)
7. Bulletti, C., Prefetto, R.A., Bazzocchi, G., Romero, R., Mimmi, P., Polli, V., Lanfranchi, G.A., Morselli Labate, A.M. and Flamigni, C. (1993). Electromechanical activities of human uteri during extra-corporeal perfusion with ovarian steroids. *Hum. Reprod.*, **8** (10), 1558–63
8. Anderson, K.E. and Ulmstem, U. (1978). Effect of nifedipine on myometrial activity and lower abdominal pain in women with primary dysmenorrhoea. *Br. J. Obstet. Gynecol.*, **85**, 142–9
9. Tabibzadeh, S.S., Kaffka, K.L., Satyaswaroop, P.G. and Kilan, P.L. (1990). IL-1 regulation of human endometrial function: presence of IL-1 receptor correlates with IL-1 stimulated PGE2 production. *J. Endocrinol. Metab.*, **70**, 1000–12
10. Bulletti, C., Iasonni, V.M., Lubicz, S., Flamigni, C. and Gurpide, E. (1986). Extracorporeal perfusion of the human uterus. *Am. J. Obstet. Gynecol.*, **154**, 683–8
11. Bulletti, C., Iasonni, V.M., Martinelli, G., Govoni, E., Tabanelli, S., Ciotti, P.M. and Flamigni, C. (1987). A 48-hour preservation of an isolated human uterus: endometrial responses to sex steroids. *Fertil. Steril.*, **47**, 122–9
12. Anderson, K.E. (1982). Pharmacological inhibition of uterine activity. *Acta Obstet. Gynecol. Scand.*, Suppl 108, 17–23
13. De Vries, K., Lyons, E.A., Ballard, G., Levi, C.S. and Lindsay, D.J. (1990). Contractions of the inner third of the myometrium. *Am. J. Obstet. Gynecol.*, **162**, 679–82
14. Salamanca, A. and Beltran, E. (1995). Subendometrial contractility in menstrual phase visualized by transvaginal sonography in patients with endometriosis. *Fertil. Steril.*, **64**, 193–5
15. Schulman, H., Duvivier, R. and Blattner, P. (1983). The uterine contractility index: a research and diagnostic tool in dysmenorrhea. *Am. J. Obstet. Gynecol.*, **145**, 1049–58.
16. Fitz Simmonds, J., Stahl, R., Gocial, B. and Shapiro, S. S. (1987). Spontaneous abortion and endometriosis. *Fertil. Steril.*, **47**, 696–8
17. Yusoff, D. (1995). Pharmacological stimulation of uterine contractions. *Semin. Perinatol.*, **19**, 73–83
18. Brosens, I.A. (1994). New principles in the management of endometriosis. *Acta Obstet. Gynecol. Scand.*, **159**, 18–21
19. Mahesh, V.B., Brann, D.W. and Hendry, L.B. (1996). Diverse modes of action of progesterone and its metabolites. *J. Steroid Biochem. Mol. Biol.*, **56**, 209–19

Growth factors in proliferative regulation of endometrium

M. Taga, T. Takahashi and H. Minaguchi

Introduction

The uterus is comprised of heterogeneous cell populations that respond uniquely to estrogen and progesterone; the proliferation of luminal and glandular epithelia occurs in response to estrogen stimulation, whereas stromal cell proliferation is dependent upon progesterone and estrogen[1]. Sex steroid hormones cause transformation of stromal cells into decidual cells and their further proliferation. Thus the endometrial tissue undergoes dynamic changes anatomically and functionally during the menstrual cycle as well as during pregnancy under the influence of sex steroid hormones. It has been thought that the actions of sex steroid hormones in the endometrium are partly mediated through several kinds of growth factors which are locally produced in the site where they have biological effect. Autocrine/paracrine regulation of endometrial growth by growth factor as a mediator is proposed[2–4]. Extensive evidence exists that stromally derived mediators can promote epithelial proliferation and differentiation in steroid hormone responsive tissues. However, there is no definitive evidence for the involvement of growth factor in the decidual transformation. In this article, we report a role of growth factor in cell proliferative regulation of endometrium with special reference to decidualization.

Materials and methods

Endometrial tissues in the proliferative phase and secretory phase were collected from endocrinologically normal patients with leiomyoma who underwent hysterectomy. Pseudopregnant endometria were also obtained from hypermenorrheic patients with leiomyoma who underwent hysterectomy after treatment with mestranol and norethisterone for several weeks to stop genital bleeding before the operation. Decidua of 5–7 weeks' gestation were obtained in artificial abortions. Primary culture of human endometrial stromal cells with or without medroxyprogesterone acetate was employed. We also used non-pregnant mouse uterus for the experiment of epithelial cell growth regulation by estrogen and growth factor.

The gene expressions of epidermal growth factor (EGF), transforming growth factor-α (TGF-α), platelet-derived growth factor (PDGF) and keratinocyte growth factor (KGF) in these tissues or cells were analyzed by reverse transcriptase-polymerase chain reaction (RT-PCR), Northern blot hybridization and *in situ* hybridization. Receptor binding for each growth factor was also investigated by Scatchard analysis. The effect of growth factors on DNA synthesis was studied by [^{3}H]thymidine incorporation into primary cultured cells.

Results and discussion

Cell proliferative regulation by growth factor in epithelium

Before discussing a cell proliferative regulation by growth factor in decidual transformation, we report briefly our experimental results on cell proliferative regulation in epithelium by

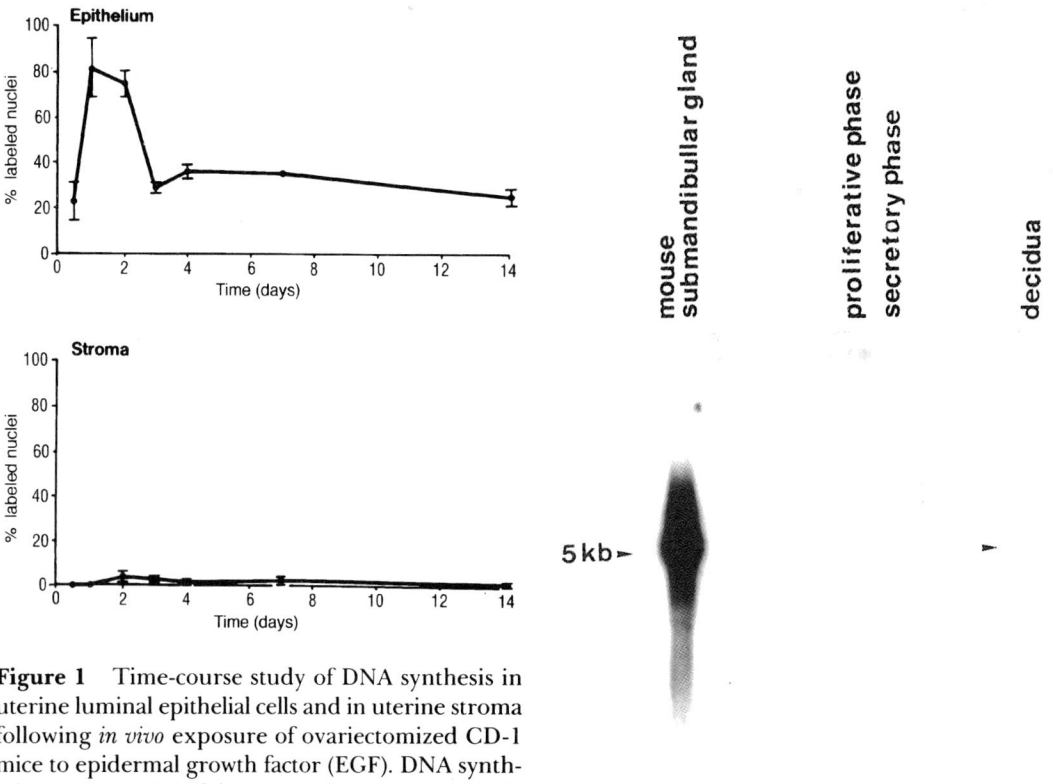

Figure 1 Time-course study of DNA synthesis in uterine luminal epithelial cells and in uterine stroma following *in vivo* exposure of ovariectomized CD-1 mice to epidermal growth factor (EGF). DNA synthesis was quantitated by autoradiographic analysis of [^{3}H]thymidine-labeled nuclei following kidney-capsule implantation of EGF-containing pellets

Figure 2 Northern blot hybridization of poly(A)+ RNA from proliferative and secretory phase human endometria, human decidua of 8 weeks' gestation and mouse submandibular gland. The arrows indicate the migration of the 5-kb human prepro-epidermal growth factor (EGF) mRNA and 4.8-kb mouse submandibular gland EGF mRNA

growth factor in mouse uterus. In an autoradiographic experiment in ovariectomized mouse uterus, EGF significantly increased DNA synthesis in mouse uterine luminal epithelial cells. Figure 1 shows the comparison of the capacity of DNA synthesis by EGF between epithelium and stroma. The DNA synthesis in epithelium was 20-fold greater than that in stroma.

When we look at the effect of antibody to growth factor on DNA synthesis in uterine epithelial cells in estrogen-treated mouse, both anti-EGF antibody and anti-TGF-α antibody sig-nificantly inhibited estrogen-induced epithel-ial proliferation in ovariectomized mouse uterus.

These results indicate that EGF and TGF-α play a major role in the cell proliferative regulation in uterine epithelium as a mediator of estrogen action.

Cell proliferative regulation by growth factor in stromal decidualization in human

Gene expressions of growth factor in human endometrium/decidua Figure 2 shows Northern blot hybridization of poly(A)+ RNA from proliferative and secretory phase human endometria, human decidua of 6–8 weeks' gestation and mouse submandibular gland. The arrows indicate the migration of the 5-kilobase (kb) human prepro-EGF mRNA and 4.8-kb mouse sub-mandibular gland EGF mRNA, which is illustrated in the left lane. No transcript was detected in proliferative and secretory phase endometria, whereas a transcript of 5 kb was detected in decidua from 6–8 weeks' gestation, which was in agreement with the size of human prepro-EGF mRNA previously reported.

Northern blot hybridization of poly(A)+ RNA from the cultured endometrial stromal cells with or without 1 µmol/l medroxyprogesterone acetate for 28 days *in vitro* revealed that a transcript of 5 kb was detected in *in vitro* medroxyprogesterone acetate-induced decidual cells, while no transcript was found in endometrial stromal cells cultured without medroxyprogesterone acetate (Figure 3).

To specify the localization of the EGF-producing cells in human decidua, *in situ* hybridization was performed using digoxygenin-labeled EGF cRNA in the section of human decidua from 8 weeks' gestation (Figure 4). Immunostaining was intense in the stromal cells of decidual tissue, confirming the synthesis of EGF in these cells. Figure 4 also shows that decidual cells with EGF mRNA were not distributed homogeneously, but were scattered heterogeneously.

The results of Northern blotting and *in situ* hybridization suggest that endometrial stromal cells are the major source of the EGF mRNA, which increases during the process of decidualization. The expression of EGF protein was observed in the stromal cells cultured with medroxyprogesterone acetate, whereas it was not detected in the cells cultured without medroxyprogesterone acetate.

As mentioned earlier, TGF-α showed a biological action similar to EGF in epithelial cell proliferation. In order to investigate whether TGF-α also has the same profile as EGF in the decidualization process, we analyzed TGF-α mRNA in human endometrium and decidua by Northern blotting. Similar to EGF, no transcript was detected in proliferative and secretory endometria, whereas a transcript of 4.8 kb, which was in agreement with the size of human prepro-TGF-α mRNA previously reported, was clearly detected in decidua from

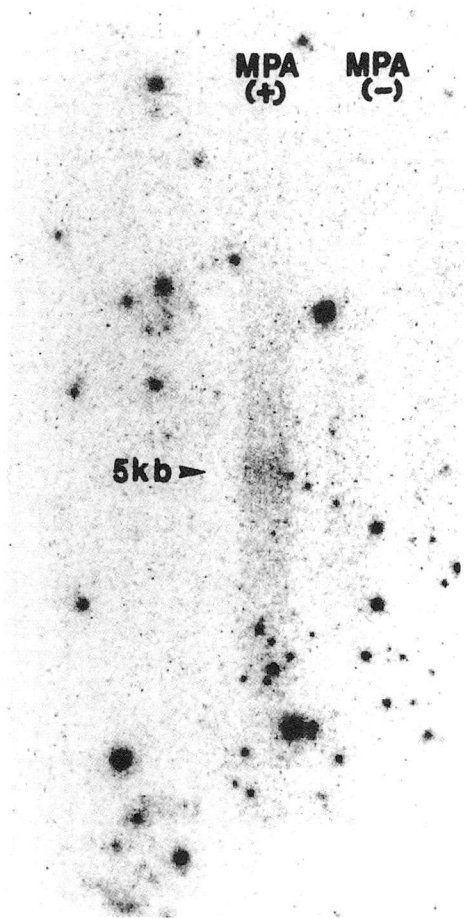

Figure 3 Northern blot hybridization of poly(A)+ RNA from the stromal cells cultured *in vitro* with or without 1 µmol/l medroxyprogesterone acetate (MPA) for 28 days. The 5-kb human prepro-epidermal growth factor (EGF) mRNA was observed in the MPA(+) lane

6–8 weeks' gestation. As with EGF, a transcript of 4.8-kb TGF-α mRNA was detected in *in vitro* medroxyprogesterone acetate-induced decidual cells, while no transcript was found in endometrial cells cultured without medroxyprogesterone acetate.

The levels of prolactin in the supernatants of culture medium during the culture of endometrial stromal cells with 1 µmol/l medroxyprogesterone acetate increased in proportion

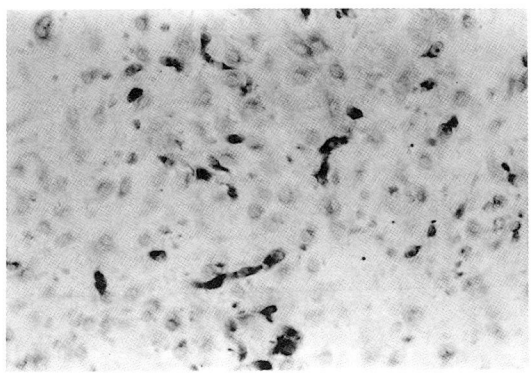

Figure 4 *In situ* hybridization of prepro-epidermal growth factor (EGF) mRNA. The section of human decidua from 8 weeks' gestation was hybridized with digoxygenin-labeled EGF cRNA. Stromal cells with intense hybridization were observed

to the duration of culture, confirming that medroxyprogesterone acetate induced decidualization. These results indicate that, like EGF, the gene expression of TGF-α increases in accordance with the degree of stromal decidualization.

Keratinocyte growth factor, also called FGF-7, was originally purified from human embryonic fibroblasts and detected in some stroma cell lines. While other growth factors such as EGF and TGF-α induce cell proliferation and cytodifferentiation not only in epithelial cells but also in fibroblasts, KGF secreted from mesenchymal fibroblasts plays a very unique role acting on only epithelial cells in a paracrine fashion. The assessment of the involvement of KGF in the regulation of endometrial function is therefore important for a better understanding of endometrial physiology, with epithelial–mesenchymal interaction being crucial to uterine function. Although the presence of KGF mRNA was reported in stromal cells of the monkey endometrium[5], there are few reports on the gene expression of KGF and its change during the menstrual cycle or during pregnancy in the human endometrium. Using RT-PCR and Northern blot hybridization, we therefore investigated the KGF mRNA in the human endometrium and its quantitative change in different sex steroid hormone environments such as proliferative phase, secretory phase, pseudopregnancy and early pregnancy.

After 1 μg of total RNA from endometria in secretory phase, proliferative phase, decidua of 7 weeks' gestation, decidua of 9 weeks' gestation and pseudopregnancy were reverse transcribed and amplified for 40 cycles by PCR using specific human KGF primers, we detected the 196-bp expected DNA band in all samples examined, demonstrating that KGF mRNA exists in these tissues.

In order to further clarify the quantitative change in KGF mRNA during decidualization, we performed Northern blot analysis with ^{32}P-labeled KGF cDNA in human endometria and decidua. The mRNA of 2.4 kb and about 5 kb were detected in each sample. The mRNA of 2.4 kb in secretory phase endometrium was 10-fold greater than that in proliferative phase endometrium. Similarly, decidua and pseudopregnant endometrium had 5–10-fold and 3–4-fold greater KGF mRNA, respectively, compared with proliferative phase endometrium. The densities of the 5-kb mRNA were almost the same among these samples. The signal in these blots with a cDNA probe for β–actin after washing out the KGF probe confirmed equivalent quantity of RNA among all lanes.

Platelet-derived growth factor (PDGF) is a dimeric protein in which the subunit peptide chains are bonded by a disulfide bridge. Although the cell proliferative effect of PDGF on the endometrial stromal cells has been reported[6], there is no report on the biological significance of PDGF in the regulation of human decidual cell function.

As for the gene expression of the PDGF subunit in human decidual cells, after RT-PCR of 40 cycles amplification, we detected the 413-bp expected DNA band of the PDGF-A subunit and the 334-bp expected DNA band of the PDGF-B subunit. These findings demonstrate that both PDGF-A and PDGF-B subunit mRNA exist in the human decidua from early pregnancy.

Table 1 Change in EGF receptor in human endometrium/decidua

	K_d (mol/l)	B_{max} (fmol/mg protein)
Proliferative phase	0.88×10^{-9}	35
Secretory phase	0.81×10^{-9}	22
Psuedopregnancy	0.85×10^{-9}	62
Early pregnancy	0.95×10^{-9}	108

Table 2 Change in EGF receptor in endometrium during *in vitro* decidualization

Duration of culture (days)		K_d (mol/l)	B_{max} (sites/cell)
0		0.70×10^{-9}	2.2×10^{-4}
14	MPA (+)	0.86×10^{-9}	11×10^{-4}
14	MPA (−)	1.0×10^{-9}	3.8×10^{-4}
28	MPA (+)	0.88×10^{-9}	34×10^{-4}
28	MPA (−)	0.70×10^{-9}	4.0×10^{-4}

MPA, medroxyprogesterone acetate

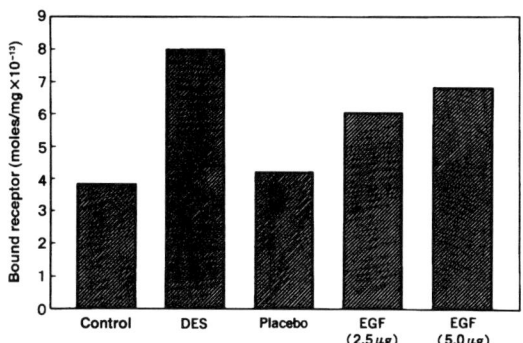

Figure 5 Epidermal growth factor (EGF), diethylstilbestrol (DES) or placebo were administered *in vivo* to ovariectomized mouse uterus. The level of bound receptor of progesterone in the uterus was determined and is shown here compared with control

Growth factor receptor in human endometrium/decidua Scatchard plots for specific EGF binding in homogenates of mid-proliferative and mid-secretory phase endometria, pseudopregnant endometrium and decidua from early pregnancy revealed that the plots in these four tissues were linear with a single component. As shown in Table 1, the maximum number (B_{max}) of EGF binding sites for homogenates of pseudopregnant or pregnant decidua was much higher than that of non-pregnant endometrium, indicating that the amount of EGF/TGF-α receptor increases during decidualization. The dissociation constant values (K_d) of the EGF/TGF-α receptor were almost similar among these tissues.

Scatchard plot analysis was also performed for the specific binding of EGF on the endometrial stromal cells cultured with or without medroxyprogesterone acetate. The definite difference in B_{max} of the EGF receptor was not found in the cultured cells when they were cultured without medroxyprogesterone acetate, regardless of the duration of culture. However, culture with medroxyprogesterone acetate significantly increased B_{max} in accordance with the duration of culture and hence decidualization (Table 2). As with decidual tissues, the K_d values remained unchanged in cultured cells, with a linear profile with a single component.

By Scatchard plot analysis of the binding of [^{125}I]PDGF dimer to each PDGF-AA and PDGF-BB ligand, we demonstrated that decidual cells had a specific PDGF receptor with a single component. Comparison of the K_d values for PDGF receptor showed that PDGF-AA dimer ligand had an 8-fold higher affinity than PDGF-BB.

The induction of progesterone receptor by estrogen is important for implantation and the maintenance of pregnancy. While it has been reported that EGF has a stimulatory effect on progesterone receptor in the endometrium *in vitro*, the data is not available for the EGF *in vivo* action on uterine progesterone receptor. *In vivo* administration of EGF increased progesterone receptor in mouse uterus, which was equivalent to the estrogen or diethylstilbestrol action (Figure 5).

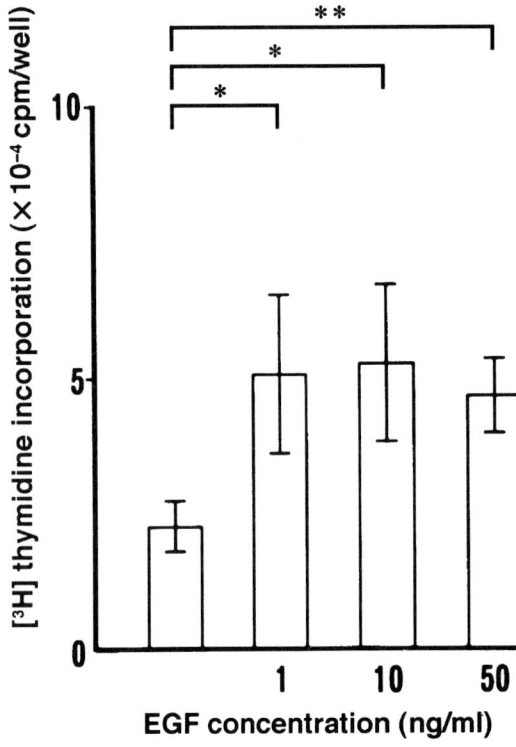

Figure 6 Mean (± SEM) changes in [³H]thymidine incorporation in the culture of non-pregnant decidualized endometrium with epidermal growth factor (EGF) at the concentrations indicated. $*p < 0.025$; $**p < 0.005$

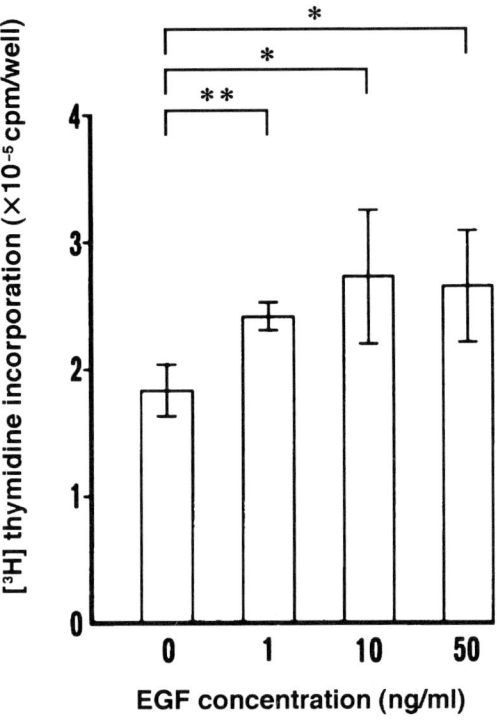

Figure 7 Mean (± SEM) changes in [³H]thymidine incorporation in the culture of early pregnant human decidua with epidermal growth factor (EGF) at the concentrations indicated. $*p < 0.025$; $**p < 0.005$

Cell proliferative effect of growth factor in human endometrium/decidua In [³H]thymidine incorporation in the culture of non-pregnant decidualized cells, EGF had a significantly stimulatory effect on DNA synthesis in non-pregnant decidualized endometrium (Figure 6) as well as in pregnant decidual cells (Figure 7). Similarly, TGF-α showed a stimulatory effect on decidual cell proliferation in early pregnancy (Figure 8).

Each PDGF dimer, PDGF-AA, PDGF-AB and PDGF-BB, stimulated [³H]thymidine incorporation in a dose-dependent manner when they were added individually to the quiescent decidual cells cultured in serum-free medium. Comparing the magnitude of [³H]thymidine incorporation among three

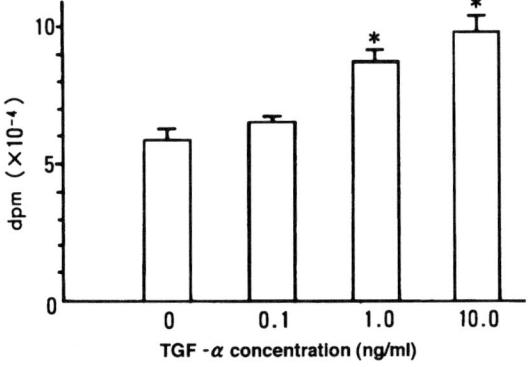

Figure 8 Mean (± SEM) dpm of [³H]thymidine incorporation in the culture of early pregnant human decidual cells with transforming growth factor (TGF)-α at the concentrations indicated (three wells for each TGF-α concentration in the representative experiment from four different decidual tissues). $*p < 0.01$ compared with control

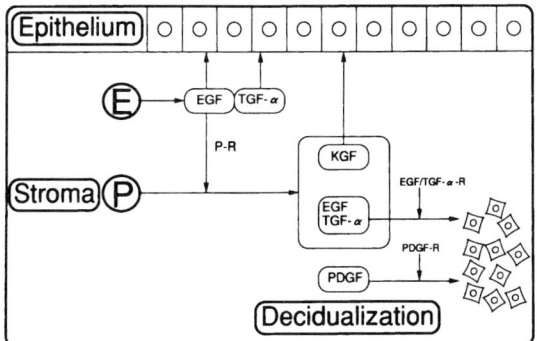

Figure 9 Schematic illustration of roles of growth factors in cell proliferative regulation in the uterus. E, estrogen; P, progesterone; EGF, epidermal growth factor; TGF-α, transforming growth factor-α; KGF, keratinocyte growth factor; PDGF, platelet-derived growth factor; -R, receptor

PDGF dimers at several concentrations, PDGF-AB and PDGF-BB had a significantly greater [^{3}H]thymidine incorporation than PDGF-AA at the concentrations of 1 ng/ml and 10 ng/ml.

In conclusion, taken together with our findings in this experiment that gene expression, receptor binding, and DNA synthesis increase during the decidualization process, EGF and TGF-α could be involved in mediating progesterone-induced uterine decidual cell growth similar to estrogen-mediated uterine luminal and glandular epithelium proliferation. PDGF and KGF, which are mesenchymal growth factors, also play a role in decidual or epithelial cell proliferation. Decidual cell formation and proliferation may thus be self-amplified by progesterone, partly via the action of growth factors in an autocrine/paracrine fashion. This is a prerequisite for decidualization, because decidual formation requires rapid cell proliferation. This is schematically illustrated in Figure 9.

Acknowledgements

The authors would like to thank Dr Sakakibara, Dr Kida, Dr Saji, Dr Matsui, Mrs Kurogi and Mrs Suyama in the Department of Obstetrics and Gynecology at the Yokohama City University School of Medicine, and Dr Nelson and Dr McLachlan in National Institutes of Health, USA for their collaboration in this study.

References

1. Huet-Hudson, Y.M., Andrews, G.K. and Dey, S.K. (1989). Cell type-specific localization of c-myc protein in the mouse uterus: modulation by steroid hormones and analysis of the peri-implantation period. *Endocrinology*, **125**, 683–90
2. Huet-Hudson, Y.M. Chkraborty, C., De, S.K., Suzuki, Y., Andrews, G.K. and Dey, S.K. (1990). Estrogen regulates synthesis of EGF in mouse uterine epithelial cells. *Mol. Endocrinol.*, **4**, 510–23
3. Murphy, L.J., Murphy, L.C. and Friesen, H.G. (1987). Estrogen induces insulin-like growth factor I expression in the rat uterus. *Mol. Endocrinol.*, **1**, 445–50
4. Diaugustine, R.P., Petrusez, P., Bell, G.I., Brown, C.F., Korach, K.S., McLachlan, J.A. and Teng, C.T. (1988). Influence of estrogens on mouse uterine epidermal growth factor precursor protein and messenger ribonucleic acid. *Endocrinology*, **122**, 2355–63
5. Koji, T., Chedid, M., Rubin, J.S., Slayden, O.D., Csaky, K.G., Aaronson, S.A. and Brenner, R.M. (1994). Progesterone-dependent expression of keratinocyte growth factor mRNA in stromal cells of the primate endometrium: keratinocyte growth factor as a progestomedin. *J. Cell. Biol.*, **125**, 393–401
6. Surrey, E.S. and Halme, J. (1991). Effect of platelet-derived growth factor on endometrial stromal cell proliferation *in vitro*: a model for endometriosis? *Fertil. Steril.*, **56**, 672–9

Apoptosis in normal endometrium and adenomyosis

Y. Otsuki, K. Ueki, M. Ueki, H. Yamashita, K. Matsumoto, E. Daikoku, Y. Fukuda, R. Hayashi, K. Nakamura, K. Nakao, O. Marukawa and Y. Ito

Introduction

Menses is generally regarded as ischemic necrosis of the functional layer caused by contraction of spiral arteries, depending on ovarian hormone levels[1]. A recent electron microscopic study[2], however, demonstrated the appearance of apoptotic bodies in the late secretory phase. We have also reported the relationship between the appearance of apoptotic endometrial glandular cells and the expression of bcl-2 protein blocking apoptosis[3]. Therefore, uterine endometrium is an attractive tissue for studying cell death especially apoptosis. Recently, various hormone drugs have become available for endometriosis externa, and the differences in response to these drugs has not yet been made clear.

This study was designed to clarify the mode of cell death in normal endometrium throughout the cycle, and in adenomyosis treated with or without hormone therapy, using immunohistochemistry and electron microscopy.

Patients and methods

Tissue samples

Normal endometrium and myometrium were collected from 34 women undergoing hysterectomy who had normal menstrual cycles and who had received no hormone therapy for at least three cycles before surgery. The samples were obtained from the fundus within the uterine cavity. Uterine samples for the study of adenomyosis were obtained from 24 women undergoing hysterectomy, some of whom received no hormone therapy (10 cases as control), and some of whom were administered danazol (Tokyo Tanabe Co. Ltd, Japan; six cases) or gonadotropin-releasing hormone (GnRH) agonist (buserelin acetate, Hoechst Pharmaceuticals & Chemicals, Tokyo, Japan; and leuprorelin acetate, Takeda Chemical Industries Ltd; eight cases).

Immunohistochemistry and electron microscopy

Parts of the fresh tissue samples were rapidly frozen in acetone with dry ice and embedded in Tissue Mount (Chiba Medical Inc., Japan). The frozen blocks were cut serially into 6-μm thick sections with a cryotome at −30 °C. Serial cryosections placed on poly-L-lysin-treated glass slides were lightly fixed in 4% paraformaldehyde, transferred to 0.1 mol/l phosphate buffer (pH 7.4), and then immunostained with an indirect immunoperoxidase technique. The antibodies used in this study were MoAb 100 against human bcl-2 protein, anti FasD antibody against Fas antigen, and both anti-Fas-L antibody against Fas ligand and anti-ICE p10 antibody against the active form of interleukin-1-β-converting enzyme (ICE) (Santa Cruz Biotechnology Inc., CA, USA), both antiestrogen receptor and progesterone receptor antibodies (Abbott Lab., Chicago, USA). Following incubation with the primary monoclonal antibody for 1 h at room temperature (24 °C), the sections were washed and incubated with goat anti-mouse secondary antibody conjugated to horseradish peroxidase (Dako, Denmark) for 3 h at room temperature. Peroxidase activity was revealed by exposing the sections to 3′,3′-diaminobenzidine tetrahydroxychloride (DAB; Sigma, MO, St. Louis, USA) solution. The sections were counterstained with 1% methyl green. The remaining surgical tissue samples were used for electron microscopy. Materials were fixed in a solution containing 0.05% glutaraldehyde, 4% paraformaldehyde, and cut into serial sections (40–60 μm thick) on a microslicer at 4 °C. Then the specimens were stained by the indirect immunoperoxidase technique, as described above for cryostat sections. After post-fixation with 1% osmium tetroxide in 0.1 mol/l phosphate buffer (pH 7.4) for 1 h, they were embedded in Epon 812 (Taab Lab., Berkshire, UK) and stained with 1% uranyl acetate in 70% ethanol. Ultrathin sections (60–80 nm thick) were examined using an electron microscope.

Results

Strong bcl-2 immunoreactivity was observed in the glandular epithelium in the proliferative to early secretory phases. The bcl-2 immunoreactivity of glandular epithelium increased as uterine glands extend from the functional layer to the basal layer (Figure 1). At high magnification, the bcl-2 was detected throughout the cytoplasm of the cells, in contrast to that of estrogen receptor and progesterone receptor in the nucleus. Endometrial samples from the late secretory to menstrual phases revealed no immunostaining for bcl-2 in all specimens examined. This bcl-2 expression pattern was similar to that of estrogen receptors and progesterone receptors throughout the menstrual cycle. Endometrial stromal cells also exhibited positive staining with anti-bcl-2 antibody, but the immunostaining pattern was not evaluated according to stage of the menstrual cycle because the stromal cell population is very heterogeneous[4]. The myometrium revealed the

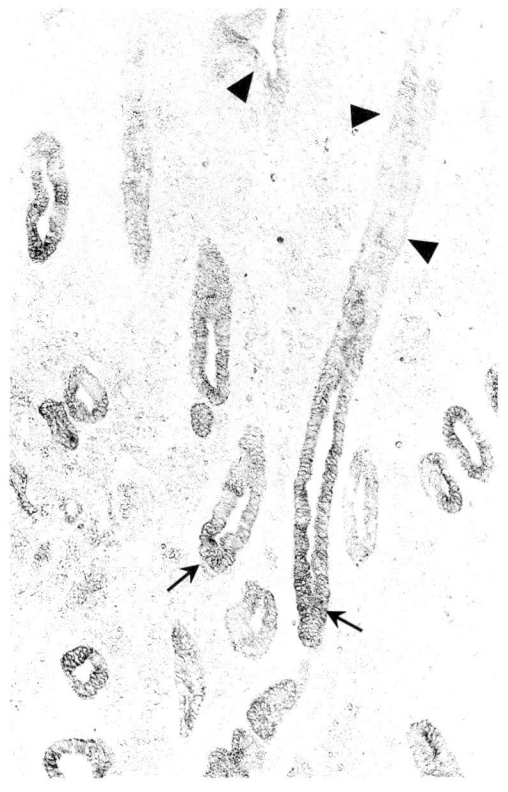

Figure 1 The immunostaining for anti-bcl-2 antibody in the endometrium in the late proliferative phase. Note the intense staining in the basal glandular cells (arrows) in contrast to the weak staining in the upper glandular cell (arrowhead). Magnification ×65

constant expression of bcl-2 as well as estrogen receptor throughout the cycle, in contrast to the endometrial glandular cells. The expressions of Fas antigen and Fas ligand were observed on the luminal cell membranes of glandular cells at the secretory phase but not at the proliferative phase, although Fas ligand was also expressed on the surface of lymphocytes in the endometrium throughout the cycle. The active form of ICE was expressed in the cytoplasm of glandular cells only at the secretory phase. Control sections failed to exhibit specific staining when the first antibody was replaced with phosphate-buffered saline or normal goat serum.

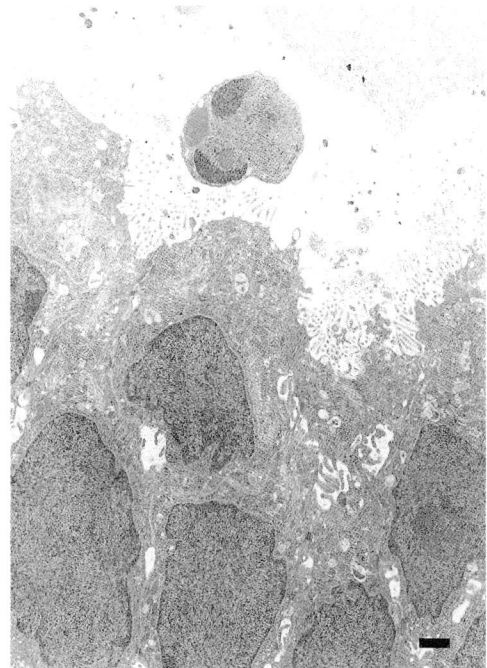

Figure 2 Electron micrograph of glandular cells in the late secretory phase. An apoptotic body showing typical chromatin condensation is observed in the uterine cavity. The bar represents 1 μm. Magnification ×3595

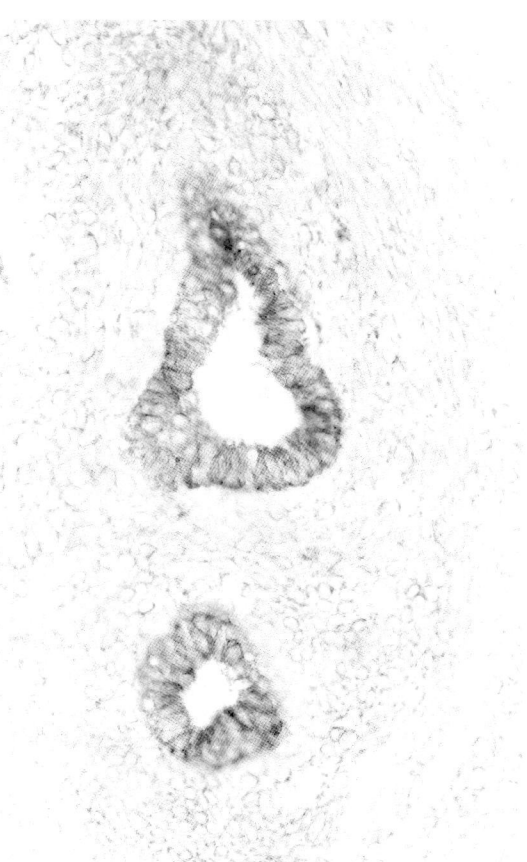

Figure 3 The immunostaining for anti-bcl-2 antibody in ectopic endometrium of adenomyosis without hormone therapy, in the secretory phase. The ectopic endometrial glandular cells strongly express bcl-2 protein, as well as surrounding smooth muscle cells in myometrium. Magnification ×607

Ultrastructurally, some glandular cells were greatly reduced in volume and rounded in shape, and the nuclear chromatin was often condensed and confluent in the late secretory phase. These apoptotic cells were gradually pushed towards the lumen and removed from the epithelium into the lumen as apoptotic bodies (Figure 2), or were engulfed and digested by adjacent glandular cells.

In adenomyosis in the control group, the most interesting finding was that all specimens showed intense expressions of both bcl-2 protein and estrogen receptor in the ectopic endometrium independently of menstrual phase (Figure 3). The expression of Fas antigen and Fas ligand in adenomyosis showed no significant tendency and varied with the cases.

In contrast, the endometrium of the danazol group revealed the suppression of bcl-2 expression, as well as of estrogen receptor and progesterone receptor. Ultrastructural characteristic findings in the endometrium of the danazol group were the destruction of organella such as mitochondria in the cytoplasm rather than nuclear changes (Figure 4). However, chromatin condensation of nuclei and the appearance of apoptotic bodies were only observed in some of the cases. The endometrium in the GnRH agonist group showed the tendency of the intense expression of bcl-2 and estrogen receptor, and these expressions were similar to those in the control group, although the expression of Fas

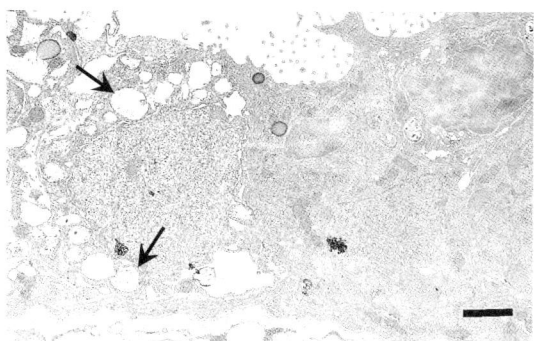

Figure 4 Electron micrograph of the glandular cells in a case administered with 600 mg/day danazol for 5 months. The cytoplasm is characterized by degenerative mitochondria (arrows) and vacuoles (arrowheads). The bar represents 1 μm. Magnification ×6180

antigen was different from that in the control group and was relatively preserved in most cases of the GnRH agonist group. The predominant ultrastructural changes in the GnRH agonist group were the presence of dilated and fused rough endoplasmic reticulum and nuclei with severe chromatin condensation, although the other organella showed no marked degeneration (Figure 5). The increased chromatin condensation and appearance of apoptotic bodies were the common findings in the GnRH agonist group (Figure 6). No essential differences in results between buserelin acetate and leuprorelin acetate were noted morphologically and biologically.

Discussion

We have clearly demonstrated the cyclic expression of bcl-2 protein in human endometrial glandular cells, showing a peak at the proliferative phase. The bcl-2 expression in endometrial glandular cells was in good correlation with that of estrogen and progesterone receptor, suggesting regulation of bcl-2 expression by these steroid hormones. This speculation might be strengthened by the

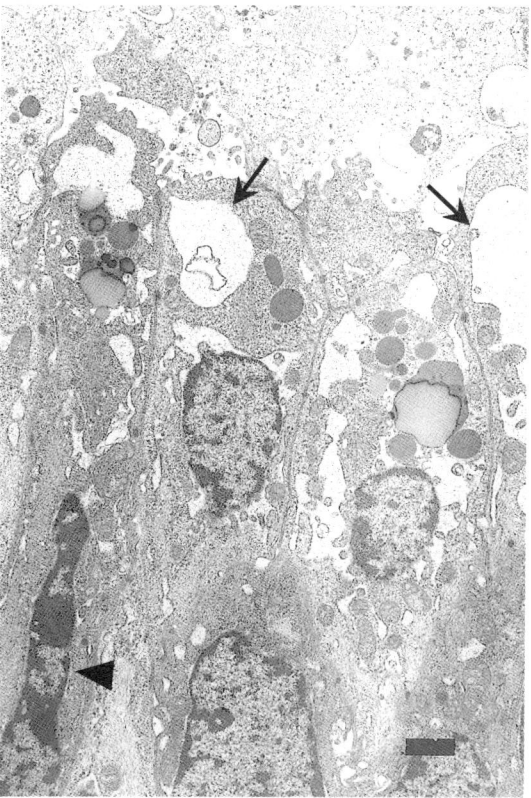

Figure 5 Electron micrograph of the glandular cells in a case injected with 3.75 mg/month leuprorelin acetate for 6 months. Note the dilated and fused rough endoplasmic reticulum (arrows) in the cytoplasm and the nuclei with severe heterochromatin or chromatin condensation (arrowhead). The bar represents 1 μm. Magnification ×5795

evidence that several estrogen hormone receptor binding motif-like sequences are found within the *bcl-2* promoter[5,6], and supported by recent studies showing bcl-2 expression associated with positive estrogen receptor in breast cancer[7,8]. Therefore, *bcl-2* gene is expressed, followed by increased *bcl-2* messenger RNA, and then the bcl-2 protein produced blocks apoptosis, when estrogen–estrogen receptor complex is bound to the *bcl-2* promoter in the proliferative phase. The most interesting finding was that the disappearance of bcl-2 expression in glandular

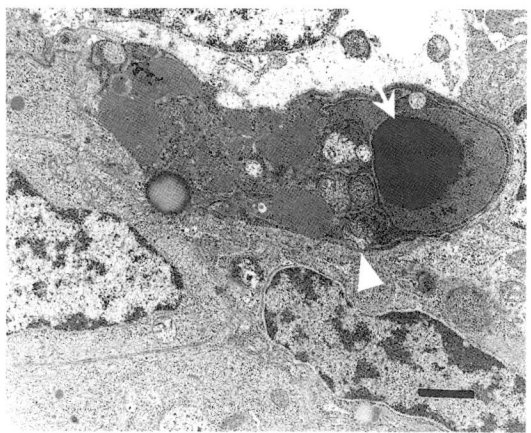

Figure 6 Electron micrograph of the glandular cells in a case administered with 900 μg/day buserelin acetate for 6 months. An ectopic glandular cell possesses a typical peripheral mass of chromatin (arrow) and organella such as mitochondria (arrowheads) are relatively preserved morphologically. The bar represents 1 μm. Magnification × 7542

cells in the late secretory phase was consistent with the appearance of apoptotic cells in the same phase. The disappearance of bcl-2 prior to massive cell death in the menstrual phase suggests that *bcl-2* plays an important role in regulating cell death of glandular epithelial cells, mainly in the functional layer, because bcl-2 protein expression in the functional layer was inferior to that in the basal layer, ranging from proliferative to early secretory phases. Since *bcl-2* is able to exert its biological activity to block apoptotic cell death in different lineages of cells such as lymphoid and neuronal cells[9–11], it is likely that *bcl-2* is functional in a similar fashion in endometrial epithelial cells.

It is well known that apoptosis is mainly mediated by several cell membranous receptors such as Fas and T-cell receptor and ICE is a common mediator in several signal transductions of apoptosis[12]. Moreover, bcl-2 blocks the upstream site of ICE in signal transductions of apoptosis, as reported by Gagliardini and colleagues[13]. Therefore, glandular cells in human endometrium may escape from apoptosis in the presence of bcl-2 in the proliferative phase but undergo apoptosis mediated by such a Fas-Fas-ligand system in the absence of bcl-2 in the secretory phase. From the above mentioned findings, apoptosis in human endometrium plays an important role in atrophy and fragility of endometrium, and then facilitates the removal of the functional layer in cooperation with the following necrosis.

This study clearly reveals several noteworthy findings in adenomyosis, although little is known of biological characteristics in adenomyosis. Firstly, adenomyosis in the control group constantly expresses bcl-2. Secondly, bcl-2 as well as estrogen receptor and progesterone receptor, is suppressed in the danazol group, although the expression of bcl-2 is preserved in the GnRH agonist group. Thirdly, the ultrastructural characteristic findings are the degeneration of organella in the danazol group, and markedly dilated rough endoplasmic reticulum, severe chromatin condensation and the appearance of apoptotic bodies in the GnRH agonist group. Therefore, the cell death of ectopic endometrial glands might be mainly necrosis in the danazol group, and apoptosis in the GnRH agonist group.

From the above-mentioned description, several biological and morphological differences between the danazol and GnRH agonist groups are elucidated in this study of adenomyosis, although it remains for further study to account for the paradoxical findings of strong bcl-2 expression and appearance of apoptotic cells observed in the GnRH agonist group.

Acknowledgements

The authors gratefully acknowledge the surgeons in Osaka Medical College, Dr K. Hamada, Dr R. Araki and Dr T. Tsurunaga in Takatsuki Red Cross Hospital, and Dr H. Kamegai and Dr Y. Suzuki in Koka Public Hospital, who allowed us to collect the tissue in theater. We also thank Dr D. Mason of the

John Radcliffe Hospital, Oxford, UK and Dr T. Koji from Nagasaki University, Japan, for providing anti-bcl-2 and anti-Fas antibodies, respectively. This work was supported in part by a Grant-in-Aid for General Scientific Research from the Ministry of Education, Science and Culture in Japan (No. 50140166).

References

1. Fawcett. D.W. (1986). Female reproductive system. In Bllom, E. and Fawcett, D.W. (eds.) *A Textbook of Histology*, pp. 879–83. (Philadelphia: W. B. Saunders)
2. Hopwood, D. and Levison, D.A. (1975). Atrophy and apoptosis in the cyclical human endometrium. *J. Pathol.*, **119**, 159–66
3. Otsuki, Y., Misaki, O., Sugimoto, O., Ito, Y., Tsujimoto, Y. and Akao, Y. (1994). Cyclic *bcl-2* gene expression in human endometrium during the menstrual cycle. *Lancet*, **344**, 28–9
4. Van Voorhis, B.J., Huettner, P.C., Clark, M.R. and Hill, J.A. (1990). Immunohistochemical localization of prostaglandin H synthetase in the female reproductive tract and endometriosis. *Am. J. Obstet. Gynecol.*, **163**, 57–62
5. Tsujimoto, Y. and Croce, C.M. (1986). Analysis of the structure, transcripts, and protein products of *bcl-2*, the gene involved in human follicular lymphoma. *Proc. Natl. Acad. Sci. USA*, **83**, 5214–18
6. Adachi, M. and Tsujimoto, Y. (1990). Potential, Z-DNA elements surrounded the breakpoints of chromosome translocation within the 5' flanking region of *bcl-2* gene. *Oncogene*, **5**, 1653–7
7. Johnston, S.R., MacLennan, K.A., Sacks, N.P., Salter, J., Smith, I.E. and Dowsett, M. (1994). Modulation of Bcl-2 and Ki-67 expression in oestrogen receptor-positive human breast cancer by tamoxifen. *Eur. J. Cancer*, **30A**, 1663–9
8. Leek, R.D., Kaklamanis, L., Pezzella, F., Gatter, K.C. and Harris, A.L. (1994). Bcl-2 in normal human breast and carcinoma, association with oestrogen receptor-positive, epidermal growth factor receptor-negative tumors and *in situ* cancer. *Br. J. Cancer*, **69**, 135–9
9. Vaux, D.L., Weissman, I.L. and Kim, S.K. (1992). Prevention of programmed cell death in *Caenorhabditis elegans* by human bcl-2. *Science*, **258**, 1955–7
10. Tsujimoto, Y. (1989). Stress-resistance conferred by high level of bcl-2a protein in human B lymphoblastoid cell. *Oncogene*, **4**, 1331–6
11. Garcia, I., Martinou, I., Tsujimoto, Y. and Martinou, J.C. (1992). Prevention of programmed cell death of sympathetic neurones by the *bcl-2* proto-oncogene. *Science*, **258**, 303–4
12. Yaun, J., Shaham, S. and Ledoux, S. (1993). The *C. elegans* cell death gene ced-3 encodes a protein similar to mammalian interleukin-1β converting enzyme. *Cell*, **75**, 641–52
13. Gagliardini, V., Fernandez, P. and Lee, R. K. (1995). Prevention of vertebrate neuronal death by the *crm*A gene. *Science*, **263**, 826–8

Heterotransplanted human endometrium in SCID mice in comparison with nude mice

D. Aoki, Y. Katsuki, Y. Shibutani, Y. Udagawa, Y. Yoshimura and S. Nozawa

Introduction

Many attempts have been made to elucidate the pathogenesis of endometriosis and to evaluate the therapeutic ability of new drugs against endometriosis by autotransplantation of endometrium in various laboratory animals. However, it is still difficult to predict exactly the *in vivo* effect of drugs on human endometrium and endometriosis through such animal studies because human heterotransplants are often rejected immunologically, even in nude mice.

Severe combined immunodeficiency (SCID) mice are congenitally deficient in T- and B-lymphocyte function because of some impairment of the lymphocyte differentiation process[1,2]. Recently, these mice have been reported to receive human normal tissues as well as tumorous ones more easily than nude mice[2].

Therefore, in this study we compared the endometrial tissues transplanted into SCID mice with those transplanted into nude mice to establish an experimental system especially useful for long-term evaluation of heterotransplanted human endometrial tissues.

Materials and methods

Human normal endometrial and myometrial specimens were obtained from uteri removed due to benign diseases such as myoma, ovarian tumor and adenomyosis. The myometrium and endometrium were separately removed from each specimen by gentle scraping and were maintained in sterilized medium-199 until transplanted.

Take rate of endometrial and myometrial transplants

The endometrial specimens in late secretory phase were cut into 2-mm cubes. One piece was gently inserted into the subcutaneous space of each mouse under intraperitoneal anesthesia with pentobarbital sodium. Fifteen female SCID mice weighing 14–25 g (Central Institute for Experimental Animals, Kawasaki, Japan; and Clea Japan, Tokyo, Japan), and 15 female BALB/c nude mice weighing 16–22 g (Clea Japan) each received a transplant. Of these mice, 10 SCID and 10 nude mice were used for transplantation of the endometrium, and the remaining ones received myometrium. The transplant-bearing mice were maintained for 10 weeks and then were sacrificed by exsanguination under ether anesthesia. Immediately after the euthanasia, each transplanted graft was excised, fixed in 10% buffered formalin, and embedded in paraffin. Sections of 4 μm in thickness were stained with hematoxylin and eosin for examination of the histology of the isolated graft and subcutaneous layer.

Take rates of the transplant were expressed as the number of mice carrying a measurable graft out of total number grafted in each group. The transplant size was measured every 2 weeks after transplantation. In brief, the subcutaneous transplant was imaged non-invasively by ultrasonography using an echo camera (SSD-650, Aloka, Tokyo, Japan) equipped with a 10-MHz in-line sector scanner probe (ASU-32WL-10, Aloka). Two rectangular diameters (a, b), and the thickness (c) of the

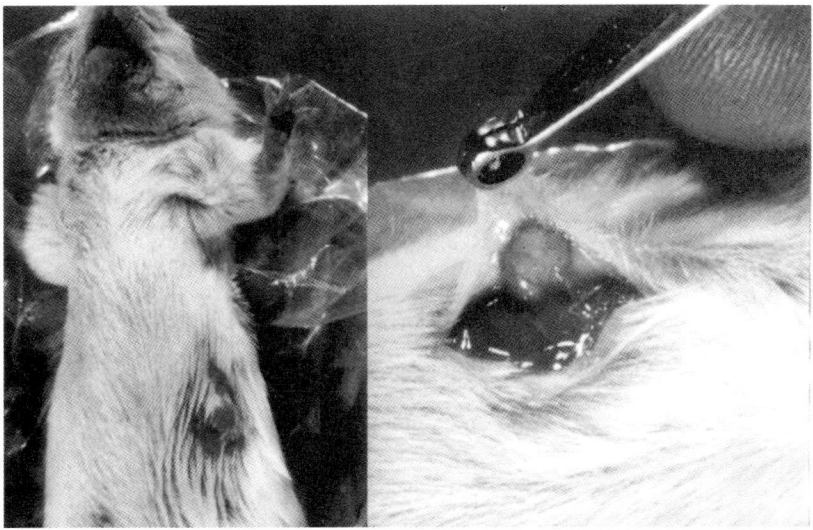

Figure 1 A severe combined immunodeficient (SCID) mouse carrying a human endometrial heterotransplant at 10 weeks after grafting. Left panel, note the graft at the right lateral abdominal region; right panel, a palpable, well-vascularized transplant is observed under the cutis of the mouse

transplant were measured on the ultrasonic image. The transplant size was expressed as the product of a, b and c.

Time-serial quantitative and morphological study of the transplanted grafts

Three SCID mice at the diestrus stage of the estrus cycle were used as the recipients of endometrial specimen. Each mouse received eight subcutaneous transplants in eight positions along a flank, or at the distal and proximal positions of the frontal and hind regions of both the left and right lateral abdominal walls. The sizes of the transplants were measured by ultrasonography on days 1, 2, 4, 7, 14, 28, 42 and 56 after grafting. One transplant from each mouse was isolated on every measurement day. After the last measurement at day 70, the remaining transplants were isolated. The isolated transplants were fixed in 10% buffered formalin and embedded in paraffin. Sections of 4 μm in thickness were stained with hematoxylin and eosin for morphological investigation. Additionally, the ability of cell proliferation was immunohistochemically examined by staining with anti-proliferating cell nuclear antigen (PCNA) antibody. The sites positive for the antibody were visualized by the peroxidase-conjugated streptoavidin–biotin complex method (LSAB kit, Dako, Santa Barbara, CA, USA).

Results

Take rate of endometrial and myometrial transplants

Heterotransplants of human endometrium and myometrium were accepted in SCID mice for at least 10 weeks after grafting (Figure 1). The survival rate up to 10 weeks after grafting was 100%. However, among nude mice, two of ten carrying the endometrium had no palpable transplant even at 2 weeks after grafting, so the take rate at 2 weeks was 80%. Thereafter, the take rate of endometrium and myometrium in nude mice gradually decreased to 40% at 10 weeks (Table 1).

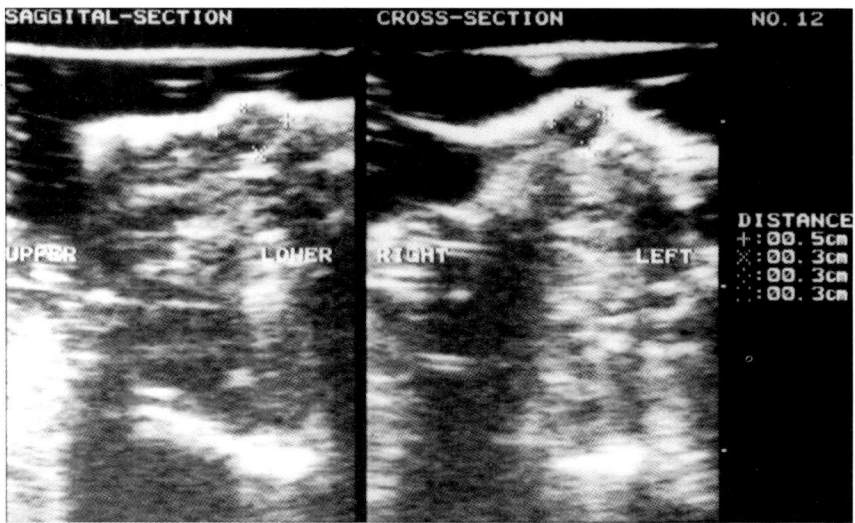

Figure 2 Ultrasonic image of an endometrial transplant in a SCID mouse. The transplant is clearly seen as a dark, subcutaneous area. Left panel, sagittal section image; right panel, cross-sectional image

Table 1 Take rates (number of mice with surviving graft divided by number of mice grafted) of human endometrium and myometrium in SCID mice and nude mice

	Take rate				
	2 weeks	4 weeks	6 weeks	8 weeks	10 weeks
Endometrium					
SCID mice	10/10	10/10	10/10	10/10	10/10
Nude mice	8/10	8/10	7/10	5/10*	4/10**
Myometrium					
SCID mice	5/5	5/5	5/5	5/5	5/5
Nude mice	5/5	5/5	4/5	3/5	2/5

*$p < 0.05$, **$p < 0.01$ compared with SCID group at corresponding time (χ^2 test)

The transplant size in all of the SCID mice was measurable by ultrasonography throughout the experimental period (Figure 2). These results were confirmed by measurement of transplant size with vernier calipers after isolation at 10 weeks. The transplant size measured by ultrasonography just before isolation from the mice revealed a significant correlation ($r = 0.915$, $p < 0.01$) with size as measured by vernier calipers immediately after isolation. The slope of the regression line was 1.017 (Figure 3). The intra- and interobserver variabilities for ultrasonography in this study were 4.5 and 6.3%, respectively.

Time-serial quantitative and morphological study of the transplanted grafts

After the transplantation into each strain of mouse, the size observed ultrasonographically increased linearly from day 1 to 7, and reached the maximum at day 7. It then decreased until day 14 and afterwards remained stable at least up to day 70 (Figures 4 and 5). Since the estrus cycle stages in the recipient mice cycled normally but the transplant size did not differ according to the estrous cycle, the transplant size seemed to depend rather on the time elapsed after the transplantation.

Morphological findings were as follows. On day 1, the transplanted endometrial glandular cells in the SCID mouse appeared viable, although degenerative changes were observed

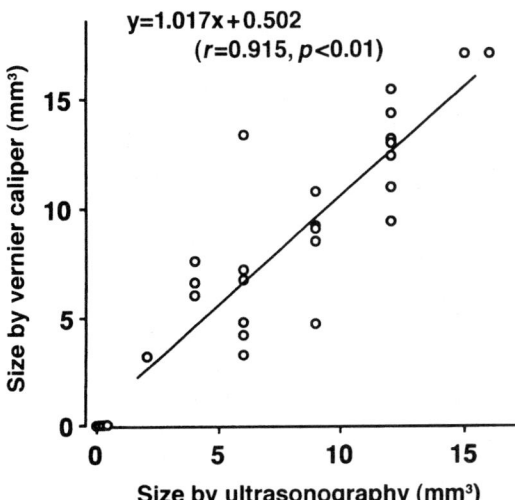

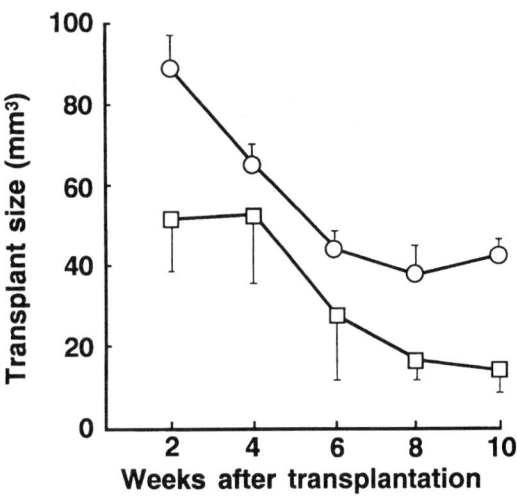

Figure 3 Relation between the *in vivo* endometrial transplant size measured non-invasively by ultrasonography at 10 weeks after grafting and the size of the same tissues measured by vernier calipers immediately after their isolation. Each point represents an individual measurement

Figure 5 Changes in volume of human myometrial transplants after grafting into the two strains of mice. Each point represents the mean ± SEM of two to five mice that carried a transplant. Transplants were grafted subcutaneously into SCID mice (○) and nude mice (□)

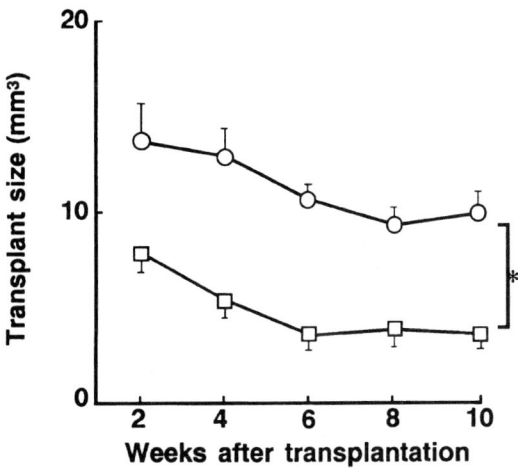

Figure 4 Changes in volume of human endometrial transplants after grafting into two strains of mice. Each point represents the mean ± SEM of four to ten mice that carried a transplant. Transplants were grafted subcutaneously into SCID mice (○) and nude mice (□). *$p < 0.01$ compared with nude mice

in the central part of the transplant (Figure 6). On days 2 and 4, there was an intensive infiltration of inflammatory cells, mainly neutrophils, and vascularization. On days 4 and 7, the remaining glandular epithelial cells in some microscopic fields seemed to have become associated with those of adjoining glandulae, suggesting epithelial cell rearrangement (Figure 6). At the same time, a number of PCNA-positive nuclei were observed in both the epithelial and interstitial cells (Figure 6). On day 14, we observed various sizes of glandulae of almost round shape surrounded by epithelial cells along with stromal cells (Figure 6). At this time, there were few PCNA-positive nuclei. The morphological aspects at this time were reproduced in a similar manner up to day 70.

Discussion

The transplants from human endometrium were completely accepted by the SCID mice,

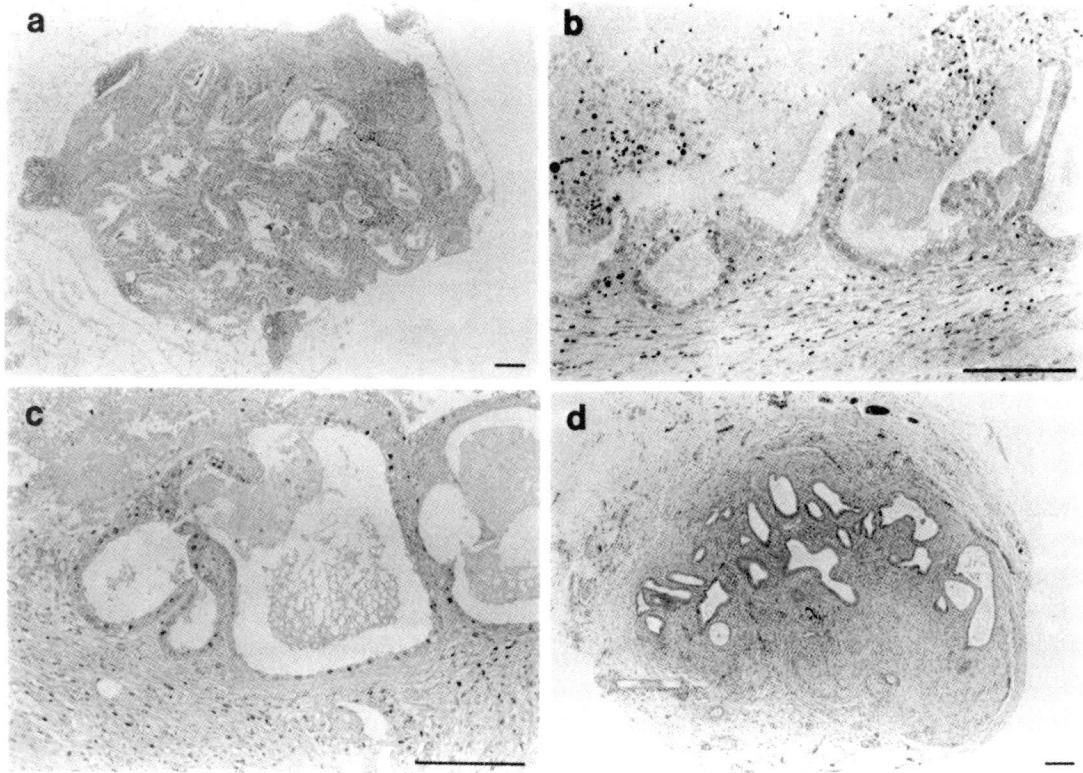

Figure 6 Photomicrographs of cross-sections of human endometrial transplants from the same endometrial source 1 day (a), 7 days (b and c), and 14 days (d) after transplantation into SCID mice (a, b and d, stained with hematoxylin and eosin; c stained with anti-PCNA antibody). The bar represents 150 μm in each case

and were ultrasonographically measurable for size for at least 10 weeks after transplantation. These mice also completely accepted the human myometrial transplants. In contrast, a lower number (40%) of the nude mice, developed as an experimental animal suitable for heterotransplantation of tissues from other species because of the deficiency of T-lymphocyte function[3], accepted human endometrial transplants in this study, in agreement with previous reports[4,5]. It has been reported that nude mice have strong natural killer activity, which serves as the dominant resistance activity against heterotransplanted tumorous tissues[6]. Suppression of natural killer activity experimentally induced in nude mice led to the stimulation of tumor cell growth[7]. We earlier reported that SCID mice showed a lower natural killer activity than nude mice and that there was sufficiently good correlation between the transplant size and the natural killer activity in SCID and nude mice, and nude mice treated with anti-asialo GM_1[7], a suppressor of natural killer activity[8]. Natural killer-mediated immunity is thus suggested to play an important role in the response to heterografts of human normal endometrium in SCID and nude mice.

The transplant size was volumetrically measurable by ultrasonography. Using this apparatus, we could monitor a transplant under the cutis and distinguish it clearly even when it was only a 1-mm cube. Additionally, our data revealed that the values obtained by ultrasonography could substitute for those exactly measured with vernier calipers. The advantageous points of this method using ultrasonography are: the method is available for a sequential measurement in one recipient; it is non-invasive; and it is applicable for measurement of many implants at one time. Therefore, this method is useful for long-term evaluation of the tissue transplanted under the cutis.

We additionally evaluated the survival process and stability of human endometrial transplants in SCID mice. The time-serial ultrasonic and morphological studies demonstrated that the transplant first exhibited an increase in size because of inflammation as seen morphologically. We consider these responses to be predominantly non-specific immunological reactions against extraneous matter in mice deficient in T- and B-cell functions. The remaining glandular epithelial cells and stromal cells then rearranged themselves, and the reconstituted glandulae showed some cystic features. At the stage of the rearrangement, several endometrial glandular cells were clearly positive for PCNA, suggesting that they showed a proliferative activity. These changes in the size and in the histological findings of the transplants terminated by 2 weeks after transplantation. Afterwards, the transplant seemed to be stable up to at least 10 weeks.

These results indicate that the non-invasive ultrasonographic device used in this study enables the sequential measurement of transplant size and that this system using SCID mice may be suitable to maintain human endometrial tissue for a long-term study. Thus, this method may be promising for evaluation of drug or hormonal effects on endometrium, even though a long time is required until their appearance.

References

1. Phillips, R.A., Jewett, M.A. and Gallie, B.L. (1989). Growth of human tumors in immunodeficient SCID mice and nude mice. *Curr. Top. Microbiol. Immunol.*, **152**, 259–63
2. Murphy, W.J., Kumar, V. and Bennett, M. (1989). Immunobiology of bone marrow transplantation: studies using SCID mice. *Curr. Top. Microbiol. Immunol.*, **152**, 251–8
3. Wortis, H.H. (1971). Immunologic responses of nude mice. *Clin. Exp. Immunol.*, **8**, 305–17
4. Bergqvist, A., Jeppsson, S., Kullander, S. and Ljungberg, O. (1985). Human endometrium transplanted into nude mice: histologic effects of various steroid hormones. *Am. J. Pathol.*, **119**, 336–44
5. Zamah, N.M., Dodson, M.G., Stephens, L.C., Buttram, V.C., Besch, P.K. and Kaufman, R.H. (1984). Transplantation of normal and ectopic human endometrial tissue into athymic nude mice. *Am. J. Obstet. Gynecol.*, **149**, 591–7
6. Kiessling, R., Klein, R., Pross, E. and Wigzell, H. (1975). Natural killer cells in the mouse. II. Cytotoxic cells with specificity of the killer cells. *Eur. J. Immunol.*, **5**, 117–21
7. Aoki, D., Katsuki, Y., Shimizu, A., Kakinuma, C. and Nozawa, S. (1994). Successful heterotransplantation of human endometrium in SCID mice. *Obstet. Gynecol.*, **83**, 220–8
8. Habu, S., Fukui, H., Shimamura, K., Kasai, M., Nagai, Y., Okumura, K. and Tamaoki, N. (1981). *In vivo* effects of anti-asialo GM$_1$. 1. Reduction of NK activity and enhancement of transplanted tumor growth in nude mice. *J. Immunol.*, **127**, 34–88

Section 3

Immunology

Immunomodulation of endometriotic implant growth and protein production

W.B. Nothnick and M.W. Vernon

Introduction

Endometriosis and the immune system

Endometriosis is a disease that occurs primarily in menstruating women and is characterized by pelvic pain and infertility. Classically defined as the presence of endometrial glands and stroma remote from the uterine cavity, endometriosis represents one of the major pathologies seen by gynecologists and infertility specialists today. Despite the high frequency with which the disease is encountered, the pathophysiology of the disease still remains unclear. One theory for the development of endometriosis suggests an aberrant immune system as a causative factor. Studies have demonstrated that women with endometriosis have altered cell-mediated immunity[1-5], which could allow translocated endometrial cells to implant and progress. Additionally, women with endometriosis have also been shown to have altered humoral immunity[6-13], increased macrophage numbers[14] and increased macrophage activational status[15,16]. Major secretory products of activated macrophages are cytokines. Therefore, it is not surprising that several cytokines have been detected in elevated concentrations in the peritoneal fluid of women with endometriosis[17-21]. It is postulated that a consequence of the elevated peritoneal fluid cytokine levels in women with endometriosis is the infertility associated with the disease and that cytokines elicit this adverse effect on fertility at multiple loci[22].

Cytokines and the endometriotic implant

In addition to reducing fertility, cytokines may also have an effect on the endometriotic implant. Cytokines are known modulators of endometrial tissue function[23] and, because implant tissue is derived from once eutopic endometrium, cytokines may be capable of inducing biological effects on the endometriotic tissue. Ectopic endometrial tissue exhibits several biochemical deviations as compared to eutopic endometrial tissue. For example, endometriotic implants and uterine endometrial tissue differ in their steroid receptor content[24], steroid responsiveness[24,25], epidermal growth factor receptor[26] and epidermal growth factor content[27], and prostaglandin production[28]. In addition, Sharpe and Vernon have identified two unique groups of polypeptides that are synthesized by endometriotic tissue but not by eutopic endometrium[29] (see Figure 1). These proteins, originally identified based on their molecular weight (M_r) and isoelectric point (pI), were termed endometriosis protein-I or Endo-I ($M_r = 40$–55, pI = 4.0–5.2) and endometriosis protein-II or Endo-II ($M_r = 28$–32, pI = 7.5–9.0).

The production of Endo-II as well as endometriotic implant growth have been shown to be associated with macrophage activation/cytokine production. Specifically, Nothnick and colleagues[30] have demonstrated that administration of the immunosuppressive agent pentoxifylline to rats with surgically induced endometriosis induced a decrease in implant

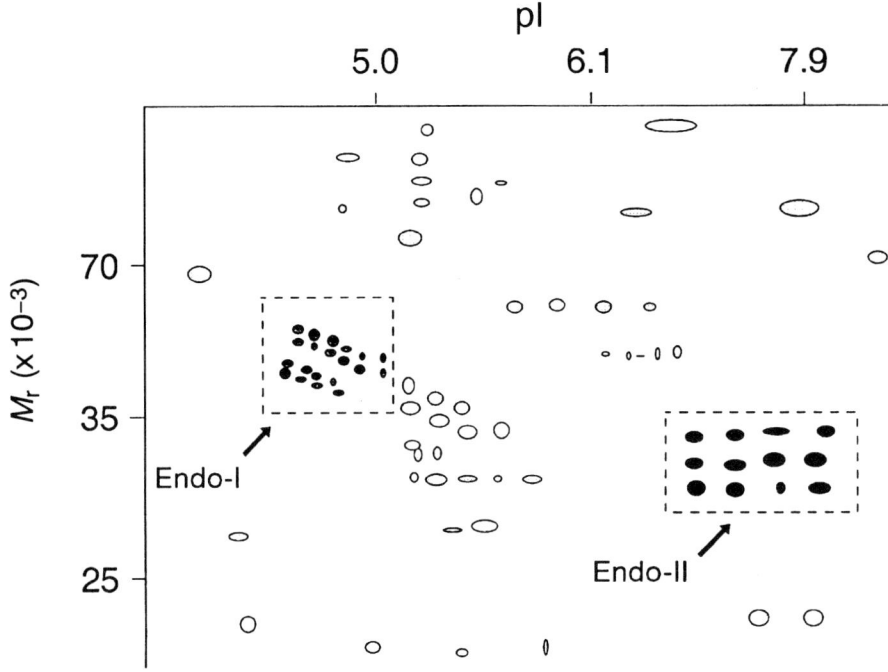

Figure 1 Schematic representation of secretory proteins of rat endometriotic implant tissue. The presence of the implant-specific proteins Endo-I ($M_r = 40$–55; pI = 4.0–5.2) and Endo-II ($M_r = 28$–32; pI = 7.5–9.0) are indicated

Endo-II production and that administration of the immunostimulatory agent lipopolysaccharide (LPS) could augment Endo-II production. In addition, pentoxifylline induced a rapid regression of endometriotic implant tissue and this pentoxifylline-induced regression was not associated with a reduction in systemic estrogen or progesterone concentrations, or reproductive cyclicity. Lastly, implant production of Endo-I was unaffected by either pentoxifylline or LPS administration. Taken together, these findings are interpreted to suggest that cytokines can modulate endometriotic implant growth and the production of endometriotic implant-specific proteins.

The role of the peritoneum in implant-specific protein production

In the rat model for surgically induced endometriosis the endometrial tissue is sutured upon mesenteric/peritoneal tissue adjacent to an arterial cascade of the small intestine. Used as a control tissue in the experiments by Nothnick and co-workers[30], mesenteric tissue which contained the arterial cascades of the small intestine was shown to produce copious amounts of Endo-I. Therefore, it is tempting to speculate that it is the blood vessels of the implant and/or the underlying blood vessels to which the implant is initially sutured which are responsible for Endo-I production and not the endometrial stromal or glandular tissue components of the implant. Although the implant-specificity of Endo-I may be uncertain, evidence suggests that endometriotic implant growth and Endo-II production is affected by the elevated peritoneal fluid levels of cytokines associated with the disease. One question that still remains unanswered is whether the cytokines act directly upon the implant to modulate these parameters or whether they act upon the peritoneal tissue

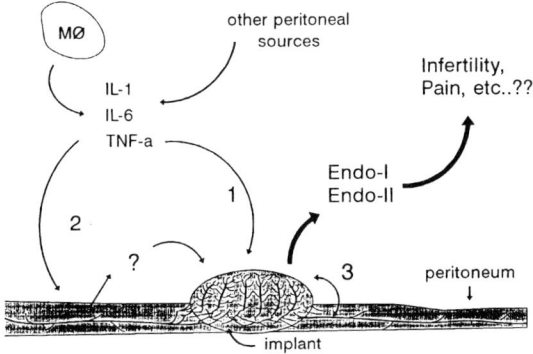

Figure 2 Diagrammatic representation of potential mechanisms for endometriotic implant-specific protein production. Three potential pathways/mechanisms for Endo-I and Endo-II production are postulated. (1) Elevated cytokine levels of macrophage (Mφ) and/or other peritoneal cell origin may directly stimulate ectopic endometriotic implant production of these proteins; (2) elevated cytokines may act upon the peritoneum to stimulate secretion of secondary mediators, which may then stimulate implant Endo-I and Endo-II production; or (3) cell-to-cell contact of ectopic endometrial tissue with peritoneal tissue may result in the latter inducing the former to produce the implant-specific proteins

which in turn influences endometriotic implant growth and Endo-II production. *In vitro* studies by Sharpe and colleagues[31] have demonstrated that co-culture of peritoneal mesothelial cells with uterine stromal cells resulted in the aggregation of the stromal cells, whereas co-culture of peritoneal subserosal cells with uterine epithelial cells induced a compact, irregular morphology of the uterine epithelial cells. This study suggested that the altered morphology of the uterine cell types may be coupled with the histological and biochemical asynchrony between eutopic and ectopic endometrial tissue and thus may play a role in Endo-I and Endo-II production by the implant. This notion of a peritoneal tissue influence on ectopic endometrial tissue biochemistry is also supported by the well documented findings that interactions between mesenchymal and epithelial cells play vital roles in embryonic development[32,33]. The possibility exists that there are several mechanisms for Endo-I and Endo-II production; these mechanisms are summarized in Figure 2. Elevated levels of cytokines originating from macrophages and/or other peritoneal cells may directly stimulate the production by the ectopic endometriotic implant of these proteins (pathway 1). Alternatively, the elevated cytokines may act upon the peritoneum to stimulate secretion of secondary mediators which may then stimulate implant Endo-I and Endo-II production (pathway 2). A third possibility would be the cell-to-cell contact of ectopic endometrial tissue with peritoneal tissue, resulting in the latter inducing the former to produce the implant-specific proteins (pathway 3). To evaluate these potential mechanisms in the production of the endometriotic implant-specific proteins, the following series of experiments was performed.

Materials and methods

Animals

We chose to examine whether the immunostimulatory agent LPS could induce eutopic endometrial production of Endo-II, thereby demonstrating that a physical interaction between peritoneal and endometrial tissue components of the endometriotic implant are not required for production of the implant-specific group of proteins. Mature female Sprague-Dawley rats (250 g; Harlan, Indianapolis, IN) were housed in an environmentally controlled room with a light:dark cycle of 14:10 h under the care and supervision of a licensed veterinarian. All animal procedures for these experiments were approved by the University of Kentucky Institutional Animal Care and Use Committee (IACUC). Rats were allowed a 2-week acclimatization period on the vivarium before any procedures were performed. Following this period, vaginal cytology was examined daily for 2 weeks and only those rats exhibiting regular estrous cycles were included in the study.

Treatment protocol and peritoneal fluid collection

Lipopolysaccharide (LPS; *Salmonella enteritidis*) was obtained from Sigma Chemical Co. (St. Louis, MO). On the first morning of proestrus after the initial 2-week cycling period, animals were injected intraperitoneally with either LPS ($n = 8$; 200 μg/kg body weight) or an equal volume of phosphate-buffered saline (PBS; $n = 7$). Animals were sacrificed 48 h later by ether overdose and vaginal cytology was noted. All animals were in the estrus to diestrus-1 stage of their reproductive cycle at the time of sacrifice. Peritoneal fluid was collected by instillation of 3 ml of PBS into the peritoneal cavity, the peritoneal area was gently massaged and fluid was removed using a 1-ml tuberculin syringe. Peritoneal fluid was then centrifuged at 1875g for 10 min at 4°C to remove cellular debris and stored at −20°C until analyzed for interleukin-1β (IL-1β) content.

Interleukin-1β quantitation

IL-1β concentrations were assessed to verify LPS bioactivity. Peritoneal fluid concentrations of IL-1β were quantitated by an enzyme-linked immunosorbent assay kit (Cistron Corp., Pinebrook, NJ). Samples were assayed in duplicate with 100 μl of each sample used according to the specifications of the manufacturer. The inter- and intra-assay coefficients of variation were 6.5% and 5.0%, respectively.

Serum steroid quantitation

To verify that treatment induction of implant-specific proteins occurred independently of serum steroid levels, serum progesterone and estrogen levels were quantitated. Steroid levels were measured by solid-phase ^{125}I-radio-immunoassays (Diagnostic Products Corp., Los Angeles, CA) previously validated in our laboratory[30]. All samples were analyzed in duplicate with the use of 100 μl of each serum sample; the detection limits of the assays were approximately 0.05 ng/ml (progesterone) and 4.0 pg/ml (estrogen). The inter- and intra-assay coefficient of variation for progesterone was 8.0% and 4.7%, respectively, and 6.4% and 5.3%, respectively, for estrogen.

Tissue culture

At sacrifice, uteri were removed and dissected to expose the luminal surface of the epithelial layer. Also at this time, mesenteric tissue containing the arterial cascades of the small intestine was removed and prepared for tissue culture. Tissues were cultured by separately placing samples (100 mg of each tissue type) in minimal essential media (MEM; Gibco, Grand Island, NY) devoid of methionine for 1 h at 37°C. Samples were then transferred to flasks containing 3 ml of MEM with 30 μCi/ml L-[^{35}S]methionine (NEN, Boston, MA). Tissues were cultured for 24 h at 37°C on a rocking platform in a gaseous atmosphere of 50% nitrogen, 45% oxygen and 5% carbon dioxide, as previously described[29,30]. Incubation was terminated by centrifugation of the medium, which was subsequently dialyzed for 24 h.

Two-dimensional polyacrylamide gel electrophoresis

All supplies for electrophoresis were purchased from BioRad Laboratories (Richmond, CA) unless otherwise noted. Two-dimensional polyacrylamide gel electrophoresis (2D-PAGE) was performed as previously described[29,30]. Briefly, 1.5×10^6 cpm of non-dialyzable radioactivity was dissolved in

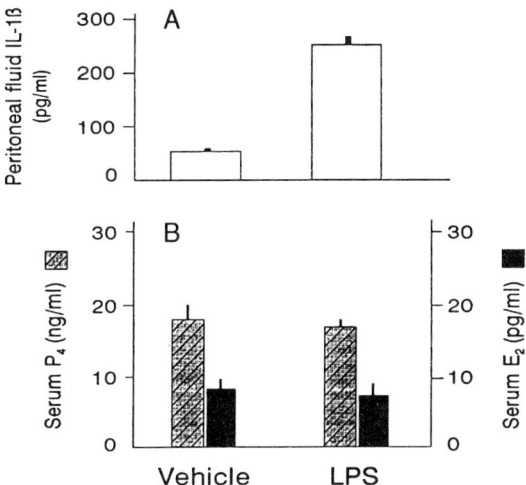

Figure 3 Peritoneal fluid interleukin-1β (IL-1β) and serum steroid concentrations in treated and untreated rats. Peritoneal fluid and serum were collected, and IL-1β (A) and steroid concentrations (B) were determined as described in *Materials and methods*. Values represent the mean ± SEM for vehicle- ($n = 7$) and LPS-treated ($n = 8$) animals. P_4, progesterone; E_2, estrogen; LPS, lipopolysaccharide

5 mmol/l K_2CO_3 containing 9.4 mol/l urea, 2% (v/v) Nonidet P-40 and 0.5% (w/v) dithiothreitol (Sigma) and applied to each first-dimension isoelectric focusing gel (IEF). A mixture of ampholines (Pharmacia Biotechnology Inc., Piscataway, NJ) was utilized to create a pH gradient of 3.0 to 9.0 for the IEF gel. The polyacrylamide (12%) second-dimension slab gels were impregnated with Amplify (Amersham, Arlington Heights, IL), dried and exposed to Kodak XAR-5 film (Sigma) for 5 days (uterus) or 2 days (mesenteric tissue) at –70 °C.

Histological preparations

Approximately 50 mg of uterine tissue was obtained at the time of sacrifice from each animal. Tissues were histologically examined by being fixed *in toto* in 10% neutral-buffered formalin. Tissues were then embedded in paraffin, serially sectioned at 7 μm and counterstained with hematoxylin and eosin, as previously described[30].

Results

All LPS-treated animals had significantly higher IL-1β peritoneal fluid concentrations than vehicle-treated animals, indicating that LPS induced cytokine production (Figure 3A). Furthermore, no differences in serum steroid levels were associated with the elevated IL-1β levels (Figure 3B). Two-dimensional electrophoretic analysis of uterine protein production revealed that uteri from both vehicle- and LPS-treated animals synthesized and released hundreds of similar proteins. However, the most striking difference in uterine protein production between vehicle- and LPS-treated animals was the production of Endo-II by uteri of LPS-treated animals (Figure 4). Specifically, conditioned uterine media from four of the eight LPS-treated animals contained the entire group (consisting of 12 individual isovariant proteins) of Endo-II proteins, whereas the remaining four of eight uterine samples contained 6–9 individual isovariant proteins (vehicle-treated uteri contained 2–4 individual isovariant proteins). Induction of uterine Endo-II production was not associated with either an alteration in uterine weight or necrosis of the tissue, as no differences in these parameters were noted between treatment groups (data not shown).

In assessing the specificity of Endo-I production, it was found that uterine conditioned media from neither vehicle- nor LPS-treated animals contained Endo-I, suggesting that this protein may not be of uterine origin and may not be regulated by immune cell secretions (Figure 4). The specificity of Endo-I production was further questioned by the finding that mesenteric tissue containing the

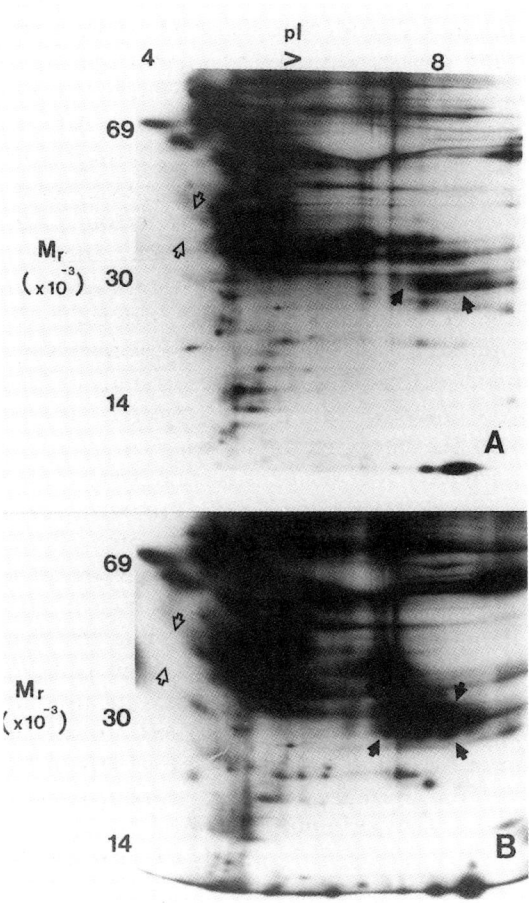

Figure 4 Representative two-dimensional SDS-PAGE fluorograph of L-[^{35}S]methionine-labeled secretory proteins from uterine tissue obtained from animals treated with either vehicle (A) or lipopolysaccharide (LPS) (B). Animals were treated and tissues were obtained and then cultured, and protein synthesis was assessed by 2D-PAGE, as described in *Materials and methods*. Open and filled arrows indicate the presence or absence of the endometriotic implant-specific proteins Endo-I ($M_r = 40$–55; pI = 4.0–5.2) and Endo-II ($M_r = 28$–32; pI = 7.5–9.0), respectively. Similar protein separation patterns were obtained from seven of seven uteri of vehicle-treated animals and four of eight LPS-treated animals. The protein separation patterns of uteri from the remaining four animals contained 6–9 individual Endo-II protein isovariants

arterial cascades of the small intestines (used as a control) from vehicle-treated animals produced copious amounts of this protein (Figure 5A). Furthermore, the production of Endo-I by this mesenteric tissue appeared to be independent of immune cell secretions, as LPS had no effect on Endo-I production (Figure 5B). Lastly, mesenteric tissue containing the arterial cascades of the small intestines produced a portion of proteins in the Endo-II group of proteins. The production of these proteins was independent of LPS administration (Figure 5), suggesting that the immunostimulatory effect of LPS on uterine Endo-II production is a tissue-specific event.

Discussion

It is demonstrated in the current study that uterine tissue can be induced by the immunostimulatory agent LPS to produce the endometriotic 'implant-specific' protein, Endo-II. These findings indicate that uterine tissue is capable of responding to LPS or LPS-induced compounds such as cytokines. Furthermore, the immunostimulatory induction of eutopic uterine Endo-II production indicates that the peritoneum does not play a vital role in the induction of endometriotic implant Endo-II synthesis, at least through a cell-to-cell contact mechanism. Although it has been demonstrated in the present and in previous studies[30] that immunostimulation can induce ectopic and eutopic endometrial production of Endo-II, the question that still remains unanswered is what is the function of Endo-II? Recently, Sharpe-Timms and colleagues[34] have shown that Endo-II shows a high degree of amino acid sequence homology with the tissue inhibitor of metalloproteinase-1 (TIMP-1). TIMP-1 functions not only as a regulator of matrix metalloproteinase activity[35], but also as a growth factor[36,37] and regulator of angiogenesis[38–40], thereby indicating that the role of Endo-II/TIMP-1 in the pathophysiology of endometriosis may be multifunctional. Recently, Nothnick and colleagues[41] have demonstrated that peritoneal fluid from women with endometriosis contains elevated TIMP activity compared to peritoneal fluid from women without the disease, further implicating TIMPs in the pathophysiology of endometriosis. Lastly, TIMP-1 production is stimulated in a variety of cell types by cytokines such as tumor necrosis factor[42] and interleukin-1[43]. Therefore, the identification of Endo-II as TIMP-1, the modulation of TIMP-1 by cytokines and the elevated levels of peritoneal fluid cytokines in women with endometriosis further lend support to the involvement of immune cell secretions in the pathophysiology of endometriosis.

The current study also demonstrates that Endo-I is a major product of mesenteric tissue which contains the arterial cascades of the small intestine and that the production of Endo-I by this tissue is not influenced by immunostimulatory agents such as LPS. This finding suggests that Endo-I may not be implant-specific. We further speculate that Endo-I is produced by the vascular tissue of the implant and not the uterine component, as eutopic uterine tissue did not produce Endo-I but mesenteric arterial tissue did. Further evidence suggesting that Endo-I may not be an implant-specific protein is the finding by Nothnick and co-workers of a group of proteins displaying a similar electrophoretic separation pattern to that of Endo-I which was detected in the peritoneal fluid of women with and without endometriosis[44]. Lastly, Sharpe-Timms and colleagues have recently demonstrated that Endo-I shows a high degree of amino acid and cDNA sequence homology with haptoglobin[45]. Haptoglobin is a major serum protein, which functions in the acute phase response to inflammation[46]. Although haptoglobin is normally found in the circulation, the possibility exists that elevated levels of this protein may be associated with endometriosis. Nothnick and co-workers[44] have shown that, qualitatively, peritoneal fluid from women with endometriosis contains a greater number of 'Endo-I like' proteins compared to peritoneal fluid from

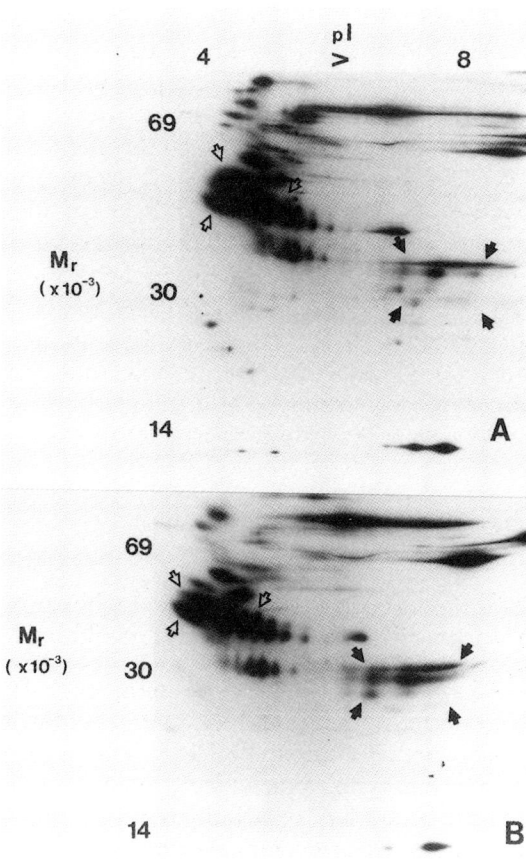

Figure 5 Representative two-dimensional SDS-PAGE fluorograph of L-[35S]methionine-labeled secretory proteins from mesenteric tissue containing the arterial cascades of the small intestines obtained from animals treated with either vehicle (A) or lipopolysaccharide (LPS) (B). Animals were treated and tissues were obtained and then cultured, and protein synthesis was assessed by 2D-PAGE, as described in *Materials and methods*. Open and filled arrows indicate the presence or absence of the endometriotic implant-specific proteins Endo-I ($M_r = 40$–55; pI = 4.0–5.2) and Endo-II ($M_r = 28$–32; pI = 7.5–9.0), respectively. Films were exposed for 2 days in contrast to the 5 days for uterine tissue (Figure 4). Similar protein separation patterns were obtained for all other mesenteric samples analyzed from animals in each treatment group

women without the disease. It is possible that, much like during the acute phase response, the development of endometriosis results in tissue damage (implantation of the ectopic endometrial tissue), which in turn signals the production of Endo-I/haptoglobin. Specifically, cytokines such as interleukin-1, tumor necrosis factor and interleukin-6 have been implicated in the acute phase response[46], and these cytokines are also elevated in the peritoneal fluid of women with endometriosis[17-20] (as a result of tissue damage?). These cytokines are then postulated to increase hepatic production of acute phase response proteins such as haptoglobin[46]. Therefore, much like Endo-II/TIMP-1, the production of Endo-I/haptoglobin by the endometriotic implant further strengthens the active role of cytokines in the pathophysiology of endometriosis.

As alluded to earlier, the original identification of Endo-I and Endo-II as implant-specific proteins undoubtedly raised the possibility of the development of markers for the (non-invasive) detection/diagnosis of endometriosis. Although it now appears that both Endo-I (haptoglobin) and Endo-II (TIMP-1) are anything but specific (as these are two abundant serum proteins), the possibility of their use as diagnostic tools still exists. Aberrant production (either elevated or suppressed compared to production in women without endometriosis) of Endo-I/haptoglobin and/or Endo-II/TIMP-1 may provide useful diagnostic/prognostic information. The production of these proteins at inappropriate times of the reproductive cycle (ovulation, embryo implantation) may contribute to the infertility associated with the disease. Thus, both Endo-I/haptoglobin and/or Endo-II/TIMP-1 may still play clinically relevant roles in the pathophysiology of endometriosis.

The findings that endometriotic implant Endo-II production and endometriotic implant growth can be suppressed by pentoxifylline may also be of clinical importance. Pentoxifylline has been shown to suppress cytokine production[47,48] and reverse the

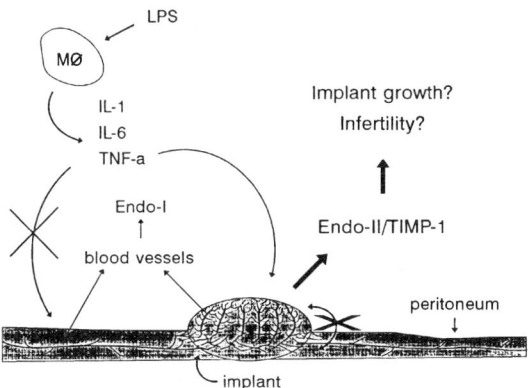

Figure 6 Working model for Endo-I and Endo-II production. We hypothesize that Endo-I is produced by arterial tissue of both the peritoneal tissue and of the endometriotic implant, suggesting that this protein may not be implant-specific. In contrast, we hypothesize that the uterine tissue of the endometriotic implant synthesizes Endo-II and that this production is stimulated by activated macrophage (Mφ) products such as cytokines

infertility associated with endometriosis[49]. In addition, the pentoxifylline-induced suppression of endometriotic tissue growth appears to be independent of systemic steroid concentrations[30]. These data, taken together, suggest that pentoxifylline could: (1) suppress endometriotic implant growth; (2) suppress implant Endo-II/TIMP-1 production; (3) suppress peritoneal fluid cytokine production; and (4) reverse the infertility associated with endometriosis, all via a steroid-independent mechanism. The ability of pentoxifylline to eliminate these symptoms/characteristics of endometriosis without disrupting reproductive cyclicity[30] would provide several benefits over current treatment regimens.

Summary and conclusion

Our working model for the mechanism of endometriotic implant-specific protein production is depicted in Figure 6. We hypothesize that cytokines, most likely of activated macrophage origin, directly stimulate the endometriotic implant production of EndoII. Furthermore, we believe that interaction between the endometriotic implant and the underlying peritoneum is not essential for the production of this protein. Lastly, we have presented compelling evidence to support the hypothesis that Endo-I is not solely an endometriotic 'implant-specific' protein, but in fact is a major secretory product of mesenteric tissue containing the arterial cascades of the small intestine as well. Taken together, our data support an active role for the immune system/cytokines in the growth and protein production of the endometriotic implant. In addition, our previous work, which demonstrated that pentoxifylline can induce a regression of endometriotic tissue independent of serum steroid production, warrants further investigation into the use of immunosuppressive agents as future therapies for the management of endometriosis. Furthermore, we feel that the recent identification of the implant-specific protein Endo-I as haptoglobin and the identification of Endo-II as TIMP-1 will undoubtedly provide new insight into the pathophysiology of the disease. Application of these findings in conjunction with today's molecular techniques will allow us to make progress in the study of a disease that has hindered patients, physicians and researchers over the past several decades.

References

1. Dmowski, W.P., Steele, R.W. and Baker, G.F. (1981). Deficient cellular immunity in endometriosis. *Am. J. Obstet. Gynecol.*, **141**, 377–83
2. Steele, R.W., Dmowski, W.P. and Marmer, D.J. (1984). Immunologic aspects of human endometriosis. *Am. J. Reprod. Immunol.*, **6**, 33–41
3. Oosterlynck, D.J., Cornillie, F.J., Waer, M., Vandeputte, M. and Koninckx, P.R. (1992). The natural killer activity of peritoneal fluid lymphocytes is decreased in women with endometriosis. *Fertil. Steril.*, **58**, 292–5
4. Kanzaki, H., Sheng-Wang, H.S., Kariya, M. and Mori, T. (1992). Suppression of natural killer cell activity by sera from patients with endometriosis. *Am. J. Obstet. Gynecol.*, **167**, 257–61
5. Oosterlynck, D.J., Meuleman, C. and Waer, M. (1992). Peritoneal fluid inhibits natural killer activity *in vitro*. *Am. J. Reprod. Immunol.*, **27**, 54–9
6. Badawy, S.Z., Cuenca, V., Stitzel, A., Jacobs, R.B.D. and Tomar, R.H. (1984). Autoimmune phenomena in infertile patients with endometriosis. *Obstet. Gynecol.*, **63**, 271–5
7. Gleicher, N., El-Roeiy, A., Confino, E. and Friberg, J. (1987). Abnormal autoantibodies in endometriosis: is endometriosis an autoimmune disease? *Obstet. Gynecol.*, **70**, 115–22
8. Kreiner, D., Fromowitz, F.B., Richardson, D.A. and Kenigsberg, D. (1986). Endometrial immunofluorescence associated with endometriosis and pelvic inflammatory disease. *Fertil. Steril.*, **46**, 243–5
9. Mathur, S., Peress, M.R., Williamson, H.O., Youmans, C.D., Maney, S.A., Garvin, A.J., Rust, P.F. and Fudenberg, H.H. (1982). Autoimmunity to endometrium and ovary in endometriosis. *Clin. Exp. Immunol.*, **50**, 259–66
10. Saifuddin, A., Buckley, C.H. and Fox, H. (1983). Immunoglobulin content of the endometrium in women with endometriosis. *Int. J. Gynecol. Pathol.*, **2**, 255–63
11. Startseva, N.V. (1980). Clinico-immunological aspects of genital endometriosis. *Akush. Ginekol. (Mosk).*, **3**, 23–6
12. Weed, J.C. and Arguembourg, P.C. (1980). Endometriosis: can it produce an autoimmune response resulting in infertility? *Clin. Obstet. Gynecol.*, **23**, 885–91
13. Wild, R.A. and Shivers, C.A. (1985). Antiendometrial antibodies in patients with endometriosis. *Am. J. Reprod. Immunol. Microbiol.*, **8**, 84–6
14. Haney, A.F., Muscato, J.J. and Weinberg, J.B. (1981). Peritoneal fluid cell populations in infertility patients. *Fertil. Steril.*, **35**, 696–8
15. Halme, J., Becker, S., Hammond, M.G. and Raj, S. (1983). Increased activation of pelvic

15. macrophages in infertile women with mild endometriosis. *Am. J. Obstet. Gynecol.*, **145**, 333–7
16. Halmes, J., Becker, S. and Wing, R. (1984). Accentuated cyclic activation of peritoneal macrophages in patients with endometriosis. *Am. J. Obstet. Gynecol.*, **148**, 85–90
17. Fakih, H., Baggett, B., Holtz, G., Tsang, K.Y., Lee, J.C. and Williamson, H.O. (1992). Interleukin-1: a possible role in the infertility associated with endometriosis. *Fertil. Steril.*, **47**, 213–17
18. Mori, H., Sawairi, M., Nakagawa, M., Itoh, N., Wada, K. and Tamaya, T. (1992). Expression of interleukin-1 (IL-1) messenger ribonucleic acid (mRNA) and IL-1 receptor mRNA in peritoneal macrophages from patients with endometriosis. *Fertil. Steril.*, **57**, 535–42
19. Punnonen, J., Teisala, K., Ranta, H., Bennett, B. and Punnonen, R. (1996). Increased levels of interleukin-6 and interleukin-10 in the peritoneal fluid of patients with endometriosis. *Am. J. Obstet. Gynecol.*, **174**, 1522–6
20. Eisermann, J., Gast, M.G., Pineda, J., Odem, R.R. and Collins, J.L. (1988). Tumor necrosis factor in peritoneal fluid of women undergoing diagnostic laparoscopic surgery. *Fertil. Steril.*, **50**, 573–9
21. Koyama, N., Matsuura, K. and Okamura, H. (1993). Cytokines in the peritoneal fluid of patients with endometriosis. *Int. J. Gynaecol. Obstet.*, **43**, 45–50
22. Muse, K.N. (1987). Endometriosis and infertility. In Wilson, E. (ed.) *Endometriosis*, pp. 91–110. (New York: Liss)
23. Tabibzadeh, S. (1991). Human endometrium: an active site of cytokine production and action. *Endocr. Rev.*, **12**, 272–90
24. Lessey, B.A., Metzger, D.A., Haney, A.F. and McCarty, K.S. (1989). Immunohistochemical analysis of estrogen and progesterone receptors in endometriosis: comparison with normal endometrium during the menstrual cycle and the effect of medical therapy. *Fertil. Steril.*, **51**, 409–15
25. Vierikko, P., Kauppila, A., Ronnberg, L. and Vihko, R. (1985). Steroidal regulation of endometriosis tissue: lack of induction of 17β-hydroxysteroid dehydrogenase activity by progesterone, medroxyprogesterone acetate or danazol. *Fertil. Steril.*, **43**, 218–24
26. Megela, C, Balducci, M., Bulletti, C., Galassi, A., Jasonni, V.M. and Flamigni, C. (1991). Tissue factors influencing growth and maintenance of endometriosis. *Ann. NY Acad. Sci.*, **622**, 257–65
27. Haining, R.E.B., Cameron, I.T., Van Papendorp, C., Davenport, A.P., Prentice, A., Thomas, E.J. and Smith, S.K. (1991). Epidermal growth factor in human endometrium: proliferative effects in culture and immunocytochemical localization in normal and endometriotic tissues. *Hum. Reprod.*, **6**, 1200–5
28. Vernon, M.W., Beard, J.S., Graves, K. and Wilson, E.A. (1986). Classification of endometriotic implants by morphologic appearance and capacity to synthesize prostaglandin F. *Fertil. Steril.*, **46**, 801–6.
29. Sharpe, K.L. and Vernon, M.W. (1993). Polypeptides synthesized and released by rat endometriotic tissue differ from those of uterine endometrium in culture. *Biol. Reprod.*, **48**, 1334–40
30. Nothnick, W.B., Curry, T.E. Jr and Vernon, M.W. (1994). Immunomodulation of rat endometriotic implant growth and protein production. *Am. J. Reprod. Immunol.*, **31**, 151–62
31. Sharpe, K.L., Zimmer, R.L., Khan, R.S. and Penney, L.L. (1992). Proliferative and morphogenic changes induced by the coculture of rat uterine and peritoneal cells: a cell culture model for endometriosis. *Fertil. Steril.*, **58**, 1220–9
32. Cuhna, G.R., Chung, L.W.K., Shannon, J.M. and Reese, B.A. (1980). Stromal–epithelial interactions in sex differentiation. *Biol. Reprod.*, **22**, 19–42
33. Cunha, G.R., Shannon, J.M., Tahuchi, O., Fuji, H. and Meloy, B.A. (1983). Epithelial–mesenchymal interactions in hormone induced development. In Sawyer, R.H. and Fallon, J.F. (eds.) *Epithelial–Mesenchymal Interactions in Development*, pp. 51–74. (New York: Praeger Publishers)
34. Sharpe-Timms, K.L., Penney, L.L., Zimmer, R.L., Wright, J.A., Zhang, Y. and Surewicz, J. (1995). Partial purification and amino acid sequence analysis of endometriosis protein-II (Endo-II) reveals homology with tissue inhibitor of metalloproteinase-1 (TIMP-1). *J. Clin. Endocrinol. Metab.*, **80**, 3784–7
35. Woessner, J.F. Jr (1991). Matrix metalloproteinases and their inhibitors in connective tissue remodeling. *FASEB J.*, **5**, 2145–54
36. Bertaux, B., Hornebeck, W., Eisen, Z.A. and Dubertret, L. (1991). Growth stimulation of

human keratinocytes by tissue inhibitors of metalloproteinases. *J. Invest. Dermatol.*, **97**, 679–85.

37. Hayakawa, T., Yamashita, K., Tanazawa, K., Uchijima, E. and Iwata, K. (1992). Growth promoting activity of tissue inhibitor of metalloproteinase-1 (TIMP-1) for a wide range of cells. A possible new growth factor in serum. *FEBS Lett.*, **298**, 29–32

38. Johnson, M.D., Kim, H.-R.C., Chesler, L., Tsao-Wu, G., Bouck, N. and Polverini, P.J. (1994). Inhibition of angiogenesis by tissue inhibitor of metalloproteinase. *J. Cell. Physiol.*, **160**, 194–202

39. Takigawa, M., Nishida, Y., Suzuki, F., Kishi, J., Yamashita, K. and Hayakawa, T. (1990). Induction of angiogenesis in chick yolk-sac membrane by polyamines and its inhibition by tissue inhibitors of metalloproteinases (TIMP and TIMP-2). *Biochem. Biophys. Res. Commun.*, **171**, 1264–71

40. Moses, M.A., Sudhalter, J. and Langer, R. (1990). Identification of an inhibitor of neovascularization from cartilage. *Science*, **248**, 1408–10

41. Nothnick, W.B., Cooke, R.G. III and Kennedy, J.L. III (1996). Elevated tissue inhibitors of metalloproteinase activity in the peritoneal fluid of women with endometriosis. Presented at the *52nd Annual Meeting of the American Society for Reproductive Medicine*, November, Boston

42. Chua, C.C. and Chua, B.H. (1990). Tumor necrosis factor alpha induces mRNA for collagenase and TIMP-1 in human skin fibroblasts. *Conn. Tissue Res.*, **25**, 161–70

43. Murphy, G., Reynolds, J.J. and Werb, Z. (1985). Biosynthesis of the tissue inhibitor of metalloproteinase by human fibroblasts in culture. Stimulation by 12-*O*-tetradecanoylphorbol 13-acetate and interleukin-1 in parallel with collagenase. *J. Biol. Chem.*, **260**, 3079–82

44. Nothnick, W.B., Curry, T.E. Jr, Muse, K.N., London, S.N. and Vernon, M.W. (1994). Detection of a unique 32 kD protein in the peritoneal fluid of women with endometriosis. *Fertil. Steril.*, **61**, 288–93

45. Sharpe-Timms, K.L., Zhang, Y.L. and Surewicz, K. (1996). Amino acid sequence and cDNA sequence analyses of endometriosis protein-I (Endo-I) reveal homology with haptoglobin-related protein. Presented at the *52nd Annual Meeting of the American Society for Reproductive Medicine*, November, Boston

46. Sigal, L.H. (1994). The acute phase response to inflammation. In Sigal, L.H. and Ron, Y. (eds.) *Immunology and Inflammation: Basic Mechanisms and Clinical Consequences*, pp. 287–302. (New York: McGraw-Hill)

47. Strieter, R.M., Reick, D.G., Ward, P.A., Spengler, R.N., Lynch, J.P. III, Larrick, J. and Kunkel, S.L. (1988). Cellular and molecular regulation of tumor necrosis factor-alpha production by pentoxifylline. *Biochem. Biophys. Res. Commun.*, **155**, 1230–6

48. Sullivan, G.W., Carper, H.T., Novick, W.J. Jr and Mandell, G.L. (1988). Inhibition of the inflammatory action of interleukin-1 and tumor necrosis factor (alpha) on neutrophil function by pentoxifylline. *Infect. Immun.*, **56**, 1722–9

49. Steinleitner, A., Lambert, H., Suarez, M., Serpa, N. and Roy, S. (1991). Immunomodulation in the treatment of endometriosis-associated subfertility: use of pentoxifylline to reverse the inhibition of fertilization by surgically-induced endometriosis in a rodent model. *Fertil. Steril.*, **56**, 975–9

Endometrial immunology in endometriosis

P. Miron, M.-H. Lachapelle and D.C. Roy

As in recurrent abortion[1], the hypothesis of immunological dysregulation has been raised by several authors to explain the pathogenesis of endometriosis. Cellular immunity, mostly the cytotoxic activity of peripheral and peritoneal natural killer cells (NK) against endometrial cells, is clearly decreased in cases of endometriosis. Moreover, an increased resistance of endometrial cells to the NK-mediated cytotoxicity has equally been reported[2,3].

Our research was designed to elucidate the immunological mechanisms involved, at the endometrial level, in endometriosis. More specifically, the purposes of our study were to compare: (1) the immunophenotypic profile of T and B lymphocytes, NK cells and monocytes in endometrial stroma; and (2) the major histocompatibility complex (MHC) class I expression on glandular endometrial cells in women with or without endometriosis.

Methods

The profiles of endometrial leukocytes and peripheral blood mononuclear cells (PBMC) were studied in patients with or without endometriosis by means of flow cytometry. Endometrial leukocytes were isolated and analyzed by a previously described methodology[4]. PBMC were prepared by Ficoll–hypaque centrifugation gradient, as previously described[5].

The enriched leukocyte fractions, retrieved from endometrial biopsies and peripheral blood, were marked with a panel of monoclonal antibodies (CD3, CD4, CD8, CD14, CD16, CD20, CD45, CD56) and then analyzed by flow cytometry on a FACScan® machine, with the use of standard techniques[6]. MHC class I expression on glandular endometrial cells was also studied, by both flow cytometry and immunohistochemistry.

Results

We found that the immunophenotypic profile of endometrial leukocytes of women with endometriosis differed from that of controls. In women with endometriosis, a significant decrease in endometrial T lymphocytes was observed, while endometrial NK cells and B lymphocytes were significantly increased ($p < 0.05$). No difference was seen in any peripheral blood lymphocyte subsets between women with or without endometriosis.

With the use of flow cytometry, MHC class I surface antigen was found to be overexpressed in women with endometriosis, compared to women without endometriosis. Similar results were obtained with immunohistochemistry staining.

Our results clearly demonstrate an immunological endometrial dysregulation in women with endometriosis. Of particular interest, in this study, is the increased percentage of NK cells in the endometrial stroma and the overexpression of MHC class I antigen on fresh glandular endometrial cells of women with endometriosis. Over recent years, a negative-signaling model has been proposed, to explain the molecular mechanisms underlying target cell MHC class I and NK cell interaction, in which NK cells would have two types of surface receptor[7]. One, known as the NKR-P1 receptor, triggers killing by NK cells. The activation of these cells to kill normal cells through this receptor would be prevented by a second receptor, which recognizes self MHC class I molecules. Recent reports have shown that MHC class I molecules, when expressed on the target cell surface, can down-regulate NK killing. In the human, several receptors for MHC class I, such as GL183, CD94 and EB6, have been described on the NK cell surface[8]. Semino and co-workers[9], in a recent publication, were also able to demonstrate that cultured endometrial cells, expressing decreased levels of MHC class I with time, could be lysed more efficiently than freshly isolated cells, expressing a 'normal' level of HLA molecules.

In conclusion, it is very tempting to postulate that the endometrial resistance to NK cells found in endometriosis is directly related to an overexpression of MHC class I surface antigen on glandular endometrial cells. It remains to be proven if this overexpression of MHC class I in endometriosis is genetically linked or is up-regulated *in vivo* by extrinsic immune or inflammatory stimuli such as interferon-α, -β and -γ, tumor necrosis factor and lymphotoxin, cytokines known to increase the levels of expression of MHC class I molecules.

References

1. Lachapelle, M.H., Miron, P., Hemmings, R. and Roy, D.C. (1996). Endometrial T, B, and NK cells in patients with recurrent spontaneous abortion. *J. Immunol.*, **156**, 4027–34
2. Oosterlynck, D.J., Meuleman, C., Waer, M., Vandeputte, M. and Koninckx, P.R. (1992). The natural killer activity of peritoneal fluid lymphocytes is decreased in women with endometriosis. *Fertil. Steril.*, **58**, 290
3. Oosterlynck, D.J., Cornillie, F.J., Waer, M., Vandeputte, M. and Koninckx, P.R. (1991). Women with endometriosis show a defect in natural killer activity resulting in a decreased cytotoxicity to autologous endometrium. *Fertil. Steril.*, **56**, 45
4. Lachapelle, M.-H., Miron, P., Hemmings, R., Baron, C. and Roy, D.C. (1996). Flow-cytometric characterization of hematopoietic cells in non-pregnant human endometrium. *Am. J. Reprod. Immunol.*, **35**, 5–13
5. Boyum, A. (1968). Isolation of mononuclear cells and granulocytes from human blood. *Scand. J. Clin. Lab. Invest.*, **21**, 77
6. Roy, D.C., Tantravahi, R., Murray, C., Dear, K., Gorgone, B. and Anderson, K.C. (1990). Natural history of mixed chimerism after bone marrow transplantation with CD6-depleted allogeneic marrow: a stable equilibrium. *Blood*, **75**, 296–304
7. Carbone, E., Terrazzano, G., Colonna, M., Tuosto, L., Piccolella, E., Franksson, L., Palazzolo, G., Pérez-Villar, J.J., Fontana, S., Kärre, K. and Zappacosta, S. (1996). Natural killer clones recognize specific soluble HLA class I molecules. *Eur. J. Immunol.*, **26**, 683–9
8. Moretta, A., Vitale, M., Sivori, S., Bottino, C., Morelli, L., Augugliano, R. *et al.* (1990). Human natural killer cell receptors for HLA class I molecules. Evidence that the Kp43 (CD94) molecule functions as receptor for HLA-B alleles. *J. Exp. Med.*, **94**, 545–55
9. Semino, C., Semino, A., Pietra, G., Mingari, M.C., Barocci, S., Venturini, P.L., Ragni, N. and Melioli, G. (1995). Role of major histocompatibility complex class I expression and natural killer-like T cells in the genetic control of endometriosis. *Fertil. Steril.*, **64**, 909–16

Peritoneal macrophages: a possible role in infertility associated with mild endometriosis

R. Honda, K. Matsuura, Y. Fukumatsu, C. Onoda and H. Okamura

Introduction

The cause of infertility in patients with minimal and mild endometriosis is not clearly understood. Several studies have demonstrated that endometriosis is associated with the activation of peritoneal macrophages[1,2]. In our previous study[3], human peritoneal macrophages were divided into four subtypes according to the localization of endogenous peroxidase activity, namely resident, exudate, exudate-resident and peroxidase-negative macrophages. We also reported that the total number and the proportion of exudate type of macrophages in peritoneal fluid of patients with endometriosis were significantly increased compared with those in patients with uterine leiomyoma[4]. In this study, to investigate the significance of peritoneal macrophages in patients with endometriosis, we examined the effects of peritoneal macrophages on fertilization and embryonic development in a mouse *in vitro* fertilization (IVF) model by using a co-culture method.

Materials and methods

Peritoneal macrophage preparation

Peritoneal macrophages were harvested by irrigation of the peritoneal cavity of adult female (C57BL/6 × DBA)F1 mice (Japan SLC, Shizuoka, Japan) with 5 ml of RPMI 1640 medium 24 h after intraperitoneal injection of either saline or thioglycolate to collect resident and exudate macrophages, respectively.

After the cells were washed twice in RPMI 1640, they were plated at a density of 1.0×10^6 cells/well in a four-well dish (Nunc). After 1 h incubation at 37 °C to allow macrophages to adhere to the bottom of the culture dishes, the cultures were washed twice with human tubal fluid (HTF) medium to remove non-adherent cells. HTF medium (1 ml) supplemented with 3 mg/ml of bovine serum albumin (BSA) was then added for co-culturing.

Mouse *in vitro fertilization*

Four- to 6-week-old (C57BL/6 × DBA)F1 female mice (Japan SLC) were superovulated with a 5 IU intraperitoneal injection of equine chorionic gonadotropin (ECG; Serotropin, Teikoku Zouki, Tokyo, Japan), followed 48 h later by an intraperitoneal injection of 5 IU of human chorionic gonadotropin (hCG, HCG; Mochida Pharmaceutical, Tokyo, Japan). Sixteen hours after the hCG injection, the mice were killed by cervical dislocation and their oviducts were dissected. The cumulus masses containing oocytes were exposed to HTF medium containing 1 mg/ml hyaluronidase for 1 min to dissociate the cumulus cells. The cumulus-free oocytes were then washed twice in HTF medium and allocated to either a control group (medium alone) or co-culture groups.

Mature (C57BL/6 × DBA)F1 male mice (Japan SLC) were killed by cervical dislocation; their cauda epididymi were dissected and placed in HTF medium supplemented with

Table 1 Effect of homologous peritoneal macrophages (Mφ) on in vitro fertilization in the mouse

	No. of oocytes	No. of two-cell embryos (%)
Control (HTF only)	125	112 (89.6)
Co-culture with resident Mφ	141	99 (70.2)*
Co-culture with exudate Mφ	150	84 (56.0)*†

HTF, human tubal fluid; *$p < 0.05$ compared with control; †$p < 0.05$ compared with resident Mφ co-culture group

Table 2 Effect of homologous peritoneal macrophages (Mφ) on embryonic development in vitro

	No. of two-cell embryos	No. of blastocysts (%)
Control (HTF only)	112	43 (38.4)
Co-culture with resident Mφ	99	60 (60.6)*
Co-culture with exudate Mφ	84	57 (67.9)*

HTF, human tubal fluid; *$p < 0.01$ compared with control

3 mg/ml BSA. After incision of the tissue, spermatozoa were allowed to disperse into the medium and were then incubated for 90 min at 37°C under 5% CO_2 in air. The oocytes were inseminated with motile spermatozoa (final concentration of 50×10^4 cells/ml). Twenty-four hours after insemination, the fertilization rates were calculated by determining the number of normal-appearing two-cell embryos. Embryonic development was observed every 24 h up to 96 h after insemination with an inverted microscope. The percentage of embryos developing normally was calculated on the basis of the fertilization rate.

Results

A total of 416 oocytes were allocated to either control or co-culture in three consecutive experiments. The fertilization rate (total number of two-cell embryos per total number of oocytes, counted 24 h after insemination) in three groups is shown in Table 1. The fertilization rates in the co-culture groups were significantly lower than that in the control group ($p < 0.05$). In the co-culture with exudate macrophages, the fertilization rate was significantly lower than that in co-culture with resident macrophages ($p < 0.05$). Although the fertilization rates in the co-culture groups were significantly lower than that in the control group, the rates of development from the two-cell stage to the blastocyst stage (total number of blastocysts per total number of two-cell embryos) were significantly higher in the co-culture groups ($p < 0.01$) (Table 2).

Discussion

Since peritoneal macrophages have access to the oviducts through peritoneal fluid, the micro-environment in which fertilization and embryonic development occur may be influenced either directly or indirectly by these cells. In our previous study, the total number and the proportion of exudate type of macrophages in peritoneal fluid of patients with endometriosis were significantly increased compared with those in the patients with uterine leiomyoma.

Exudate macrophages, showing peroxidase activity only in cytoplasmic granules, are thought to be an activated type of peritoneal macrophage[4]. They exudate from peripheral blood into the peritoneal cavity with higher phagocytic activity according to the pathological conditions. In animal experiments, exudate macrophages are also recovered from peritoneal lavage after stimulation of the peritoneal cavity by intraperitoneal injection of chemical substances such as thioglycolate.

In this study, peritoneal macrophages had an adverse influence on the fertilization process, with exudate macrophages especially having a stronger adverse effect on fertilization. Peritoneal macrophages have been shown to phagocytize and degrade spermatozoa *in vitro*, and they may cause infertility in patients with endometriosis by increasing activity of phagocytosis[5]. It is possible that such phagocytosis and degeneration also contributed to the lower fertilization rate in our co-culture groups. It has been shown that the increase of the cytokine levels, produced by activated macrophages, in the peritoneal fluid of patients with endometriosis may contribute to infertility. In our previous study[6], there was no inhibitory effect of interleukin-1, interleukin-5 and interleukin-6 on fertilization and embryonic development.

The current study therefore suggests that peritoneal macrophages directly impair the process of fertilization. On the other hand, the present study showed that peritoneal macrophages enhance mouse embryonic development at an early stage *in vitro*. It is not well understood how they extend their beneficial effect to embryonic development. It is thought that peritoneal macrophages may release specific or non-specific embryotrophic substances that enhance the metabolism of embryos.

References

1. Halme, J., Becker, S., Hammond, M.G., Raj, M.H.G. and Raj, S. (1983). Increased activation of pelvic macrophages in infertile women with mild endometriosis. *Am. J. Obstet. Gynecol.*, **145**, 333–7
2. Fakih, H., Baggett, B., Holtz, G., Tsang, K., Lee, J.C. and Williamson, H.O. (1987). Interleukin-1: a possible role in the infertility associated with endometriosis. *Fertil. Steril.*, **47**, 213–17
3. Miyamura, S., Okamura, H., Naito, M. and Takahashi, K. (1987). Ultracytochemical localization of peroxidase activity in human peritoneal macrophages. *J. Clin. Electron Microsc.*, **20**, 449–50
4. Fukumatsu, Y., Katabuchi, H., Miyamura, S., Matsuura, K., Naito, M., Takahashi, K. and Okamura, H. (1989). Ultracytochemical observations of endogenous peroxidase activity of peritoneal macrophages in patients with endometriosis. In *Proceedings of XIIIth World Congress on Fertility and Sterility*, Vol. IV, pp. 67–73. (Carnforth: Parthenon)
5. Muscato, J.J., Haney, A.F. and Weinberg, J.B. (1982). Sperm phagocytosis by human peritoneal macrophages: a possible cause of infertility in endometriosis. *Am. J. Obstet. Gynecol.*, **144**, 503–10
6. Yang, G.Y., Matsuura, K., Honda, R., Fukumatsu, Y., Kawano, T. and Okamura, H. (1993). Effect of human recombinant interleukins on *in vitro* fertilization and early embryonic development of mouse. *Jpn. J. Fertil. Steril.*, **38**, 91–5

Effect of autoantibodies on embryo implantation

19

W.P. Dmowski

Introduction

In 1980, Weed and Arguembourg[1] demonstrated with immunofluorescence the presence of IgG and C3 deposits in the endometrial tissues from women with endometriosis, but not from healthy controls. This indirect evidence for antigen–antibody reaction led them to the following hypothesis. In women with endometriosis, endometriotic antigens in the peritoneal cavity stimulate the immune system to produce anti-endometrial autoantibodies. These autoantibodies subsequently react with endometrial antigens in the uterine cavity leading to implantation failure and increased frequency of miscarriages (Figure 1). Subsequent studies from several laboratories demonstrated a high frequency of anti-endometrial antibodies, as well as antibodies directed against cell-derived antigens and the presence of other autoimmune phenomena in women with endometriosis. An association between abnormal autoantibodies and reproductive failure has been demonstrated by investigators studying recurrent spontaneous abortions, intrauterine growth retardation, fetal death and unexplained infertility. Simultaneously, the development of *in vitro* fertilization–embryo transfer (IVF–ET) technology has allowed investigation and better understanding of the sequential steps in human reproduction, implicating the anti-implantation effect as the mechanism of autoantibody action. Thus although the specific effect of the autoantibodies on the reproductive function is still unclear, the data accumulated during the past 15 years provide evidence in support of the hypothesis of Weed and Arguembourg.

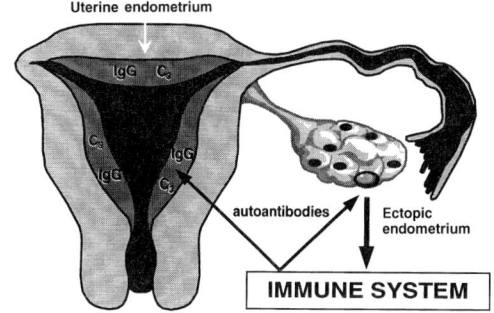

Figure 1 Autoimmune phenomena in endometriosis; findings and hypothesis of Weed and Arguembourg[1]

Anti-endometrial autoantibodies in endometriosis

The first report indicating the presence of anti-endometrial antibodies in the circulation is credited to Mathur and colleagues[2]. These authors, using passive hemagglutination techniques, demonstrated circulating anti-endometrial and anti-ovarian antibodies in women with endometriosis. Subsequently, other investigators using immunofluorescence, immunodiffusion, immunoelectrophoresis, immunohistochemistry, immunoblotting, enzyme-linked immunosorbent assay (ELISA) and cell ELISA techniques confirmed the initial study and over 30 reports have been published, only one of which is contradictory[3]. The latter study can probably be dismissed because of numerous technical problems[4]. The autoantibodies of IgG, IgM and IgA isotypes have been identified in the endometrium (both eutopic and ectopic), circulation and peritoneal fluid as well as other body fluids. There is, however, no agreement as to the frequency of anti-endometrial antibodies in women with endometriosis and in normal controls, and the selection of the subject populations seems to play a significant role. Using an indirect immunofluorescence technique and monolayer cultures of an endometrial carcinoma cell line, Wild and associates reported that the sensitivity of their assay was as high as 83%, and the specificity 76%[5].

The circulating anti-endometrial antibodies seem to bind to eutopic as well as ectopic endometrium[6], and to the cytoplasm of the epithelial but not stromal cells[7]. Interestingly, these autoantibodies bind to the endometrial cells from healthy women and from endometriosis patients, and to the cultured cell lines. Wild and associates demonstrated that this binding is a specific antigen–antibody reaction mediated by F(ab′)$_2$ fragment[8]. Several investigators have attempted to identify endometrial antigens which are the targets for the anti-endometrial antibodies. It appears that anti-endometrial autoantibodies bind to multiple antigens present in the endometria of both healthy women and women with endometriosis (non-specific antigens). There are also specific antigens identified only in the endometria from women with endometriosis. Molecular weights of the specific antigens seem quite variable, according to different investigators. Mathur and associates identified several with molecular weights 26, 34, 42, 82, 94, 110, 120 and 140 kDa[9,10]. Rajkumar and colleagues[11] isolated one specific antigen of molecular weight 34 kDa, Gorai and colleagues[12] three of molecular weights 26, 34 and 42 kDa, Kim and associates[13] three of molecular weights 71, 92 and 103 kDa, and Odukoya and colleagues[6] two of molecular weights 60 and 66 kDa. The most recent report from Mathur and colleagues suggests that there may be two specific antigens of molecular weights 64 and 72 kDa, and homology with α2-Heremans Schmidt (HS) glycoprotein and transferrin[14]. Both of these proteins are constituents of the normal endometria, but the antibodies were most likely produced against genetically or microbially altered antigen molecules.

Most investigators agree that the circulating anti-endometrial antibody levels do not change significantly during the menstrual cycle and that there is no effect of the stage of the disease. A report by Fernandez-Shaw and colleagues[15] suggests that the prevalence of anti-endometrial antibodies may be higher in women with endometriosis and infertility than in those with endometriosis and no fertility problems.

Autoantibodies against cell-derived antigens in endometriosis

The presence of abnormal antibodies against structural cell elements in women with endometriosis was first reported by Gleicher and associates[16]. Subsequently over 20 reports from six different laboratories confirmed high prevalence of such autoantibodies in the circulation, and in the peritoneal and other body fluids of affected women. Although most of the investigators studied only one or two of the possible antibodies, most commonly lupus anticoagulant, anti-cardiolipin or anti-nuclear antibodies, there is a rationale for evaluation of a complete panel[17]. Such a panel includes IgG, IgA and IgM isotypes of antibodies directed against seven phospholipids (cardiolipin, phosphatidyl-serine, phosphatidyl-glycerol, phosphatidyl-ethanolamine, phosphatidyl-inositol, phosphatidic acid and phosphatidyl-choline), five histone subfractions (H1, H2A, H2B, H3, H4) and the nucleus (ssDNA, dsDNA, poly(I), poly(dT)). There is no agreement as to the prevalence of these autoantibodies in women with and without endometriosis.

Although in the original study by Gleicher and colleagues[16], two-thirds of women with endometriosis had some type of autoantibody anomaly, the prevalence of individual autoantibodies varied from 7.5 to 45.5%. Several studies evaluated the effect of the cycle phase on autoantibody positivity, but none was demonstrated. The effect of stage, however, is not entirely clear. Kilpatrick and colleagues[18] found no differences in the mean anti-cardiolipin antibody levels in different stages of endometriosis. Gleicher and colleagues[16] and Taylor and associates[19], on the other hand, demonstrated decreasing prevalence and decreasing levels of abnormal autoantibodies with increasing stage of the disease. Several studies indicate that antibodies against cell-derived antigens, similarly to anti-endometrial antibodies, may be more prevalent if endometriosis is associated with infertility.

Other autoimmune phenomena in endometriosis

In addition to the antibodies listed above and directed against cell-derived antigens or endometrial tissues, other autoimmune phenomena have also been described in endometriosis. Fernandez-Shaw and colleagues[15] reported circulating anti-endothelial antibodies which reacted with vascular endothelium in the endometrium as well as in other tissues. Taylor and associates[19] reported a higher prevalence of autoantibodies to ribonucleoproteins in endometriosis than in controls. Other investigators observed autoantibodies against organs (organ-specific) or tissues (tissue-specific), such as ovary, thyroid, skeletal and smooth muscle. There is, however, no agreement as to the presence or frequency of such antibodies[6]. A recent publication by D'Cruz and colleagues[20] reports higher prevalence and an association with infertility of autoantibodies to carbonic anhydrase in women with endometriosis as compared to normal controls. A decrease in the *in vitro* IgG production in advanced, as opposed to early endometriosis has been reported by Gebel and co-workers[21]. This is an interesting finding, in view of the already-mentioned higher levels of abnormal autoantibodies in early stages of the disease reported by other investigators. Circulating levels of CA-125 antigen are increased in endometriosis, but not to the same extent as in ovarian neoplasia. There are, however, contradictory data on immunoglobulin and complement concentrations in the peripheral circulation of women with endometriosis.

Multiple autoantibodies against different tissues indicate polyclonal B cell activation, and prompted Gleicher and associates[16] to consider endometriosis as a form of an autoimmune disease. In addition to polyclonal B cell activation, endometriosis shares with autoimmune diseases several other characteristics such as multi-organ involvement, familial occurrence with possible genetic basis, female preponderance, tissue damage and association with other autoimmune diseases. There is, however, no data to support the concept that autoantibodies play a role in the pathogenesis of endometriosis. Danazol, an agent effective in the treatment of endometriosis, is known to suppress abnormal autoantibodies in several autoimmune diseases. Treatment with danazol lowers abnormal autoantibodies in endometriosis and may also improve reproductive performance[22–24].

Autoantibodies and reproductive function

Endometriosis can only be diagnosed by a direct visualization of the endometriotic lesions or by biopsy of suspicious areas. Several reports indicate that subclinical, microscopic endometriosis may frequently escape clinical diagnosis. Some of such patients with infertility problems may then be included in the category of 'unexplained infertility'. It is, therefore, not a surprise that several investigators identified higher prevalence and higher levels of abnormal autoantibodies in unexplained infertility as compared to normal controls[25–27]. In women with autoimmune diseases such as systemic lupus erythematosus, the presence of abnormal autoantibodies has been associated with high pregnancy wastage. In healthy women with abnormal autoantibodies, there is also a high incidence of reproductive failure. Recurrent spontaneous abortions, intrauterine growth retardation, intrauterine fetal death, and pregnancy-induced hypertension leading to pre-eclampsia have all been reported. In such patients, thrombosis in placental vessels and thrombocytopenia are a frequent finding. These conditions in otherwise healthy women without evidence of an autoimmune disease have variously been referred to as lupus anticoagulant syndrome (LACS)[28], reproductive autoimmune failure syndrome (RAFS)[29], anti-cardiolipin syndrome (ACLS)[30] or anti-phospholipid syndrome (APLS)[31]. It appears that all acronyms may refer to the same subclinical form of the autoimmune disease affecting reproductive performance. It is unclear at this time what is the role of autoantibodies in this condition and what is the mechanism of anti-fertility effects. It has been suggested that autoantibodies induce thrombosis in spiral arteries of the endometrium and in the placenta causing infarctions and decreased blood supply to the conceptus[32]. Others have proposed that abnormal autoantibodies, especially of the anti-phospholipid group, bind to the trophoblast and alter its function[33]. Several studies indicate that treatment with glucocorticoids, which presumably suppress abnormal autoantibodies, as well as anti-coagulant therapy such as aspirin and heparin, may improve reproductive performance in affected patients[17].

Effect of abnormal autoantibodies on *in vitro* fertilization success rates

The development and popularization of Assisted Reproductive Technologies during the past 15 years has led to better understanding of the human reproductive function and has allowed new insights into various aspects of infertility. Studies of different *in vitro* fertilization (IVF) cycle parameters provide information on specific phases of the reproductive process such as the response to gonadotropin stimulation, oocyte development, egg and sperm interaction, early embryo development and implantation. The most inefficient step in this process is embryo implantation with implantation rates per embryo seldom exceeding 10–15%. In evaluating abnormal autoantibodies in patients undergoing IVF, several investigators have reported a high prevalence of autoantibodies in failed IVF cycles[34–38]. El-Roeiy and associates[34] demonstrated a higher concentration of autoantibodies in the follicular fluids than in sera. The initial concern that the IVF procedures may somehow lead to the development of abnormal autoantibodies was, however, not substantiated. Fisch and colleagues[36], who measured anti-phospholipid antibodies before, during and after the IVF cycle, indicated that although the IVF patients had higher levels of autoantibodies than normal controls, there was no change in the autoantibody level as a result of the IVF cycle. On the other hand, several studies have demonstrated that the presence of autoantibodies affects IVF outcome. Birkenfeld and colleagues[37] reported that 18 of 56 patients (32%) who failed IVF-embryo transfer (IVF-ET) were autoantibody-positive, as compared to none of 14 who conceived with IVF and seven of 69 (10%) in the unselected group of new IVF candidates. Geva and associates[38] went a step further. They measured several autoantibodies in a group of 21 women who had chemical, but no clinical pregnancies as a result of the IVF cycle. The prevalence of autoantibodies in this group was 33.3% as compared to none of 21 women who conceived and delivered with the IVF and embryo transfer treatment. These data clearly suggest anti-implantation effects of abnormal autoantibodies.

This anti-implantation effect of abnormal autoantibodies appears to be reversed by treatment. Birkenfeld and colleagues[37] reported that seven of 15 autoantibody-positive patients who had previously failed IVF-ET conceived during a subsequent IVF-ET cycle while on treatment with prednisone and aspirin. In another study, Sher and colleagues[39] reported that treatment with aspirin and heparin increased the pregnancy rate per transfer in autoantibody-positive women from 16 to 49%.

Effect of endometriosis on *in vitro* fertilization success rates

The procedures performed during the IVF-ET cycle correct or identify most of the mechanisms of infertility implicated in endometriosis. Aspiration of the eggs with laparoscopically or sonographically guided needle, *in vitro* fertilization, early embryonic development in the laboratory, and ultimately transfer of the developing embryos into the female reproductive system, all IVF-ET related procedures, correct for or identify problems caused by endocrine or ovulatory dysfunction, abnormal fertilization, failure of early embryonic development, or abnormal ovum pick-up or transport. Thus one would expect IVF pregnancy rates to be comparable in patients with and without endometriosis.

Indeed, according to most of the reports, IVF pregnancy rates seem to be at least as high in endometriosis as in other diagnostic entities. It is generally agreed that there is no adverse effect of the disease on patients' response to stimulation or the number of eggs retrieved. An exception may be advanced endometriosis, where several investigators have reported fewer follicles and lower numbers of eggs retrieved[40–43]. It is likely that women with advanced disease, especially after repeated ovarian resections, produce fewer follicles and fewer eggs. There is also a general consensus that endometriosis does not adversely affect the fertilization process, although lower fertilization rates in early endometriosis have been noted by some[43]. The majority of published reports indicate that neither endometriosis nor its stage adversely affect IVF pregnancy rates. Nevertheless, two recent reports suggest lower pregnancy and lower implantation rates in endometriosis as compared to tubal disease[43,44]. One of these studies implicated poor quality of the embryos as a cause of implantation failure. The authors reported that in their oocyte donation program the lowest implantation rate (7%) was noted when embryos originated from oocytes retrieved from women with endometriosis[44]. In contrast, implantation rates were 16% for embryos derived from oocytes of fertile donors. In the other report the implantation rate was much lower in stage I and II (2.8%) as opposed to stage III and IV endometriosis (5.5%) and tubal factor infertility (8.1%)[43].

It is unclear whether, and if so to what extent, endometriosis affects the implantation rates. The results of contradictory reports need to be interpreted with caution, taking into account the design of each study and patient selection. In a recent study of 239 consecutive oocyte recipients, there was no apparent difference in the implantation rates in the presence of endometriosis ($n = 55$, implantation rate 12%) or in its absence ($n = 184$, implantation rate 13%)[45]. However, the autoantibody status was not tested in this study. It is possible that abnormal autoantibodies in follicular fluids may affect fertilization *in vitro* and early embryo development, and may interfere with subsequent implantation. This concept is supported by a recent report indicating that anti-phospholipid antibodies bind to mouse pre-embryos[46]. If so, the practice of repeated washing and cumulus–corona cell removal during egg collection at some laboratories may explain similar fertilization rates, embryo development and implantation rates in endometriosis and tubal disease[47].

In our experience, the overall IVF pregnancy rates are similar in endometriosis and other diagnostic entities, and there is no effect of the stage of the disease[48]. However, the differences become apparent when the autoantibody status is considered. We recently analyzed IVF cycle parameters including pregnancy rates in women with endometriosis who were autoantibody positive or negative[48]. There was no difference between the groups in any of the cycle parameters including response to ovarian stimulation, number of

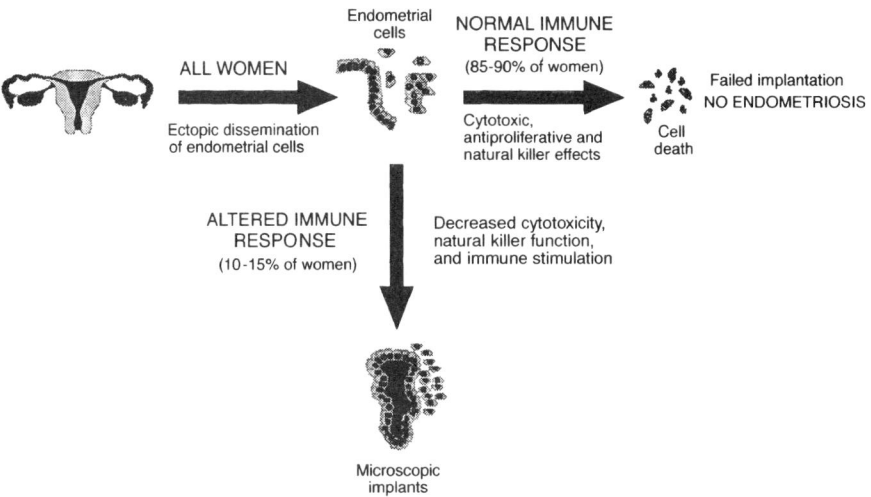

Figure 2 Immune system and endometriosis; the role of the immune response in the development of the disease

follicles produced, number of eggs retrieved, percentage fertilized or number of embryos transferred. There was, however, a significant difference in the pregnancy rates: 22.9% in autoantibody-positive and 45.7% in auto-antibody-negative patients. At the time of IVF-ET some patients had evidence of active disease, while others did not. As expected, active disease was more common in the auto-antibody-positive than in the autoantibody-negative group (80% vs. 36%). Some patients in this study received corticosteroids during the IVF cycle, on an empirical basis to improve the IVF success rates. It is interesting to note that all patients with endometriosis who had three or more autoantibodies and conceived were on corticosteroid treatment. When pregnancy rates were analyzed according to the autoantibody status and the use of corticosteroids, the rationale for the use of these steroids in auto-antibody-positive patients became quite apparent. Autoantibody-positive patients undergoing IVF were more likely to conceive if they were taking corticosteroids. On the other hand, there was no effect of corticosteroids in autoantibody-negative patients.

Conclusions

We can conclude from this review that the hypothesis originally proposed by Weed and Arguembourg[1] still remains valid. The data that have accumulated during the past 15 years indicate that endometriosis is frequently associated with autoimmune phenomena which may lead to infertility and reproductive failure. The exact mechanism through which abnormal autoantibodies affect reproductive performance is unclear, but the data strongly suggest an adverse effect on the embryo, its implantation and subsequent trophoblast development. There is no evidence, however, to indicate that autoimmune phenomena play a role in the pathogenesis of endometriosis.

Studies from our Institute and from other laboratories suggest that endometriosis develops as a result of the specific alteration in the immune response and that autoantibody production is a secondary phenomenon in response to ectopic endometrial growth[49]. According to this concept, endometrial cells are displaced outside of the uterine cavity during menses in all women. In about 85 to 90% of women, these cells are removed from the

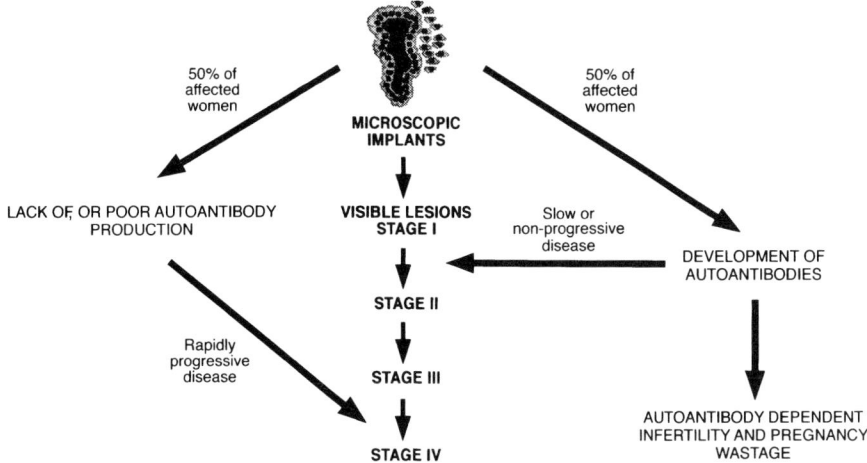

Figure 3 Immune system and endometriosis; the role of autoantibodies in progression of endometriosis and in reduced reproductive performance

ectopic locations by the normally functioning immune system (Figure 2). In about 10 to 15% of women, because of the genetic predisposition or environmental effects, the immune system is unable to remove the misplaced endometrial cells and allows their implantation, leading to endometriosis. Endometriotic cells in ectopic locations stimulate abnormal autoantibody production by B cells in about 50 to 60% of women with endometriosis (Figure 3). These autoantibodies bind to eutopic as well as ectopic endometrial cells. Available data indicate that by binding to the ectopic endometrium, autoantibodies initiate the inflammatory and cytotoxic effect which may limit the progression of endometriosis. Thus the higher the autoantibody concentration, the less invasive is the disease. At the same time, abnormal autoantibodies bind to the eutopic endometrium, also causing cell destruction and leading to failure of embryo implantation, infertility and recurrent miscarriages.

References

1. Weed, J.C. and Arguembourg, P.C. (1980). Endometriosis: can it produce an autoimmune response resulting in infertility? *Clin. Obstet. Gynecol.*, **23**, 885–93
2. Mathur, S., Peress, M.R., Williamson, H.O., Youmans, C.D., Maney, S.A., Garvin, A.J., Rust, P.F. and Fudenberg, H.H. (1982). Autoimmunity to endometrium and ovary in endometriosis. *Clin. Exp. Immunol.*, **50**, 259–66
3. Switchenko, A.C., Kauffman, R.S. and Becker, M. (1991). Are there antiendometrial antibodies in sera of women with endometriosis? *Fertil. Steril.*, **56**, 235–41
4. Wild, R.A., Shivers, C.A. and Medders, D. (1992). Detection of antiendometrial antibodies in patients with endometriosis: methodological issues. *Fertil. Steril.*, **58**, 518–21
5. Wild, R.A., Hirisave, V., Podczaski, E.S., Coulam, C., Shivers, C.A. and Satyaswaroop, P.G. (1991). Autoantibodies associated with endometriosis: can their detection predict presence of the disease? *Obstet. Gynecol.*, **77**, 927–31
6. Odukoya, O.A., Wheatcroft, N., Wetman, A.P. and Cooke, I.D. (1995). The prevalence of endometrial immunoglobulin G antibodies in patients with endometriosis. *Hum. Reprod.*, **10**, 1214–19

7. Wild, R.A., Satyaswaroop, P.G. and Shivers, A.C. (1987). Epithelial localization of antiendometrial antibodies associated with endometriosis. *Am. J. Reprod. Immunol.*, **13**, 62–5
8. Wild, R.A., Medders, D. and Zhang, R. (1991). F(ab')$_2$ segment is the active component of immunoglobulin G autoantibody generation in patients with endometriosis. *Fertil. Steril.*, **56**, 900–3
9. Mathur, S., Chihal, H.J., Homm, R.J., Garza, D.E., Rust, P.F. and Williamson, H.O. (1988). Endometrial antigens involved in the autoimmunity of endometriosis. *Fertil. Steril.*, **50**, 860–3
10. Mathur, S., Garza, D.E. and Smith, I.F. (1990). Endometrial autoantigens eliciting immunoglobulin (Ig)G, IgA, and IgM responses in endometriosis. *Fertil. Steril.*, **54**, 56–63
11. Rajkumar, K., Malliah, V. and Simpson, C.W. (1992). Identifying the presence of antibodies against endometrial antigens. A preliminary study. *J. Reprod. Med.*, **37**, 552–6
12. Gorai, I., Ishikawa, M., Onose, R., Hirahara, F. and Minaguchi, H. (1993). Antiendometrial autoantibodies are generated in patients with endometriosis. *Am. J. Reprod. Immunol.*, **29**, 116–23
13. Kim, J.G., Kim, C.W., Moon, S.Y., Chang, Y.S. and Lee, J.Y. (1995). Detection of antiendometrial antibodies in sera of patients with endometriosis by dual-colored, double-labeling immunohistochemical method and Western blot. *Am. J. Reprod. Immunol.*, **34**, 80–7
14. Mathur, S.P., Zhou, G.X., Arnaud, P., Jiang, H., Butler, W.J. and Zhang, H. (1996). Antibodies to endometrial transferrin and alpha 2-Heremans Schmidt (HS) glycoprotein in patients with endometriosis. *Am. J. Reprod. Immunol.*, **35**, 483–94
15. Fernandez-Shaw, S., Hicks, B.R., Yudkin, P.L., Kennedy, S., Barlow, D.H. and Starkey, P.M. (1993). Anti-endometrial and anti-endothelial autoantibodies in women with endometriosis. *Hum. Reprod.*, **8**, 310–15
16. Gleicher, N., El-Roeiy, A., Confino, E. and Friberg, J. (1987). Is endometriosis an autoimmune disease? *Obstet. Gynecol.*, **70**, 115–22
17. Gleicher, N., Pratt, D. and Dudkiewicz, A. (1993). What do we really know about autoantibody abnormalities and reproductive failure: a critical review. *Autoimmunity*, **16**, 115–40
18. Kilpatrick, D.C., Haining, R.E.B. and Smith, S.S.K. (1991). Are cardiolipin antibody levels elevated in endometriosis? *Fertil. Steril.*, **55**, 436–7
19. Taylor, P.V., Maloney, M.D., Campbell, J.M., Skerrow, S.M., Nip, M.M., Parmar, R. and Tate, G. (1991). Autoreactivity in women with endometriosis. *Br. J. Obstet. Gynaecol.*, **98**, 680–4
20. D'Cruz, O.J., Wild, R.A., Haas, G.G. Jr and Reichlin, M. (1996). Antibodies to carbonic anhydrase in endometriosis: prevalence, specificity, and relationship to clinical and laboratory parameters. *Fertil. Steril.*, **66**, 547–56
21. Gebel, H., Braun, D.P., Rotman, C., Rana, N. and Dmowski, W.P. (1993). Mitogen induced production of polyclonal IgG is decreased in women with severe endometriosis. *Am. J. Reprod. Immunol.*, **29**, 124–30
22. Chihal, H.J., Mathur, S., Holtz, G.L. and Williamson, H.O. (1986). An endometrial antibody assay in the clinical diagnosis and management of endometriosis. *Fertil. Steril.*, **46**, 408–11
23. El-Roeiy, A., Dmowski, W.P., Gleicher, N., Radwanska, E., Harlow, L., Binor, Z., Tummon, I. and Rawlins, R.G. (1988). Danazol but not gonadotropin-releasing hormone agonists suppresses autoantibodies in endometriosis. *Fertil. Steril.*, **50**, 864–71
24. Ota, H., Maki, M., Shidara, Y., Kodama, H., Takahashi, H., Hayakawa, M., Fujimori, R., Kushima, T. and Ohtomo, K. (1992). Effects of danazol at the immunologic level in patients with adenomyosis, with special reference to autoantibodies: a multi-center cooperative study. *Am. J. Obstet. Gynecol.*, **167**, 481–6
25. Gleicher, N., El-Roeiy, A., Confino, E. and Friberg, J. (1989). Reproductive failure because of autoantibodies: unexplained infertility and pregnancy wastage. *Am. J. Obstet. Gynecol.*, **160**, 1376–85
26. Taylor, P.V., Campbell, J.M. and Scott, J.S. (1989). Presence of autoantibodies in women with unexplained infertility. *Am. J. Obstet. Gynecol.*, **161**, 377–9
27. Kim, C.H., Cho, Y.K. and Mok, J.E. (1996). The efficacy of immunotherapy in patients who underwent superovulation with intrauterine insemination. *Fertil. Steril.*, **65**, 133–8
28. Gleicher, N. and Friberg, J. (1985). IgM gammopathy and the lupus anticoagulant syndrome in habitual aborters. *J. Am. Med. Assoc.*, **253**, 3278–81
29. Gleicher, N. and El-Roeiy, A. (1988). The

reproductive autoimmune failure syndrome (RAFS). *Am. J. Obstet. Gynecol.*, **159**, 223–7
30. Hughes, G.R., Harris, N.N. and Gharavi, A.E. (1986). The anticardiolipin syndrome. *J. Rheumatol.*, **13**, 486–9
31. Mackworth-Young, C.G. (1990). Anti-phospholipid antibodies: more than just a disease marker. *Immunol. Today*, **11**, 60–5
32. Feinstein, D.I. (1985). Lupus anticoagulant, thrombosis and fetal loss. *N. Engl. J. Med.*, **313**, 1348–50
33. Rote, N.S. (1996). Antiphospholipid antibodies and recurrent pregnancy loss. *Am. J. Reprod. Immunol.*, **35**, 394–401
34. El-Roeiy, A., Gleicher, N., Friberg, J., Confino, E. and Dudkiewicz, A. (1987). Correlation between peripheral blood and follicular fluid autoantibodies and impact on *in vitro* fertilization. *Obstet. Gynecol.*, **70**, 163–9
35. Fisch, B., Rikover, Y., Shohat, L., Zurgil, N., Tadir, Y., Ovadia, J., Witz, I.P. and Yron, I. (1991). The relationship between *in vitro* fertilization and naturally occurring antibodies: evidence for increased production of antiphospholipid autoantibodies. *Fertil. Steril.*, **56**, 718–24
36. Fisch, B., Fried, S., Manor, Y., Ovadia, J., Witz, I.P. and Yron, I. (1995). Increased antiphospholipid antibody activity in *in-vitro* fertilization patients is not treatment-dependent but rather an inherent characteristic of the infertile state. *Am. J. Reprod. Immunol.*, **34**, 370–4
37. Birkenfeld, A., Mukaida, T., Minichiello, L., Jackson, M., Kase, N.G. and Yemini, M. (1994). Incidence of autoimmune antibodies in failed embryo transfer cycles. *Am. J. Reprod. Immunol.*, **31**, 65–8
38. Geva, E., Yaron, Y., Lessing, J.B., Yovel, I., Vardinon, N., Burke, M. and Amit, A. (1994). Circulating autoimmune antibodies may be responsible for implantation failure in *in vitro* fertilization. *Fertil. Steril.*, **62**, 802–6
39. Sher, G., Feinman, M., Zouves, C., Kuttner, G., Maassarani, G., Salem, R., Matzner, W., Ching, W. and Chong, P. (1994). High fecundity rates following *in-vitro* fertilization and embryo transfer in antiphospholipid antibody seropositive women treated with heparin and aspirin. *Hum. Reprod.*, **9**, 2278–83
40. Chillik, C.F., Acosta, A.A., Garcia, J.E., Perera, S., Van Uem, J.F., Rosenwaks, Z. and Jones, H.W. Jr (1985). The role of *in vitro* fertilization in infertile patients with endometriosis. *Fertil. Steril.*, **44**, 56–61
41. Matson, P.L. and Yovich, J.L. (1986). The treatment of infertility associated with endometriosis by *in vitro* fertilization. *Fertil. Steril.*, **46**, 432–4
42. Dlugi, A.M., Loy, R.A., Dieterle, S., Bayer, S.R. and Seibel, M.M. (1989). The effect of endometriosis on *in vitro* fertilization outcome. *J. In Vitro Fertil. Embryo Transfer*, **6**, 338–41
43. Arici, A., Oral, E., Bukulmez, O., Duleba, A., Olive, D.L. and Jones, E.E. (1996). The effect of endometriosis on implantation: results from the Yale University *in vitro* fertilization and embryo transfer program. *Fertil. Steril.*, **65**, 603–7
44. Simon, C., Gutierrez, A., Vidal, A., de los Santos, M.J., Tarin, J.J., Remohi, J. and Pellicer, A. (1994). Outcome of patients with endometriosis in assisted reproduction: results from *in-vitro* fertilization and oocyte donation. *Hum. Reprod.*, **9**, 725–9
45. Sung, L., Mukherjee, T., Takeshige, T., Bustillo, M. and Copperman, A.B. (1996). Endometriosis is not detrimental to embryo implantation in oocyte recipients. Presented at the *43rd Annual Meeting of the Society for Gynecological Investigation*, March, Philadelphia
46. Coulam, C. (1996). Embryo as a target for APA. Presented at the *Chicago Association of Reproductive Endocrinologists Meeting*, September, Chicago
47. Olivennes, F., Feldberg, D., Hung-Ching, L., Cohen, J., Moy, F. and Rosenwaks, Z. (1995). Endometriosis: a stage by stage analysis – the role of *in vitro* fertilization. *Fertil. Steril.*, **64**, 392–8
48. Dmowski, W.P., Rana, N., Michalowska, J., Friberg, J., Papierniak, C. and El-Roeiy, A. (1995). The effect of endometriosis, its stage and activity, and of autoantibodies on *in vitro* fertilization and embryo transfer success rates. *Fertil. Steril.*, **63**, 555–62
49. Dmowski, W.P. and Braun, D.P. (1995). Immunological aspects of endometriosis. *Contemp. Rev. Obstet. Gynaecol.*, **7**, 167–71

Role of peritoneal inflammation in endometriosis associated with infertility

J.K. Halme

Inflammation in endometriosis

Endometriosis clearly is a chronic (and cyclic) inflammatory disease with the classic triad signs of inflammation present during the progression of the disease: pain, increased vascularity and scarring. Even in the absence of pain, laparoscopic observation or biopsy most often documents the presence of the other two signs in or around peritoneal implants.

In addition to the well-known physiological sources for an inflammatory response in the peritoneal environment such as retrograde flow[1], rupture of a preovulatory follicle and spermatozoa, ectopic endometrial implants provide a non-physiological source in patients with endometriosis associated with infertility (Table 1). *In situ* menstruation around the time of menses has been histologically documented. In addition, local 'breakthrough bleeding' of the ectopic endometrium may also contribute to or enhance this response[2]. In our studies we documented a highly significant increase in the presence of blood in the peritoneal fluid in women with endometriosis as compared to other women when they underwent laparoscopy during the non-perimenstrual part of their cycle[1].

In the past 15 years, abundant evidence has accumulated to document the presence of inflammation in the peritoneal cavity in endometriosis (Table 2). The volume of peritoneal fluid and its content of macrophages are significantly increased in women with mild endometriosis[3-5]. Other evidence for inflammation includes increased prostanoids[6], macrophage activation[7,8], proteolytic enzymes[7] and inflammatory cytokines such as interleukins (IL) 1–10[9-12] and tumor necrosis factor-α (TNF-α)[13] in the peritoneal fluid of patients with endometriosis and infertility. Increased vascularity in and around endometriosis lesions is a well-known phenomenon and indicates the presence of angiogenesis; this has also been confirmed by identification of angiogenic factors in the peritoneal fluid in endometriosis[13-15].

Since the macrophage is the predominant nucleated cell in the peritoneal fluid, it represents the first-line host response to an inflammatory stimulus. Attracted by chemotaxis, these cells extravasate through pores in the vessel

Table 1 Sources of inflammation in peritoneal cavity

Physiological
Retrograde menstruation
Rupture of the ovulating follicle
Sperm

Non-physiological, caused by ectopic implants
In situ menstruation
In situ breakthrough bleeding
Altered response – secretion

Table 2 Signs of inflammation in peritoneal cavity in endometriosis

Increased fluid volume
Increased number and activation of macrophages
Increased release of proteolytic enzymes
Increased secretion of inflammatory cytokines
Increased angiogenesis
Scarring

wall to enter the peritoneal cavity[16]. Both autocrine and paracrine mechanisms are thought to be involved in the cell–cell communication and modification of the cellular interactions. Inflammatory cytokines such as transforming growth factor-β (TGF-β) and interleukins mediate such interactions. In addition, growth factors may provide a mitogenic stimulus for fibroblasts, leading to adhesion formation. Many growth factors, including platelet-derived growth factor (PDGF), fibroblast growth factor (FGF), epidermal growth factor (EGF) and TGF-α and -β have also been shown to be mitogenic for endometrial cells, thus providing a potential stimulus for the growth of ectopic endometrium[17,18].

As a reflection of the inflammatory environment, increased peritoneal fluid volume appears to have a detrimental impact on fecundability. Syrop and Halme[19] found that in patients with endometriosis it took a significantly longer time to achieve pregnancy for those patients with peritoneal fluid volume exceeding 12 ml as compared to those with less fluid. Hormonal suppression of menstrual function by progestin has been shown to result in a significant decrease in both fluid volume and content of macrophages[20].

In view of these data it appears quite likely that endometriosis is associated with an inflammatory exudate in the peritoneal compartment. What, then, are the possible mechanisms by which these inflammatory changes negatively impact on the reproductive process?

Adverse effects on reproduction

Several lines of evidence have accumulated in recent years to document, by direct experiments in various test systems, the fact that peritoneal fluid from patients can possess reproductive toxicity. Generally, these studies require gametes or tissues from other species for testing, except in the case of human sperm function, human semen being readily available.

Of interest are the studies by Suginami and co-workers[21,22], who developed an *in vitro* test of tubal function by utilizing the fimbriae of golden hamsters; they standardized conditions in which the fimbriae captured oocyte–cumulus complexes from superovulated mice. Peritoneal fluid from endometriosis patients appeared to contain inhibitory activity (ovum capture inhibitor, OCI). The source of this activity is not known, but OCI appears to be a large heat-labile protein and its activity in peritoneal fluid is reduced by treatment with danazol.

Peritoneal macrophages that constitute the vast majority of nucleated cells in the peritoneal fluid have been implicated through various mechanisms in mediation of adverse effects on the reproductive process. The direct phagocytosis of sperm, cellular cytotoxicity or release of harmful secretory products by these cells have been investigated.

It is clear that macrophages are primarily responsible for the physiological phagocytosis of cellular debris, including sperm, in the peritoneal fluid. In view of this, several studies have attempted to find evidence for abnormal or increased sperm phagocytosis in the peritoneal fluid of patients with endometriosis[2,23–26]. To date, out of five studies addressing this issue, three found increased phagocytosis compared with the situation in patients without endometriosis[23,24,26].

The ready availability of murine embryos and their widespread use in the quality control of media in embryology laboratories have made it possible to test the effects of peritoneal fluid or macrophage-conditioned media on the *in vitro* development of mouse embryos. Alternatively, *in vivo* models (mouse and rabbit) have been used for this purpose. A total of nine such studies are available in the literature; five of these demonstrate toxic effects on embryo development and four do not[27–34] (see Table 3). The reasons for these discrepant findings are unclear, and well-founded doubts can be raised about the lack of sensitivity of the murine embryo model in prediction of toxicity towards human embryos. For obvious reasons, human embryos are not and will not be easily available for testing purposes.

Since peritoneal fluid or the Fallopian tube immersed in the fluid are the sites where fertilization occurs[23], several studies have addressed the issue of sperm toxicity in patients with endometriosis. Effects of peritoneal fluid or peritoneal macrophage conditioned media from patients have been studied on sperm motility, sperm velocity or zona-free hamster egg penetration (Table 4).

A total of 15 studies have been published between 1982 and 1996[35–49]. Out of these, 13 studies have demonstrated a significant degree of sperm toxicity, whereas only two studies have shown no increased toxicity in endometriosis as compared to that in patients with unexplained infertility, in those with adhesions, or in fertile women (Table 5). In the first of the studies that did not demonstrate toxicity we used heat-treated peritoneal fluid and it has been subsequently shown that the sperm toxicity of peritoneal fluid is heat-labile[39].

In the most recent study on the subject Aeby and co-workers[49] quite convincingly demonstrated that peritoneal fluid from patients with minimal endometriosis significantly decreased both the mean swimming velocity and zona-free hamster egg penetration of normal sperm. With all these data taken into consideration, it thus appears that, indeed, sperm toxicity is the most important mechanism by which the local inflammatory environment in endometriosis negatively impacts on reproduction.

Possible mediators of infertility

In order to identify the specific substance(s) responsible for anti-fertility effects, attempts have been made to test several cytokines, secretory products of either macrophages or lymphocytes, directly for adverse effects *in vitro*. Haimovici and associates[29] tested various concentrations of IL-1, interferon-γ (IFN-γ), IL-2 and TNF and found significant embryotoxicity only with TNF and IFN-γ. IL-1 and IL-2 were not found to exhibit such an effect by Schneider and colleagues[30]. These

Table 3 Embryo toxicity in endometriosis? Studies with peritoneal fluid or macrophage medium

Toxicity demonstrated	No toxicity seen
Morcos et al. (1985)[27]	Schneider et al. (1989)[30]
Hahn et al. (1986)[28]	Awadalla et al. (1987)[25]
Haimovici et al. (1987)[29]	Prough et al. (1990)[31]
Prough et al. (1991)[32]	Dodds et al. (1992)[33]
Taketani et al. (1992)[34]	

Table 4 Types of sperm toxicity demonstrated in peritoneal fluid in endometriosis

Reduced sperm motility/velocity
Reduced acrosome loss
Reduced ovum binding/penetration
Reduced fertilization

Table 5 Sperm toxicity in endometriosis? Studies with peritoneal fluid or macrophage medium

Toxicity demonstrated	No toxicity seen
Oak et al. (1985)[36]	Halme and Hall (1982)[35]
Chacho et al. (1986)[37], (1987)[39]	Leach et al. (1990)[42]
Burke (1987)[38]	
Sueldo et al. (1987)[40]	
Eisermann et al. (1989)[41]	
Coddington et al. (1992)[43]	
Curtis et al. (1993)[44]	
Drudy et al. (1994)[45]	
Arumugam (1994)[46]	
Zullo et al. (1994)[47]	
Tasdemir et al. (1995)[48]	
Aeby et al. (1996)[49]	

two compounds appear, therefore, unlikely to be responsible for deleterious effects, although a preliminary study had so suggested[9].

TNF-α and IFN-γ remain the two cytokines exhibiting gamete toxicity present in the peritoneal fluid of patients with endometriosis. Virtually no information is available about interferon levels in peritoneal fluid, but three of four studies have detected TNF-α-related cytotoxicity in peritoneal fluid in patients with endometriosis[13,41,50,51]. It has also been demonstrated that the spermotoxic activity in peritoneal fluid was directly proportional to the level of TNF-α measured in the fluid samples. Total motility, sperm velocity and zona-free hamster egg penetration were all affected in a dose-dependent fashion[50].

Summary

In summary, there is considerable evidence for the presence of a chronic inflammatory peritoneal environment in patients with endometriosis. The inflammation is not restricted to the tissue surrounding the ectopic implants, since significant changes have been found in the cellular and chemical composition of the peritoneal fluid in these patients. These changes appear to include pronounced gametotoxic properties, predominantly on sperm, that contribute to the reduced fecundability in endometriosis.

References

1. Halme, J., Hammond, M.G., Hulka, J.F., Raj, S.J. and Talbert, L.M. (1984). Retrograde menstruation in healthy women and in patients with endometriosis. *Obstet. Gynecol.*, **64**, 151–4
2. Halme, J., Becker, S. and Wing, R. (1984). Accentuated cyclic activation of peritoneal macrophages in patients with endometriosis. *Am. J. Obstet. Gynecol.*, **148**, 85–90
3. Drake, T.S., Metz, S.A., Grunert, G.M. and O'Brien, W.F. (1980). Peritoneal fluid volume in endometriosis. *Fertil. Steril.*, **34**, 280–3
4. Haney, A.F., Muscato, J.J. and Weinberg, J.B. (1982). Peritoneal fluid cell populations in infertility patients. *Fertil. Steril.*, **35**, 696–9
5. Syrop, C.H. and Halme, J. (1987). Cyclic changes of peritoneal fluid parameters in normal and infertile patients. *Obstet. Gynecol.*, **69**, 416–18
6. Syrop, C.H. and Halme, J. (1987). Peritoneal environment and infertility. *Fertil. Steril.*, **48**, 1–9
7. Halme, J., Becker, S., Hammond, M.G., Raj, M.H. and Raj, S. (1983). Increased activation of pelvic macrophages in infertile women with mild endometriosis. *Am. J. Obstet. Gynecol.*, **145**, 333–7
8. Halme, J., Becker, S. and Haskill, S. (1987). Altered maturation and function of peritoneal macrophages: possible role in pathogenesis of endometriosis. *Am. J. Obstet. Gynecol.*, **156**, 783–9
9. Fakih, H., Baggett, B., Holtz, G., Tsang, K.-Y., Lee, J.C. and Williamson, H.O. (1987). Interleukin-1: a possible role in the infertility associated with endometriosis. *Fertil. Steril.*, **47**, 211–15
10. Buyalos, R.P., Funari, V.A., Azzizz, R., Watson, J.M. and Martinez-Maza, O. (1992). Elevated interleukin-6 levels in peritoneal fluid in patients with pelvic pathology. *Fertil. Steril.*, **58**, 302–6
11. Ryan, I.P., Tseng, J.F., Schriock, E.D. and Khorram, O. (1995). Interleukin-8 concentrations are elevated in peritoneal fluid of women with endometriosis. *Fertil. Steril.*, **63**, 929–32
12. Punnonen, J., Teisala, K., Ranta, H., Bennett, B. and Punnonen, R. (1996). Increased levels of interleukin-6 and interleukin-10 in the peritoneal fluid of patients with endometriosis. *Am. J. Obstet. Gynecol.*, **174**, 1522–6
13. Halme, J. (1989). Release of tumor necrosis factor-alpha by human peritoneal macrophages *in vivo* and *in vitro*. *Am. J. Obstet. Gynecol.*, **161**, 1718–25
14. Oosterlynck, D.J., Meuleman, C., Sobis, H., Vandeputte, M. and Koninckx, P.R. (1993). Angiogenic activity of peritoneal fluid from women with endometriosis. *Fertil. Steril.*, **59**, 778–82
15. McLaren, J., Prentice, A., Sharnock-Jones, D.S. and Smith, S.K. (1996). Vascular endothelial growth factor (VEGF) concentrations are

elevated in peritoneal fluid of women with endometriosis. *Hum. Reprod.*, **11**, 220–3
16. Halme, J., Becker, S. and Haskill, S. (1987). Altered maturation and function of peritoneal macrophages: possible role in pathogenesis of endometriosis. *Am. J. Obstet. Gynecol.*, **156**, 783–9
17. Halme, J., White, C., Kauma, S., Estes, J. and Haskill, S. (1988). Peritoneal macrophages from patients with endometriosis release growth factor activity *in vitro*. *J. Clin. Endocrinol. Metab.*, **66**, 1044–9
18. Hammond, M.G., Oh, S.T., Anners, J., Surrey, E.S. and Halme, J. (1993). The effect of growth factors on the proliferation of human endometrial stromal cells in culture. *Am. J. Obstet. Gynecol.*, **168**, 1131–8
19. Syrop, C.H. and Halme, J. (1986). A comparison of peritoneal fluid parameters of infertile patients and the subsequent occurrence of pregnancy. *Fertil. Steril.*, **46**, 631–5
20. Weinberg, J.B. and Haney, A.F. (1988). Reduction of the intraperitoneal inflammation associated with endometriosis by treatment with medroxyprogesterone acetate. *Am. J. Obstet. Gynecol.*, **159**, 450–4
21. Suginami, H., Yano, K., Watanabe, K. and Matsuura, S. (1986). A factor inhibiting ovum capture by the oviductal fimbria present in endometriosis peritoneal fluid. *Fertil. Steril.*, **46**, 1140–6
22. Suginami, H. and Yano, K. (1988). An ovum capture inhibitor (OCI) in endometriosis peritoneal fluid: an OCI related membrane responsible for fimbrial failure of ovum capture. *Fertil. Steril.*, **50**, 648–53
23. Muscato, J.J., Haney, A.F. and Weinberg, J.B. (1982). Sperm phagocytosis by human peritoneal macrophages: a possible cause of infertility in endometriosis. *Am. J. Obstet. Gynecol.*, **144**, 503–10
24. London, S.N., Haney, A.F. and Weinberg, J.B. (1985). Macrophages and infertility: enhancement of human macrophage-mediated sperm killing by antisperm antibodies. *Fertil. Steril.*, **43**, 274–8
25. Awadalla, S.G., Friedman, C.I., Haq, A.U. and Roh, S.I. (1987). Local peritoneal factors: their role in infertility associated with endometriosis. *Am. J. Obstet. Gynecol.*, **157**, 1207–14
26. Samejima, T., Masuzaki, H., Tshimaru, T. and Yamabe, T. (1989). Activity of peritoneal macrophages in endometriosis. *Asia-Oceanic J. Obstet. Gynecol.*, **15**, 175–81
27. Morcos, R.N., Gibbons, W.E. and Findley, W.E. (1985). Effect of peritoneal fluid on *in vitro* cleavage of 2 cell mouse embryos: possible role in infertility associated with endometriosis. *Fertil. Steril.*, **44**, 678–83
28. Hahn, D.W., Carraher, R.P. and Foldesy, R.G. (1986). Experimental evidence for failure to implant as a mechanism of infertility associated with endometriosis. *Am. J. Obstet. Gynecol.*, **155**, 1109
29. Haimovici, A.F., Hill, J.A. and Anderson, D.J. (1987). The effects of soluble products of activated lymphocytes and macrophages on blastocyst implantation events *in vitro*. *Biol. Reprod.*, **44**, 69–75
30. Schneider, E.G., Armant, D.R., Kupper, T.S. and Polan, M.L. (1989). Absence of a direct effect of recombinant interleukins and cultured peritoneal macrophages on early embryonic development in the mouse. *Biol. Reprod.*, **40**, 825–33
31. Prough, S.G., Aksel, S., Gilmore, S.M. and Yeoman, R.R. (1990). Peritoneal fluid fractions from patients with endometriosis do not promote two-cell mouse embryo growth. *Fertil. Steril.*, **54**, 927–30
32. Prough, S.G., Aksel, S., Yeoman, R.R. and Wiebe, R.H. (1991). Peritoneal fluid from patients with unexplained infertility inhibits growth of 2-cell mouse embryos. *Int. J. Fertil.*, **13**, 17–20
33. Dodds, W.G., Miller, F.A., Friedman, C.I., Lisko, B., Goldberg, J.M. and Kim, M.H. (1992). The effect of preovulatory peritoneal fluid from cases of endometriosis on murine *in vitro* fertilization, embryo development, oviduct transport and implantation. *Am. J. Obstet. Gynecol.*, **166**, 219–24
34. Taketani, Y., Kuo, T.-M. and Mizuno, M. (1992). Comparison of cytokine levels and embryo toxicity in peritoneal fluid in infertile women with untreated and treated endometriosis. *Am. J. Obstet. Gynecol.*, **167**, 265–70
35. Halme, J. and Hall, J.L. (1982). Effect of pelvic fluid from endometriosis patients on human sperm penetration of zona-free hamster ova. *Fertil. Steril.*, **37**, 573–6
36. Oak, M.K., Chantler, E.N., Vaughan-Williams, C.A. and Elstein, M. (1985). Sperm survival studies in peritoneal fluid from infertile women with endometriosis and unexplained infertility. *Clin. Reprod. Fertil.*, **3**, 297–303
37. Chacho, K.J., Chacho, M.S., Andresen, P.J.

and Scommegna, A. (1986). Peritoneal fluid in patients with and without endometriosis: prostanoids and macrophages and their effect on the spermatozoa penetration assay. *Am. J. Obstet. Gynecol.*, **154**, 1290–9
38. Burke, R.K. (1987). Effects of peritoneal washings from women with endometriosis on sperm velocity. *J. Reprod. Med.*, **32**, 743–6
39. Chacho, K.J., Andresen, P.J. and Scommegna, A. (1987). The effect of peritoneal incubates on the spermatozoa assay. *Fertil. Steril.*, **48**, 694–6
40. Sueldo, C.E., Lambert, H., Steinleitner, A., Rathwick, G. and Swanson, J. (1987). The effect of peritoneal fluid from patients with endometriosis on murine sperm–oocyte interaction. *Fertil. Steril.*, **48**, 678–83
41. Eisermann, J., Register, K.B., Strickler, R.C. and Collins, J.L. (1989). The effect of tumor necrosis factor on human sperm motility *in vitro*. *J. Androl.*, **10**, 270–4
42. Leach, R.E., Arneson, B.W., Ball, G.D. and Ory, S.J. (1990). Absence of entisperm antibodies and factors influencing sperm motility in the cul-de-sac fluid of women with endometriosis. *Fertil. Steril.*, **53**, 351–3
43. Coddington, C.C., Oehninger, S., Cunningham, D.S. and Hansen, K. (1992). Peritoneal fluid from patients with endometriosis decreases sperm binding to the zona pellucida in the hemizona assay: a preliminary report. *Fertil. Steril.*, **57**, 783–6
44. Curtis, P., Lindsay, P., Jackson, A.E. and Shaw, R.W. (1993). Adverse effects on sperm movement characteristics in women with minimal and mild endometriosis. *Br. J. Obstet. Gynaecol.*, **100**, 165–9
45. Drudy, L., Lewis, S.E., Barry-Kinsella, C., Harrison, R.F. and Thompson, W. (1994). The influence of peritoneal fluid from patients with minimal stage or treated endometriosis on sperm motility parameters using computer-assisted semen analysis. *Hum. Reprod.*, **9**, 2418–23
46. Arumugam, K. (1994). Endometriosis and infertility: raised ion concentration in the peritoneal fluid and its effect on the acrosome reaction. *Hum. Reprod.*, **9**, 1153–7
47. Zullo, F., Corea, D., Torano, P. and Placco, C. (1994). Sperm–peritoneal fluid incubation test: influence of a GnRH agonist treatment. *Acta Eur. Fertil.*, **25**, 291–3
48. Tasdemir, M., Tasdemir, I., Kodama, H. and Tanaka, T. (1995). Effect of peritoneal fluid from infertile women with endometriosis on ionophore-stimulated acrosome loss. *Hum. Reprod.*, **10**, 2419–22
49. Aeby, T.C., Huang, T. and Nakayama, R.T. (1996). The effect of peritoneal fluid from patients with endometriosis on human sperm function *in vitro*. *Am. J. Obstet. Gynecol.*, **174**, 1779–85
50. Eisermann, J., Gast, M.J., Pineda, J., Odem, R.R. and Collins, J.L. (1988). Tumor necrosis factor in peritoneal fluid of women undergoing laparoscopic surgery. *Fertil. Steril.*, **50**, 573–9
51. Vercellini, P., De Benedetti, R., Rossi, E. and Colombo, A. (1993). Tumor necrosis factor in plasma and peritoneal fluid of women with and without endometriosis. *Gynecol. Obstet. Invest.*, **36**, 39–41

Resident leukocytes in endometriosis

C.A. Witz, N.A. Klein and R.S. Schenken

Introduction

Factors regulating the histogenesis and growth of endometriosis are poorly understood. Hormonal influences, although clearly playing an important role, do not fully account for the variable growth patterns of endometriotic tissue. Recent reports suggest that, in addition to hormonal factors, peripheral and/or peritoneal fluid leukocytes and their secretory products are involved in regulating the growth of ectopic endometrium[1-3]. However, the peritoneal fluid environment cannot completely explain the variability of growth and invasiveness of individual implants in the same patient. This suggests that local factors may also be instrumental in modulating the growth and progression of ectopic endometrium.

Leukocytes comprise up to 25% of the cell population of endometrium. The majority of these cells are T lymphocytes and macrophages[4,5]. They are found as isolated cells scattered throughout the stroma, as lymphoid aggregates bordering the basalis epithelium, and within glandular and surface epithelium[5,6]. Recent studies have suggested the cytokine products from these leukocytes play an important role in regulating the differentiation and proliferative activity of eutopic endometrium. For example, the macrophage secretory products, interleukin-1 and interleukin-6, inhibit endometrial stromal cell proliferation *in vitro*[7,8]. Likewise, γ-interferon, produced predominantly by activated T lymphocytes, has been shown to inhibit the proliferation of endometrial epithelial cells *in vitro*[9]. Our initial study was designed to characterize the resident leukocyte population and proliferation activity of endometriosis and to compare the findings with those of eutopic endometrium. Subsequently, others have confirmed and extended our findings.

Materials and methods

Tissue collection

Endometriotic tissue was obtained from women undergoing surgery for pelvic pain or infertility, in the proliferative phase of the menstrual cycle. Superficial peritoneal implants ($n = 24$), appearing as raised reddish nodules, and tissue from ovarian endometriomas ($n = 5$) were examined. Control tissue consisted of eutopic endometrium obtained in the proliferative ($n = 19$) or secretory ($n = 25$) phase. Specimens were collected by aspiration biopsy, curettage, or from extirpated uteri for non-endometrial pathology. Tissue was snap-frozen in liquid nitrogen and stored at −70°C. Serial 4-μm sections were placed on glycine-coated slides, air-dried and fixed for 5 min in acetone at 4°C. Sections were transferred to Tris-buffered saline (TBS; 0.1 mol/l, pH 7.4) prior to routine staining with hematoxylin and eosin or immunostaining.

Histology

Sections from each specimen were stained with hematoxylin and eosin. Eutopic endometria were dated according to criteria of Noyes and Hertig[10].

Immunocytochemistry

Sections were first stained for surface antigen CD45 (leukocyte common antigen; AMAC Inc., Westbrook, ME, USA), CD3 (T-cell marker; DAKO Corporation, Carpinteria, CA, USA), or CD11c (tissue macrophage marker; DAKO). These antibodies have been characterized previously[11–14]. In subsequent studies to characterize cell subpopulations and activation status, we used monoclonal antibodies to CD4 (T-helper-inducer cells; DAKO), CD8 (T cytolytic-suppressor cells; DAKO), CD22 (B-cells; DAKO), CD56 (natural killer cells; DAKO) and VLA-1 (activated T-cells; T Cell Science Inc., Cambridge, MA, USA). Briefly, slides were incubated at 37°C with normal horse serum followed by mouse monoclonal antibody, biotinylated anti-mouse secondary antibody, and finally, avidin–biotin peroxidase complex (Vectastain®; Vector Laboratories Inc., Burlingame, CA, USA). Slides were then reacted in a mixture of diaminobenzidine and hydrogen peroxide, which yielded a brown reaction product. Primary antibodies were used at a dilution of 1:50, and secondary antibody at 1:200. Positive controls consisted of cytospin preparations of peripheral blood leukocytes. Negative controls were prepared by substituting non-immune mouse serum at equivalent protein concentrations for the primary antibody.

Quantitation and statistics

Sections were examined under oil immersion. The concentration of positively stained stromal cells was determined by examining a minimum of 500 cells. Isolated diaminobenzidine-reacted cells that were not involved with lymphoid aggregates were counted as positive. The results are expressed as the percentage of positively stained cells. Comparisons of these values in ectopic endometrium, eutopic secretory endometrium, and eutopic proliferative endometrium were performed, using a one-way analysis of variance (ANOVA). Bartlett's test was used to determine the homogeneity of variances. Logarithmic transformation was performed when appropriate. The statistical analysis was performed using the computer program Minitab (Minitab Inc., State College, PA, USA) on an Apple personal computer (Apple Computer Inc., Cupertino, CA, USA). When significant differences among the groups were identified with ANOVA, the Student–Newman–Keuls and Tukey's tests were employed to compare individual groups. The critical value of the studentized range was provided by a standard text of statistical tables[15].

Results

Histological characteristics

Hematoxylin- and eosin-stained sections of eutopic endometrium revealed normal proliferative and secretory endometrium. No specimen revealed hyperplasia, endometritis, or other histological evidence of endometrial pathology. Similarly stained sections of endometriotic tissue revealed atrophic or proliferative endometrial glands and stroma. All sections of endometriotic tissue also contained surrounding fibrotic tissue and variable amounts of hemosiderin.

Resident leukocyte population in eutopic endometrium

Cells labeled with CD45, CD3 or CD11c were identified by their plasma membrane reactivity (Figure 1). Eutopic endometrium contained CD45+ cells scattered throughout the stroma as well as aggregates of these cells found primarily in the basalis adjacent to glands. Many of the scattered cells were closely juxtaposed to the basement membrane of the glandular epithelium. In addition, occasional CD45+ cells were found within the glandular and surface epithelium. Staining with CD3 and CD11c revealed that the

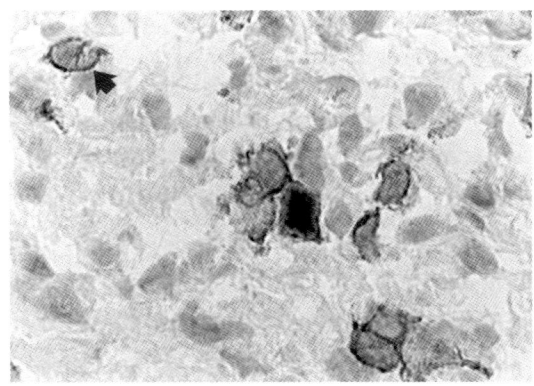

Figure 1 Photomircrograph of ectopic endometrium stained for leukocyte common antigen CD45 (dark plasma membrane reactivity, arrow)

Table 1 Proportion of scattered stromal cells staining for lymphoid cell antigens. Data are expressed as means ± SEM

Tissue type	CD45+ (%)	CD3+ (%)	CD11c+ (%)
Proliferative endometrium ($n = 8$)	7.5 ± 0.8	6.4 ± 0.7	3.8 ± 0.3
Secretroy endometrium ($n = 13$)	11.1 ± 1.2	5.0 ± 0.6	4.5 ± 0.3
Endometriosis ($n = 17$)	19.0 ± 1.4*	9.9 ± 0.8*	9.3 ± 1.0

*$p < 0.02$ compared with proliferative and secretory endometrium

majority of the CD45+ cells represented T-cells and macrophages, as has been previously shown by others[4,5,16,17]. The proportions of CD11c+ and CD3+ cells appeared to remain relatively constant throughout the menstrual cycle. In contrast, there was a rise in the number of total CD45+ cells in the mid- to late secretory phase.

Resident leukocyte populations in endometriosis

Endometriotic tissue contained significantly higher proportions of scattered stromal CD45+, CD3+ and CD11c+ cells as compared with eutopic endometrium in either the proliferative or secretory phase ($p \leq 0.02$, Table 1). There were no significant differences between peritoneal implants and endometriomas in the proportions of cells expressing each marker. Rare CD45+ cells were found within the endometriotic glandular epithelium. Only occasional implants contained lymphoid aggregates located near the glands.

Resident leukocyte subpopulations

There was no significant difference in the concentration of B lymphocytes. A posteriori comparison between the individual groups revealed that in the stroma of ectopic endometria, there was a significantly higher concentration of CD4+ cells than in proliferative and secretory eutopic endometria (6.2% vs. 2.6%, $p < 0.01$, and 6.2% vs. 2.5%, $p < 0.01$, respectively). Likewise, compared to proliferative and secretory eutopic endometria, endometriosis contained significantly more CD8+ cells (6.4% vs. 3.1%, $p < 0.01$, and 6.4% vs. 2.6%, $p < 0.01$, respectively) and VLA-1 positive cells (4.7% vs. 3.0%, $p < 0.05$, and 4.7% vs. 1.6%, $p < 0.01$, respectively). There was a significantly greater concentration of VLA-1 positive cells in endometrium during the proliferative compared to the secretory phase (3.0% vs. 1.6%, $p < 0.05$). In addition, ectopic endometrium contained significantly fewer natural killer cells than did proliferative and secretory endometrium ($p < 0.05$).

Controls

Peripheral blood leukocytes expressed each of the markers as brown membrane staining with diaminobenzidine. All sections stained with non-immune mouse serum in place of the primary antibody were negative for plasma membrane staining.

Comments

These data establish the presence of resident leukocytes in endometriotic tissue. As in eutopic endometrium, the majority of these cells are T-cells and macrophages. The presence of lymphocytes and macrophages in normal endometrium, both scattered and in aggregates, has been well-documented[4,5,16,18,19]. The present study demonstrates that scattered T-cells (CD3+) and macrophages (CD11c+) in endometriosis are present in higher concentrations than in normal endometrium. However, lymphoid aggregates are less common in endometriotic tissue. We have further characterized the subpopulation of T-cells. The results demonstrate that there is an increased concentration of both T4 (helper/inducer) and T8 (cytolytic/suppressor) cells in the stroma of ectopic endometrium compared to both proliferative and secretory phase eutopic endometrium. In addition, the stroma of ectopic endometrium contains an increased population of activated, VLA-1-positive T-cells, compared to secretory endometrium. In eutopic endometrium, there were no cycle-dependent differences seen in the concentration of T4 and T8 cells. Tabibzadeh[6] found similar numbers of VLA-1 positive T-cells throughout the cycle, but we observed a greater number of activated T-cells in proliferative endometrium than in secretory endometrium.

Since our original studies, several other groups have reported leukocyte populations in endometrium and endometriosis. Oosterlynck and colleagues studied endometriotic tissue specimens obtained from women during the proliferative ($n = 9$) or luteal phase ($n = 6$) of their cycles[20]. Consistent with our findings, T-cells and macrophages were the most common subpopulation. The CD4/CD8 ratio in their study was 0.8, whilst that in our study was 0.9. Both B-cells and natural killer cells were infrequently seen. No differences between the proliferative and secretory phases were apparent.

Jones and colleagues performed a comprehensive study of the leukocyte population in eutopic and ectopic endometrium across all stages of the menstrual cycle[21]. T-cells and macrophages were again the major leukocyte component of endometriotic lesions. B-cells and natural killer cells were rare. Interestingly, there was no variation in leukocyte numbers with menstrual cycle phase in ectopic endometrium. Consistent with our original work, the concentration of T-cells and macrophages was increased in ectopic endometrium as compared to eutopic endometrium when tissue was obtained during the proliferative or early secretory phase. In the late secretory phase, no differences between ectopic and eutopic endometrium were noted except that the population of granulated cells was lower in endometriotic tissue. The authors also observed no difference in leukocyte populations in eutopic endometrium of women with and without endometriosis.

This latter observation is inconsistent with a recent publication[22] demonstrating a significantly increased expression of T-cells, macrophages, adhesion molecules and HLA antigens in eutopic endometrium of women with endometriosis. However, only 10 women with endometriosis were compared with 42 infertile controls. Furthermore, the stage of cycle was not reported in patients with endometriosis. Another observation was that danazol (400 mg/day for 4 months) significantly suppressed the expression of $\gamma\delta$ T-cell receptors, CD2, and the major histocompatability antigens HLA-ABL and HLA-DR. The significance of these observations remains to be established.

In conclusion, there is an increasing body of data confirming that endometriotic tissue contains a higher concentration of T-cells and macrophages. It appears that the increased concentration is similar to that of premenstrual endometrium and that endometriotic tissue leukocyte populations do not vary during the menstrual cycle.

Acknowledgements

We appreciate the constructive comments of Dr S. Tabibzadeh and gratefully acknowledge the assistance of Ms Irma Garcia in the preparation of this manuscript.

References

1. Halme, J., White, C., Kauma, S., Estes, J. and Haskill, S. (1988). Peritoneal macrophages from patients with endometriosis release growth factor activity *in vitro*. *J. Clin. Endocrinol. Metab.*, **66**, 1044–9
2. Oosterlynck, D.J., Cornillie, F.G., Waer, M., Vandeputte, M. and Koninckx, P.R. (1991). Women with endometriosis show a defect in natural killer activity resulting in a decreased cytotoxicity to autologous endometrium. *Fertil. Steril.*, **56**, 45–51
3. Surrey, E.S. and Halme, J. (1991). Effect of platelet-derived growth factor on endometrial stromal cell proliferation *in vitro*: a model for endometriosis? *Fertil. Steril.*, **56**, 672–9
4. Kamat, B.R. and Isaacson, P.G. (1987). The immunocytochemical distribution of leukocytic subpopulations in human endometrium. *Am. J. Pathol.*, **127**, 66-73
5. Marshall, R.J. and Jones, D.B. (1988). An immunohistochemical study of lymphoid tissue in human endometrium. *Int. J. Gynecol. Pathol.*, **7**, 225–35
6. Tabibzadeh, S. (1990). Evidence of T-cell activation and potential cytokine action in human endometrium. *J. Clin. Endocrinol. Metab.*, **71**, 645–9
7. van Le, L., Oh, S., Anners, J.A., Rinehart, C.A. and Halme, J. (1992). Interleukin-1 inhibits growth of normal endometrial stromal cells. *Obstet. Gynecol.*, **80**, 405–9
8. Zarmakoupis, P., Rier, S., Maroulis, G. and Becker, J. (1995). Inhibition of endometrial cell proliferation by interleukin-6. *Hum. Reprod.*, **10**, 2395–9
9. Tabibzadeh, S.S., Satyaswaroop, P.G. and Potu, N.R. (1988). Antiproliferative effect of interferon-γ in human endometrial epithelial cells *in vitro*: potential local growth modulatory role in endometrium. *J. Clin. Endocrinol. Metab.*, **67**, 131–8
10. Noyes, R.W. and Hertig, A.T. (1955). Dating the endometrial biopsy. *Fertil. Steril.*, **1**, 3–25
11. Gerdes, J., Lemke, H., Baisch, H., Wacker, H.H., Schwab, U. and Stein, H. (1984). Cell cycle analysis of a cell proliferation-associated human nuclear antigen defined by the monoclonal antibody Ki-67. *J. Immunol.*, **133**, 1710–15
12. Warnke, R.A., Gatter, K.C., Falini, B., Hildreth, P., Woolston, R.E., Pulford, K., Cordell, J.L., Cohen, B., De Wolf-Peeters, C. and Mason, D.Y. (1983). Diagnosis of human lymphoma with monoclonal anti-leukocyte antibodies. *N. Engl. J. Med.*, **309**, 1275–81
13. Tunnacliff, A., Olsson, C., Traunecker, A., Krissanhsen, G.W., Karjalainen, K. and Del La Hera, A. (1989). T32.2 The majority of CD3 epitopes are conferred by the epsilon chain. In Knapp, W. *et al.* (eds.) *Leukocyte Typing IV. White Cell Differentiation Antigens*, pp. 295–6. (Oxford, New York, Tokyo: Oxford University Press)
14. Lanier, L.L., Arnaout, M.A., Schwarting, R., Warner, N.L. and Ross, G.D. (1985). PI150/95, third member of the LFA-1/CR3 polypeptide family identified by anti-Leu-M5 monoclonal antibody. *Eur. J. Immunol.*, **15**, 713–18
15. Rohlf, F.J. and Sokal, R. (1981). *Statistical Tables*, pp. 133–7. (New York: W.H. Freeman and Company)
16. Bulmer, J.N., Lunny, D.P. and Hagin, S.V. (1988). Immunohistochemical characterization of stromal leukocytes in non-pregnant human endometrium. *Am. J. Reprod. Immunol. Microbiol.*, **17**, 83–90
17. Tabibzadeh, S. (1991). Induction of HLA-DR expression in endometrial epithelial cells by endometrial T-cells: potential regulatory role of endometrial T-cells *in vivo*. *J. Clin. Endocrinol. Metab.*, **73**, 1352–9
18. Tabibzadeh, S. (1990). Proliferative activity of lymphoid cells in human endometrium throughout the menstrual cycle. *J. Clin.*

Endocrinol. Metab., **70**, 437–43

19. Morris, H., Edwards, J., Tiltman, A. and Emms, M. (1985). Endometrial lymphoid tissue: an immunohistological study. *J. Clin. Pathol.*, **38**, 644–52
20. Oosterlynck, D.J., Cornillie, F.J., Waer, M. and Koninckx, R.P. (1993). Immunohistochemical characterization of leucocyte subpopulations in endometriotic lesions. *Arch. Gynecol. Obstet.*, **253**, 197–206
21. Jones, R.K., Bulmer, J.N. and Searle, R.F. (1996). Immunohistochemical characterization of stromal leukocytes in ovarian endometriosis: comparison of eutopic and ectopic endometrium with normal endometrium. *Fertil. Steril.*, **66**, 81–9
22. Ota, H., Igarashi, S., Hayakawa, M., Matsui, T., Tanaka, H. and Tanaka, T. (1996). Effect of danazol on the immunocompetent cells in the eutopic endometrium in patients with endometriosis: a multicenter cooperative study. *Fertil. Steril.*, **65**, 545–51

Cytokines in peritoneal fluid from women with active endometriosis

T. Harada, F. Taniguchi, T. Iwabe, Y. Onohara, M. Tanikawa and N. Terakawa

Introduction

Endometriosis is an enigmatic disease with poorly understood pathogenesis. A cause-and-effect relation between minimal or mild endometriosis and infertility is also unclear[1]. A recent hypothesis suggests that peritoneal fluid in women with endometriosis contains an increased number of activated macrophages that secrete a variety of local products, also known as cytokines[2]. Cytokines have been implicated in the control of implantation and the growth of endometrial cells outside the uterus[3,4]. Cytokines are also believed to be related to infertility in women with endometriosis. It has been shown that peritoneal fluid from women with endometriosis inhibits mouse embryo growth[5].

Peritoneal endometriosis can be classified as red, black or white lesions. Red-colored lesions are known to be an active form of endometriosis, because vascularization and mitotic activity are shown to be most prominent in these lesions[6].

In this study, we measured the peritoneal fluid levels of interleukin-6 and interleukin-8 and investigated the correlations between peritoneal fluid levels of these cytokines and the size and the number of red active endometriotic lesions. The effects of interleukin-6 on the development of single-cell mouse embryos and of interleukin-8 on the growth of human eutopic and ectopic stromal cells were also evaluated.

Materials and methods

Subjects

Peritoneal fluid was obtained from 38 Japanese women of reproductive age who underwent laparoscopy for infertility work-up or laparoscopic cystectomy for ovarian chocolate cysts. All laparoscopic procedures were performed under general anesthesia between days 5 and 30 of the menstrual cycle. Of the 38 patients studied, 19 patients had pelvic endometriosis and 19 patients were free of endometriosis.

Endometriosis was staged according to the criteria of the revised American Fertility Society (AFS) classification system, by laparoscopic inspection of the pelvis[7]. Observations and surgical procedures were recorded on video tape. We assessed the size and the number of all active non-pigmented lesions at the laparoscopy and on the video tapes. Active lesions were identified according to the criteria of Jansen and Russell[8] and Wiegerinck and associates[9]. Individual active lesions, such as red flame-like lesions, gland-like lesions and red vesicles were scored on a 4-point scale according to the revised AFS scoring system: 0, no active endometriosis; 1, active lesion(s) < 1 cm; 2, active lesion(s) 1–3 cm; 4, active lesion(s) > 3 cm.

Collection and isolation of samples

Peritoneal fluid was obtained via a laparoscopic cannula immediately after the introduction of the laparoscope. Aspiration was performed under direct visualization from the posterior cul-de-sac and anterior vesicouterine fold. We recorded the total fluid volume obtained. Fluid samples were centrifuged at $800\,g$ for 10 min at 4 °C, to separate the cell pellet and the supernatant. The cell-free supernatant was then stored at −70 °C until assayed.

Assays

The concentrations of interleukin-6 and interleukin-8 were determined using specific sandwich enzyme-linked immunosorbent assays (R & D Systems, Minneapolis, MN, USA). The detection limits of the assays were 0.1 pg/ml for interleukin-6 and 10 pg/ml for interleukin-8. The intra-assay variations were less than 5%.

Embryo collection and culture

Female 5–6-week-old B6C3F1 mice were superovulated by intraperitoneal injection of 7.5 IU pregnant mares' serum gonadotropin (Peamex, Sankyo Zoki Co. Ltd., Tokyo, Japan); 7.5 IU of human chorionic gonadotropin (hCG, Pregnyl, N.V. Organon, Tokyo, Japan) was administered 48 h later. Immediately after injection of hCG, the females were mated with males of the same strain. Single-cell embryos were collected from the oviducts after 20 h and washes in HEPES-buffered human tubal fluid (HTF) medium containing 1 mg/ml of bovine serum albumin (BSA) (Fraction V, Sigma Chemical Co., St Louis, MO, USA)[10]. The embryos were cultured in HTF medium containing 50 or 100 pg/ml of human recombinant interleukin-6 (Chinese hamster ovary (CHO) cell derived, Genzyme, Cambridge, MA, USA). A monoclonal antibody against interleukin-6 (monoclonal mouse antihuman interleukin-6, Genzyme) was used to neutralize the specific effects of interleukin-6.

Isolation and culture of eutopic and ectopic endometrial stromal cells

Eutopic and ectopic endometrial tissues were collected from patients who underwent hysterectomy and laparoscopic cystectomy of endometrioma, respectively. Stromal cells were collected from tissue samples according to the method of Osteen and associates[11]. In brief, the endometrial tissues were minced and digested with collagenase, and then serially filtered through nylon mesh with apertures of 40–70 µm to trap the glandular epithelium. The filtered fraction was separated further from epithelial cell clumps by differential sedimentation at unit gravity. Stromal cells were cultured in Dulbecco Modified Eagle's Medium/Ham's F-12 (DMEM/F-12) supplemented with 10% fetal bovine serum (FBS). We used the stromal cells in culture after first passage.

Thymidine incorporation

The activity of DNA synthesis was determined by tritiated thymidine incorporation in the cells. Twenty-thousand cells per well were placed in 24-well dishes. After culture for 72 h, the medium was replaced by DMEM/F-12 with 2% FBS. Interleukin-8 (UBI, human recombinant endothelial interleukin-8, 77 amino acids, concentration range 0–200 pg/ml) and 2 µCi of methyl-tritiated thymidine (Amersham, TRK120, specific activity 3.77 GBq/mg) were added and cultured for an additional 24 h. DNA was extracted by cell lysis with sodium hydroxide, and radioactivities were measured by scintillation counting.

Statistical analysis

The clinical data are presented as the group mean ± SE. Because the cytokine data were not normally distributed, they were analyzed using non-parametric analysis (Mann–Whitney test). Correlation analysis with concentrations of cytokines and scores of active lesions were performed using linear regression analysis. The data on embryo development was analyzed using the χ^2 test. Analysis of variance (ANOVA) was used for comparison between multiple data in the thymidine incorporation experiment. A p value of < 0.05 was regarded as statistically significant.

Results

Interleukin-6 and interleukin-8 levels

There were significant differences in peritoneal fluid levels of interleukin-6 and interleukin-8 between women with and without endometriosis (Table 1).

There were significant positive correlations between peritoneal fluid concentrations of log-transformed interleukin-6 and interleukin-8 and active lesion scores ($R = 0.74$, $y = 0.23x + 1.02$, $p < 0.01$ for interleukin-6; $R = 0.55$, $y = 61.2x - 15.2$, $p < 0.05$ for interleukin-8). The peritoneal fluid concentrations of interleukin-6 and interleukin-8 increased as the score of active lesions increased.

Effect of interleukin-6 on mouse embryo development

The addition of 50 and 100 pg/ml of human recombinant interleukin-6 significantly inhibited blastocyst formation in single-cell mouse embryos. The adverse effect of interleukin-6 was neutralized by the addition of the anti-interleukin-6 antibody (0.1 µg/ml) (Figure 1).

Effect of interleukin-8 on the proliferation of eutopic and ectopic endometrial cells

Thymidine incorporation by eutopic endometrial stromal cells was significantly increased by the addition of 50–200 pg/ml of interleukin-8 (Figure 2). Addition of interleukin-8 also stimulated thymidine incorporation by ectopic endometrial cells (Figure 3).

Discussion

Peritoneal fluid levels of interleukin-6 and interleukin-8 were increased in patients with active endometriosis in the present study. The addition of human recombinant interleukin-6 to the culture medium suppressed the rate of blastocyst formation of mouse embryos. The results suggest that increased peritoneal fluid levels of cytokines may contribute to infertility by adversely affecting embryonic development. On the other hand, interleukin-8 stimulated the growth of both eutopic and ectopic endometrial cells. This angiogenic cytokine may have a role in the progression of endometriosis.

Peritoneal endometriosis is classified into red, white or black lesions[6]. Vascularization[6] and metabolic activities[12] are most pronounced in red lesions. These early lesions invade the extracellular matrix[13]. We therefore classified

Table 1 Levels of interleukin-6 and interleukin-8 in peritoneal fluid obtained from women at laparoscopy. Values are given as means ± SE

	Interleukin-6 (pg/ml)	Interleukin-8 (pg/ml)
Without endometriosis	22 ± 4	36 ± 13
With endometriosis	104 ± 49*	133 ± 41*

*$p < 0.05$ compared with controls

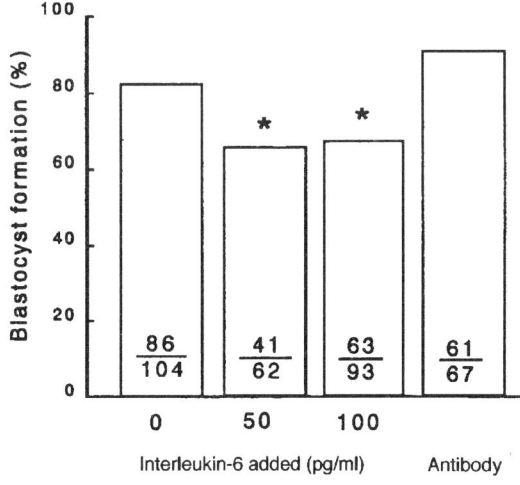

Figure 1 Effects of interleukin-6 and an anti-interleukin-6 antibody on blastocyst formation of single-cell mouse embryos. The numbers within the bars indicate the numbers of blastocyst/single-cell embryos. *$p < 0.05$ compared with control

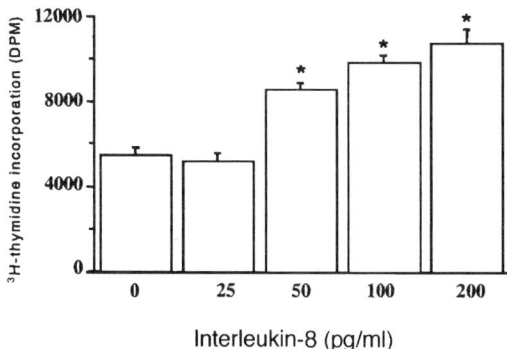

Figure 2 Effects of interleukin-8 on the proliferation of eutopic endometrial stromal cells. DPM, degradation per minute. $*p < 0.01$ compared with control. Values are given as means ± SE

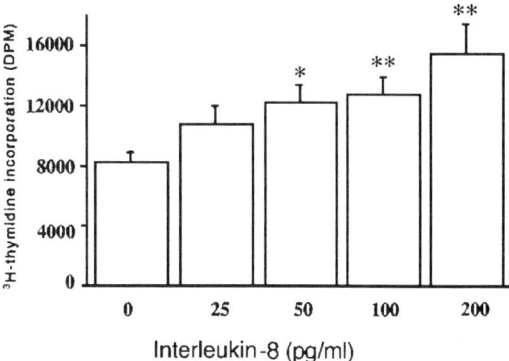

Figure 3 Effects of interleukin-8 on the proliferation of ectopic endometrial stromal cells. DPM, degradation per minute. $*p < 0.05$, $**p < 0.01$ compared with control. Values are given as means ± SE

red lesions as active lesions. The present results suggest that an increased number of red-colored lesions is correlated with elevated concentrations of cytokines in the peritoneal fluid.

Interleukin-6 is a multifunctional cytokine involved in the regulation of the immune response, hematopoiesis and inflammation. It is produced in response to infection or injury by a variety of cell types, including monocytes, lymphocytes, fibroblasts, endothelial cells and keratinocytes[14]. The peritoneal fluid level of interleukin-6 is increased in women with pelvic pathology[15]. Interleukin-8 is a potent angiogenic agent and a chemoattractant for neutrophils. Ryan and colleagues reported that interleukin-8 concentrations are elevated in peritoneal fluid of women with endometriosis[16]; our data are consistent with this. Interleukin-8 may be important for the progression of endometriosis, because angiogenesis is an important step in the establishment of endometriosis.

Interleukin-6 and interleukin-8 in peritoneal fluid are secreted from peritoneal leukocyte components, including the monocytes and macrophages. Macrophages, which are present in the peritoneal cavity, are potent producers of cytokines[4,17]. Recent data suggest that endometrial cells present in peritoneal endometriotic implants may be another important source of interleukin-6[18]. The present results also suggest that peritoneal implants, particularly the so-called 'red' lesions, may be a source of these cytokines. Immunohistochemical studies are needed to provide direct evidence of expression of interleukin-6 and interleukin-8 by these tissues.

In conclusion, the present results show that cytokines, which are increased in peritoneal fluid associated with active endometriotic lesions, may have essential roles in the pathogenesis of endometriosis.

References

1. Mio, Y., Toda, T., Harada, T. and Terakawa, N. (1992). Luteinized unruptured follicle in the early stages of endometriosis as a cause of infer-tility. *Am. J. Obstet. Gynecol.*, **167**, 271–3
2. Ramey, J.W. and Archer, D.F. (1993). Peritoneal fluid: its relevance to the development of endo-metriosis. *Fertil. Steril.*, **60**, 1–14
3. Oosterlynck, D.J., Meuleman, C., Sobis, H., Vandeputte, M. and Koninckx, P.R. (1993). Angiogenic activity of peritoneal fluid from

women with endometriosis. *Fertil. Steril.*, **59**, 778–82
4. Halme, J. (1989). Release of tumor necrosis factor-alpha by human peritoneal macrophages *in vivo* and *in vitro*. *Am. J. Obstet. Gynecol.*, **161**, 1718–25
5. Prough, S.G., Aksel, S., Gilmore, S.M. and Yeoman, R.R. (1990). Peritoneal fluid fractions from patients with endometriosis do not promote two-cell mouse embryo growth. *Fertil. Steril.*, **54**, 927–30
6. Nissole, M., Casanas-Roux, F., Anaf, V., Mince, J.M. and Donnez, J. (1993). Morphometric study of the stromal vascularization in peritoneal endometriosis. *Fertil. Steril.*, **59**, 681–4
7. The American Fertility Society (1985). Revised American Fertility Society classification of endometriosis: 1985. *Fertil. Steril.*, **43**, 351–2
8. Jansen, R.P. and Russell, P. (1986). Nonpigmented endometriosis: clinical, laparoscopic, and pathologic definition. *Am. J. Obstet. Gynecol.*, **155**, 1154–9
9. Wiegerinck, M.A.H.M., Van Dop, P.A. and Brosens, I.A. (1993). The staging of peritoneal endometriosis by the type of active lesion in addition to the revised American Fertility Society classification. *Fertil. Steril.*, **60**, 461–4
10. Harada, T., Tanikawa, M., Iwabe, T., Onohara, Y., Mio, Y. and Terakawa, N. (1992). Measurement of uptake and incorporation of nucleic acid precursors by preimplantation mouse embryos after development *in vivo* and *in vitro*. *J. Assist. Reprod. Genet.*, **9**, 551–6
11. Osteen, K.G., Hill, G.A., Hargrove, J.T. and Gorstein, F. (1989). Development of a method to isolate and culture highly purified populations of stromal and epithelial cells from human endometrial biopsy specimens. *Fertil. Steril.*, **52**, 965–72
12. Vernon, M.W., Beard, J.S., Graves, K. and Wilson, E.A. (1986). Classification of endometriotic implants by morphologic appearance and activity to synthesize prostaglandin F. *Fertil. Steril.*, **46**, 801–6
13. Spuijbroek, M.D.E., Dunselman, G.A.J., Menheere, P.P.C.A. and Evers, J.L.H. (1992). Early endometriosis invades the extracellular matrix. *Fertil. Steril.*, **58**, 929–33
14. Kishimoto, T. (1989). The biology of interleukin-6. *Blood*, **74**, 1–10
15. Buyalos, R.P., Funari, V.A., Azziz, R., Watson, J.M. and Martinez-Maza, O. (1992). Elevated interleukin-6 levels in peritoneal fluid of patients with pelvic pathology. *Fertil. Steril.*, **58**, 302–6
16. Ryan, I.P., Tseng, J.F., Schirock, E.D., Khorram, O., Landers, D.V. and Taylor, R.N. (1995). Interleukin-8 concentrations are elevated in peritoneal fluid of women with endometriosis. *Fertil. Steril.*, **63**, 929–32
17. Bauer, J., Ganter, U., Geuger, T., Jacobshagen, U., Hirano, T., Matsuda, T. *et al.* (1988). Regulation of interleukin-6 expression in cultured human blood monocyte and monocyte-derived macrophages. *Blood*, **72**, 1134–40
18. Rier, S.E., Zamakoupis, P.N., Hu, X. and Becker, J.L. (1995). Dysregulation of interleukin-6 responses in ectopic endometrial stromal cells: correlation with decreased soluble receptor levels in peritoneal fluid of women with endometriosis. *J. Clin. Endocrinol. Metab.*, **80**, 1431–7

Heat shock proteins and endometriosis

H. Ota, S. Igarashi, J. Hatazawa and T. Tanaka

Introduction

Heat shock proteins (HSPs) are a highly conserved group of proteins found in all organisms. Increased synthesis of these proteins occurs in response to many environmental stresses, including temperature changes, inflammation and fever, viral infections and so forth[1]. Principally, they play an essential role as molecular chaperons in the folding of newly synthesized proteins in cells[2]. Increased HSP synthesis has also been found following T-lymphocyte activation with mitogens and cytokines. Further studies suggest that HSPs are directly or indirectly involved with the immune system, through antigen processing, antigen presentation or as peptide-binding proteins. Moreover, it has been reported that subsets of γδT cells, which are a minor T-cell subset in peripheral blood and do not recognize HLA antigens, can recognize HSP65 and HSP70 as specific antigens[3], working as a ligand of γδT cells.

Numerous reports have suggested that endometriosis is associated with changes in the immune system. Immunohistochemical studies have revealed an increased deposition of immunoglobulins and complement components in the endometrium of patients with endometriosis[4-6]. Not only humoral alterations, but also cellular abnormalities are found in the endometrial stroma, namely, an increased number of macrophages, T cells or B cells[7-9]. Additional findings were strong expression of HLA antigens and adhesion molecules in glandular cells[10]. Of particular interest was the increased number of γδT cells in the stroma of endometrium[9].

These facts prompted us to investigate if HSPs have any role in the abnormal immune response observed in endometriosis and adenomyosis. We immunohistochemically studied the localization of HSPs in eutopic endometrium. Furthermore, we investigated the effect of danazol on the expression of HSPs in eutopic endometrium of patients with endometriosis and adenomyosis.

Materials and methods

The subjects consisted of women who were treated at the Department of Obstetrics and Gynecology at Akita University Hospital. They were divided into three groups: the fertile control group, the endometriosis group which included women with laparoscopically diagnosed disease, and the adenomyosis group, in which women who underwent hysterectomy were diagnosed as having adenomyosis histologically, while 21 adenomyosis women treated with danazol were diagnosed based on the presence of an enlarged uterus without leiomyoma (over goose-egg size; approximately $\geq 180\,g$), magnetic resonance imaging and CA125 levels ($\geq 50\,U/ml$) in peripheral blood. All adenomyosis patients fulfilled the diagnostic criteria. Fertile controls consisted of women in the proliferative phase and in the secretory phase. All the controls were parous women with clear male factor infertility. None of the controls had identifiable endometriosis or adenomyosis.

Before the operation or treatment with danazol, endometrial tissue was obtained either in the proliferative or secretory phase. These tissues were obtained in accordance with the rules and regulations of the institution and after approval of the institutional review board. The menstrual cycle of the patients was estimated by endometrial dating according to the method of Noyes and co-workers[11].

The patients were treated with danazol (400 mg) orally twice a day, from the 1st day of the cycle, for 4 months. Endometrial tissue was obtained again 2 months after the beginning of the administration. Those with leiomyoma or abnormal endometrial histology were excluded.

The monoclonal antibodies for all HSPs were purchased from StressGen Biotechnologies Co., Victoria, BC, Canada. The dilution used for the staining was ×200. The endometrial tissue samples were cut into blocks (approximately 1 cm³), embedded in optimal cutting temperature compound (Sakura Finetek USA, Torrance, CA, USA) and snap-frozen in liquid nitrogen immediately after curettage or hysterectomy. Serial cryostat 4-μm sections of tissue were cut and stained with hematoxylin and eosin to identify the endometrial glands. The sections were stained using the peroxidase–antiperoxidase (PAP) method as reported previously[10].

Evaluation was performed in ten non-overlapping fields of view per biopsy in a systematic random sampling pattern (magnification ×400). Since preliminary studies revealed that stromal cells in the functionalis of the endometrium during both the proliferative and secretory phases were negative or very weakly positive for each HSP, only glandular cells in endometriotic tissue were evaluated for staining. Surface epithelium, stromal cells, lymphocytes and vascular endothelial cells in the eutopic and/or ectopic endometria were not examined. Staining was evaluated using an evaluation nomogram as reported previously[10]. In brief, each section was graded from 1+ to 3+ according to the frequency of positive cells and intensity of staining in the endometrial glands. The sections were ranked from 1 to 5 according to the evaluation nomogram.

Statistical analysis of the evaluation nomogram score in each group among the three groups was performed by the Kruskal–Wallis test. The score differences between the proliferative and secretory phases in the control group were analyzed by the Mann–Whitney test. The score differences between those before and after danazol treatment were analyzed by the Wilcoxon test. The data were regarded as significant if $p < 0.05$.

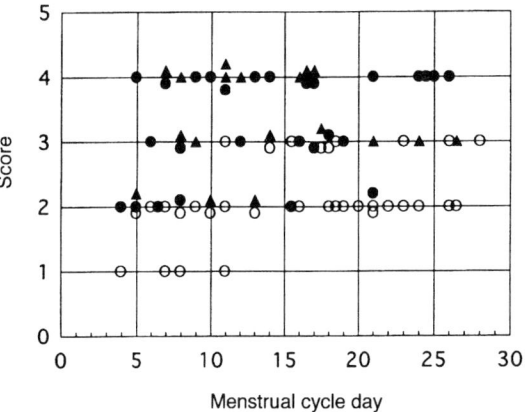

Figure 1 Evaluation nomogram score of HSP27 throughout the menstrual cycle. Open circles, fertile controls; filled circles, endometriosis patients; filled triangles, adenomyosis patients

Results

During the normal menstrual cycle, the scores for HSP27, HSP60 and HSP70 were significantly higher in the secretory phase than those in the proliferative phase, as shown in Figures 1, 2 and 3. As for HSP27, there were significant differences among the three groups in both of the two phases. That is, the score was higher in adenomyosis and endometriosis compared with the control group. Furthermore, there was a significant difference regarding the mean score for HSP70 among the three groups in the proliferative phase, whereas no difference was found in the secretory phase. The scores for HSP60 tended to be higher in adenomyosis and endometriosis. When each score for HSP27, HSP60 or HSP70 was plotted sequentially with the dating after ovulation, no cyclical changes were found within the phase.

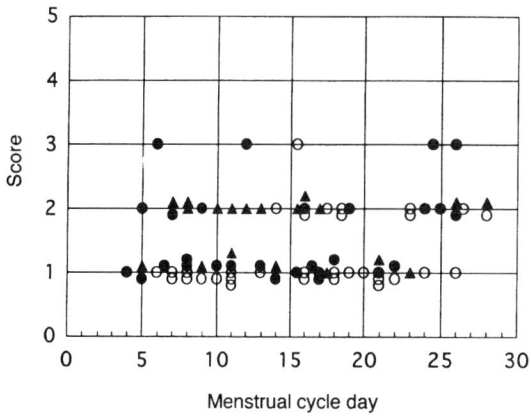

Figure 2 Evaluation nomogram score of HSP60 throughout the menstrual cycle. Open circles, fertile controls; filled circles, endometriosis patients; filled triangles, adenomyosis patients

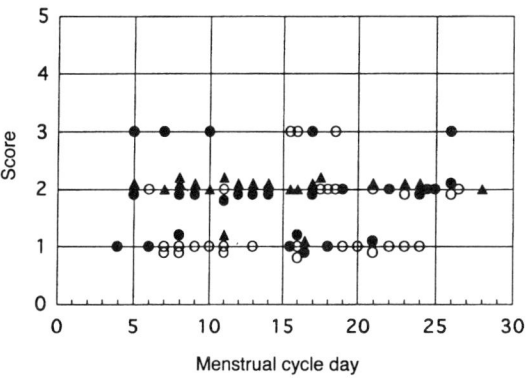

Figure 3 Evaluation nomogram score of HSP70 throughout the menstrual cycle. Open circles, fertile controls; filled circles, endometriosis patients; filled triangles, adenomyosis patients

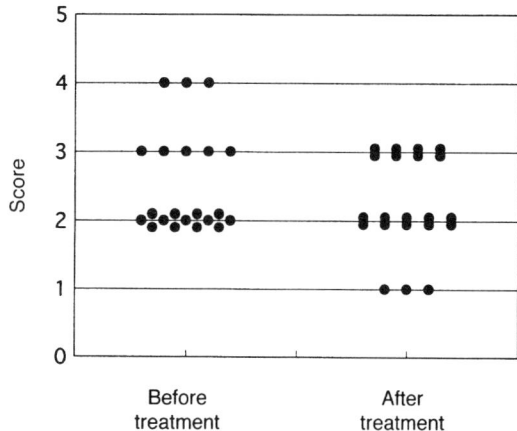

Figure 4 Evaluation nomogram score of HSP27 before and during danazol treatment in the adenomyosis patients

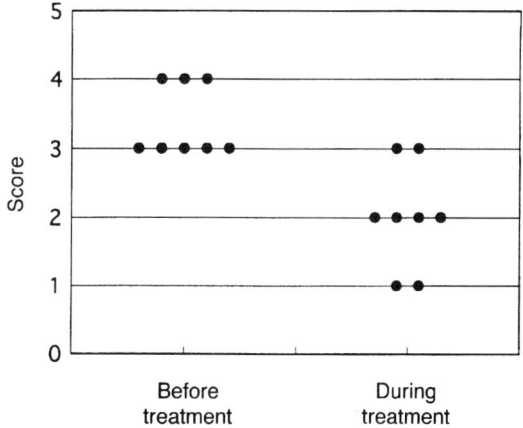

Figure 5 Evaluation nomogram score of HSP27 before and during danazol treatment in the higher group (score ≥ 3) of the adenomyosis patients

Treatment with danazol for 2 months significantly decreased the score for HSP27 in adenomyosis, as shown in Figure 4. Since the mean scores for HSP27 in adenomyosis exceeded the control score, they were divided into two groups, the higher group (score ≥ 3) and the normal group (score ≤ 2), and variations in score after danazol treatment were analyzed. In the higher group, the scores were significantly reduced after 2 months of treatment, while in the normal group the scores did not vary (Figure 5 and 6). Similar changes in the scores for HSP60 and HSP70 were noted during danazol treatment (data not shown).

Positive expression of HSP27, HSP60 and HSP70 in glandular cells was detected mainly in the cytoplasm and partly in the nucleus and membrane, as shown in Figure 7. There were no obvious changes in the distribution of the proteins between eutopic and ectopic endometrium, nor between before and during danazol treatment.

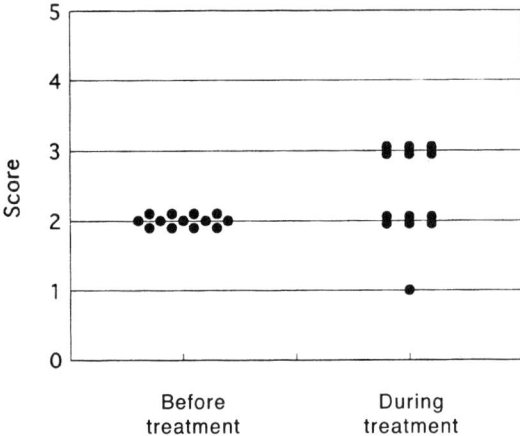

Figure 6 Evaluation nomogram score of HSP27 before and during danazol treatment in the normal group (score ≤ 2) of the adenomyosis patients

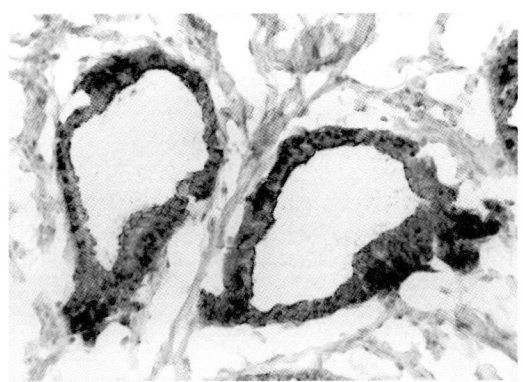

Figure 7 Stained cells for HSP27 in the eutopic endometrium in endometriosis. Evaluation nomogram score was 4 (×116)

Discussion

Endometriosis is an enigmatic disease, since it is associated with numerous changes in the immune system, without showing any apparent autoimmune phenomena. A series of immunohistochemical studies of humoral or cellular alterations regarding various antigens found on the glandular cells suggested the presence of systemic immunological alterations in endometriosis and adenomyosis[5,9,10,12].

The present study clearly demonstrated an increased expression of HSP27 regardless of the menstrual phase and HSP70 in the proliferative phase in patients with endometriosis and adenomyosis. In human cells, the constitutively expressed HSP27 is cytoplasmic and often observed concentrated in a perinuclear zone[13]. The role of HSP27 is not fully understood. It has been reported that HSP27 participates as a molecular chaperon in the folding of newly synthesized proteins in cells[13]. The protein is phosphorylated in response to a large variety of stimuli. Such stimuli include heat shock, cytokines, growth factors and so forth. Thus, the increase in intracellular HSP27 through phosphorylation may be implicated in the immune response mediated by macrophages and/or T cells. The second possibility is that HSP27 might be involved in hormonal action. It is reported that in the absence of estrogen, estrogen receptor is present in an inactive form in the cytoplasm. Once estrogen goes inside the cells and binds to its receptor, the estrogen receptor complex dissociates HSP90 and becomes active, and redistributes inside the nucleus[14]. It is well known that danazol inhibits the secretion of ovarian estrogen. Furthermore, Fuqua and co-workers[15] reported that in a cultured human breast cancer cell line the treatment with estrogen increased the amount of HSP27. Since the expression of HSP27 in the present study was reduced during danazol treatment, it is possible that the protein might have a role in the activation process of estrogen.

It has been reported that HSPs vary in accordance with the menstrual cycle. For example, HSP27 and HSP60 increased progressively during the late proliferative and early secretory phases, and diminished in the mid- to late secretory and menstrual phases[16]. On the other hand, it has also been reported that HSP70 is expressed more markedly in the mid- to late secretory phases than in the proliferative phase[17]. In the present study, the scores for all HSPs in the control group were significantly higher in the secretory phase than those in the proliferative phase, which agree in part with data of previous reports.

There has been several studies indicating that HSPs are deeply involved in various autoimmune diseases. For example, anti-HSP60 antibody has been detected in synovial fluid of patients with rheumatoid arthritis[18]. There is a study showing that in infertile women, including those with endometriosis, HSP70 is strongly expressed compared with controls, although the number of endometriosis cases studied was very few[19]. It is well documented that patients with endometriosis and adenomyosis are frequently positive for autoantibodies, particularly to phospholipids. Yet, little is known about a possible association between autoantibodies and HSPs.

The effect of danazol in autoimmune disorders is interesting. It seems quite likely that danazol modulates immunological functions *in vivo*. It has been reported that treatment with danazol in patients with endometriosis reduced various autoantibodies for phospholipids in peripheral blood and improved fertility[20]. We have also reported a similar reduction of autoantibodies by danazol in a time-dependent manner in patients with adenomyosis[8]. From these studies, it is quite probable that danazol can affect not only serum factors, but can also improve the microenvironment of endometrium in uterus. For example, immunohistochemical studies revealed that the administration of danazol for 2 months inhibited the number of $\gamma\delta T$ cells, CD2-positive cells and the expression of HLA antigens and adhesion molecules, near to control levels in patients with endometriosis and adenomyosis[9,10]. In the present study, the scores of HSPs decreased to control levels after treatment with danazol for 2 months, which implies the modulatory action of the agent. These findings indicate that danazol modulates surface antigens in glandular cells, involving intracellular molecules such as HSPs. In conclusion, it would be necessary to further clarify the involvement of HSPs in abnormal immune response in endometriosis and adenomyosis.

Acknowledgement

This work was supported in part by an educational grant from Tokyo Tanabe Pharmaceutical Co. Ltd (Tokyo, Japan).

References

1. Jacquier-Sarlin, M.R., Fuller, K., Dinh-Xuan, A.T., Richard, M.-J. and Polla, B.S. (1994). Protective effects of HSP70 in inflammation. *Experientia*, **50**, 1031–8
2. Feige, U. and Mollenhauer, J. (1992). Multi-author reviews: heat shock proteins. *Experientia*, **48**, 621–2
3. Beagley, K.W., Fujihashi, K., Black, C.A., Lagoo, A.S., Yamamoto, M., McGhee, J.R. and Kiyono, H. (1993). The *Mycobacterium tuberculosis* 71-kDa heat shock protein induces proliferation and cytokine secretion by murine gut epithelial lymphocytes. *Eur. J. Immunol.*, **23**, 2049–52
4. Weed, J.C. and Arquembourg, P.C. (1980). Endometriosis: can it produce an autoimmune response resulting in infertility? *Clin. Obstet. Gynecol.*, **23**, 885–93
5. Kreiner, D., Fromowitz, F.B., Richardson, D.A. and Kenigsberg, D. (1986). Endometrial immunofluorescence associated with endometriosis and pelvic inflammatory disease. *Fertil. Steril.*, **46**, 243–6
6. Ota, H. and Maki, M. (1990). Content of immunoglobulin G and complement components C3 and C4 in endometriotic tissue or endometrium in women with adenomyosis or endometriosis. *Med. Sci. Res.*, **18**, 727–8
7. Witz, C.A., Montoya, I.A., Dey, T.D. and Schenken, R.S. (1994). Characterization of lymphocyte subpopulations and T cell activation in endometriosis. *Am. J. Reprod. Immunol.*, **32**, 173–9
8. Ota, H., Igarashi, S., Hayakawa, M., Matsui, T., Tanaka, H. and Tanaka, T. (1996). Effect of danazol on the immunocompetent cells in the

eutopic endometrium in patients with endometriosis: a multicenter co-operative study. *Fertil. Steril.*, **65**, 545–51
9. Ota, H., Igarashi, S. and Tanaka, T. (1996). Expression of γδT cells and adhesion molecules in endometriotic tissue in patients with endometriosis and adenomyosis. *Am. J. Reprod. Immunol.*, **35**, 477–82
10. Ota, H. and Igarashi, S. (1993). HLA-DR expression in endometriotic tissue in patients with endometriosis and adenomyosis. *Fertil. Steril.*, **60**, 834–8
11. Noyes, R.W., Hertig, A.T. and Rock, J. (1950). Dating the endometrial biopsy. *Fertil. Steril.*, **1**, 3–25
12. Lessey, B.A., Castelbaum, A.J., Sawin, S.W., Buck, C.A., Schinnar, R., Bilker, W. and Strom, B.L. (1994). Aberrant integrin expression in the endometrium of women with endometriosis. *J. Clin. Endocrinol. Metab.*, **79**, 643–9
13. Arrigo, A.-P. and Landy, J. (1994). *The Biology of Heat Shock Proteins and Molecular Chaperones*, pp. 335–73. (New York: Cold Spring Harbor Laboratory Press)
14. Pratt, W.B. (1993). The role of heat shock proteins in regulating the function, folding, and trafficking of the glucocorticoid receptor. *J. Biol. Chem.*, **268**, 21455–8
15. Fuqua, S.A.W., Blum-Salingaros, M. and McGuire, W.L. (1989). Induction of the estrogen-related '24 K' protein by heat. *Cancer Res.*, **49**, 1668–73
16. Tabibzadeh, S., Kong, Q.F., Satyaswaroop, P.G. and Babaknia, A. (1996). Heat shock proteins in human endometrium throughout the menstrual cycle. *Hum. Reprod.*, **11**, 633–40
17. Koshiyama, M., Konishi, I., Nanbu, K., Nanbu, Y., Mandai, M., Komatsu, S., Yamamoto, S., Mori, T. and Fujii, S. (1995). Immunohistochemical localization of heat shock proteins HSP70 and HSP90 in the human endometrium: correlation with sex steroid receptors and Ki-67 antigen expression. *J. Clin. Endocrinol. Metab.*, **80**, 1106–12
18. Yang, X.-D. and Feige, U. (1992). Heat shock proteins in autoimmune disease. From causative antigen to specific therapy? *Experientia*, **48**, 650–6
19. Nip, M.M.C., Miller, D., Taylor, P.V., Gannon, M.J. and Hancock, K.W. (1994). Expression of heat shock protein 70 kDa in human endometrium of normal and infertile women. *Hum. Reprod.*, **9**, 1253–6
20. El-Roeiy, A., Dmowski, W.P., Gleicher, N., Radwanska, E., Harlow, L., Binor, Z., Tummon, I. and Rawlins, R.G. (1988). Danazol but not gonadotropin-releasing hormone agonists suppresses autoantibodies in endometriosis. *Fertil. Steril.*, **50**, 864–71

Section 4

Regulatory mechanisms, growth factors and cell adhesion molecules in the pathogenesis of endometriosis

Establishment of a permanent human endometriosis-derived cell line (FbEM-1)

J. Bouquet de Jolinière, M. Doussau, M. Canis, M. Levardon and J. Gogusev

Introduction

Mechanisms controlling development, growth and differentiation of endometriosis have not been well defined so far. Several hypotheses including endometrial cell reflux, celomic metaplasia, embryonic cell rests and immunological theories have been proposed[1,2]. It is noteworthy that ovarian steroids, estrogen in particular, serve as the primary mitogenic stimulus for successful growth of the ectopic endometriotic cells[3]. Several studies have demonstrated that endometriotic implants contain lower concentrations of estrogen and progesterone receptor proteins than those found in normal endometrium[4,5]. In this context, endometriosis has not been reported in prepubertal or premenarchal women[6]. However, this disease can be diagnosed in postmenopausal patients with high estrogen levels and in patients treated with hormonal therapy for gonadal dysgenesis[1]. In general, the concentration of estrogen and progesterone receptors detected in endometriosis implants is usually lower than that in eutopic endometrium[7,8]. In certain circumstances, steroid receptors are not detectable in endometriotic implants[7–9]. Based on the observation that the growth of endometriotic tissue is stimulated by estrogens and inhibited by progesterone in most patients[1], induction of hypoestrogenism using gonadotropin-releasing hormone (GnRH) analogs generally results in temporary involution but not complete regression of the endometriotic implants[10]. These observations suggest that although ovarian steroids stimulate endometrial cell growth, additional mechanisms must be involved in controlling endometriotic cellular proliferation[1].

In this report, we describe the establishment of a permanent human cell line FbEM-1, derived from peritoneal endometriotic implants from a patient with endometriosis. This cell line was isolated by serial passages, giving rise to a spontaneously proliferating cell line, which was characterized by immunocytochemical and cytogenetic techniques. The results presented demonstrate that the FbEM-1 cells share certain immunological markers expressed in the normal endometrium and therefore may be extremely useful for studying the role of the hormone polypeptides and their receptors in the dynamics and etiology of the endometriotic disease.

Materials and methods

Source of endometriosis cell

A 29-year-old woman with an echogenic adnexal mass detected on ultrasonography was recruited for the possible retrieval of endometrioma biopsies at surgery. The patient was first treated with GnRH agonist therapy and followed for several months before surgery. Since pain and ovarian mass persisted, laparoscopy was performed detecting severe endometriosis designated as stage IVd according to the American Fertility Society (AFS) classification[11].

Cell preparation and culture

Endometriosis cultures were prepared from biopsies of both peritoneal implants and from the cellular material from the 'chocolate cyst' fluid, as previously described[12], with some modifications. Briefly, the fragments were rinsed, minced and digested with collagenase (2 mg/ml) at 37°C in 5% CO_2 for 60 min. Epithelial glands were separated from stromal cells, blood cells and debris by serial filtration using narrow gauge sieves (45 μm). Thereafter the glands were washed from the sieves and allowed to proliferate in Dulbecco's modified Eagle medium (Life Technologies Ltd., UK) supplemented with 10% fetal calf serum and antibiotics. In a separate experiment, stromal cells from the endometriotic peritoneal implants were plated and allowed to adhere to the culture flasks; thereafter blood cells and debris were removed by rinsing. Stromal-like cell cultures were established in parallel using the cellular material from the fibrous part of the endometrioma wall, following the same culture procedures.

Immunocytochemistry

To determine whether the FbEM-1 cells retained phenotypically specific epithelial markers related to normal endometrial cells, we performed immunocytochemistry using a panel of specific antibodies (Table 1). For immunostaining, cytocentrifuge smears of proliferating FbEM-1 cells were fixed in either 4% paraformaldehyde or cold acetone (10%), rinsed in phosphate-buffered saline and incubated with the primary antibody. Monoclonal (Moabs) and/or polyclonal antibodies were revealed using rabbit anti-mouse or goat anti-rabbit immunoglobulin G peroxydase conjugated antibodies (Dako, Denmark) according to standard methods. Control slides were incubated with normal mouse serum to replace the specific monoclonal or polyclonal antibodies. Immunoreactivity of the antibodies was evaluated semiquantitatively as follows: (+ +) intense staining; (+) moderate staining; (+/–) weak staining; (–) staining not significantly greater than that of the control slide.

Cytogenetic analysis

Chromosomal studies were performed at three different passages. The cells were incubated in Dulbecco's modified Eagle medium supplemented with 10% fetal calf serum and colchicine (0.01 mg/ml). After 2 h the suspension was centrifuged and the cells were incubated for 30 min at 37°C in a solution containing 0.075 mol/l potassium chloride, and fixed with methanol:acetic acid (3:1). Chromosomes on air-dried slides were R-banded with 0.25% trypsin and stained with 0.5% Wright's stain.

Xenografting into nude mice

Cells were grown to confluency, trypsinized and resuspended in medium. Three nude mice (nu/nu Swiss strain, Iffa-Credo, France) were injected subcutaneously in both flanks with 10^7 cells suspended in 0.5 ml of medium. Progress of xenografts was monitored by weekly inspection during 6 months.

Results

Establishment of FbEM-1 cell line and growth characteristics

The primary cultures obtained after seeding the endometriotic glands from the peritoneal biopsies and those obtained from the chocolate cyst fluid contained mostly flat adherent cells. The mixed cell populations appeared variable in their size and in their morphology. After the first passage, the adherent cells with epithelial morphology became admixed with round cells forming clumps. Within 1 week, several small foci consisting of rather small spindle or polygonal cells appeared among the loosely proliferating epithelial-like cells and gradually increased in size. After 3–4 weeks in culture, aggregate-forming round cells growing

Table 1 Phenotype of the FbEM-1 cell line

Antibody used	Specificity	Source	Immunolabeled cells (%)
CL (5D3)	CK 8, 18, 19	Boehringer Mannheim (Germany)	60
V9	vimentin	Dako (Denmark)	30
CEA (II-7)	CEA	Dako (Denmark)	—
OC-125	CA-125	Dako (Denmark)	—
E29	EMA	Dako (Denmark)	<5
Factor VIII	vWF	Dako (Denmark)	—
IOT2	HLA class I	Immunotech (France)	40
CD3 (UCHT1)	T cells	Dako (Denmark)	—
CD20 (B-Ly)	B cells	Dako (Denmark)	—
CD45 RB	T, B, Mo, Mϕ, Gr	Dako (Denmark)	—
PR (B-30)	progesterone receptor	Santa Cruz (USA)	40
AR (C-19)	androgen receptor	Santa Cruz (USA)	<10
ER (H-20)	estrogen receptor	Santa Cruz (USA)	—
DE-R11	desmin	Dako (Denmark)	—
CIV22	collagen IV	Dako (Denmark)	—

CK, cytokeratin; CEA, carcinoembryonic antigen; CA-125, carcinoma antigen-125; EMA, epithelial membrane antigen; Gr, granulocytes

in suspension appeared which were successfully passaged at a density of 2×10^5/ml. At passage 4–5, approximately 6 weeks later, the cells began to grow rapidly, and thereafter could be serially subcultured at a dilution of 1:4 every week. These cells maintained in medium supplemented with 10% fetal calf serum grew vigorously with a mean doubling time of about 38 h in the exponential growth phase. This new cell line, designated FbEM-1, has been stably maintained for over 40 passages and the population doubling time has not varied over 12 months in culture (Figure 1). On phase contrast microscopy, the FbEM-1 cells at passage 20 and 32 continued to grow in suspension, and remained polymorphic with cytoplasmic protrusions and aggregate forming capacity (Figure 2). FbEM-1 cells have maintained a stable morphology during 2 years *in vitro* without signs of senescence, such as reduction in the rate of cell growth.

The cultured stromal cells from both endometriotic implants (StFb) and the fibrous endometrioma wall appeared as adherent fibroblast-like cells, their doubling time being approximately 9 days (Figure 1). Both endometriosis stromal cells and those from the endometrioma wall grew as elongated cells which were densely packed and which reached confluency in about 14–18 days (Figure 2). Phenotypically, cultured stromal cells were different from the FbEM-1 cells.

Cytochemical characteristics of the cell line

Results of the immunohistochemical staining of FbEM-1 cells with specific monoclonal and polyclonal antibodies are summarized in Table 1. Among the epithelial markers, cytokeratin expression remained one of the most specific characteristics at various passages. The anti-cytokeratin antibody detecting cytokeratin 8, 18 and 19 produced cytoplasmic labeling of the majority of FbEM-1 cells immunostained at passage 12 and 20 (Figure 3). Strong cytokeratin labeling was also detected in the majority of the cells derived from the autologous normal endometrium (not shown). These cells were negative for factor VIII-related antigen, indicating no contamination with endothelial cells. Unexpectedly, FbEM-1

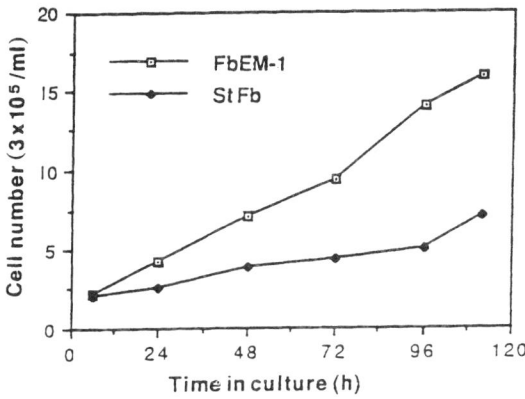

Figure 1 Growth curve of the FbEM-1 cell line at the 7th passage and stromal cell cultures (StFb) from the endometriotic implants at the same *in vitro* passage. The cells in the logarithmic growth phase were seeded at 2×10^5/ml. Each point represents the mean ± SE of triplicate cultures evaluated in two separate experiments

cells were negative or weakly immunoreactive for epithelial membrane antigen (EMA), whereas the normal endometrial cells were consistently stained. Lymphoid or monocyte/macrophage cell lineages were excluded by negative immunolabeling using antibodies against CD3, CD20 and CD45 antigens. Results of steroid receptor expression in FbEM-1 cells are also reported in Table 1. More than 40% of the cells were immunoreactive with the antiprogesterone antibody, showing a brown nuclear stain produced by the 3,3'Diaminobenzidine (DAB) colorimetric reaction (Figure 3). Conversely, less than 10% were stained with anti-androgen receptor antibody, while no positive immunostaining was obtained using specific anti-estrogen receptor antibody. Some of these phenotypic characteristics are thus consistent with a cell line of endometrial epithelial origin.

Cytogenetic findings

On karyotype analysis, the FbEM-1 cells examined at passages 8 and 20 exhibited a hypotetraploid karyotype with a modal

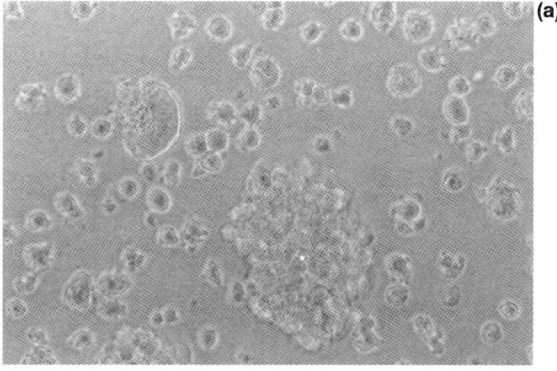

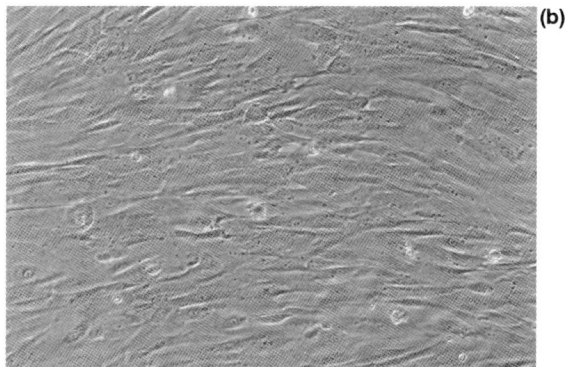

Figure 2 (a) Phase contrast photomicrograph of cultured FbEM-1 cells at passage 17. Note the presence of large polymorphic round cells growing in suspension and forming aggregates (original magnification ×600). (b) Phase contrast microscopy of 8 days culture of stromal cells from a separate endometriotic implant obtained from the same patient. Note the presence of densely packed fibroblast-like cells (original magnification ×600)

chromosome number of 61. The composite karyotype of the FbEM-1 cell line was 61 (x, +1, +2, +3, der4q+, 5q+, +7, +8, +10, −X, +15, +17, +18, +19, +20, +21). Remarkably, most of the cells contained a constant abnormality in the karyotype with the presence of an elongated long arm of chromosomes 4 and 5 (Figure 4).

Growth in nude mice

Six months after inoculation of cells, tissue from the site of injection was taken from two

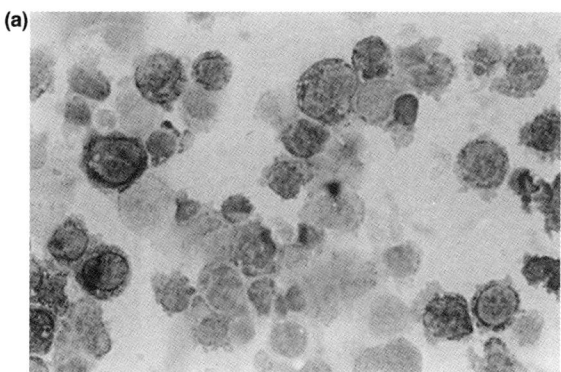

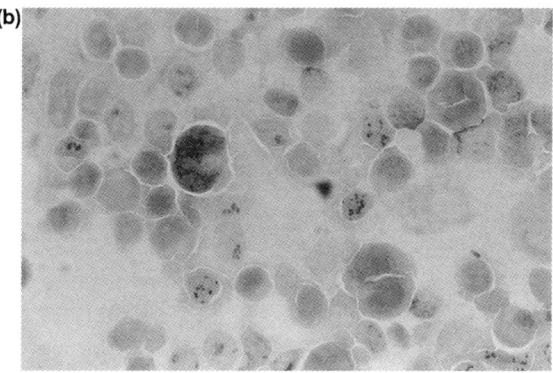

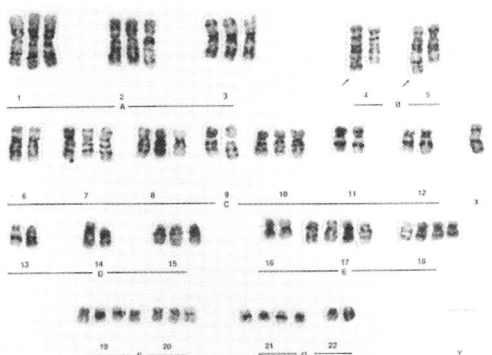

Figure 3 Immunohistochemical localization of cytokeratin (a) and progesterone receptor molecules (b) in FbEM-1 cells on cytocentrifuge smears. The cytokeratin proteins are localized exclusively in the cytoplasm while progesterone receptor is localized in the nuclei of FbEM-1 cells (original magnification ×600)

Figure 4 R-banded hypo-tetraploid karyotype of FbEM-1 cells from the 7th passage. Presence of a variety of chromosome abnormalities representing 61 chromosomes, including 4q+ and 5q+ (arrowheads)

of the animals and analyzed after hematoxylin and eosin staining. On histological analysis, no tumor growth was revealed on tissue sections, and only fibrous scar tissue remained.

Discussion

In this study we have investigated detailed morphologic and growth characteristics of a newly established human endometriosis-derived FbEM-1 cell line. The findings include excessive proliferation of rather heterogeneous small round to polygonal cells, exhibiting pleomorphism and positive immunoreactivity for vimentin, cytokeratin, progesterone and androgen receptor. Conversely, only weak cytoplasmic staining was observed with anti-EMA, whereas the CA-125 and the carcinoembryonic antigen were not detected in FbEM-1 cells. Some of these features are compatible with the expression pattern of antigenic molecules specific to cells from endometrial origin. These results are in agreement with previous studies showing that endometriosis-derived cells grown in short-term culture expressed appropriate cell-specific cytoskeletal elements including cytokeratin, vimentin, EMA and CA-125[13,14]. Concerning the pattern of steroid receptor expression, consistent nuclear immunostaining was detected for progesterone receptor in approximately 40% of the FbEM-1 cells, while estrogen receptor molecules were not found. Weak nuclear immunolabeling of androgen receptor was also present in less than 10% of FbEM1 cells. Decreased levels of estrogen and progesterone receptors in endometriotic tissue when compared to the normal endometrium have been described[7,8]. In contrast, no such differences were found between the level of expression of androgen receptors, which generally remained similar to the normal endometrial tissue[15,16]. Comparatively, variable levels of steroid receptors have been described in cultured normal endometrial cells when evaluated by the effect of different steroid drugs on their growth *in vitro*[17]. However, in a recent study it has been suggested that there were no substantial qualitative differences between the levels of estrogen receptor, prolactin and CA-125 synthesis in cultured cells from endometrioma and normal endometrium[14].

Altogether, the present results suggest that there is a differential expression of the progesterone, androgen and estrogen receptors in the FbEM-1 cells during various *in vitro* passages. Additionally, we detected similar levels of progesterone and androgen receptors and absence of estrogen receptor molecules in normal endometrial cells cultured in the same *in vitro* conditions (not shown). The failure to detect estrogen receptor in cultured FbEM-1 cells may be a result of either low sensitivity of detection, or specific regulation of estrogen and progesterone receptor protein levels during the cell cycle progression. Since it is accepted that the culture possibly modifies cell-specific protein expression, it would be of significance to determine whether the immunologically detected steroid receptors in FbEM-1 cells are biologically active. In this respect, the absence of estrogen receptors in FbEM-1 cells may provide additional information about the clinical unresponsiveness seen in 20–25% of patients submitted to different hormonal regimens[18].

The increased proliferative potential of the FbEM-1 cell line *in vitro* may be mediated directly or indirectly by the observed chromosomal changes. To our knowledge, only one study has analyzed the chromosomal structure of endometriosis after short-term culture[19]. A panel of 45 endometrial implants were investigated for cytogenetic abnormalities and showed no consistent chromosome aberrations in any of the cases. In the majority of specimens, random numerical changes involving various chromosomes were detected except in one case where an inversion of chromosome 9 has been recognized as an isolated abnormality[19]. The cytogenetic analysis of the FbEM-1 cell line has shown presence of aneuploidy.

Nevertheless, no tumorigenic effect was obtained after injection of the cells from various passages into the nude mice observed during several months. At the present time, we cannot exclude the theory that the FbEM-1 cells arose from an endometriotic focus undergoing neoplastic transformation[20]. However, characteristic chromosomal abnormalities including the 12q24 and the reciprocal translocation t(6;14) found in ovarian tumors[21] were not detected in FbEM-1 cells. In this context, it is well known that other benign tumors contain clonal chromosomal aberrations such as lipomas[22], pleomorphic adenomas[23] and meningiomas[24], and that an abnormal chromosome pattern is not always associated with malignant disorder[25]. Whether the hypotetraploid karyotype in the FbEM-1 cell line possesses a common chromosomal marker with other endometriotic lesions *in vivo* or grown *in vitro* remains to be further elucidated.

To our knowledge, establishment of a permanent human endometriosis-derived cell line has not yet been reported because the establishment is difficult and cell lines retaining the peculiar nature of the original endometriotic proliferation cannot always be obtained. Progress has long been hampered by the inability of human glandular epithelial cells to transform spontaneously *in vitro*. The cell line FbEM-1 has survived a crisis which occurred between passages 20 and 24, and has now been maintained spontaneously *in vitro* for more than 50 passages. However, although certain phenotypic characteristics of FbEM-1 cells, including cytokeratin, progesterone and androgen receptor protein expression, show similarities to the endometrial cells in culture, delineation of such parallels does not definitively identify that endometriosis arises from endometrium.

In conclusion, the FbEM-1 cell line, stably retaining a morphologically distinct nature as endometriotic proliferation *in vitro*, could be useful for multidisciplinary studies such as the line of cell differentiation, histogenesis, biological behavior and therapeutic models in human endometriosis.

References

1. Olive, D.L. and Schwartz, L.B. (1993). Endometriosis. *N. Engl. J. Med.*, **328**, 1759–69
2. Ridley, J.H. (1968). The histogenesis of endometriosis: a review of facts and fancies. *Obstet. Gynecol. Surv.*, **23**, 1–7
3. Di Zerega, G.S., Barber, D.L. and Hodgen, G.D. (1980). Endometriosis: role of ovarian steroids in initiation, maintenance and suppression. *Fertil. Steril.*, **33**, 649–53
4. Lyndrup, J., Thorpe, S., Glenthoj, A., Obel, E. and Sele, V. (1987). Altered progesterone/estrogen receptor ratios in endometriosis. *Acta Obstet. Gynecol. Scand.*, **66**, 625–9
5. Prentice, A., Randall, B.J., Weddell, A., McGill, A., Henry, L., Horne, C.H. and Thomas, E.J. (1992). Ovarian steroid receptor expression in endometriosis and in two potential parent epithelia: endometrium and peritoneal mesothelium. *Hum. Reprod.*, **7**, 1318–25
6. Gleicher, N., el-Roeiy, A., Confino, E. and Fuberg, J. (1987). Abnormal autoantibodies in endometriosis: is endometriosis an autoimmune disease? *Obstet. Gynecol.*, **70**, 115–22
7. Bergqvist, A., Rannevik, G. and Torell, J. (1981). Estrogen and progesterone cytosol receptor concentration in endometriotic tissue and intrauterine endometrium. *Acta Obstet. Gynecol. Scand.*, **101**(Suppl.), 53–8
8. Jänne, O., Kauppila, A., Kokko, E., Lantto, T., Rönnberg, L. and Vihko, R. (1981). Estrogen and progestin receptors in lesions: comparison with endometrial tissue. *Am. J. Obstet. Gynecol.*, **141**, 562–6
9. Lessey, B.A., Metzger, D.A., Haney, A.F. and McCarty, K.S. Jr (1989). Immunohistochemical analysis of estrogen and progesterone receptors in endometriosis: comparison with normal endometrium during the menstrual cycle and the effect of medical therapy. *Fertil. Steril.*, **51**, 409–15
10. Meldrun, D.R. (1985). Management of endometriosis with gonadotropin releasing hormone agonists. *Fertil. Steril.*, **44**, 581–2
11. The American Fertility Society (1985). Revised American Fertility Society classification of endometriosis. *Fertil. Steril.*, **43**, 351–2
12. Osteen, K.G., Hill, G.A., Hargrove, J.T. and Gorstein, F. (1989). Development of a method to isolate and culture highly purified populations of stromal and epithelial cells from human endometrial biopsy specimens. *Fertil. Steril.*, **52**, 965–72
13. Matthews, C.J., Redfern, C.P., Hirst, B.H. and Thomas, E.J. (1992). Characterization of human purified epithelial and stromal cells from endometrium and endometriosis in tissue culture. *Fertil. Steril.*, **57**, 990–7
14. Ryan, I.P., Schriock, E.D. and Taylor, R.N. (1994). Isolation, characterization, and comparison of human endometrial and endometriosis cells *in vitro*. *J. Clin. Endocrinol. Metab.*, **78**, 642–9
15. Punnonen, R., Pettersson, K., Vanharanta, R. and Lukola, A. (1985). Androgen, estrogen and progestin binding in cytosols of benign gynecologic tumors and tumor-like lesions. *Horm. Metab. Res.*, **17**, 607–9
16. Bergqvist, A. and Ferno, M. (1988). Steroid receptors in endometriotic tissue and endometrium assayed with monoclonal antibodies. In Genazzani, A.R., Petraglia, F., Volpe, A. and Facchinetti, F. (eds.) *Recent Research on Gynecological Endocrinology*, Vol. 1, pp. 394–9. (Carnforth, UK: Parthenon Publishing)
17. Rose, G.L., Dowsett, M., Mudge, J.E., White, J. and Jeffcoate, S.L. (1988). The inhibitory effects of danazol, danazol metabolites, gastrinone and testosterone on the growth of human endometrial cells *in vitro*. *Fertil. Steril.*, **49**, 224–8
18. Hull, M.E., Moghissi, K.S., Magyar, D.F. and Hayes, M.F. (1987). Comparison of different treatment modalities of endometriosis in infertile women. *Fertil. Steril.*, **47**, 40–4
19. Dangel, A., Medchill, M.T., Davis, G., Meloni, A.M. and Sandberg, A. (1994). Cytogenetic studies in endometriosis tissue. *Cancer Genet. Cytogenet.*, **78**, 172–4
20. Heaps, J.M., Nieberg, R.K. and Berek, J.S. (1990). Malignant neoplasms arising in endometriosis. *Obstet. Gynecol.*, **75**, 1023–8
21. Wake, N., Hreshchyshyn, M.M., Piver, S.M., Matsui, S. and Sandberg, A. (1980). Specific cytogenetic changes in ovarian cancer involving chromosomes 6 and 14. *Cancer Res.*, **40**, 4512–18

22. Sreekantaiah, C., Leong, S.P.L., Karakousis, C.P., McGee, D.L., Rappaport, W.D., Villar, H.V., Neal, D., Fleming, S., Wankel, A., Herrington, P.N., Carmona, R. and Sandberg, A.A. (1990). Cytogenetic profile of 109 lipomas. *Cancer Res.*, **51**, 422–33
23. Mark, J. and Dahlenfors, R. (1986). Cytogenetic observations in 100 human benign pleomorphic adenomas: specificity of the chromosomal aberrations and their relationship to sites of localized oncogenes. *Anticancer Res.*, **6**, 299–308
24. Zang, D.K. (1982). Cytological and cytogenetical studies on human meningioma. *Cancer Genet. Cytogenet.*, **6**, 249–74
25. Dal Cin, P. and Sandberg, A.A. (1990). Karyotypic analysis of solid tumours. In Underwood, J.C.E. (ed.) *Current Topics in Pathology*, Vol. 82, *Pathology of the Nucleus*, pp. 258–88. (Berlin: Springer-Verlag)

Expression of steroid receptors, vimentin and cytokeratin in endometriotic tissue

M. Nisolle, J. Donnez and F. Casanas-Roux

Steroid receptors

The presence of estrogen receptors (ER) and progesterone receptors (PR) has been documented both in human endometrium[1,2] and in endometriotic tissue[3-8]. Measurement of ER and PR in cytosol extracts of endometriotic implants does not permit the identification of receptors in the cells of interest. Immunohistochemical techniques with monoclonal antibodies specific to ER and PR allow direct visualization of nuclear receptor sites within individual cells, require small amounts of tissue, and permit the identification of receptors in the glandular and stromal cells.

We evaluated the ER and PR content of eutopic endometrium throughout the menstrual cycle, and of peritoneal endometriotic lesions, using a recently advanced stereographic computer technology to find out whether the concentrations of endometriotic nuclear receptors undergo cyclic changes in a similar way to normal endometrial tissue[9].

Methodology

Immunostaining quantitative analysis was performed with the computerized microscope image processor. All samples were analyzed field-by-field using the 100× immersion objective of the Axioskop light microscope (Zeiss, Oberkochen, Germany) through the charge coupled device (CCD) camera (Dage-MTI, Michigan City, IL, USA). The image features were displayed on the RGB monitor and stored for processing by the image analysis program which we created and set on the Vidas 2.1 (Kontron Bioanalyse GmBH, Eching, Germany). The program was set up in order to allow the interactive selection of the objects (positive and/or negative epithelial and stromal nuclei) for subsequent automatic measurement. The selection of the nuclei was carried out on objects in the 'gray reference image' which had to be identified before the densitometric parameters of each individual nucleus were measured: mean gray value of the nucleus and standard deviation of the gray values inside the nucleus, mean optical density of the nucleus and standard deviation of the optical densities inside the studied nucleus. In each case, the camera had to be adjusted interactively before image analysis started, in order to define the amplification factor and the reference voltage, and make possible the evaluation and comparison of the different gray level values. In each case, about 100 positive and negative nuclei at the level of the stroma and glandular epithelium, respectively, were selected on a blind basis and evaluated. The only selection criterion was the absence of superimposition of the nuclei in order to obtain the real optical density. The percentage of positive nuclei in each category of cells, epithelial and stromal respectively, was calculated. The distribution of specific staining was evaluated according to an optical density scale using the values of all the positive nuclei of a given receptor; the quantitative H-score (QH-score) was calculated as follows: QH-score $=\Sigma P_i$, where i is the optical intensity

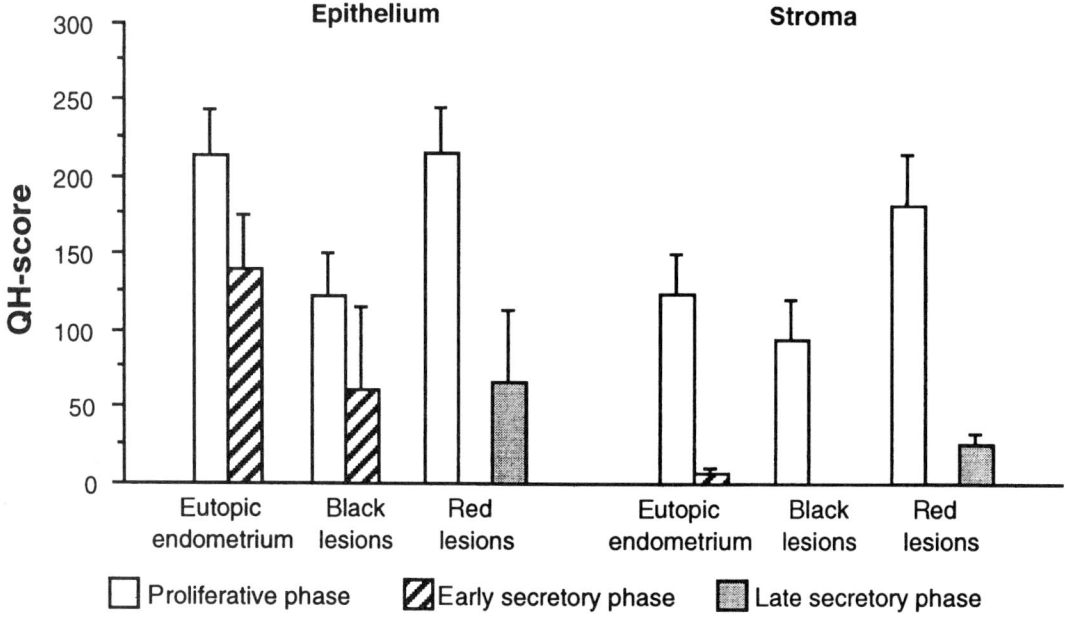

Figure 1 Estrogen receptors: mean ± SD quantitative H-score of the glandular and stromal cells in eutopic endometrium and black and red peritoneal lesions throughout the menstrual cycle

(from 0 to 3) and P is the percentage of stained cells for each given i (from 0 to 100%). The χ^2 test, the median test and the one-way analysis of variance were used for statistical analysis[10].

Results

QH-score of estrogen receptors and progesterone receptors

The results of the measurement of ER and PR content of eutopic endometrium and peritoneal endometriosis according to the QH-score are shown in Figures 1 and 2.

Eutopic endometrium The highest mean QH-scores of the ER content of epithelial and stromal nuclei (234 ± 77 and 125 ± 86, respectively) were obtained during the proliferative phase and subsequently, a significant decrease ($p < 0.001$) was noted during the early and late secretory phases. The highest QH-scores of PR content were also noted during the proliferative phase in the nuclei of the glandular epithelium and stroma (261 ± 64 and 195 ± 62, respectively) and during the early secretory phase (243 ± 93 and 192 ± 82, respectively). A significant decrease ($p < 0.001$) was observed in both types of nuclei during the late secretory phase.

Black lesions The highest mean QH-scores of ER content were also found during the proliferative phase in the epithelial nuclei (123 ± 89), as well as the stromal nuclei (94 ± 84). During the secretory phase, a significant decrease was observed in both types of nuclei. The highest QH-scores of PR content were also observed during the proliferative phase in the glandular epithelium and stroma of endometriotic implants (263 ± 69 and 198 ± 83, respectively). A decrease (not significant) in PR content occurred in the glandular epithelium during the secretory phase. A significant decrease was observed during the late secretory phase in the stroma (132 ± 120).

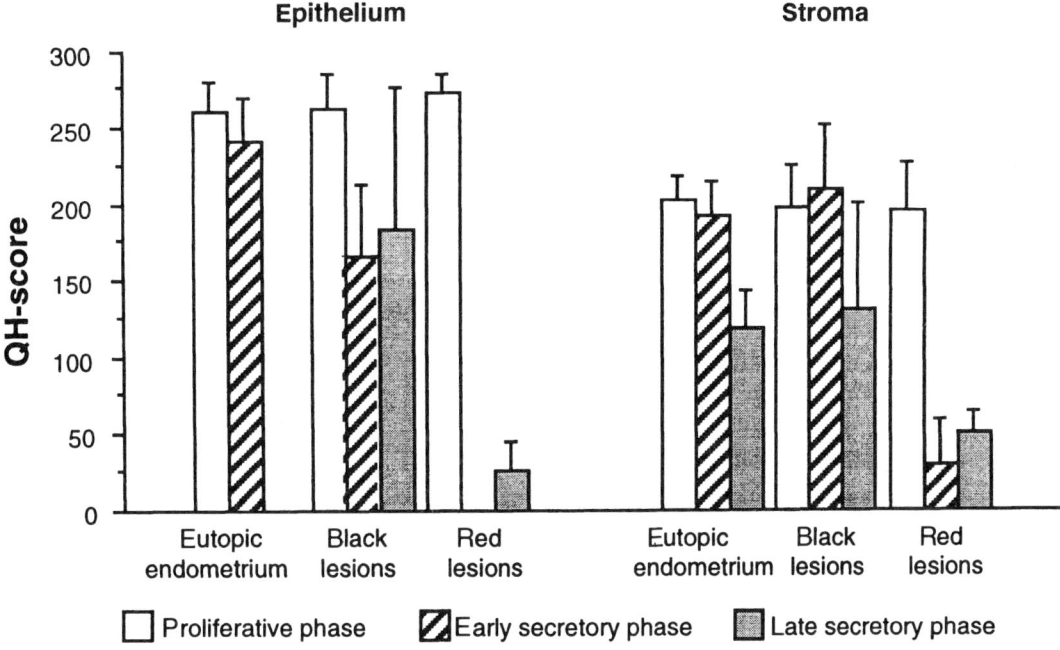

Figure 2 Progesterone receptors: mean ± SD quantitative H-score of the glandular and stromal cells in eutopic endometrium and black and red peritoneal lesions throughout the menstrual cycle

Red lesions The highest mean QH-scores of ER content were again found during the proliferative phase in the epithelial nuclei (216 ± 28), as well as the stromal nuclei (182 ± 33). During the secretory phase, a significant ($p < 0.05$) decrease was noted in both types of nuclei. The highest mean QH-scores of PR content were also observed during the proliferative phase in the glandular epithelium and stroma (273 ± 13 and 197 ± 31, respectively). During the secretory phase, a significant ($p < 0.02$) decrease in PR content also occurred in the glandular epithelium (27 ± 19) and in the stroma (51 ± 13).

Comparison between eutopic endometrium and peritoneal endometriosis

Estrogen receptors The ER content was found to be lower in the glandular epithelium of black lesions than in eutopic endometrium, but similar cyclic changes (a decrease during the secretory phase) were observed. In the stroma, the ER content and its cyclic variations were similar in eutopic and ectopic endometrium.

A similar ER content was observed in the glandular epithelium of eutopic endometrium and red lesions during the proliferative phase. During the late secretory phase, a higher QH-score was found in the glandular epithelium of red lesions. In the stroma, the ER content was similar during the proliferative phase but higher in red lesions during the late secretory phase.

Progesterone receptors The PR content was found to be similar in eutopic endometrium and black lesions, except for a significantly higher PR content observed in the glandular epithelium of black lesions during the late secretory phase.

The PR content was found to be similar in the glandular epithelium of eutopic endometrium and red lesions during the proliferative phase. A significantly higher PR content was observed in red lesions during the late secretory phase. However, when compared to black lesions, the PR content during the late secretory phase was found to be significantly lower in red lesions. In the stroma, the PR content was similar in eutopic endometrium and red lesions during the proliferative phase, but lower in red lesions during the early and late secretory phases.

Comments

Several methods have been used to measure steroid receptors in endometrium and in endometriotic tissue. In the case of hormone-ligand binding assays, which require homogenized tissue extracts, the involvement of surrounding non-target tissue reduces the level of specific binding. By contrast, immunohistochemical techniques using monoclonal antibodies specific to ER and PR have the advantage of requiring only a small amount of tissue and maintaining tissue architecture, thus allowing the assessment of the cellular distribution of receptors. But immunological methods may detect receptor molecules that are not biologically active.

In our study, immunohistochemical staining was also used but the distribution and the intensity were determined by an advanced computerized stereographic technology using image analysis. To our knowledge, a comparison of the visual H-score vs. computer image analysis for steroid receptors has only been made for breast cancer by McClellan and colleagues[11]. For each nucleus, the corresponding nuclear optical density was obtained by computerized image analysis. This method has two very clear advantages: the distinction between cell types is well defined, and the receptor content is quantitatively analyzed.

Another interesting finding was the disappearance of PR in the glandular epithelium during the late secretory phase. This can reflect its declining functional importance during early pregnancy in cell populations, whereas stroma, which becomes decidualized, would logically require receptors to support its further growth and development.

In our quantitative immunohistochemical study, cyclic changes were noted in eutopic endometrium, as well as in black lesions. Indeed, the ER content of glandular epithelium and stroma decreased significantly during the secretory phase in the same way in both ectopic and eutopic endometrium. The ER content was, however, lower in the glandular epithelium of black lesions than in eutopic endometrium. The PR content and its cyclic changes were similar in both endometrium and endometriosis, except in the glandular epithelium during the late secretory phase where a persistently high PR content was observed in black lesions. The discrepancy between the results of our study and the other studies may be due to the different assay methods used. In particular, biochemical assays which require a tissue homogenate obscure the heterogeneity of receptor content between glands and stroma, and between endometriotic implants and non-endometrial tissue. Our method is probably more objective because the observer does not have to determine the degree of staining. This distinction is automatically established using computerized image analysis.

Analyzing these data in relation to the absence of secretion in endometriotic lesions previously described, we suggested either differences in the regulation of the receptors between eutopic and ectopic endometrium, or the presence of an unknown control mechanism between the receptors and the intracellular content. Indeed, the fact that the PR do not disappear during the late secretory phase proves that in black lesions, the regulation of PR is not under the control of progesterone only. One explanation is that the tissue response which results in an alteration of the histological appearance is somewhat distal to ER and PR regulation and, therefore, more vulnerable to regulatory influences from surrounding non-endometrial tissue. Whereas the regulation of ER and PR synthesis appears to be a direct effect of estrogen and progesterone in eutopic endometrium, the proliferative and secretory effects of these steroids on endometriotic tissue appear to be, at least in part, indirect, affected by growth factors and other paracrine substances whose precise role in the regulation of endometriotic structure and function remains to be clarified.

In our study, the high PR content found in the epithelial and stromal cells of ectopic endometrium suggests a residual functional importance of both epithelium and stroma at the end of the cycle. This suggests that both epithelium and stroma play a major role in the growth and development of endometriosis. Bergqvist and Ferno[7,8] also found a higher PR content in endometriotic tissue during the luteal phase than during the follicular phase. They proposed, as an explanation of this cyclical pattern, that the hormonal regulation of endometriotic tissue is different from that of endometrium, and that PR are synthesized but not completely biologically active. In our opinion, the persistence of PR in both the epithelium and stroma of endometriotic lesions may explain the inefficacy of medical therapy[9], and the reason why peritoneal endometriosis can quickly recur after cessation of medical therapy[12]. The persistence of PR in the glandular epithelium can also account for the persistence of histologically active disease after a 6-month agonist therapy. In the stroma, the PR content is similar in both endometrium and endometriosis. In endometrium, the persistently high PR content during the secretory phase was interpreted as a sign of the functional importance of the stroma, which requires receptors to support its further growth and development during the late luteal phase. In endometriosis, a similarly high PR content in the stroma during the luteal phase strongly suggests that the stroma plays an important role in the development of endometriotic tissue.

Cytokeratin and vimentin expression

Intermediate filaments constitute a distinct fibrous network within the cytoplasm of higher eukaryotic cells, and can be divided into five subclasses, biochemically and immunologically distinct: cytokeratin characteristic of epithelial cells, vimentin that occurs in mesenchymally derived cells, desmin typical of myogenic cells, glial filaments that are found in astrocytes, and neurofilaments found in neuronal cells. The immunohistochemical identification of proteins has been widely used to determine and aid in the differential diagnosis of tumors, because tumors retain the capability to synthesize the same intermediate filaments as their parent tissues.

Several authors[13,14] have reported the coexpression of cytokeratin and vimentin in eutopic and ectopic endometrium and have not found any significant differences between the two tissues or according to the phase of the menstrual cycle.

We evaluated the coexpression of cytokeratin and vimentin in peritoneal endometriosis (black and red lesions) and in eutopic endometrium throughout the cycle. The H-score was calculated in the epithelial and stromal cells of both tissues using the equation described by McCarty and colleagues[15]. The staining was evaluated by determination of the distribution of staining within each tissue component and the intensity of the staining.

Results

Figures 3 and 4 illustrate the H-score of the cytokeratin staining and vimentin staining in the glandular epithelium and stroma of eutopic endometrium and ectopic peritoneal endometriosis throughout the cycle.

Cytokeratin

Glandular epithelium In eutopic endometrium, the cytokeratin H-score observed during the proliferative phase (111 ± 33) was significantly ($p < 0.001$) lower than that observed during the early and late secretory phases (220 ± 78 and 245 ± 64, respectively).

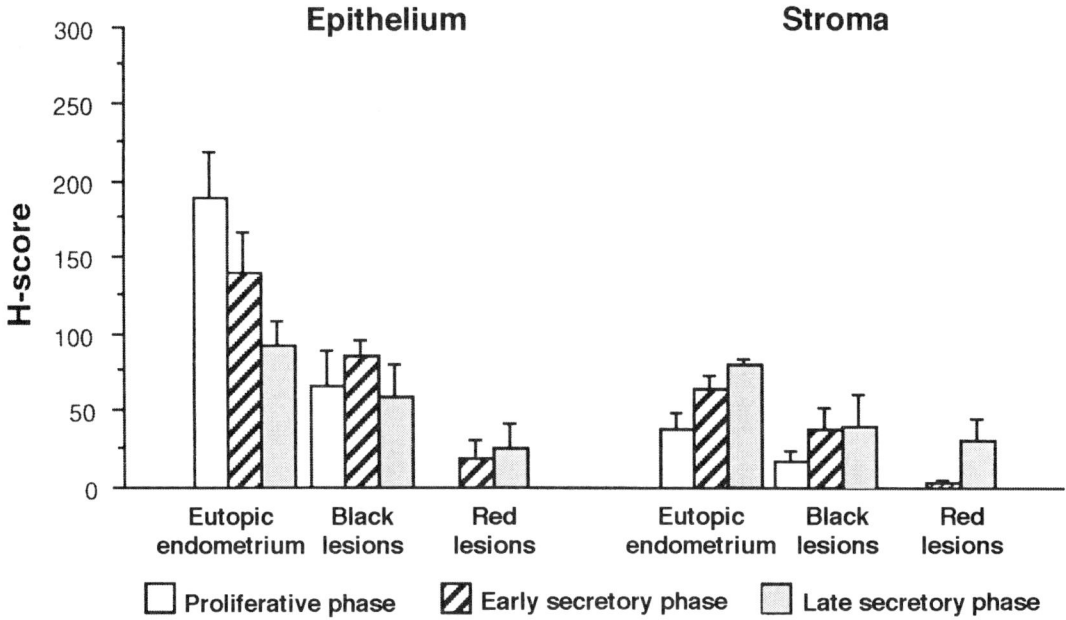

Figure 4 Vimentin: H-score (mean ± SEM) of the epithelial and stromal cells in eutopic endometrium and black and red peritoneal lesions according to the cycle phase

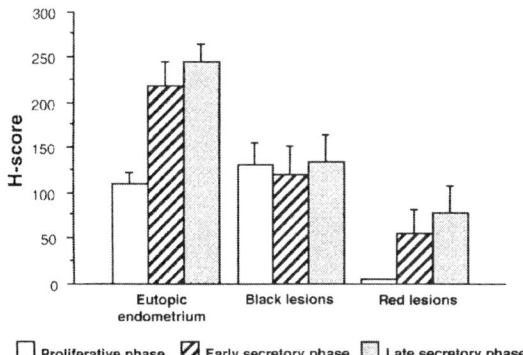

Figure 3 Cytokeratin: H-score (mean ± SEM) of the epithelial cells in eutopic endometrium and black and red peritoneal lesions according to the cycle phase

In black lesions, the cytokeratin H-score did not significantly differ during the different menstrual cycle phases: its value was 131 ± 76 during the proliferative phase, 121 ± 81 during the early secretory phase and 135 ± 59 during the late secretory phase.

In red lesions, low H-scores were observed when compared to eutopic endometrium and black lesions. The cytokeratin H-score was lower in peritoneal endometriosis than in eutopic endometrium. This difference was statistically significant during the early and late secretory phases ($p < 0.02$ and $p < 0.01$, respectively).

Stroma No cytokeratin staining was observed in the stromal cells.

Vimentin

Glandular epithelium In eutopic endometrium, the vimentin H-score was the highest during the proliferative phase (188 ± 92) compared with that observed during the early secretory phase (140 ± 84) and the late secretory phase (93 ± 49). The decrease was statistically significant during the secretory phases ($p < 0.01$). Moreover, the pattern of vimentin immunoreactivity in the epithelial cells was different according to the menstrual cycle phase. Indeed, in the proliferative glands, the immunoreaction for vimentin resulted in a fasciculated pattern of staining, whereas vimentin was strictly confined to the basal pole of the cytoplasm in the secretory glands.

In black lesions, the vimentin H-score was found not to be significantly different during the different menstrual cycle phases. Its value was 66 ± 66 during the proliferative phase, and 86 ± 22 and 60 ± 36 during the early and late secretory phases, respectively.

In red lesions, the vimentin H-score was, respectively, 20 ± 27 and 26 ± 40. No significant difference was noted between the two phases of the cycle. The vimentin H-score was significantly lower ($p < 0.005$) in red lesions when compared to black lesions during the early secretory phase. Hyperplasia was obvious in some areas, and the vimentin staining was negative in these areas. The secretory changes were then absent in the glandular epithelium. In other areas, the heterogeneity of vimentin staining was obvious. Indeed, some areas revealed a high staining intensity, although others were negative.

Stroma In eutopic endometrium, the vimentin H-score was found to be different according to the menstrual cycle phase. A significantly higher vimentin H-score was observed during the early ($p < 0.05$) and late secretory phases (65 ± 25 and 80 ± 15, respectively) ($p < 0.001$) when compared to the proliferative phase (39 ± 29).

In black lesions, the vimentin H-score was 17 ± 24 during the proliferative phase and increased up to 38 ± 32 during the early secretory phase, and to 40 ± 36 during the late secretory phase.

In red lesions, the vimentin H-score was, respectively, 4 ± 4 and 32 ± 33 during the early and late secretory phases. However, these differences were not statistically significant. When compared to black lesions, the vimentin H-score was significantly ($p < 0.05$) lower in red lesions during the early secretory phase.

Comments

Cytokeratins have proved to be useful markers of cell type and cell differentiation. The coexpression of intermediate filaments in glandular epithelial cells, as well as the consistently cytokeratin-negative stromal cells, has already been proved by several authors[13,16].

The results concerning the cyclic variations of cytokeratin and vimentin staining in eutopic endometrium are controversial. Moreover, the comparison of cytokeratin and vimentin staining between eutopic and ectopic endometrium is also a subject for discussion[13,14,16].

Although Nakamura and colleagues[14] did not observe any cyclic variations in cytokeratin staining, our study[17] demonstrated cyclic variations in eutopic endometrium: a significant increase was observed during the secretory phase which could be related to a higher degree of differentiation during this phase. The epithelial cells expressed cytokeratin but the stromal cells never did.

Strong vimentin expression was observed during the proliferative phase and the early secretory phase[17]. The significant decrease observed during the late secretory phase confirms the results of Ohwada and colleagues[18] and Nakamura and colleagues[14], but contrasts with the study of Norwitz and associates[13] and Viale and co-workers[16] who failed to demonstrate any cyclic variation. Vimentin serves a structural function in the cytoplasm. The loss of these cytoskeletal proteins in the endometrial glands can play a role in the implantation process[13] but it may also reflect a change in glandular function.

In our study, the comparison of the staining pattern revealed that peritoneal endometriosis expressed cytokeratin similarly to eutopic endometrium, but to a much lesser extent[17].

The vimentin content was also consistently lower than in eutopic endometrium. In endometriosis, it could be interpreted as a lower degree of cell differentiation. In hyperplastic endometrial lesions[19], the loss of vimentin expression in the absence of secretory changes gives rise to suspicion regarding their benign process. Similar findings (loss of vimentin expression and absence of secretory changes) were observed in areas with glandular hyperplasia found in red lesions. It is questionable to interpret these data as a factor of aggressivity as has been done in normal endometrium[19]. In our opinion, red lesions showing reduced vimentin expression represent the most 'progressive' form of peritoneal endometriosis.

References

1. Tamaya, T., Murakami, T. and Okada, H. (1986). Concentrations of steroid receptors in normal human endometrium in relation to the day of the menstrual cycle. *Acta Obstet. Gynecol. Scand.*, **65**, 195–8
2. Bouchard, P., Marraoui, J., Massai, M.R., Medalie, D.E., De Ziegler, D., Perrot-Applanat, M., Frydman, R. and Bergeron, C. (1991). Immunocytochemical localization of oestradiol and progesterone receptors in human endometrium: a tool to assess endometrial maturation. *Baill. Clin. Obstet. Gynecol.*, **5**, 107–15
3. Jänne, O., Kauppila, A., Kokko, E., Lantto, T., Rönnberg, L. and Vihko, R. (1981). Estrogen and progestin receptors in endometriosis lesions: comparison with endometrial tissue. *Am. J. Obstet. Gynecol.*, **141**, 562–6
4. Bergqvist, A., Jeppsson, S. and Ljungberg, O. (1985). Histochemical demonstration of estrogen and progesterone binding in endometriotic tissue and in uterine endometrium. *J. Histochem. Cytochem.*, **33**, 155–61
5. Lessey, B.A., Metzger, D.A., Haney, A.F. and McCarty, K.S. Jr (1989). Immunohistochemical analysis of estrogen and progesterone receptors in endometriosis: comparison with normal endometrium during the menstrual cycle and the effect of medical therapy. *Fertil. Steril.*, **51**, 409–15
6. Metzger, D.A. (1993). Cyclic changes in endometriosis implants. In Brosens, I.A. and Donnez, J. (eds.) *The Current Status of Endometriosis Research and Management*, pp. 89–108. (Carnforth, UK: Parthenon Publishing)
7. Bergqvist, A. and Ferno, M. (1993). Estrogen and progesterone receptors in endometriotic tissue and endometrium: comparison according to localization and recurrence. *Fertil. Steril.*, **60**, 63–8
8. Bergqvist, A. and Ferno, M. (1993). Oestrogen and progesterone receptors in endometriotic tissue and endometrium: comparison of different cycle phases and ages. *Hum. Reprod.*, **8**, 2211–17
9. Nisolle, M., Casanas-Roux, F., Wyns, C., De Menten, Y., Mathieu, P.E. and Donnez, J. (1994). Immunohistochemical analysis of estrogen and progesterone receptors in endometrium and peritoneal endometriosis: a new quantitative method. *Fertil. Steril.*, **62**, 751–9
10. Siegel, S. (1956). *Non Parametric Statistics for the Behavioural Sciences*. International Student Edition. (New York: McGraw Hill)
11. McClellan, R.A., Wilson, D., Leake, R., Finlay, P. and Nicholson, R.I. (1991). A multicentre study into the reliability of steroid receptor immunocytochemical assay quantification. *Eur. J. Cancer*, **27**, 711–15
12. Evers, J.L. (1987). The second-look laparoscopy for evaluation of the result of medical treatment of endometriosis should not be performed during ovarian suppression. *Fertil. Steril.*, **47**, 502–4
13. Norwitz, E.R., Fernandez-Shaw, S., Barlow, D.H. and Starkey, P.M. (1991). Expression of intermediate filament in endometrial glands changes with the onset of pregnancy and in endometriosis. *Hum. Reprod.*, **6**, 1470–3
14. Nakamura, M., Katabuchi, H., Tohya, T.R., Fukumatsu, Y., Matsuura, K. and Okamura, H. (1993). Scanning electron microscopic and immunohistochemical studies of pelvic endometriosis. *Hum. Reprod.*, **8**, 2218–26
15. McCarty, K.S. Jr, Miller, L.S., Cox, E.B., Konrath, J. and McCarty, K.S. (1985). Estrogen receptor analyses: correlation of biochemical and immunohistochemical methods using monoclonal antireceptor antibodies. *Arch. Pathol. Lab. Med.*, **109**, 716–21
16. Viale, G., Gambacorta, M., Dell'Orto, P. and Coggi, G. (1988). Coexpression of cytokeratins and vimentin in common epithelial tumours of

the ovary: an immunocytochemical study of 83 cases. *Virchows Arch. (A)*, **413**, 91–101

17. Nisolle, M., Casanas-Roux, F. and Donnez, J. (1995). Coexpression of cytokeratin and vimentin in eutopic endometrium and endometriosis throughout the menstrual cycle: evaluation by a computerized method. *Fertil. Steril.*, **64**, 69–75

18. Ohwada, M., Suzuki, M. and Tamada, T. (1990). Immunohistochemical investigation of vimentin in uterine endometrial and endocervical adenocarcinoma. *Nippon Sanka Fujinka Gakkai Zasshi*, **42**, 1237–43

19. Nakopoulou, L., Minaretzia, D., Tsionou, C. and Mastrominas, M. (1990). Value of immunohistochemical demonstration of several epithelial markers in hyperplasia and neoplastic endometrium. *Gynecol. Oncol.*, **37**, 346–53

Growth factor gene expression in endometriotic tissue

Y.M. Choi

Introduction

At present there is growing evidence suggesting that growth factors may be associated with the disease process of endometriosis. Many growth factors and their receptors have been found in eutopic endometrium, and most of them have also been demonstrated in ectopic endometrium. Several known growth factors have been shown to stimulate the proliferation of endometrial cells in culture. Experimental data indicating that estrogen modulates some growth factors or their receptors in estrogen-responsive tissues further support the concept that growth factors are involved in the disease process of endometriosis.

In the present paper, studies on growth factor gene expression in endometriotic tissue, and related findings including our own, shall be reviewed.

Epidermal growth factor and its receptor

Epidermal growth factor (EGF) has been shown to induce proliferation in endometrial cell culture[1-5]. EGF also stimulates DNA and protein synthesis in endometriotic stromal cells *in vitro*[4]. Both EGF and its receptor have been identified immunohistochemically in endometrial and endometriotic tissue. In eutopic endometrium, EGF immunoreactivity is found in stroma and/or glands, with some differences in its localization among the investigators[1,6,7]. Further studies are needed to identify the exact source(s) of EGF in endometrium, while EGF mRNA is detected in normal endometrium[8,9] and endometrial stromal cells in culture[10]. In human endometriotic tissue, EGF immunoreactivity was also detected in glandular and stromal tissue[1]. In surgically induced endometriosis in rats, the highest immunostaining of EGF was associated with inflammatory cells infiltrated among endometrial stromal cells, followed by luminal and glandular epithelial and stromal cells[11].

Immunoreactive EGF receptors have been found in the gland and stroma of endometriotic lesions as well as eutopic endometrium[12-15]. There was no difference in the intensity of staining of EGF receptors between the glands of normal endometrium and those of endometriosis[13-15].

Endometriosis implants have the mRNA that encodes EGF receptor[15]. Quantitative analysis of EGF receptor gene expression revealed that endometriotic tissue had significantly less mRNA for EGF receptor than eutopic endometrium, recalling a similarity with estrogen receptor levels in endometriotic tissue compared to eutopic endometrium[15] (Figure 1). This might explain the previous report[4] that the stimulatory effect of EGF, with respect to DNA or protein synthesis, was significantly greater in endometrial stroma than in endometriotic stroma.

Many experimental data in animals indicate that estrogen modulates EGF[16,17] and EGF receptor[18-20] in estrogen-responsive tissues including uterus. Estrogen and progesterone regulate EGF receptor levels in eutopic endometrium[21]. Recent evidence suggests that some of the physiological actions of EGF are mediated through an estrogen receptor[22].

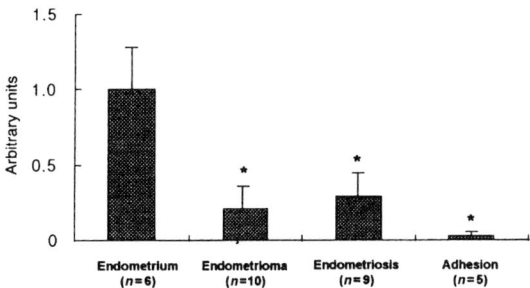

Figure 1 Relative abundance of mRNA for epidermal growth factor receptor (arbitrary units; mean ± SEM) in eutopic endometria from different phases of the menstrual cycle, cyst walls of endometriomas, endometriotic implants and pelvic adhesions. Eutopic endometrium had the highest mRNA level. *$p < 0.05$ compared with endometrium. No statistical differences were noted among cyst walls of endometriomas, endometriotic implants and pelvic adhesions. Reproduced from reference 12, with permission

Transforming growth factor-α

Transforming growth factor (TGF)-α is a protein with extensive sequence homology to EGF and acts by binding to the EGF receptor. In proliferative endometrium, TGF-α immunostaining is localized predominantly to stromal cells with no or light staining in glandular epithelium[23]. In secretory endometrium, moderate to intense staining is observed in glandular and surface epithelium and around spiral arterioles[23]. In addition, mRNA for TGF-α is detected in eutopic endometrium[24]. In surgically induced endometriosis in rats, the pattern of immunostaining for TGF-α was similar to that observed for EGF[11].

TGF-α has an effect similar to that of EGF in stimulating the proliferation of endometrial stromal cells[25,26]. TGF-α expression is also up-regulated by estrogens in a certain endometrial cancer cell line[27].

Basic fibroblast growth factor

Basic fibroblast growth factor (FGF) has an angiogenic activity as well as its mitogenic activity on human endometrial cells[5,25,26], which may be important in the implantation or maintenance of ectopic endometrium.

Basic FGF immunoreactivity is found in ectopic endometrium of women with endometriosis[28,29]. Immunoreactivity is predominantly confined to glandular epithelial cells with little or only light staining seen in stromal cells.

We have also demonstrated the expression of basic FGF mRNA by ribonuclease protection assay and two forms of FGF receptor mRNA by reverse transcriptase-polymerase chain reaction (RT-PCR) in endometriotic tissue as well as in eutopic endometrium[29,30]. We have compared the quantitative expression of basic FGF mRNA in endometriotic tissue with that in normal endometrium. The quantity of basic FGF mRNA in proliferative endometrium ($n = 7$, $1.00 ± 0.10$ arbitrary units, mean ± SEM) was similar to that in the secretory endometrium ($n = 5$, $1.18 ± 0.10$ units). The quantity of basic FGF mRNA in endometrioma ($n = 5$, $0.63 ± 0.08$ units) was about two-thirds of that found in the proliferative endometrium ($n = 5$, $1.00 ± 0.10$ units)[29] (Figure 2). Recent data showed that the concentrations of EGF and basic FGF were highly variable in the peritoneal fluid of women with or without endometriosis and did not differ significantly, and that the concentrations were so low that neither EGF nor basic FGF in peritoneal fluid could bind to its receptor[31].

We have investigated the effect of estrogen on the expression of basic FGF in human endometrial cells. When stromal cells were cultured in media containing 17β-estradiol, there was an increase in the level of basic FGF mRNA expression (unpublished data) (Figure 3). This finding further supports the hormonal regulation of basic FGF expression in endometrial tissue, as previously suggested by another investigator[32] who showed that estradiol stimulated the synthesis of basic FGF in endometrial adenocarcinoma cell lines and that this stimulation was abolished by progesterone.

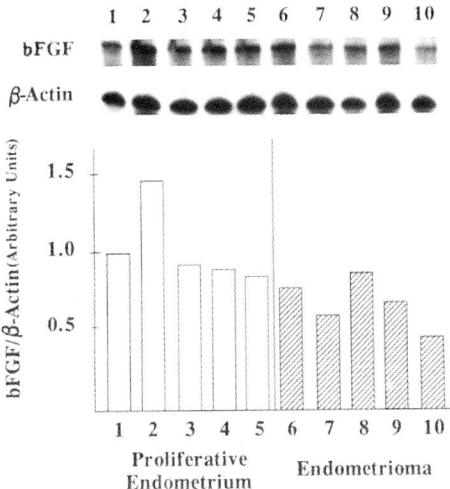

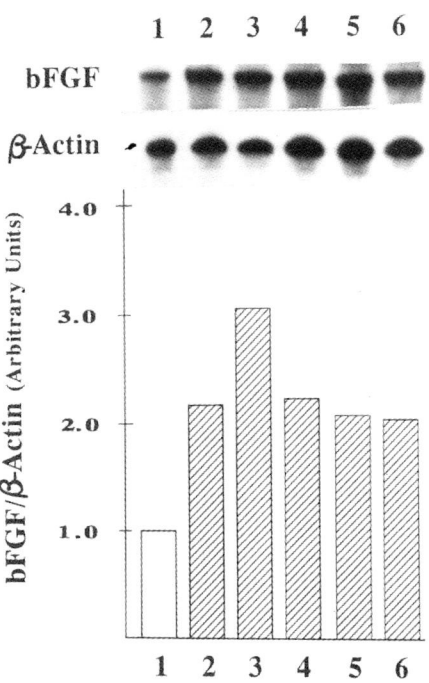

Figure 2 Expression of basic fibroblast growth factor (bFGF) mRNA in endometriomas assessed by ribonuclease protection assay. Lanes 1–5, proliferative endometrium; lanes 6–10, endometriomas. Autoradiography was carried out for 10 days for bFGF, 3 hours for β-actin. The amount of bFGF mRNA was corrected by the amount of β--actin mRNA. One arbitrary unit was defined as the mean value of bFGF mRNA in the proliferative endometrium. The amount of bFGF mRNA in endometriomas (0.63 ± 0.08 units, mean $\pm$ SEM) was two-thirds of that in the proliferative endometrium (1.00 ± 0.10 units) ($p < 0.05$)

Transforming growth factor-β

TGF-β has been proposed by some investigators as one of the growth factors which may be crucially involved in the pathogenesis of endometriotic implants[33]. TGF-β is one of the most potent chemoattractants for human monocytes[34] and an inducer of fibrosis and angiogenesis[35]. TGF-β also has striking immunoregulatory activities, as it can inhibit T lymphocyte, B lymphocyte and natural killer cell function[36]. The natural killer activity of peritoneal fluid lymphocyte is decreased in women with endometriosis[37], while TGF-β activity is increased in peritoneal fluid from women with endometriosis[38]. TGF-β is also

Figure 3 Expression of basic fibroblast growth factor (bFGF) mRNA in stromal cell cultures when incubated with various concentrations of 17β-estradiol, assessed by ribonuclease protection assay. Lane 1, no estradiol; lane 2, 10^{-8} mol/l; lane 3, 10^{-7} mol/l; lane 4, 10^{-6} mol/l; lane 5, 10^{-5} mol/l; lane 6, 10^{-4} mol/l. Stromal cells were cultured for 6 h with the above concentrations. In a representative experiment, shown in this figure, the increases in bFGF mRNA in each group compared to the control group were 114% in 10^{-8} mol/l 17β-estradiol, 204% in 10^{-7} mol/l, 120% in 10^{-6} mol/l, 103% in 10^{-5} mol/l and 102% in 10^{-4} mol/l 17β-estradiol

known to stimulate the growth of endometrial stromal cells[26].

In normal endometrium, TGF-β mRNA is equally distributed in endometrial glands and stroma, and its mRNA varies during the menstrual cycle[9,39]. Endometrial implants in surgically induced endometriosis in rats contains immunoreactive TGF-β[40]. All the cell types in the endometrial implants, with the exception of stromal cells, immunostained for TGF-β. The highest immunostaining was noted in the inflammatory cells that were infiltrated among endometriotic stromal cells and implant-associated cysts. This finding suggests the importance of endometriotic inflammatory cells in the maintenance and viability of the endometriotic implants.

Vascular endothelial growth factor

Vascular endothelial growth factor (VEGF) is a glycoprotein that promotes endothelial cell growth *in vitro*[41], and induces angiogenesis *in vivo*[42]. Unlike other classical angiogenic growth factors, functional, high-affinity receptors for VEGF are confined to vascular endothelial cells[43].

VEGF immunoreactivity is found in glandular epithelial cells of the proliferative and secretory endometrium[44,45]. VEGF mRNA is expressed in both stroma and glandular epithelium in the proliferative endometrium and in glandular epithelium in the secretory endometrium[46]. Estrogen increases VEGF mRNA expression in the rat uterus[47], and in an endometrial carcinoma cell line[46].

Very recently McLaren and colleagues[48] reported that VEGF was expressed predominantly by tissue macrophages invading ectopic endometrium with only light staining on the glandular epithelium. VEGF immunoreactivity was also found in activated peritoneal fluid macrophages. It is noteworthy that the expression of VEGF in endometriotic implants is wholly different from that of eutopic endometrium. The authors suggest that the profound angiogenesis which arises around endometriotic implants is a consequence of altered macrophage function and does not reflect angiogenic activity in the eutopic endometrium. These findings provide further evidence for the crucial role of activated macrophages in establishing and maintaining ectopic endometrium.

Conclusion

It is becoming more evident that growth factors and growth factor receptors are expressed in ectopic endometrium. Several types of growth factors, whether derived from ectopic endometrial cells or invading inflammatory cells, provide an autocrine or paracrine stimulus for stromal/epithelial cell proliferation to maintain the growth of endometriotic implants.

References

1. Haining, R.E.B., Cameron, I.T., Papendorp, C., Davenport, A.P., Prentice, A., Thomas, E.J. and Smith, S.K. (1991). Epidermal growth factor in human endometrium: proliferative effects in culture and immunocytochemical localization in normal and endometriotic tissues. *Hum. Reprod.*, **6**, 1200–5
2. Strowitzki, T., Wiedemann, R. and Hepp, H. (1991). Influence of growth factors EGF, IGF-1, and human growth hormone on human endometrial stromal cells *in vitro*. *Ann. NY Acad. Sci.*, **626**, 308–11
3. Chegini, N., Rossi, M.J. and Masterson, B.J. (1992). Platelet-derived growth factor (PDGF), epidermal growth factor (EGF), and EGF and PDGF B-receptors in human endometrial tissue: localization and *in vitro* action. *Endocrinology*, **130**, 2373–85
4. Mellor, S.J. and Thomas, E.J. (1994). The actions of estradiol and epidermal growth factor in endometrial and endometriotic stroma *in vitro*. *Fertil. Steril.*, **62**, 507–13
5. Choi, Y.M., Ku, S.Y. and Lee, J.Y. (1996). The effects of sex steroids and growth factor on the proliferation of human endometrial stromal cells. *Korean J. Obstet. Gynecol.*, **39**, 679–87
6. Hofmann, G.E., Scott, R.T. Jr, Bergh, P.A. and Deligdisch, L. (1991). Immunohistochemical

localization of epidermal growth factor in human endometrium, decidua, and placenta. *J. Clin. Endocrinol. Metab.*, **73**, 882–7

7. Chegini, N., Rossi, M.J. and Masterson, B.J. (1992). Platelet-derived growth factor (PDGF), epidermal growth factor (EGF), and EGF and PDGF β receptors in human endometrial tissue: localization and *in vitro* action. *Endocrinology*, **130**, 2373–85
8. Haining, R.E., Schofield, J.P., Jones, D.S., Rajput-Williams, J. and Smith, S.K. (1991). Identification of mRNA for epidermal growth factor and transforming growth factor-alpha present in low copy number in human endometrium using reverse transcriptase-polymerase chain reaction. *J. Mol. Endocrinol.*, **6**, 207–14
9. Murphy, L.J., Gong, Y. and Murphy, L.C. (1991). Growth factors in normal and malignant uterine tissue. *Ann. NY Acad. Sci.*, **622**, 383–401
10. Hornstein, M.D. and Yeh, J. (1992). Gene expression of transforming growth factor alpha (TGF-alpha), epidermal growth factor (EGF), and their common receptor in cultured human endometrial cells. Presented at the *3rd World Congress on Endometriosis*, Brussels, June
11. Simms, J.S., Chegini, N., Williams, R.S., Rossi, A.M. and Dunn, W.A. Jr (1991). Identification of epidermal growth factor, transforming growth factor-alpha, and epidermal growth factor receptor in surgically induced endometriosis in rats. *Obstet. Gynecol.*, **78**, 851–6
12. Melega, C., Balducci, M., Bulletti, C., Galassi, A., Jasonni, V.M. and Flamigni, C. (1991). Tissue factors influencing growth and maintenance of endometriosis. *Ann. NY Acad. Sci.*, **622**, 256–65
13. Prentice, A., Thomas, E.J., Weddell, A., McGill, A., Randall, B.J. and Horne, C.H.W. (1992). Epidermal growth factor receptor expression in normal endometrium and endometriosis: an immunohistochemical study. *Br. J. Obstet. Gynaecol.*, **99**, 395–8
14. Zhang, R., Wild, R.A., Medders, D. and Kajdacsy-Balla, A. (1993). Epidermal growth factor receptors in endometriosis. *Am. J. Gynecol. Health*, **7**, 33–7
15. Huang, J.C. and Yeh, J. (1994). Quantitative analysis of epidermal growth factor gene expression in endometriosis. *J. Clin. Endocrinol. Metab.*, **79**, 1097–101
16. DiAugstine, R.P., Pertrusz, P., Bell, G.I., Korach, K.S. and McLachlan, J.A. (1988). Influence of estrogens on mouse uterine epidermal growth factor precursor protein and messenger ribonucleic acid. *Endocrinology*, **122**, 2355–63
17. Huet-Hudson, Y.M., Chakravorty, C., De, S.K., Suzuki, Y., Andrews, G.K. and Dey, S.K. (1990). Estrogen regulates the synthesis of epidermal growth factor in mouse uterine epithelial cells. *Mol. Endocrinol.*, **4**, 510–23
18. Mukku, V.R. and Stancel, G.M. (1985). Regulation of epidermal growth factor receptor by estrogen. *J. Biol. Chem.*, **260**, 9820–4
19. Lingham, R.B., Stancel, G.M. and Loos-Mitchell, D.S. (1988). Estrogen regulation of epidermal growth factor receptor messenger ribonucleic acid. *Mol. Endocrinol.*, **2**, 230–5
20. Gardner, R.M., Verner, G., Kirkland, J.L. and Stancel, G.M. (1989). Regulation of uterine epidermal growth factor (EGF) receptors by estrogen in the mature rat and during the estrous cycle. *J. Steroid Biochem.*, **32**, 339–43
21. Taketani, Y. and Mizuno, M. (1991). Evidence for direct regulation of epidermal growth factor receptors by steroid hormones in human endometrial cells. *Hum. Reprod.*, **6**, 1365–9
22. Ignar-Trowbridge, D.M., Nelson, K.G., Bidwell, M.C., Curtis, S.W., Washburn, T.F., McLachlan, J.A. and Korach, K.S. (1992). Coupling of dual signalling pathways: epidermal growth factor action involves the estrogen receptor. *Proc. Natl. Acad. Sci. USA*, **89**, 4658–62
23. Horowitz, G.M., Scott, R.T. Jr, Drews, M.R., Navot, D. and Hoffman, G.E. (1993). Immunohistochemical localization of transforming growth factor-α in human endometrium, decidua, and trophoblast. *J. Clin. Endocrinol. Metab.*, **76**, 786–92
24. Murphy, L.J., Gong, Y., Murphy, L.C. and Bhavnani, B. (1991). Growth factors in normal and malignant uterine tissue. *Ann. NY Acad. Sci.*, **622**, 383–91
25. Irwin, J.C., Utian, W.H. and Eckert, R.L. (1991). Sex steroids and growth factors differentially regulate the growth and differentiation of cultured human endometrial stromal cells. *Endocrinology*, **129**, 2385–92
26. Hammond, M.G., Oh, S.T., Anners, J., Surrey, E.S. and Halme, J. (1993). The effect of growth factors on the proliferation of human endometrial stromal cells in culture. *Am. J. Obstet. Gynecol.*, **168**, 1131–8
27. Gong, Y., Ballejo, G., Murphy, L.C. and Murphy, L.J. (1992). Differential effects of

estrogen and antiestrogen on transforming growth factor gene expression in human adenocarcinoma cells. *Cancer Res.*, **52**, 1704–9
28. Ferriani, R.A., Charnock-Jones, D.S., Prentice, A., Thomas, E.J. and Smith, S.K. (1993). Immunohistochemical localization of acidic and basic fibroblast growth factors in normal human endometrium and endometriosis and the detection of their mRNA by polymerase chain reaction. *Hum. Reprod.*, **8**, 11–16
29. Choi, Y.M., Glatstein, I.Z., Huang, J.C., Hornstein, M.D. and Yeh, J. (1993). Expression of basic fibroblast growth factor in endometriotic tissue. Presented at the *49th Annual Meeting of the American Fertility Society*, Montreal, October.
30. Choi, Y.M., Hornstein, M.D. and Yeh, J. (1993). Gene expression of basic fibroblast growth factor and fibroblast growth factor receptor in the cultured human endometrial stromal cells. Presented at the *40th Annual Meeting of Society for Gynecologic Investigation*, Toronto, March
31. Huang, J.C., Papasakelariou, C. and Dawood, M.Y. (1996). Epidermal growth factor and basic fibroblast growth factor in peritoneal fluid of women with endometriosis. *Fertil. Steril.*, **65**, 931–4
32. Presta, M. (1988). Sex hormones modulate the synthesis of basic fibroblast growth factor in human endometrial adenocarcinoma cells: implications for the neovascularization of normal and neoplastic endometrium. *J. Cell. Physiol.*, **137**, 593–7
33. Oosterlynck, D.J. and Koninckx, P.R. (1994). Local peritoneal factors in the development of endometriosis. In Coutinho, E.M. (ed.) *Progress in the Management of Endometriosis. The Proceedings of the 4th World Congress of Endometriosis*, pp. 23–9. (New York and London: Parthenon Publishing)
34. Francis, N., Wahl, L.M., Roberts, A.B. and Sporn, M.B. (1987). Transforming growth factor type β induces monocyte chemotaxis and growth factor production. *Proc. Natl. Acad. Sci. USA*, **84**, 5788–92
35. Yang, E.Y. and Moses, H.L. (1990). Transforming growth factor β1-induced changes in cell migration, proliferation, and angiogenesis in the chicken chorioallantoic membrane. *J. Cell. Biol.*, **111**, 731–41
36. Rook, A.H., Kehrl, J.H., Wakefield, L.M., Roberts, A.B., Sporn, M.B., Burlington, D.B., Lane, L.C. and Franci, A.S. (1986). Effects of transforming growth factor β on the functions of natural killer cells: depressed cytolytic activity and blunting of interferon responsiveness. *J. Immunol.*, **136**, 3916–20
37. Oosterlynck, D.J., Meuleman, C., Waer, M., Vandeputte, M. and Koninckx, P.R. (1992). The natural killer activity of peritoneal fluid lymphocytes is decreased in women with endometriosis. *Fertil. Steril.*, **58**, 290–5
38. Oosterlynck, D.J., Meuleman, C., Waer, M. and Koninckx, P.R. (1994). Transforming growth factor-β activity is increased in peritoneal fluid from women with endometriosis. *Obstet. Gynecol.*, **83**, 287–92
39. Kauma, S., Matt, D., Strom, S., Eierman, D. and Turner, T. (1990). Interleukin-1β, human leukocyte antigen HLA-DRa, and transforming growth factor-β expression in endometrium, placenta, and placental membranes. *Am. J. Obstet. Gynecol.*, **163**, 1430–7
40. Chegini, N., Gold, L.I. and Williams, R.S. (1994). Localization of transforming growth factor beta isoforms TGF-β1, TGF-β2, and TGF-β3 in surgically induced endometriosis in the rat. *Obstet. Gynecol.*, **83**, 455–61
41. Bikfalvi, A., Sauzeau, C., Moukadiri, H., Maclouf, J., Busso, N., Bryckaert, M., Plouet, J. and Tobelem, G. (1991). Interaction of vasculotropin/vascular endothelial cell growth factor with human umbilical vein endothelial cells: binding, internalization, degradation, and biological effects. *J. Cell. Physiol.*, **149**, 50–9
42. Wilting, J., Christ, B., Bokeloh, M. and Weich, H.A. (1993). *In vivo* effects of vascular endothelial growth factor on the chicken chorioallantoic membrane. *Cell Tissue Res.*, **274**, 163–72
43. Jakeman, L.B., Winder, J., Bennett, G.L., Altar, C.A. and Ferrara, N. (1992). Binding sites for vascular endothelial growth factor are localized on endothelial cells in adult rat tissues. *J. Clin. Invest.*, **89**, 244–53
44. Li, X.F., Gregory, J. and Ahmed, A. (1994). Immunolocalisation of vascular endothelial growth factor in human endometrium. *Growth Factors*, **11**, 277–82
45. Torry, D.S., Harris, G., Holt, V., Caudle, M.R., Keenan, J.A. and Torry, R.J. (1996). Vascular endothelial growth factor expression in cycling human endometrium. *Fertil. Steril.*, **66**, 72–80
46. Charnock-Jones, D.S., Sharkey, A.M., Rajput-Williams, J., Burch, D., Schofield, J.P.,

Fountain, S.A., Boocock, C.A. and Smith, S.K. (1993). Identification and localization of alternately spliced mRNAs for vascular endothelial growth factor in human uterus and estrogen regulation in endometrial carcinoma cell lines. *Biol. Reprod.*, **48**, 1120–8

47. Cullinan-Bove, K. and Koos, R.D. (1993). Vascular endothelial growth factor/vascular permeability factor expression in the rat uterus: rapid stimulation by estrogen correlates with estrogen-induced increases in uterine capillary permeability and growth. *Endocrinology*, **133**, 829–37

48. McLaren, J., Prentice, A., Charnock-Jones, D.S., Millican, S.A., Muller, K.H., Sharkey, A.M. and Smith, S.K. (1996). Vascular endothelial growth factor is produced by peritoneal fluid macrophages in endometriosis and is regulated by ovarian steroids. *J. Clin. Invest.*, **98**, 482–9

27
Potential implications of peritoneal fluid mitogens related to proteolysis of insulin-like growth factor binding protein-3 in the pathophysiology of endometriosis

A. Lemay, M. Koutsilieris, A. Akoum and R. Maheux

Introduction

The etiology and the pathophysiology of endometriosis remain obscure. It is becoming evident that the growth of ectopic endometrial-like tissues on the peritoneum and organs of the pelvic cavity is influenced not only by sex steroid hormones but also by paracrine and autocrine factors. This paper reviews evidence for the implication of growth factors in the pathophysiology of endometriosis. The recent progress in molecular technologies has permitted collection of information concerning the expression and localization of growth factors in normal eutopic endometrium and in ectopic endometriotic lesions. Data are becoming available on growth factor expression, secretion and regulation by isolated stromal cells. The involvement of growth factors has been assessed mainly by characterization of the mitogenic activity of the peritoneal fluid bathing the peritoneal lesions. Our recent data implicate the insulin-like growth factor (IGF)/IGF binding protein-3 (IGFBP-3)/protease system where peritoneal fluid mitogenic activity is related to proteolysis of IGFBP-3. These recent observations are consistent with tissue remodeling, associating paracrine growth factors with extracellular matrix proteases expressed and secreted by endometrially derived cells.

Expression and localization of growth factors in endometriotic tissues

Several growth factors, their receptors and regulatory proteins have been identified in endometrium, and cellular localization and steroid-dependence of these proteins, as well as action of several growth modulators on endometrial cell function, have been studied[1]. A list of growth factors expressed in the endometrium is presented in Table 1. In general, endometrial growth factors have been found in both the stroma and glands, except for insulin-like growth factors (IGF) and platelet-derived growth factor (PDGF) which were not detected in glands, and acidic and basic fibroblast growth factors (FGFa, b) and vascular endothelial growth factor (VEGF) which were not found in the stroma. The expression of growth factors is increased during the secretory phase of the menstrual cycle for epidermal growth factor (EGF) and IGF-II, and during the proliferative phase for IGF-I.

Recent data also describe the tissue distribution of growth factors in endometriotic lesions. EGF and EGF-receptor have been localized by immunohistochemistry in glands and stroma of surgically induced endometriosis in the rat[2]. A similar pattern of distribution was found for transforming growth factor-α (TGF-α), whereas TGF-β was limited to

Table 1 Growth factors expressed in tissues, secreted by stromal cells and detected in peritoneal fluid

	Expression				Effect on secretion by stromal cells		Detection in peritoneal fluid	
	Endometrium		Endometriosis					
	Stroma	Gland	Stroma	Gland	Estrogens	Progestins	Control	Endometriosis
IGF-I	++	+					+	
IGF-II	+	++					+	
EGF	+	++	+	+			+	
FGFa,b		+	+	+			+	
TGF-α	++	+	+	+	decreased			
TGF-β				+			+	+++
PDGF	+				no effect	no effect		
VEGF		+	+	+	highly increased	increased	+	+++
CSF							+	++

IGF, insulin-like growth factor; EGF, epidermal growth factor; FGFa, acidic fibroblast growth factor; FGFb, basic fibroblast growth factor; TGF, transforming growth factor; PDGF, platelet derived growth factor; VEGF, vascular endothelial growth factor; CSF, colony stimulating factor; +, positive; ++, strongly positive; +++, very strongly positive

epithelial cells[3]. FGFa and FGFb were also found in glands but not in the stroma of human endometriotic lesions using both immunohistochemistry and the reverse transcriptase polymerase chain reaction (RT-PCR)[4]. However, both the stroma and the glands were found to express VEGF according to the techniques of *in situ* hybridization and Northern blot analysis[5]. The roles of these factors in comparison with those evoked in normal endometrium remain to be documented[1].

Proliferation of stromal cells and secretion of growth factors

The growth factors mentioned above have been reported to stimulate the proliferation of stromal cells prepared from eutopic endometrial tissue in culture (Table 1). Moreover, both stromal and epithelial cells secrete TGF-β into the culture medium[6]. Estrogens decrease this secretion. Stromal cells can also release VEGF which is increased by the addition of estrogens[5] and progesterone. However, there is no apparent effect of estrogens and progesterone on the release of PDGF by stromal cells. Thus stromal and epithelial cells derived from the endometrium are not only stimulated by growth factors but express and release growth factors. The secretion of at least some of these growth factors can be modified by sex steroid hormones.

Recent studies have reported the peritoneal fluid content of several growth factors including insulin-like growth factor-I (IGF-I), IGF-II, EGF, FGF, TGF-β and VEGF[7] (Table 1). The peritoneal fluid content of TGF-β, VEGF and macrophage colony stimulating factor (M-CSF) was significantly greater in endometriosis patients as compared to that of control women requesting tubal ligation and having a normal pelvis[5,8,9].

The secretion of growth factors by endometrial cells regurgitated in the pelvic cavity through the Fallopian tubes at the time of menses could therefore contribute to the development of endometriotic lesions. These factors could also come from cells of the endometriotic lesions. However, there is as yet no report of growth factors acting on or secreted by cells prepared from endometriotic lesions. These interesting observations provide first-line evidence for the eventual implication of growth factors in the development of endometriotic lesions.

Identification of peritoneal fluid mitogenic IGFBP-3 fragments

One approach to evaluating the eventual implication of growth factors in the pathophysiology of endometriosis is to characterize the mitogenic activity of the peritoneal fluid. Early studies indicated that the peritoneal fluid contains macrophage-derived growth factor(s) (MDGF). Addition of conditioned media from cultured macrophages increased [3H]thymidine incorporation in NIH-3T3 mouse embryo fibroblasts[10]. A high level of mitogenic activity was found in 68% of endometriosis patients as compared to low levels observed in 28% of controls. A similar observation also reported [3H]thymidine incorporation in endometrial stromal cells at a higher rate in endometriosis patients than in controls[11]. Addition of peritoneal fluid to culture medium also increased the number of cultured endometrial stromal cells. Interestingly this stimulatory effect was partially prevented by preincubating the cells with an anti-IGF receptor type I[12].

These results prompted our studies on the characterization of peritoneal fluid mitogenic activity. In initial experiments, NIH/3T3 (American Type Culture Collection: CRL-1658) mouse embryo fibroblasts, KLE (ATCC: CRL-1622) human endometrial adenocarcinoma cells and primary cultures of rabbit epithelial and stromal cells were used to assess the effect of individual peritoneal fluid on [3H]thymidine incorporation into cellular DNA[13]. The rate of [3H]thymidine incorporation into cellular DNA of all cell types was significantly higher compared with that in controls when increasing amounts of proteins from peritoneal fluid were added to culture media. Peritoneal fluid originating from women either with or without evidence of endometriosis demonstrated similar mitogenic properties.

A purification scheme was elaborated for the characterization of growth factors from endometrial cell types. In an initial study, peritoneal fluid was collected from women with laparoscopic evidence of endometriosis. Peritoneal fluid was retained on and eluted from carboxymethyl sepharose, heparin-sepharose, cartridges of C18 silica and reverse-phase high-performance liquid chromatography (rHPLC) columns in sequence. At the rHPLC stage, discrete protein peaks were found showing mitogenic activity for fibroblasts and rabbit endometrial epithelial cells[14]. Unfortunately, there was not enough material to achieve identification of the rHPLC-recovered material.

The purification scheme described above was applied to a larger amount of peritoneal fluid coming from women without evidence of endometriosis at laparoscopy. Stromal and epithelial cells isolated from human endometrium were used to assess the proliferative effects of peritoneal extracts. Analysis of the purified material on sodium dodecyl sulfate polyacrylamide gel electrophoresis (SDS-PAGE) revealed four protein bands with relative molecular weights of 17 000–18 000, 20 000, 25 000 and 30 000. After the first step of purification on rHPLC, we obtained the four ultraviolet peaks detected by SDS-PAGE in the eluates of the Sep-Pak column (Waters Associates, Mississanga, Canada). All four peaks contained preferential mitogenic activity on human epithelium-derived endometrial cells[15]. The peaks separated by SDS-PAGE were transferred to an Immobilon-p membrane (Amersham, Oakville, Canada) for micro-sequencing. As illustrated in Figure 1, we obtained a partial sequence for the protein bands with relative masses 17 000–18 000, 20 000, 25 000 and 29 000–30 000. The N-terminal sequences of these peptides matched the 162–171, 162–180, 162–167 and 162–171 amino acids of IGFBP-3. The common start of

```
PF: 17-18 kDa      --162-----------170-----------180
PF: 20 kDa         RY- K V D Y E S Q S T D
PF: 25 kDa         RY- K V D Y E S Q S T D T Q N F S X E X K
PF: 29-30 kDa      RY- K V D Y E S X X X X X X X X X X X X
                   RY- K V D Y E S Q S T D

human IGFBP-3      RY- K V D Y E S Q S T D T Q N F S S E S K

bovine IGFBP-3     RY- K V D Y E S Q S T D T Q N F S S E S K
porcine IGFBP-3    RY- K V D Y E S Q S T D T Q N F S S E S K

rat IGFBP-3        RY-(K)V D(Y)E S Q S T D T Q N F S S E S K
```

Figure 1 Amino acid sequence of N-terminal fragments of insulin-like growth factor binding protein-3 (IGFBP-3). PF, peritoneal fluid; NFS, potential n-linked glycosylation sites; X, residues not detected; sites of truncated rat IGFBP-3/fragments are circled

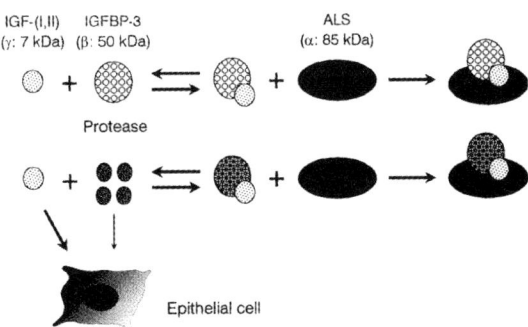

Figure 2 Insulin-like growth factor (IGF)/IGF-binding protein-3 (IGFBP-3)/protease system. IGF-I and IGF-II bind reversibly with IGFBP-3. The IGF/IGFBP-3 can also bind with the acid labile subunit (ALS) to form a large 150 kDa complex. After protease action on IGFBP-3, four fragments having masses 17–30 kDa have been identified. These fragments have direct mitogenic activity on endometrial-derived epithelial cells. IGFBP-3 proteolysis would also increase the bioavailability of IGF

these peptides isolated from the peritoneal fluid of normal women was identical to the N-terminal truncated forms of IGFBP-3 previously detected in rat serum. This part of the IGFBP-3 molecule is highly preserved in the IGFBP-3 of different species and contains N-linked glycosylation sites, suggesting an important role in the structure-function of IGFBP-3. These results indicate that the peritoneal fluid contains N-terminal fragments of the IGFBP-3 which have a mitogenic effect on primary culture of epithelial cells isolated from the human endometrium. Our results are in good agreement with the recent data from Giudice and colleagues[12] showing the presence of IGFBP-3 protease activity in the peritoneal fluid of normal women as compared to no appreciable amounts of enzyme activity in paired serum samples.

The IGF/IGFBP-3/protease system is depicted in Figure 2. As previously demonstrated in the serum of pregnant women, there is a significant proteolytic degradation of IGFBP-3 in the peritoneal fluid, giving differences in measurement of IGFBP-3 by ligand blotting and Western immunoblotting. The physiological implications of IGFBP-3 degradation by protease have been presented by Binoux and associates[16] and Lamson and colleagues[17]. Proteolysis of IGFBP-3 results in a reduction of its binding affinity for IGFs and in an increase in the dissociation rate of bound IGFs, thus increasing the bioavailability of IGFs. Our finding that N-terminal truncated fragments of IGFBP-3 have apparent direct mitogenic activity on epithelial cells derived from human endometrium suggests other mechanisms of action of the IGF system[15]. Receptors for IGFBP-3 have been found in Hs578T human breast cancer cells[18], and there could also be changes in receptor response to altered IGFBP-3. The elucidation of these putative mechanisms requires further characterization of IGFBP-3 fragments *in vitro* using cell culture systems.

Association of mitogenic and proteolytic activities of IGFBP-3

Considering the potential role of IGFBP-3 protease and our previous findings of mitogenic activity of N-terminal truncated forms of IGFBP-3 in the peritoneal fluid, it appeared pertinent to provide evidence for a probable link between the mitogenic and proteolytic activities of the peritoneal fluid. In order to

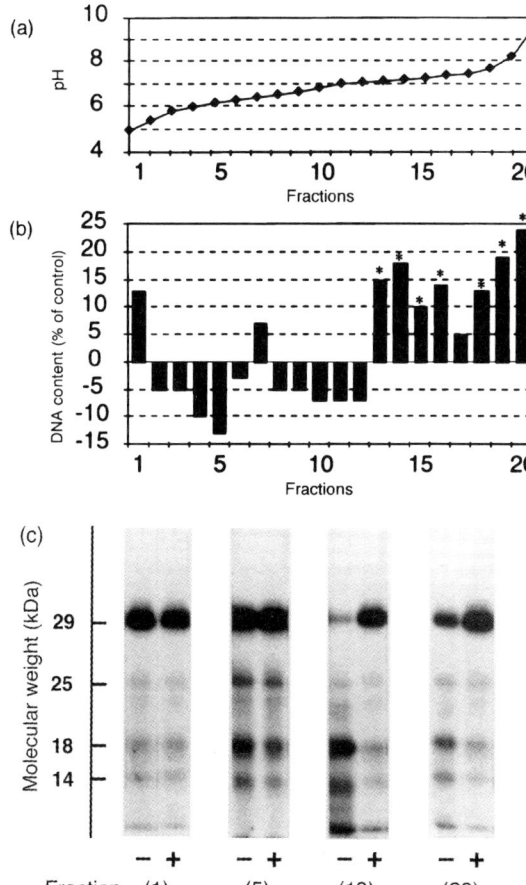

Figure 3 Mitogenic activity and insulin-like growth factor binding protein-3 (IGFBP-3) proteolysis in peritoneal fluid fractionated by isoelectric focusing. (a) pH profile, (b) mitogenic activity, $*p < 0.05$ and (c) proteolysis of IGFBP-3 following isoelectric focusing fractionation of 10 ml of peritoneal fluid from women with laparoscopic evidence of endometriosis

rapidly evaluate these two types of activity we have set up a preparative isoelectric focusing procedure.

The isoelectric focusing procedure using the Rotofor system (Bio-Rad Laboratories Canada Ltd., Mississanga, Canada) allows the separation of proteins contained in 10 ml of pooled peritoneal fluid into 20 fractions. Figure 3 illustrates the pH values and the mitogenic activity in the various fractions after an initial focusing between pH 3 and 10, and a second focusing between pH 5 and 8. A constant amount of 100 μg of proteins was used to assess the mitogenic activity in each fraction. As compared to controls containing 100 μg of BSA (bovine serum albumin), significant mitogenic activity was mainly associated with fractions corresponding to pH 7.10 ± 0.02. To evaluate the proteolytic activity, 300 μg of proteins of each fraction were incubated with 30 000 c/min of [^{125}I]-labeled IGFBP-3 in the presence or absence of diisopropylfluorophosphate (DFP) as protease inhibitor. Proteins were then separated on SDS-PAGE as shown in Figure 3. The auto-radiogram of recombinant [^{125}I]-labeled IGFBP-3 for fractions 1 and 5 indicated a strong signal for the IGFBP-3 with relative mass 29 000 and a weak signal for IGFBP-3 fragments having relative masses 14 000, 18 000 and 25 000. By contrast, in fractions 13 and 20, showing elevated mitogenic activity, there was an important decrease of the band with mass 29 000, with the appearance of strong signals mainly for the bands with masses 14 000 and 18 000. In these two fractions the proteolysis of IGFBP-3 was almost completely prevented by the addition of DFP in the incubation medium. The finding in this experiment of mitogenic activity associated with proteolysis of IGFBP-3 in common fractions is further evidence for the fact that the mitogenic activity is related to fragmentation of IGFBP-3. The possibility that the IGF system may be one of several growth factor systems in the peritoneal fluid that can stimulate endometrial cellular proliferation is supported by the data of Giudice and colleagues[12] on peritoneal fluid analysis of IGF-1, IGF-II, IGFBPs and hydrolysis of IGFBP-3. The link between proteolysis of IGFBP-3 and mitogenic activity suggests that alterations in the IGF/IGFBP-3/protease system present in the peritoneal fluid would be involved in the proliferation of ectopic implants of endometriotic cells.

IGFBP-3 protease activity which was observed initially in the serum of women with normal pregnancy[19] has already been

Table 2 Proteases expressed in tissues, secreted by stromal cells and detected in peritoneal fluid

	Expression				Effect on secretion by stromal cells			Detection in peritoneal fluid	
	Endometrium		Endometriosis						
	Stroma	Gland	Stroma	Gland	Estrogens	Progestins	Cytokines*	Control	Endometriosis
Plasminogen	+	++	+++	+		decreased			
tPA	-	+	+	-		decreased		+	++
uPA			-	++		decreased		+	++
PAI	-	+	-	-	no effect	decreased			
MMP-1		-					increased		
MMP-2							increased		
MMP-3		-			no effect	decreased	increased		
Matrilysin		+							
MMEP	+	-					increased		
TIMP-1	+	-					increased		

tPA, tissue plasminogen activator; uPA, urokinase plasminogen activator; PAI, plasminogen activator inhibitor; MMP, matrix metalloproteinase; MMEP, membrane metalloendopeptidase; TIMP, tissue inhibitor metalloprotease; *interleukin-1α and tumor necrosis factor-α; -, negative; +, positive; ++, strongly positive; +++, very strongly positive

documented in several other physiological situations such as the seminal plasma of normal men[20] and the embryonic cavities in early human pregnancy[21]. Pathological conditions have been associated with an altered IGF/IGFBP-3/protease system in the serum of patients with diabetes[22], breast cancer[23], in the cerebrospinal fluid of subjects with central nervous system tumor or meningitis[24] and in the synovial fluid of cases of arthritis[25].

Expression and secretion of proteases by endometrial cells

The observations reported above are in line with the concept that proteases coupled with growth factors are implied in tissue remodeling. It is readily apparent that several growth factors and proteases which are stored or fixed on the extracellular matrix take part in the lysis of stroma and proliferation of cells during tissue implantation and proliferation in several physiological and pathological conditions. Indeed, as indicated in Table 2, several proteases have recently been shown to be expressed in the eutopic endometrium and ectopic endometriotic implants using techniques of immunohistochemistry, in situ hybridization and Northern blot analysis[26–28]. Kallikreins 1, 2 and 3 have also been found in the endometrium by RT-PCR amplification and Southern blot analysis[29]. A recent study reports that the level of cathepsin D measured by an immunoradiometric method is significantly higher in endometriotic tissue than in endometrium[30]. Several matrix metalloproteases have been reported to be released by endometrial stromal cells in culture[31–33] (Table 2). The secretion of these proteases is generally increased by progesterone and cytokines such as interleukin-1α and tumor necrosis factor-α (TNF-α). Progesterone also increases the secretion of plasminogen activator inhibitor (PAI) and tissue inhibitor of metalloprotease-3 (TIMP-3)[34]. Endo-II, a protein released in culture media by rat endometriotic tissue was partially purified. Its amino acid sequence revealed homology with TIMP-1[35]. It is also interesting to consider that plasminogen activators have previously

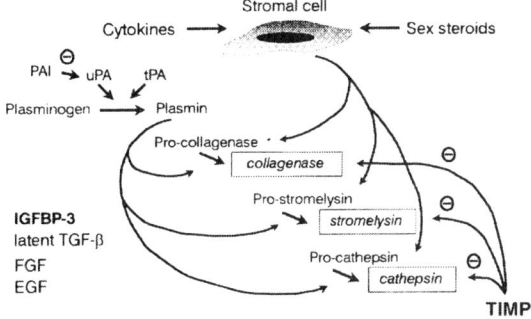

Figure 4 Extracellular matrix cascade of proteases. Cytokines and sex steroids activate and/or regulate gene coding for proteases in stromal cells. These proteases are synthesized as inactive precursors and activated by plasmin, the formation of which is triggered by urokinase or tissue activator. The proteases are inhibited by inhibitors of plasminogen activators and by tissue inhibitor of metalloproteases. Proteases, inhibitors and several growth factors are stored or bound to the extracellular matrix. They can be released during degradation of the matrix and exert proteolytic and mitogenic activities. PAI, plasminogen activator inhibitor; uPA, urokinase plasminogen activator; tPA, tissue plasminogen activator; TIMP, tissue inhibitor of metalloprotease; IGFBP-3, insulin-like growth factor binding protein-3; TGF-β, transforming growth factor-β; FGF, fibroblast growth factor; EGF, epidermal growth factor; –, negative effect

been found to be elevated in the peritoneal fluid of patients with endometriosis[36].

Our observation of an IGF/IGFBP-3/protease system in the peritoneal fluid would probably reflect tissue remodeling taking place in the peritoneal cavity. We have previously reported that urokinase-type plasminogen activator stimulates osteoblasts in PA-III cell-induced osteoblastic metastases via an IGF-1 dependent mechanism[37]. Current experiments indicate the presence of urokinase in the same fractions of peritoneal fluid containing mitogenic activity, IGFBP-3 protease and IGFBP-3 fragments (data not shown). Altogether these observations suggest that a protease cascade would be operative in the peritoneal fluid (Figure 4).

The stromal cells under the influence of cytokines and/or sex steroids release inactive protease precursors. These proteases are converted into active enzymes by plasmin deriving from the conversion of plasminogen by urokinase-type or tissue-type plasminogen activator. Plasminogen activator inhibitor and tissue inhibitor of metalloprotease act as counter regulatory factors in this situation. Further studies are required to evaluate the role of this protease cascade in the proteolysis of IGFBP-3 and its associated mitogenic activity. It is anticipated that other growth factors known to be secreted in a precursor form, such as latent IGF-β, or known to be bound to the extracellular matrix, such as FGF, would also be activated by proteases and participate in the remodeling process taking place in the pathophysiology of endometriosis.

Conclusion

Based on data in the literature and on our recent experimental observations, the mitogenic activity of the peritoneal fluid is related at least in part to an IGF/IGFBP-3/protease system. The proteolysis of IGFBP-3 is associated with increased mitogenic activity. This effect would be due to increased bioavailability of insulin-like growth factors but also to intrinsic mitogenic properties of the IGFBP-3 fragments. Further studies are required to better understand the relationship between peritoneal fluid mitogens and proteases. The actual data also indicate that the proteolysis of IGFBP-3 results from urokinase activation of plasmin and matrix metalloproteases. Other growth factors could also be activated by this cascade of proteases. These biomolecular changes in peritoneal fluid would reflect tissue remodeling involved in implantation, proliferation, differentiation, angiogenesis or adhesion formation. The eventual evaluation of alterations in growth factors and proteases appears very interesting with regard to a better understanding of the pathophysiology of endometriosis.

References

1. Giudice, L.C. (1994). Growth factors and growth modulators in human uterine endometrium: their potential relevance to reproductive medicine. *Fertil. Steril.*, **61**, 1–17
2. Simms, J.S., Chigini, N., Williams, R.S., Rossi, A.M. and Dunn, W.A. (1991). Identification of epidermal growth factor, transforming growth factor-alpha, and epidermal growth factor receptor in surgically induced endometriosis in rats. *Obstet. Gynecol.*, **78**, 850–7
3. Chegini, N., Gold, I.L. and Williams, R.S. (1994). Localization of transforming growth factor beta isoform TGF-β1, TGF-β2, and TGF-β3 in surgically induced endometriosis in the rat. *Obstet. Gynecol.*, **83**, 455–61
4. Ferriani, R.A., Charnock-Jones, D.S., Prentice, A., Thomas, E.J. and Smith, S.K. (1993). Immunohistochemical localization of acidic and basic fibroblast growth factors in normal human endometrium and endometriosis and the detection of their mRNA by polymerase chain reaction. *Hum. Reprod.*, **8**, 11–16
5. Shifren, J.L., Tseng, J.F., Zaloudek, C.J., Ryan, I.P., Meng, G., Ferrara, N., Jaffe, R.B. and Taylor, R.N. (1996). Ovarian steroid regulation of vascular endothelial growth factor in the human endometrium: implications for angiogenesis during the menstrual cycle and in the pathogenesis of endometriosis. *J. Clin. Endocrinol. Metab.*, **81**, 3112–18
6. Tan, X.M., Zhao, Y., Rossi, M.J., Abu-Rustum, R.S., Ksander, G.A. and Chegini, N. (1994). Expression of transforming growth factor-β (TGFβ) isoforms and TGFβ type II receptor messenger ribonucleic acid and protein, and the effect of TGFβs on endometrial stromal cell growth and protein degradation *in vitro*. *Endocrinology*, **135**, 450–9
7. Ramey, J.W. and Archer, D.F. (1993). Peritoneal fluid: its relevance to the development of endometriosis. *Fertil. Steril.*, **60**, 1–14
8. Oosterlynck, D.J., Meuleman, C., Waer, M. and Koninckx, P.R. (1994). Transforming growth factor-b activity is increased in peritoneal fluid from women with endometriosis. *Obstet. Gynecol.*, **83**, 287–92
9. Weinberg, J.B., Haney, A.F., Xu, F.J. and Ramakrishnan, S. (1991). Peritoneal fluid and plasma levels of human macrophage colony-stimulating factor in relation to peritoneal fluid macrophage content. *Blood*, **78**, 513–16
10. Halme, J., Kauma, W.S., Estes, J. and Haskill, S. (1988). Peritoneal macrophages from patients with endometriosis release growth factor activity *in vitro*. *J. Clin. Endocrinol. Metab.*, **66**, 1044–9
11. Surrey, E.S. and Halme, J. (1990). Effect of peritoneal fluid from endometriosis patients on endometrial stromal cell proliferation *in vitro*. *Obstet. Gynecol.*, **76**, 792–7
12. Giudice, L.C., Dsupin, B.A., Gargosky, S.E., Rosenfeld, R.G. and Irwin, J.C. (1994). The insulin-like growth factor system in human peritoneal fluid: its effects on endometrial stromal cells and its potential relevance to endometriosis. *J. Clin. Endocrinol. Metab.*, **79**, 1284–93
13. Koutsilieris, M., Allaire-Michaud, L., Fortier, M. and Lemay, A. (1991). Mitogen(s) for endometrial-like cells can be detected in human peritoneal fluid. *Fertil. Steril.*, **56**, 888–93
14. Koutsilieris, M., Niklinski, W., Frenette, G. and Lemay, A. (1993). Heparin–sepharose binding growth factors in peritoneal fluid of women with endometriosis. *Fertil. Steril.*, **59**, 93–7
15. Koutsilieris, M., Akoum, A., Lazure, C., Frenette, G., Lemay, A. and Le Groupe d'Investigation en Gynécologie (1995). N-terminal truncated forms of insulin-like growth factor binding protein-3 in the peritoneal fluid of women without laparoscopic evidence of endometriosis. *Fertil. Steril.*, **63**, 314–21
16. Binoux, M., Hossenlopp, P., Lassarre, C. and Segovia, B. (1991). Degradation of IGF binding protein-3 by proteases: physiological implications. In Spencer, E.M. (ed.) *Proceedings of the 2nd International Symposium on Insulin-like Growth Factors/Somatomedins*, pp. 329–36. (New York: Elsevier Science)
17. Lamson, G., Giudice, L.C., Cohen, P., Liu, F., Gargosky, S., Muller, H.L., Oh, Y., Wilson, K.F., Hintz, R.L. and Rosenfeld, R.G. (1993). Proteolysis of IGFBP-3 may be a common regulatory mechanism of IGF action *in vivo*. *Growth Regul.*, **3**, 91–5
18. Oh, Y., Muller, H.L., Lamson, G. and Rosenfeld, R.G. (1993). Insulin-like growth factor (IGF)-independent action of IGF-binding protein-3

in Hs578T human breast cancer cells. *J. Biol. Chem.*, **268**, 14964–71

19. Giudice, L.C., Farrell, E.M., Pham, H., Lamson, G. and Rosenfeld, R.G. (1990). Insulin-like growth factor binding proteins in maternal serum throughout gestation and in the puerperium: effects of a pregnancy-associated serum protease activity. *J. Clin. Endocrinol. Metab.*, **71**, 806–16

20. Cohen, P., Graves, H.C.P., Peehl, D.M., Kamarei, M., Giudice, L.C. and Rosenfeld, R.G. (1992). Prostate-specific antigen (PSA) is an insulin-like growth factor binding protein-3 protease found in seminal plasma. *J. Clin. Endocrinol. Metab.*, **75**, 1046–53

21. Nonoshita, L.D., Wathen, N.C., Dsupin, B.A., Chard, T. and Giudice, L.C. (1994). Insulin-like growth factors (IGFs), IGF-binding proteins (IGFBPs), and proteolyzed IGFBP-3 in embryonic cavities in early human pregnancy: their potential relevance to maternal–embryonic and fetal interactions. *J. Clin. Endocrinol. Metab.*, **79**, 1249–55

22. Bang, P., Brismar, K. and Rosenfeld, R.G. (1994). Increased proteolysis of insulin-like growth factor-binding protein-3 (IGFBP-3) in non-insulin-dependent diabetes mellitus serum, with elevation of a 29 kilodalton (kDa) glycosylated IGFBP-3 fragment contained in the approximately 130- to 150-kDa ternary complex. *J. Clin. Endocrinol. Metab.*, **78**, 1119–27

23. Frost, V.J., Helle, S.I., Lonning, P.E., van der Strappen, J.W.J. and Holly, J.M.P. (1996). Effects of treatment with megestrol acetate, aminoglutethimide, or foremstane on insulin-like growth factor (IGF) I and II, IGF-binding proteins (IGFBPs) and IGFBP-3 protease status in patients with advanced breast cancer. *J. Clin. Endocrinol. Metab.*, **81**, 2216–21

24. Muller, H.L., Oh, Y., Gargosky, S.E., Lehrnbecher, T., Hintz, R.L. and Rosenfeld, R.G. (1993). Concentrations of insulin-like growth factor (IGF)-binding protein-3 (IGFBP-3), IGF, and IGFBP-3 protease activity in cerebrospinal fluid of children with leukemia, central nervous system tumor, or meningitis. *J. Clin. Endocrinol. Metab.*, **77**, 1113–19

25. Matsumoto, T., Gargosky, S.E., Iwasaki, K. and Rosenfeld, R.G. (1996). Identification and characterization of insulin-like growth factors (IGFs), IGF-binding proteins (IGFBPs), and IGFBP proteases in human synovial fluid. *J. Clin. Endocrinol. Metab.*, **81**, 150–5

26. Rodgers, W.H., Osteen, K.G., Matrisian, L.M., Navre, M., Giudice, L.C. and Gorstein, F. (1993). Expression and localization of matrilysin, a matrix metalloproteinase, in human endometrium during the reproductive cycle. *J. Obstet. Gynecol.*, **168**, 253–60

27. Head, J.R., MacDonald, P.C. and Casey, M.L. (1993). Cellular localization of membrane metalloendopeptidase (enkephalinae) in human endometrium during the ovarian cycle. *J. Clin. Endocrinol. Metab.*, **76**, 769–76

28. Fernandez-Shaw, S., Marshall, J.M., Hicks, B., Barlow, D.H. and Starkey, P.M. (1995). Plasminogen activators in ectopic and uterine endometrium. *Fertil. Steril.*, **63**, 45–51

29. Clements, J. and Mukhtar, A. (1994). Glandular kallikreins and prostate-specific antigen are expressed in the human endometrium. *J. Clin. Endocrinol. Metab.*, **78**, 1536–9

30. Bergqvist, A., Ferno, M. and Mattson, S. (1996). A comparison of cathepsin D levels in endometriotic tissue and in uterine endometrium. *Fertil. Steril.*, **65**, 1130–4

31. Rawdanowicz, T.J., Hampton, A.L., Nagase, H., Woolley, D.W. and Salamonesen, L.A. (1994). Matrix metalloproteinase production by cultured human endometrial stromal cells: identification of interstitial collagenase, gelatinase-A, gelatine-B, and stromelysin-1 and their differential regulation by interleukin-1α and tumor necrosis factor-α. *J. Clin. Endocrinol. Metab.*, **79**, 530–6

32. Casslen, B., Nordengren, J., Gustavsson, B., Nilbert, M. and Lund, L.R. (1995). Progesterone stimulates degradation of urokinase plasminogen activator (u-PA) in endometrial stromal cells by increasing its inhibitor and surface expression of the u-PA receptor. *J. Clin. Endocrinol. Metab.*, **80**, 2776–84

33. Martelli, M., Capana, A. and Bischof, P. (1993). Sécrétion des matrixines par l'endomètre humain. *Gynecol. Obstet.*, **1**, 200–13

34. Higuchi, T., Kanzaki, H., Nakayama, H., Fujomoto, M., Hatayama, H., Kojima, K., Iwai, M., Mori, T. and Fujita, J. (1995). Induction of tissue inhibitor of metalloproteinase 3 gene expression during *in vitro* decidualization of human endometrial stromal cells. *Endocrinology*, **136**, 4973–81

35. Sharpe-Timms, K.L., Penney, L.L., Zimmer, R.L., Wright, J.A., Zhang, Y. and Surewicz, K.

(1995). Partial purification and amino acid sequence analysis of endometriosis protein-II (Endo-II) reveals homology with tissue inhibitor of metalloproteinase-1 (TIMP-1). *J. Clin. Endocrinol. Metab.*, **80**, 3784–7

36. Astedt, B. and Nordenskjold, F. (1984). Plasminogen activators in endometriosis. *Acta Obstet. Gynecol. Scand.* **123** (Suppl.), 23–4

37. Koutsilieris, M., Frenette, G., Lazure, C., Lehoux, J.-G., Govindan, M.V. and Plychornakos, C. (1993). Urokinase-type plasminogen activator: a paracrine factor regulating the bioavailability of IGFs in PA-III cell-induced osteoblastic metastases. *Anticancer Res.*, **13**, 481–6

Role of hepatocyte growth factor and its receptor *c-met* in pathogenesis of endometriosis

J. Sugawara, T. Fukaya, T. Murakami, H. Yoshida and A. Yajima

Introduction

Endometriosis is a common gynecological disease which has been associated with infertility or chronic pelvic pain. The natural history and the pathogenesis of endometriosis have been poorly understood. Recently active remodeling of endometriotic lesions has been observed in women with endometriosis[1,2]. The local factor(s) that regulates the remodeling of lesions remains unknown. The role of growth factors in the remodeling has been evaluated in the present study.

Hepatocyte growth factor (HGF) has been recognized as a strong mitogen for primary cultured rat hepatocytes[3,4]. Recent studies have demonstrated HGF to be a mesenchymal-derived pleiotropic factor that mediates mesenchymal–epithelial interactions, acting as a mitogen, motogen and morphogen of various epithelial cells[3–5]. HGF has been strongly considered as a specific factor for the regeneration or reconstruction of various tissues. The proto-oncogene *c-met* encoded protein has been identified as the receptor of HGF[6,7]. Over-expression of *c-met* oncogene has been associated with the carcinogenesis of several cancers[8,9].

In the present study, we investigate the expression of HGF and *c-met* in endometriotic lesions and the biological effects of HGF on cultured endometrial cells.

Materials and methods

RT-PCR and Southern blot hybridization

Peritoneal biopsy specimens ($n = 18$) were obtained at the time of laparoscopy for infertility or benign gynecological disease. Ten of the 18 patients had pelvic endometriosis on histological examination. Four of the 10 endometriotic specimens were recognized as red lesions and six specimens were typical black lesions. Eight normal peritoneal biopsies were obtained from the pouch of Douglas. Two normal peritoneal specimens were obtained from patients with endometriosis. Polyadenylated RNA was purified and reverse transcribed (RT) to cDNA. The HGF and *c-met* cDNA was subjected to 45 cycles of polymerase chain reaction (PCR) using primers specific for human HGF and *c-met*. Each primer gives a fragment length of 278 base pairs for HGF, and 294 base pairs for *c-met*. For the internal control, cDNA was also amplified by 35 cycles of PCR with β-actin primers, and the 368 base pair fragments were obtained. If genomic DNA contaminated the mRNA preparation, we obtained 500 base pair fragments. Southern blot hybridization was performed to confirm each specific fragment.

Immunohistochemistry for *c*-met

Peritoneal biopsy specimens ($n = 20$) were obtained at laparoscopy for infertility or benign gynecological disease. Ten of the 20 patients had pelvic endometriosis on histological diagnosis. Six of these 10 biopsy specimens were red lesions and four were typical black lesions. Ten normal peritoneal tissues were obtained from the pouch of Douglas. Immunohistochemical staining was performed with Histofine SAB-PO kits (Nichirei, Tokyo, Japan). The primary antibody used in this study was a polyclonal antibody against human c-MET (Santa Cruz Biotech, CA, USA), at a dilution of 1:20. The staining of nuclei was performed in 1% methyl green.

Cell isolation and culture

Endometrial biopsy specimens were obtained at the time of laparoscopy or laparotomy performed for benign gynecological diseases from ten Japanese women who were in the proliferative phase of the menstrual cycle. The latter information was confirmed by the date of the last menstrual period and a histologic examination. All patients had regular menstrual cycles and none of them had undergone hormonal treatment prior to surgery. Their ages ranged from 20 to 40 years. All biopsy specimens were collected at the Tohoku University Hospital between June 1995 and July 1996, with the permission of the local ethics committee. Informed consent was also obtained from each patient. The endometrial biopsy specimens were immediately placed in an ice cold, 1:1 mixture of Dulbecco Modified Eagle's Medium and Ham's F-12 (DMEM/F-12), GIBCO BRL, Grand Island, NY) and transported to the laboratory. Tissues were dissociated as reported by Smith and Kelly[10], with some modifications. The characteristics of isolated cells were determined by cell morphology and immunocytochemistry using specific antibodies for cytokeratin, vimentin, factor VIII and CD45 (DAKO).

Proliferation assay

To determine the mitogenic effects of HGF on cultured endometrial epithelial cells, we performed the MTT assay. Isolated epithelial cells were placed in 96-well multichamber dishes (Becton Dickinson, NJ, USA) at a density of 10^4 cells per well. After 24 h incubation, culture media were replaced with serum-free medium for 24 h. Epithelial cells were treated with serum-free medium with or without recombinant HGF (SIGMA, MO, USA) for 24 h. MTT assay was performed on triplicate samples[11]. Using this method, colored crystals were produced within the viable cells, extracted with Triton X-100 overnight, and the absorbance at 540 nm was measured using a microplate reader. This absorbance was closely linked with the thymidine incorporation assay[11].

Migration assay

Cell motility was investigated by migration assay with the Boyden's chamber technique. Polycarbonate filters (cell culture inserts, 8 μm pore size; Becton Dickinson) were used in this study. Epithelial cells purified from eutopic endometrium in medium containing 1% fetal bovine serum were seeded in the upper chambers and after the cells were attached to the filters, HGF was added to the lower chambers. After 24 h incubation, the upper surfaces of the chambers were scraped and washed with phosphate-buffered saline. The chambers were then fixed and stained with Diff-Quick (International Reagents Corp. Kobe, Japan) and the number of migrated cells were determined using a computerized image analysis system (LUZEX, NIRECO, Tokyo, Japan). Cell counts were performed in three randomly selected areas (magnification × 100) for triplicate samples.

Three-dimensional cell culture

A three-dimensional cell culture system was established as follows. Epithelial cell suspensions were mixed with ECM gels (MATRIGEL, Becton Dickinson) in 24-well culture dishes, and two-fold DMEM/F12 containing 2.5%

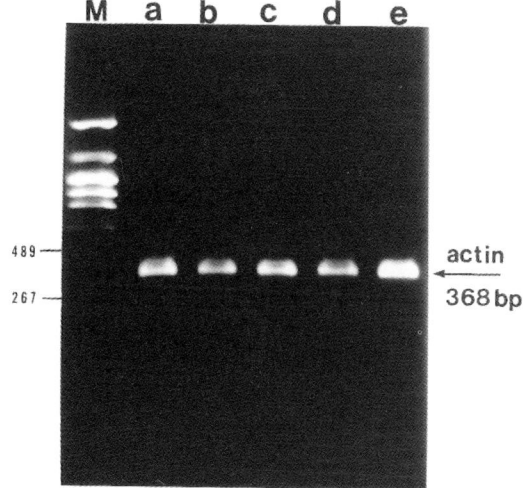

Figure 1 Ethidium bromide staining of RT-PCR products for the β-actin gene. PCR for the β-actin gene primers showed that the amount and quality of mRNA was not significantly different in (a) positive control, (b) red lesions, (c) typical black lesions, (d) normal peritoneum from patients with endometriosis and (e) normal peritoneum from patients without endometriosis

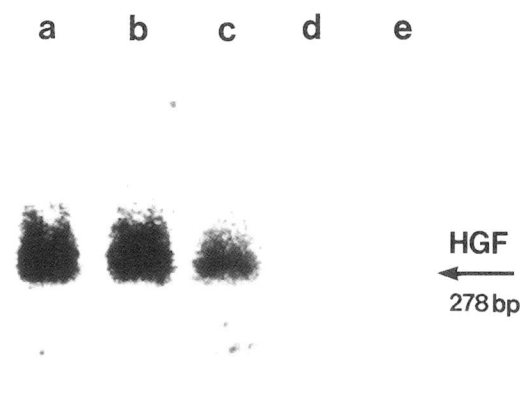

Figure 2 Southern blot analysis for RT-PCR products of HGF. HGF gene expression was detected in all specimens with endometriotic lesions. No expression of the HGF gene was found in normal peritoneum with or without endometriosis. (a) positive control, (b) red lesions, (c) typical black lesions, (d) normal peritoneum from patients with endometriosis and (e) normal peritoneum from patients without endometriosis

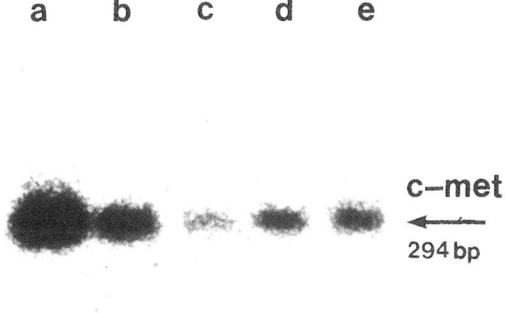

Figure 3 PCR products of the c-*met* gene were detected in all endometriotic lesions and normal peritoneum. (a) positive control, (b) red lesions, (c) typical black lesions, (d) normal peritoneum from patients with endometriosis and (e) normal peritoneum from patients without endometriosis

fetal bovine serum with or without HGF was added and cultured for 3 weeks. Morphological changes with or without lumen formation were analyzed by counting 100-cell clusters in three randomly selected areas (magnification × 100) and the percentages of clusters which formed epithelial lumens were counted with phase contrast light microscopy. To determine the histological characteristics of clusters, gels were fixed and embedded in paraffin, sectioned at 1 μm and stained with hematoxylin and eosin.

Enzyme-linked immunosorbent assay for HGF

Purified stromal cells from patients with ($n = 6$) and without ($n = 5$) endometriosis were cultured in 24-well multichamber culture dishes in DMEM/F12 supplemented with 2.5% fetal bovine serum, 100 U/ml penicillin, 100 μg/ml streptomycin and 2.5 μg/ml amphotericin B. All patients with endometriosis had active lesions (red lesions). Cell cultures were performed in triplicate. After 48 h incubation, culture supernatants were collected and duplicate samples were analyzed with the HGF ELISA kit (Institute of Immunology, Tokyo, Japan).

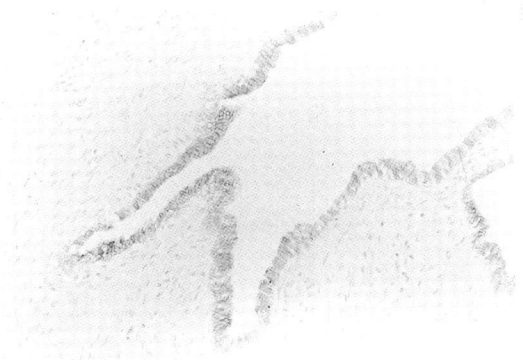

Figure 4 Immunohistochemical staining of pelvic endometriotic lesions. Immunohistochemistry was performed with the use of the polyclonal antibody for c-MET. Magnification was ×200

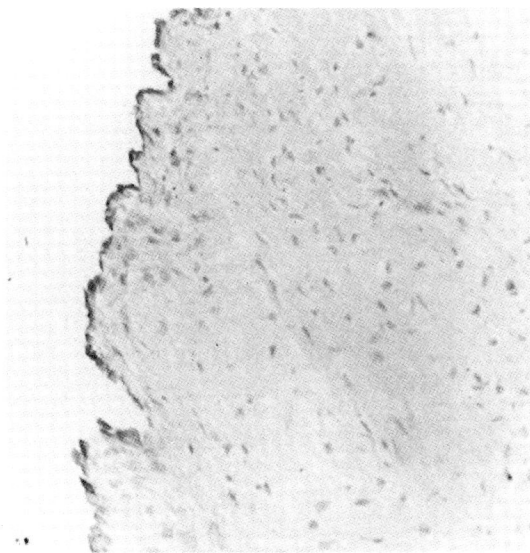

Figure 5 Immunohistochemical staining of normal peritoneum obtained from patients without endometriosis. Immunohistochemistry was performed using a c-MET polyclonal antibody. Magnification was ×200

Results

RT-PCR and Southern blot hybridization

All samples demonstrated amplification of the β-actin gene with no genomic DNA contamination (Figure 1). HGF gene expression was detected in all specimens with endometriotic lesions. No expression of the HGF gene was found in normal peritoneum with or without endometriosis (Figure 2). PCR products of the c-*met* gene were detected in all endometriotic lesions and normal peritoneum (Figure 3).

Immunohistochemistry for c-met

Positive staining was observed in the cytoplasm of ectopic endometrial epithelial cells (Figure 4) and peritoneal mesothelial cells (Figure 5).

Characterization of isolated cells

Isolated endometrial epithelial and stromal cells were determined morphologically by phase-contrast microscopy. Epithelial cells formed colonies and spread out gradually and showed polygonal cells with obvious epithelial morphology. Stromal cells showed the spindle shaped, fibroblast-like morphology. The characterization of isolated cells was further determined by immunocytochemistry for cytokeratins, vimentins, factor VIII and CD45 (data not shown). Epithelial cells were positively stained for cytokeratins, whereas stromal cells were positive for vimentins. By immunocytochemistry for factor VIII and CD45, contaminations of endothelial cells and leukocytes were shown to be less than 1%.

Proliferation assay

Mitogenic effects of HGF on cultured epithelial cells were determined by MTT assay. The addition of 10 ng/ml and 50 ng/ml HGF resulted in a significant increase in absorption at 540 nm as seen in Figure 6. This absorption was closely linked with the thymidine incorporation assay. HGF stimulates proliferation of endometrial epithelial cells in a dose-dependent manner.

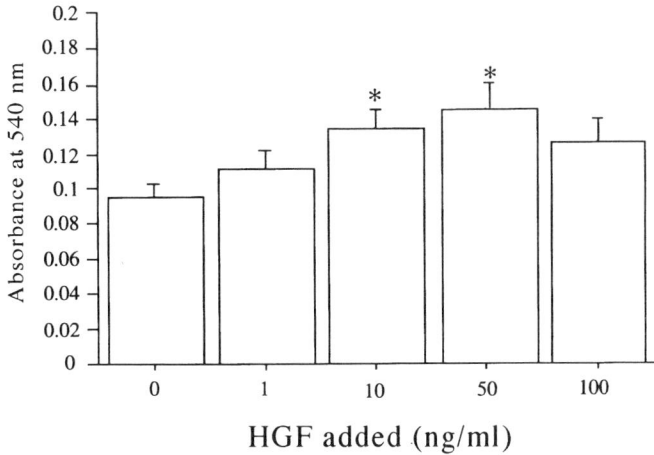

Figure 6 Mitogenic effects of hepatocyte growth factor (HGF) on cultured endometrial epithelial cells were analyzed with MTT assay. The addition of HGF resulted in significant increase in absorption at 540 nm. Results are presented as mean ± SE. *$p < 0.05$, Mann-Whitney U-test, compared with control

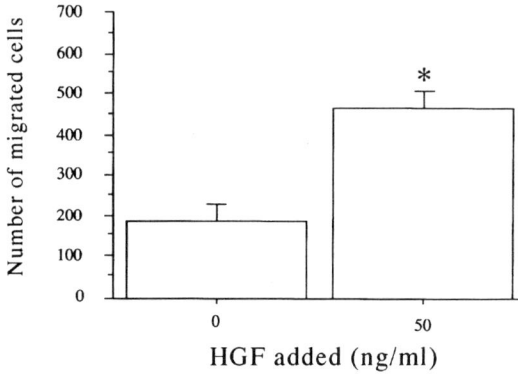

Figure 7 Cell migration of endometrial epithelial cells was determined with Boyden's chamber technique. The addition of hepatocyte growth factor (HGF) resulted in a significant increase of migrated cells. Results are presented as mean number of cells (± SE). *$p < 0.05$, Mann-Whitney U-test, compared with control

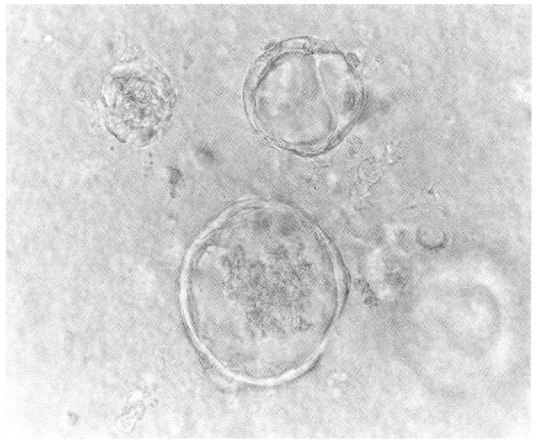

Figure 8 Phase-contrast microscopy of endometrial epithelial cells cultured in Matrigel. Cells formed cell clusters and showed lumen formation. Magnification was ×200

Migration assay

Motogenic effects of HGF on epithelial cells were determined using the Boyden's chambers technique. As seen in Figure 7, the addition of 50 ng/ml HGF in the lower chambers resulted in a significant increase of migrated cells. When HGF was added to the upper chambers, migrated cells were not observed in the lower chambers (data not shown). From these observations, it is concluded that HGF shows chemotactic activity on cultured endometrial epithelial cells.

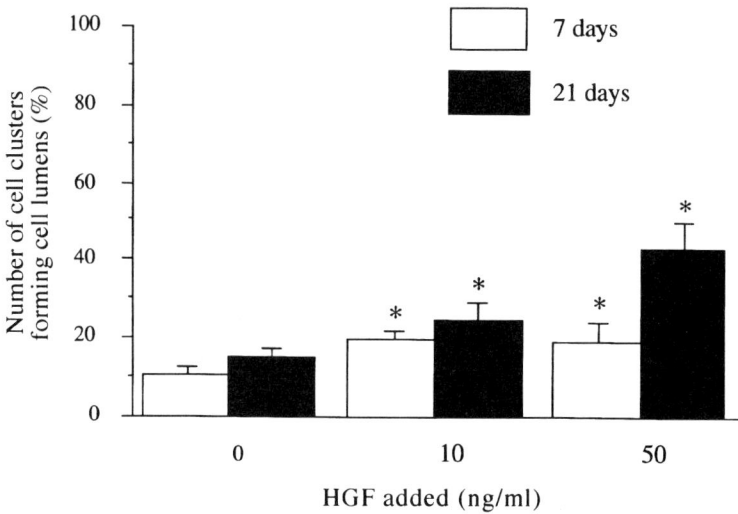

Figure 10 The rate of lumen formation was analyzed by counting 100-cell clusters in three randomly selected areas with phase-contrast microscopy. Results are presented as mean ± SE. *$p < 0.05$, Mann-Whitney U-test, compared with control. HGF, hepatocyte growth factor

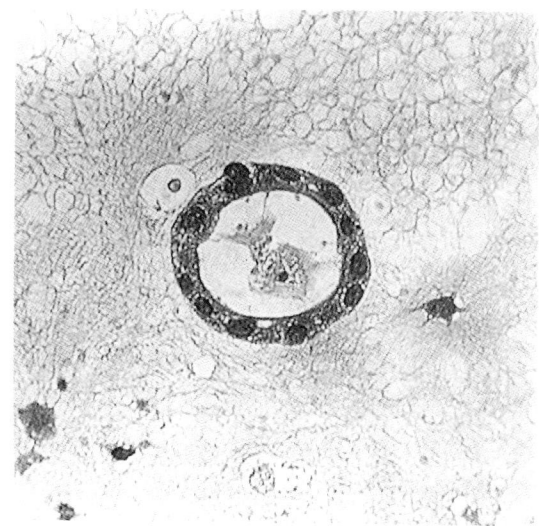

Figure 9 Hematoxylin and eosin staining resulted in obvious epithelial morphology with epithelial lumens. Magnification was ×200

cell clusters and showed lumen formation as seen in Figure 8. The hematoxylin and eosin stain resulted in obvious epithelial morphology with epithelial lumens (Figure 9). Lumen formation was stimulated by the addition of 50 ng/ml HGF in culture medium (Figure 10). HGF showed morphological effects on endometrial epithelial cells.

Enzyme-linked immunosorbent assay for HGF

Isolated endometrial stromal cells showed spindle shaped, fibroblast-like morphology. Production of HGF by stromal cells from eutopic endometrium of patients with endometriosis was significantly higher than in controls (Figure 11). The mean values are presented, and as the quantity of HGF was not normally distributed, non-parametric statistical analyses were performed.

Three-dimensional cell culture

In the three-dimensional cell culture system, cultured endometrial epithelial cells formed

Discussion

The natural history and the pathogenesis of endometriosis have been poorly understood.

Role of hepatocyte growth factor in endometriosis

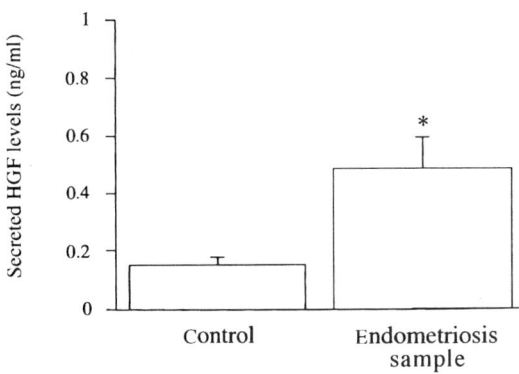

Figure 11 Secretion of hepatocyte growth factor (HGF) by endometrial stromal cells cultured for 48 h in medium containing 2.5% fetal bovine serum. Cell cultures were performed in triplicate, and duplicate supernatants were analyzed with enzyme immunoassay. Results are presented as mean ± SE. *$p < 0.05$, Mann-Whitney U-test, compared with control

Recent reports have revealed that active remodeling of endometriotic lesions has been observed. Local factors that regulate endometriotic lesions remain unknown.

In the present study, HGF mRNA was detected only in endometriotic lesions, whereas its receptor c-*met* mRNA was detected in both endometriotic lesions and normal peritoneum. By immunohistochemistry for c-*met*, HGF receptor was shown to be present in ectopic endometrial epithelial cells and peritoneal mesothelial cells. Recent studies suggest that HGF stimulates proliferation of cultured endometrial epithelial cells and superficial epithelialization of epithelial cells cultured on Matrigel, and HGF may be important for endometrial reconstruction and growth[12]. These observations suggest that HGF may also regulate the reconstruction and growth of endometriotic lesions. Although the origin of endometriotic cells remains uncertain, there were close similarities between eutopic and ectopic endometrial cells *in vitro*[13]. In this study we demonstrated the role of HGF in reconstruction and growth of endometriotic lesions.

From the results of the MTT assay for cultured epithelial cells, HGF was shown to stimulate proliferation of these cells in a dose-dependent manner. These results indicate that HGF has mitogenic effects on cultured endometrial epithelial cells. HGF is known as a scatter factor which acts as a motogen for various epithelial cells[14,15]. In this study, we demonstrated motogenic effects on cultured endometrial epithelial cells using Boyden's chamber technique.

The source of HGF remains unknown, but HGF has been known as a mesenchymal-derived factor, and peritoneal macrophages may produce HGF. It has been documented that peritoneal macrophages are increased and activated[16,17], and it is possible that these cells act as a chemoattractant for endometrial epithelial cells. From these results, it can be concluded that HGF stimulates the migration of endometrial epithelial cells in retrograde menstrual flow and this may be a key to the theory of implantation or the invasiveness of endometriotic lesions. To determine the morphological effects of HGF, we established a three-dimensional cell culture system. Isolated epithelial cells were cultured in Matrigel, and these cells formed cell clusters and gradually showed lumen formation. HGF added to the culture medium stimulates formation of epithelial lumens and HGF may be an important factor which regulates reconstruction or regeneration of endometrial glandular elements.

As mentioned above, it is also possible that endometrial stromal cells may produce HGF. By enzyme-linked immunosorbent assay for HGF, stromal cells were shown to produce detectable levels of HGF. Surprisingly, significantly increased levels of HGF were observed in stromal cells from patients with endometriosis. In recent years, many investigators have observed that peritoneal macrophages were increased and activated[16,17] and several inflammatory cytokines were elevated in peritoneal fluid of women with endometriosis[18-20]. Recent reports have also suggested that inflammatory changes are observed in eutopic endometrium of women with endometriosis[21,22]. Tseng and colleagues[23] reported that interleukin-6 secretion is up-regulated in eutopic endometrial stromal cells from women with endometriosis. Interleukin-1 and -6 responsive elements were located in the transcription initiation site of the human HGF gene[24,25], and the HGF gene is activated transcriptionally by these cytokines[26]. These observations suggest that up-regulated secretion of HGF by stromal cells of patients with endometriosis may be the effect of inflammatory changes of eutopic endometrium. From another viewpoint, up-regulation of HGF by endometrial stromal cells is an intrinsic factor in patients with endometriosis, and inflammatory changes may activate the secretion of HGF.

In conclusion, hepatocyte growth factor may play an important role in the regulation of endometriotic lesions, and increased secretion of HGF by stromal cells from eutopic endometrium of patients with endometriosis may be a key to clarifying the pathogenesis of endometriosis. Further investigation is necessary for prevention and therapy of this enigmatic disease.

References

1. Hoshiai, H., Ishikawa, M., Sawatari, Y., Noda, K. and Fukaya, T. (1993). Laparoscopic evaluation of the onset and progression of endometriosis. *Am. J. Obstet. Gynecol.*, **169**, 714–19
2. Wiegerlinck, M.A.H.M. and Van Dop, P.A. (1993). The staging of peritoneal endometriosis by the type of active lesion in addition to the revised American Fertility Society classification. *Fertil. Steril.*, **60**, 461–4
3. Nakamura, T., Nishizawa, T., Hagiya, M., Seki, T., Shimonishi, M., Sugimura, A., Tashiro, K. and Shimizu, S. (1989). Molecular cloning and expression of hepatocyte growth factor. *Nature (London)*, **342**, 440–3
4. Matsumoto, K. and Nakamura, T. (1992). Hepatocyte growth factor: molecular structure, roles in liver regeneration, and other biological functions. *Crit. Rev. Oncogenesis*, **3**, 27–54
5. Di Renzo, M.F., Narshimhan, R.P., Olivero, M., Bretti, S., Giordano, S., Medico, E., Gaglia, P., Zara, P. and Comoglio, P.M. (1991). Expression of the Met/HGF receptor in normal and neoplastic human tissues. *Oncogene*, **6**, 1997–2003
6. Bottaro, D.P., Rubin, J.S., Falleto, D.L., Chan, A.M., Kmiecik, T.E., Vande Woude, G.F. and Aaronson, S.A. (1991). Identification of the hepatocyte growth factor receptor as the c-*met* proto-oncogene product. *Science*, **251**, 802–4
7. Dean, M., Park, M., Le Beau, M.M., Robins, T.S., Diaz, M.O., Rowly, J.D., Blair, D.G. and Vande Woude, G.F. (1985). The human *met* oncogene is related to the tyrosine kinase oncogenes. *Nature (London)*, **318**, 385–8
8. Di Renzo, M.F., Olivero, M., Ferro, S., Prat, M., Bongarzone, I., Pielotti, M. and Comoglio, P.M. (1992). Overexpression of the c-MET/HGF receptor gene in human thyroid carcinoma. *Oncogene*, **7**, 2549–53
9. Di Renzo, M.F., Olivero, M., Katsaros, D., Crepaldi, T., Gaglia, P., Zola, P., Sismondi, P. and Comoglio, P.M. (1994). Overexpression of the MET/HGF receptor in ovarian cancer. *Int. J. Cancer*, **58**, 658–62
10. Smith, S.K. and Kelly, R.W. (1987). The effect of estradiol-17β and actinomycin D on the release of PGF and PGE separated cells of human endometrium. *Prostaglandins*, **34**, 553–60
11. Mosmann, T. (1983). Rapid colorimetric assay for cellular growth and survival: application to proliferation and cytotoxicity assays. *J. Immunol. Meth.*, **65**, 55–63
12. Negami, A., Sasaki, H., Kawakami, Y., Kamitani, N., Kotsuji, F., Tominaga, T. and Nakamura, T. (1995). Serum human hepatocyte growth factor in human menstrual cycle and pregnancy: novel serum marker of regeneration and reconstruction of human endometrium. *Horm. Res.*, **44**, 42–6
13. Matthews, C.J., Redfern, C.P.F., Hirst, B.H. and Thomas, E.J. (1992). Characterization of human purified epithelial and stromal cells from endometrium and endometriosis in

tissue culture. *Fertil. Steril.*, **57**, 990–7
14. Furlong, R.A., Takehara, T., Taylor, W.G., Nakamura, T. and Rubin, J.S. (1991). Comparison of biological and immunochemical properties indicates that scatter factor and hepatocyte growth factor are indistinguishable. *J. Cell Sci.*, **100**, 173–7
15. Konishi, T., Takehara, T., Tsuji, T., Ohsato, K., Matsumoto, K. and Nakamura, T. (1991). Scatter factor from human embryonic lung fibroblasts is probably identical to hepatocyte growth factor. *Biochem. Biophys. Res. Commun.*, **180**, 765–73
16. Haney, A.F., Muscato, J.J. and Weinberg, J.B. (1981). Peritoneal fluid cell populations in infertility patients. *Fertil. Steril.*, **35**, 696–8
17. Halme, A.F., Becker, S., Hammond, M.G., Raj, M.H.G. and Raj, S. (1983). Increased activation of pelvic macrophages in infertile women with mild endometriosis. *Am. J. Obstet. Gynecol.*, **145**, 333–7
18. Eisermann, J., Gast, M.J., Pineda, J., Odem, R.R. and Collins, J.L. (1988). Tumor necrosis factor in peritoneal fluid of women undergoing laparoscopic surgery. *Fertil. Steril.*, **50**, 573–9
19. Taketani, Y., Kuo, T.M. and Miguro, M. (1992). Comparison of cytokine levels and embryo toxicity in peritoneal fluid in infertile women with untreated and treated endometriosis. *Am. J. Obstet. Gynecol.*, **167**, 765–70
20. Fakih, H., Baggett, B., Holtz, G., Tsang, K.-Y., Lee, J.C. and Williamson, H.O. (1987). Interleukin-1: a possible role in the infertility associated with endometriosis. *Fertil. Steril.*, **47**, 213–17
21. Leiva, M.C., Hasty, L.A. and Lytte, C.R. (1994). Inflammatory changes of the endometrium in patients with minimal-to-moderate endometriosis. *Fertil. Steril.*, **62**, 967–72
22. Akoum, A., Hebert, J., Lemay, A., Le group d'investigation en gynecologie and Brunet, C. (1995). Secretion of monocyte chemotactic protein-1 by cytokin-stimulated endometrial cells of women with endometriosis. *Fertil. Steril.*, **63**, 322–8
23. Tseng, J.F., Ryan, I.P., Milam, T.D., Murai, J.T., Schriock, E.D., Landers, D.V. and Taylor, R.N. (1996). Interleukin-6 secretion *in vitro* is upregulated in ectopic and eutopic endometrial stromal cells from women with endometriosis. *J. Clin. Endocrinol. Metab.*, **81**, 1118–22
24. Seki, T., Hagiya, M., Shimonishi, M., Nakamura, T. and Shimizu, S. (1991). Organization of the human hepatocyte growth factor-encoding gene. *Gene*, **102**, 213–19
25. Miyazawa, K., Kitamura, A. and Kitamura, N. (1991). Structural organization and the transcription initiation site of the human hepatocyte growth factor gene. *Biochemistry*, **30**, 9170–6
26. Matsumoto, K., Okazaki, H. and Nakamura, T. (1992). Up-regulation of hepatocyte growth factor gene expression by interleukin-1 in human skin fibroblasts. *Biochem. Biophys. Res. Commun.*, **188**, 235–43

Progesterone and transforming growth factor-β co-mediate matrix metalloproteinase expression in a model of endometriosis

29

K.G. Osteen, K.L. Bruner, L.I. Gold and E. Eisenberg

Introduction

While being a complex and persistent disease, endometriosis is rather simply defined as the growth of functionally active endometrial glands and stroma at an extrauterine site. Endometriosis is most frequently found within the pelvic cavity and rarely occurs at extrapelvic sites. Nevertheless, several pathophysiological mechanisms must be evoked to account for the full spectrum of the presentation of this disease[1]. Several etiologies have been proposed for the development of endometriosis including celomic metaplasia of cells lining the peritoneum, development of steroid-sensitive embryonic cell rests and impairment of cellular immunity. However, most incidences of the disease appear to be linked to the oldest theory of endometriosis, the extrauterine implantation of endometrial tissue entering the peritoneal cavity through the Fallopian tubes at the time of menstruation[2,3]. Support for this metastatic theory is provided by the observation that women who have had endometrial fragments introduced into the peritoneal space either accidentally during uterine surgery[4,5] or experimentally[6] can develop endometriosis. The disease may affect as many as 10–15% of all women of reproductive age in the United States and as many as 35% of infertile women may suffer from endometriosis[7]. While malignant transformation of endometriotic lesions occurs only rarely, endometriosis is an invasive and persistent disease, and complications such as bowel obstruction and inflammation can become life-threatening. Additionally, pelvic sites of endometriosis contribute to numerous gynecological disorders in addition to infertility, including pelvic pain, dysmenorrhea, dyspareunia, uterine retroversion and abnormal bleeding. Clearly, the disease of endometriosis presents a challenging problem for the clinician and a better understanding of the cellular mechanisms which lead to the onset of this condition may provide important clues for therapy development.

A role for ovarian steroids in the pathophysiology of endometriosis has been recognized for some time, and evidence continues to accumulate suggesting a clinical correlation between a woman's estrogen exposure and the development of this disease. For example, women who delay childbirth and thus have many uninterrupted menstrual cycles are more likely to develop endometriosis than women who have had multiple pregnancies[8]. A similar epidemiology has been reported for endometriosis in primates undergoing continuous menstrual cycling in captivity compared with free-ranging females[9]. Alternatively, lifestyle activities which decrease endogenous estrogen levels in women such as smoking and strenuous exercise are correlated with less frequent development of this disease[10]. Interestingly, it has been reported that endometriotic lesions contain aromatase, an enzyme necessary for estrogen synthesis, which may enhance estrogen-mediated growth in ectopic tissues[11]. In contrast to the agonistic role of estrogen, progesterone exposure appears to provide women with a significant degree of protection against development of this disease. Regression of endometriotic lesions has been observed during pregnancy where elevated levels of progesterone can oppose the action of estrogen[12], and progestin therapy has been used to treat the disease in the absence of pregnancy[13]. Nevertheless, the interactive role of steroids on endometriosis is not completely understood, and depending on the site of growth, the response of individual ectopic lesions to steroids can be quite variable. While steroids appear necessary for the maintenance of endometriotic lesions[14], receptors for either estrogen or progesterone are often reduced or defective at ectopic sites of endometriosis[15-17].

Endometriotic lesions atrophy in the absence of steroidal support, but the ultimate control of cell behavior in tissues within the reproductive tract is not achieved by steroids alone, but rather through the co-ordinated actions of steroids and locally produced members of several growth factor families[18]. Cell–cell communication is critical to the overall regulation of the normal endometrium[19], and emerging studies indicate that disruption of paracrine communication may be a component of the pathophysiology of endometriosis[20]. For example, estrogen effects on endometrial function can be mediated via the secondary action of epidermal growth factor (EGF)[21] and both EGF and EGF receptors have been found in ectopic lesions of endometriosis[16,22]. In vitro studies have demonstrated that EGF, but not estrogen, can induce proliferation of cells obtained from endometriotic lesions[23,24]. Compared to estrogen-mediated paracrine communication, the nature of secondary messengers of progesterone action in the endometrium or in lesions of endometriosis is less clear. Members of the transforming growth factor-β (TGF-β) family, however, can inhibit cell growth via autocrine or paracrine mechanisms in numerous reproductive tissues[18]. In the human endometrium, TGF-$β_1$ is abundant and appears to be the principal isoform produced by epithelial cells, while both TGF-$β_1$ and TGF-$β_2$ have been localized to the stroma[25-27]. The expression and activity of members of the TGF-β family can vary considerably within tissues depending on the effects of other locally produced cytokines or even in response to changes in structural architecture[28]. Surgically induced endometriotic lesions in a rodent (rat) model express immunoreactive TGF-β suggesting that this growth factor family could play a role in the disease as well as with adhesion formation which often accompanies endometriotic lesions[29]. In the human disease, increased levels of TGF-β have been measured in the peritoneal fluid of women with endometriosis compared to normal controls[30]. Little additional information has been reported to date in regard to the expression or action of TGF-β in the disease endometriosis.

In addition to the trophic effects of steroids and growth factors on the growth and differentiation of endometrium and endometriotic lesions, biomolecules associated with tissue repair and establishment of tissue structure must be considered. For example, specific cellular and biochemical mechanisms must exist by which relatively normal endometrial tissue, deposited in the peritoneal cavity of some women can establish and maintain ectopic implantation sites. Establishment of early implantation sites of endometriosis is associated with breakdown and remodeling of the extracellular matrix (ECM)[31]. The ECM is composed of a variety of rather stable and interactive biomolecules, and to break down, remodel or repair these molecules requires the concerted action of specific enzymes known as matrix metalloproteinases (MMPs). The MMPs are a multi-gene family of enzymes that are classified based on ECM substrate specificity[32]. MMPs are highly regulated at the transcriptional level by a variety of regulatory agents which are active in the reproductive tract including steroids, growth factors and oncogenes[33,34]. In addition to transcriptional regulation, MMPs require activation of pro-enzymes following secretion and can also be regulated by a group of broadly expressed natural inhibitors known as tissue inhibitors of metalloproteinases (TIMPs). At present, four TIMP molecules have been described: TIMP-1, TIMP-2, TIMP-3 and TIMP-4[35–37]. Given the dynamic nature of the menstrual cycle, it is not surprising that a number of MMPs have been detected in the endometrium[38,39]. Members of the stromelysin class of MMPs appear to be under the most stringent endocrine control in the endometrium and their mRNAs are expressed in a cycle stage-specific manner in association with endometrial growth and during tissue breakdown and repair at the time of menstruation[38,40]. Our research group determined that expression of MMPs of the stromelysin family is quite low during the secretory phase as tissue exposure to progesterone increases. Interestingly, the suppression of the epithelial-specific MMP, matrilysin, requires the secondary action of TGF-β which is secreted by endometrial stromal cells in response to progesterone[41], while the effects of TGF-β on stromal-specific MMPs is currently unclear. As progesterone levels drop during the last days of the menstrual cycle, mRNAs for all the stromelysins are widely expressed in regions of tissue breakdown. The co-operative action of steroids and growth factors appears to maintain a proper balance between expression of MMPs and their tissue inhibitors during the normal menstrual cycle. The expression of MMPs in menstrual endometrium as well as the continued growth-related expression of these enzymes suggests a cell mediated mechanism by which menstrual tissue might be able to establish ectopic sites of endometriosis. We present here studies which suggest an interactive role for progesterone and TGF-β in the regulation of endometrial MMP expression as well as in the development of ectopic lesions in an experimental model of endometriosis.

Materials and methods

Tissue procurement

Endometrial tissues for organ culture were obtained from a population of normal women with a pipelle suction curette from the fundus region of the uterus during the proliferative interval (days 9–12) of the menstrual cycle. Endometriotic samples for tissue culture were obtained from patients undergoing ablation surgery during the proliferative phase of the menstrual cycle. Endometrial and endometriotic tissues for immunohistochemical analysis were obtained from the pathology archives at Vanderbilt University Hospital, Nashville, TN, USA. The use of human tissue was approved by Vanderbilt University's Institutional Review Board and Committee for the Protection of Human Subjects.

Organ culture system

Endometrial and endometriotic tissues for organ culture were dissected into uniform fragments of 1–2 mm, and 8–10 fragments were assigned to each treatment group within culture inserts (Millipore®, Bedford, MA, USA) containing phenol red-free Dulbecco's Modified Eagle's Medium/Ham's F-12 (DMEM/F-12) supplemented with ITS+ (Collaborative Biomedical Products, Bedford, MA, USA) and ExCyte (Miles Scientific, Kankakee, IL, USA). Organ cultures were maintained at 37 °C in a humidified chamber containing 95% air and 5% CO_2 in the presence of either 10 nmol/l estradiol, 1 nmol/l estradiol and 500 nmol/l progesterone, or 1 nmol/l estradiol and 2 ng/ml TGF-β (TGF-β$_1$; R & D Systems, Minneapolis, MN, USA).

Immunohistochemistry

The expression of TGF-β isotypes in endometrium versus endometriotic tissues was determined using polyclonal antisera directed against TGF-β_1 and TGF-β_2 as previously described[26]. These antisera, produced in rabbits immunized with synthetic peptides, showed no cross-reactivity on Western blot analysis. Deparaffinized, formalin-fixed sections of normal endometrium or lesions of endometriosis were pre-incubated with blocking solution (Tris-buffered saline (TBS) with 0.1% Bovine serum albumin (BSA) and 1% normal serum) for 20 min at room temperature (22–24 °C) and incubated overnight at 4 °C with a dilution of antisera in blocking solution. The slides were washed with TBS, and antibody complexes were detected using a streptavidin–biotin complex kit. Enzyme activity was visualized using a 3,3'-diaminobenzidene tetrahydrochloride solution which resulted in a brown precipitate. After three washes in TBS, the slides were counterstained with hematoxylin and cover slipped using Permount (Fisher Scientific, Norcross, GA, USA). Normal preimmune serum was used as a negative control.

TGF-β radioreceptor assay

TGF-β activity was measured in media collected from organ cultures of normal endometrium versus endometriotic tissue by radioreceptor assay (RRA) utilizing AKR-2B (clone 84A) cells and [^{125}I]TGF-β. This RRA does not discriminate among isotypes of TGF-β, but is highly sensitive for identifying TGF-β activity in medium collected from tissue cultures. The AKR-2B cells were plated at a density of 5×10^4 cells/well in a 24-well tissue culture plate and allowed to attach overnight. The cells were then washed with phosphate-buffered saline (PBS) containing 0.1% BSA and incubated at room temperature on a rotating platform with binding buffer (11.9% HEPES, 7.5% NaCl, 0.3% KCl, 1.2% $MgSO_4$, 0.1% $CaCl_2$, and 2% BSA, pH 7.5). After incubation, the binding buffer was removed and fresh buffer plus the acid-treated culture media and 0.05 ng [^{125}I]TGF-β was added for another 2 h. Non-specific binding was determined for each sample in the presence of excess TGF-β. After the final incubation, the cells were washed with PBS and the bound radioactivity was extracted with PBS containing 0.5% Triton-X 100 (Sigma Chemical Co., St. Louis, MO, USA).

SDS-PAGE

Prostromelysin-1 and promatrilysin proteins were detected in the conditioned media collected from organ cultures of endometrial and endometriotic tissue after an 18-h labeling period with [^{35}S]methionine. The amount of protein-bound ^{35}S was determined by trichloroacetic acid precipitation, and 5×10^5 precipitable counts were selectively immunoprecipitated with rabbit polyclonal antibodies against rat stromelysin and human matrilysin as previously reported[34]. The antibody complexes were removed with Protein-A Sepharose (Sigma Chemical Co., St. Louis, MO, USA), the samples were run on a 12% acrylamide gel and results were documented by autoradiography.

Nude mouse endometriosis model

Five-week-old ovariectomized athymic (nude) mice were housed in sterile cages in rooms maintained at 26.7 °C with a 12-h light/12-h dark cycle. All housing materials, food and water were autoclaved prior to use. Prior to any invasive procedure, the mice were anesthetized by Metafane® inhalation (Pitman-Moore, Mundelein, IL, USA). The mice received sterile 60-day-release capsules of 1.5 mg estradiol, inserted at a site just below the scapula, from 24 h to 2 weeks prior to injection of endometrial tissue. The tissue was injected with an 18-gauge needle into the peritoneal space, just below the umbilicus. Ten to 12 days later, the mice were sacrificed and necropsied for signs of endometriotic-like disease.

Table 1 Immunohistochemical localization of TGF-β_1 and TGF-β_2

Tissue	TGF-β_1		TGF-β_2	
	Glands	Stroma	Glands	Stroma
Normal proliferative endometrium	++	+	+	+
Endometriosis	+++	++	++	+++

+, weakly positive; ++, moderately positive; +++, strongly positive. TGF-β_1 is most strongly expressed in glandular epithelium while TGF-β_2 is most strongly expressed in the stroma. Relative to normal endometrium, endometriotic tissues consistently expressed both TGF-β isoforms more strongly

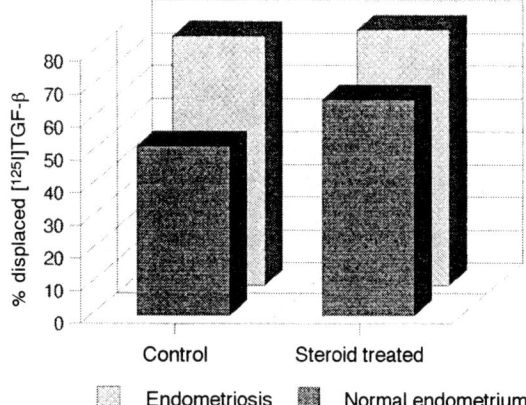

Figure 1 Transforming growth factor-β (TGF-β) radioreceptor assay. Normal proliferative endometrium and endometriotic tissue were maintained in steroid-free media or media containing estradiol (1 nmol/l) and progesterone (500 nmol/l) for 24 h. TGF-β activity was determined in acid treated conditioned media by displacement of [^{125}I]TGF-β in AKR-2B cells. In normal endometrium, elevated levels of TGF-β were observed following steroid treatment. Higher levels of TGF-β activity were consistently found in media from endometriotic tissue cultures, but little steroid regulation was observed

Results and discussion

Transforming growth factor-β expression in the disease endometriosis

In the normal endometrium the loss of MMP expression during the secretory phase occurs in conjunction with a rise in TGF-β levels[25,41] and TIMP-1 expression[38]. In a previous study our laboratory determined that both TGF-β_1 and TGF-β_2 proteins increase within the endometrium following the ovulatory rise in circulating progesterone *in vivo* and that the message levels for each TGF-β isotype increase in response to progesterone treatment *in vitro*[25,41]. In the current study we demonstrate that human endometriotic lesions express TGF-β isotypes at a higher level than observed in normal endometrium. Using isotype specific antibodies, immunohistochemical analysis revealed expression of both TGF-β_1 and TGF-β_2 within endometriotic lesions. For each isotype, levels of TGF-β expression were higher in endometriotic lesions compared to eutopic tissues during the proliferative stage of the menstrual cycle (Table 1). Additionally, endometriotic tissues maintained *in vitro* as short-term organ cultures secreted elevated levels of TGF-β-like activity into culture media compared to similar cultures of normal proliferative phase endometrial tissues (Figure 1). Together, these observations of abundant *in vivo* TGF-β expression as well as *in vitro* TGF-β secretion in lesions of endometriosis versus normal endometrium agree with the report of elevated TGF-β levels in peritoneal fluid of women with endometriosis[30]. These observations also suggest that the association of TGF-β expression with the action of progesterone in the normal endometrium may be somehow disrupted in ectopic sites of endometrial tissue growth. The steroidal control of expression and action of TGF-β in the disease endometriosis remains poorly understood but may play a significant role in the pathophysiology of this disease.

A model for the study of MMP expression in endometriosis

Our laboratory has demonstrated that both progesterone and TGF-β are important mediators of the suppression of endometrial MMPs following growth-related processes which require ECM remodeling. However, matrix degrading enzymes may contribute to the pathophysiological processes leading to the initial establishment of endometriosis by mediating the implantation of retrograde menstrual tissues. Matrix degradation has been documented in women during the early stages of endometriosis development[31]. To explore the role of endometrial MMP expression in the establishment of ectopic lesions of endometriosis, our laboratory developed a nude mouse model which appears to reflect many of the cellular dynamics of the human disease. Using an approach similar to that described by Zamah and colleagues[42], an experimental model system was developed in which human endometrial tissue, obtained during the proliferative stage of the menstrual cycle can be treated *in vitro* with trophic agents and subsequently injected into the peritoneal space of ovariectomized nude mice[20,43]. Using this model, endometrial tissue treated with estrogen secretes MMPs *in vitro* and subsequently establishes ectopic lesions in approximately 95% of recipient nude mice while suppression of MMP secretion by progesterone treatment *in vitro* essentially eliminates the subsequent development of lesions in recipient animals[20]. The involvement of MMPs in establishment of human lesions in this animal model was confirmed by treatments of tissue and recipient animals with an inhibitor of MMP action, TIMP-1, which significantly reduced lesion establishment[43]. The ability of progesterone treatment to block establishment of ectopic lesions by endometrial tissue in this experimental model suggests that regulation of MMP expression may provide a treatment strategy for women with endometriosis. Additionally, since we have linked progesterone-mediated suppression of an epithelial-specific MMP to the secondary action of TGF-β[41], it would seem logical to explore the role TGF-β might independently play in this model of experimental endometriosis. For this study we obtained endometrial tissue during the proliferative phase of the menstrual cycle when MMPs are expressed *in vivo* and treated the tissue *in vitro* with TGF-β. As shown in Figure 2, exposure of endometrial tissue to TGF-β in organ culture suppresses secretion of both matrilysin and stromelysin-1. Subsequently, we tested whether treatment of endometrial tissues with TGF-β, prior to injection of the tissue into nude mice, might also prevent lesion formation in a manner similar to that previously observed following progesterone treatment. We were rather surprised to find that mice receiving endometrial tissue treated with TGF-β developed ectopic lesions at a similar rate to tissue treated with estrogen (Table 2).

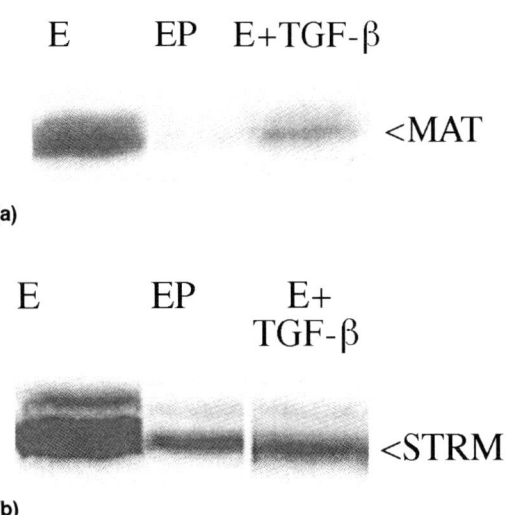

Figure 2 Regulation of matrix metalloproteinases in organ culture. Tissue from proliferative phase endometrium was maintained as organ cultures for 24 h in the presence of 10 nmol/l estradiol (E), 1 nmol/l estradiol plus 500 nmol/l progesterone (EP) or 1 nmol/l estradiol and 2 ng/ml TGF-β$_1$. Promatrilysin (MAT) and prostromelysin-1 (STRM) protein were detected in the conditioned media after a 20-h labeling with [^{35}S]methionine by selective immunoprecipitation, followed by SDS-PAGE and autoradiography. Promatrilysin (a) and prostromelysin-1 (b) secretion are suppressed following either progesterone or TGF-β treatment

Table 2 Effect of TGF-β on the ability of human endometrial tissue to establish lesions in nude mice

Tissue treatment	Animal treatment	No. with lesions	Total no. of animals	% with lesions
Estradiol	Estradiol	14	15	95.6
Estradiol/ progesterone	Estradiol	0	10	0
Estradiol/ TGF-β	Estradiol	13	14	92.9

Proliferative phase organ cultures of human endometrium were cultured *in vitro* for 24 h in the presence of 10 nmol/l estradiol, 1 nmol/l estradiol and 500 nmol/l progesterone, or 1 nmol/l estradiol and 2 ng/ml TGF-β$_1$. The mice had previously been implanted with a subcutaneous pellet containing estradiol

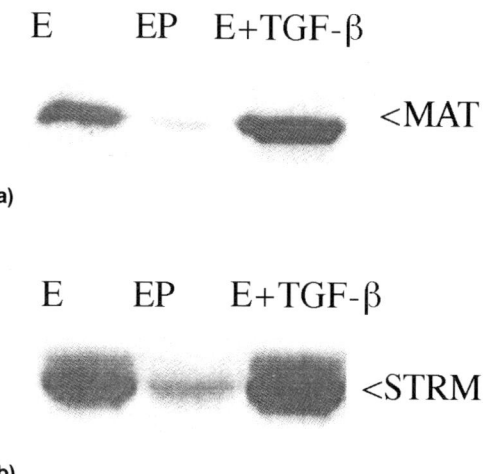

Figure 3 Transient regulation of matrix metalloproteinases in organ culture by transforming growth factor-β (TGF-β). Tissue from proliferative phase endometrium was maintained as organ cultures for 24 h in the presence of 10 nmol/l estradiol (E), 1 nmol/l estradiol plus 500 nmol/l progesterone (EP) or 1 nmol/l estradiol and 2 ng/ml TGF-β$_1$. The cultures were subsequently maintained for an additional 24 h in media containing no steroid or growth factor. Promatrilysin (MAT) and prostromelysin-1 (STRM) protein were detected in the conditioned media after a 20-h labeling with [^{35}S]methionine by selective immunoprecipitation, followed by SDS-PAGE and autoradiography. Although both pro-matrilysin (a) and prostromelysin-1 (b) remain suppressed in tissues cultured for 24 h with progesterone, re-expression of these proteins is noted in tissues treated with TGF-β

In order to examine the lack of effect of TGF-β treatment in our experimental model, we examined further the dynamics of MMP secretion in organ cultures of endometrial tissues treated with progesterone versus TGF-β. Examination of MMP secretion in explants over 72 h of culture revealed that while initial exposure of tissue to TGF-β resulted in suppression of MMP secretion, the suppressive effect was transient and MMP secretion rebounded after 72 h of culture (Figure 3). In contrast to TGF-β treatment, progesterone treatment maintained a suppressive effect on MMP secretion over the 72-h period examined even after removal of the steroid *in vitro* (Figure 3). From these studies, we have concluded that TGF-β can, in concert with progesterone, suppress endometrial MMP expression and secretion; however, TGF-β does not replace the overall effects of progesterone and cannot independently prevent ectopic lesions in an experimental model of endometriosis.

Summary

Although ovarian steroids are clearly necessary for the regulation of endometrial function, the importance of local paracrine factors such as TGF-β is also becoming apparent. Subtle changes in either the steroidal or cytokine milieu can have a dramatic effect on cellular behavior in reproductive tissues. Growth factors such as TGF-β can also mediate steroid-independent actions especially in response to disruptions in the tissue environment[44,45]. The studies described here suggest that TGF-β cannot duplicate fully the action of progesterone in the suppression of endometrial MMPs and thus cannot independently prevent an endometriotic-like disease in nude mice. Additionally, our findings of elevated TGF-β in endometriotic lesions would indicate that

TGF-β may contribute to the progression of this disease[27,29,30]. TGF-β levels are normally elevated in response to the action of progesterone in the endometrium[34] and contribute to the suppression of matrilysin[41]. Our results in this study indicate that an altered cellular response may occur in endometrial tissues exposed to elevated TGF-β in the absence of progesterone since MMP expression rebounds following TGF-β treatment alone. Such a possibility is also supported by an aberrant expression pattern of matrilysin in endometriotic lesions[43]. Matrilysin expression is suppressed by TGF-β in normal endometrium[41] but not in endometriotic lesions even though TGF-β levels are elevated. Although studies are yet to be forthcoming which definitively show an involvement of MMPs in the development and/or progression of endometriosis in humans, numerous studies provide circumstantial evidence that this is indeed the case[20,31,43,46]. As we begin to develop a better understanding of the roles of both steroids and growth factors in the normal regulation of endometrial MMPs and the misregulation seen in endometriosis, we will likely gain new insight into not only the disease but also into the development of better treatment strategies.

References

1. Mahmood, T.A. and Templeton, A. (1990). Pathophysiology of mild endometriosis: review of literature. *Hum. Reprod.*, **5**, 765–84
2. Sampson, J.A. (1927). Peritoneal endometriosis due to menstrual dissemination of endometrial tissues into the peritoneal cavity. *Am. J. Obstet. Gynecol.*, **14**, 422–69
3. Ishimaru, T. and Masuzaki, H. (1991). Peritoneal endometriosis: endometrial tissue implantation as a primary etiologic mechanism. *Am. J. Obstet. Gynecol.*, **165**, 210–14
4. Ridley, J.H. (1968). The histogenesis of endometriosis. A review of facts and fancies. *Obstet. Gynecol. Surv.*, **20**, 1–35
5. Sorensen, S.S., Andersen L.F. and Lose, G. (1994). Endometriosis by implantation: a complication of endometrial ablation. *Lancet*, **343**, 1226
6. Ridley, J.H. and Edwards, I.K. (1958). Experimental endometriosis in the human. *Am. J. Obstet. Gynecol.*, **76**, 783–90
7. Cramer, D.W. (1987). Epidemiology of endometriosis in adolescents. In Wilson, E.A. (ed.) *Endometriosis*, p. 5. (New York: Alan Liss Inc.)
8. Halme, J. and Stovall, D. (1995). Endometriosis and its medical management. In Wallach, E.E. and Zacur, H.A. (eds.) *Reproductive Medicine and Surgery*, p. 695–710. (St. Louis: Mosby)
9. Ami, Y., Suzaki, Y. and Goto, N. (1993). Endometriosis in *Cynomolgus* monkeys retired from breeding. *J. Vet. Med. Sci.*, **55**, 7–11
10. Cramer, D.W., Wilson, E., Stillman, R.J., Berger, M.J., Belisle, S., Schiff, I., Albrecht, B., Gibson, M., Stadel, B.V. and Schoenbaum, S.C. (1986). The relation of endometriosis to menstrual characteristics, smoking and exercise. *J. Am. Med. Assoc.*, **255**, 1904–8
11. Noble, L.S., Simson, E.R., Johns, A. and Bulun, S.E. (1996). Aromatase expression in endometriosis. *J. Clin. Endocrinol. Metab.*, **87**, 174–9
12. Ramzy, I. (1989). Pathology. In Schenken, R.S. (ed.) *Endometriosis: Contemporary Concepts and Clinical Management*, p. 60. (Philadelphia: J.B. Lippincott Company)
13. Olive, D.L. (1989). Medical treatment: alternatives to danazol. In Shenken, R.S. (ed.) *Endometriosis: Contemporary Concepts and Clinical Management*, p. 192. (Philadelphia: J.B. Lippincott Company)
14. Dizerega, G.S., Barber, D.L. and Hodgen, G.D. (1980). Endometriosis: role of steroids in initiation, maintenance and suppression. *Fertil. Steril.*, **33**, 649–53
15. Lessey, B.A., Metzger, D.A., Haney, A.F. and McCarty, K.S. Jr (1989). Immunohistochemical analysis of estrogen and progesterone receptors in endometriosis: comparison with normal endometrium during the menstrual cycle and the effect of medical therapy. *Fertil. Steril.*, **49**, 229–35

16. Melega, C., Balducci, M., Bulletti, C., Galassi, A., Jasonni, V. and Flamigni, C. (1991). Tissue factors influencing growth and maintenance of endometriosis. In Bulletti, C. and Gurpide, E. (eds.) *The Primate Endometrium, Ann. NY Acad. Sci.*, **622**, 256–65
17. Metzger, D.A., Szpak, C.A. and Haney, A.F. (1993). Histologic features associated with hormonal responsiveness of ectopic endometrium. *Fertil. Steril.*, **59**, 83–8
18. Anderson, T.L., Gorstein, F. and Osteen, K.G. (1990). Stromal–epithelial cell communication, growth factors and tissue regulation. *Lab. Invest.*, **62**, 519–21 (Editorial)
19. Giudice, L.C. Dsupin, B.A. and Irwin, J.C. (1992). Steroid and peptide regulation of insulin-like growth factor-binding proteins secreted by human endometrial stromal cells is dependent on stroma differentiation. *J. Clin. Endocrinol. Metab.*, **75** (5), 1235–41
20. Osteen, K.G., Bruner, K.L., Sierra-Rivera, E., Keller, N.R. and Eisenberg, E. (1996). Interleukin-1α opposes progesterone suppression of matrix metalloproteinases in an endometriosis model. Abstract presented at *Society for the Study of Reproduction*, July, London, Ontario, Canada
21. Tomooka, Y., Di Augustine, J.A. and McLachlan, J.A. (1986). Proliferation of mouse uterine epithelial cells *in vitro*. *Endocrinology*, **118**, 1011–18
22. Haining, R.E., Cameron, I.T. and van Papendorp, C. (1991). Epidermal growth factor in human endometrium: proliferative effects in culture and immunocytochemical localization in normal and endometriotic tissues. *Hum. Reprod.*, **8**, 2211–17
23. Mellor, S.J. and Thomas, E.J. (1994). The action of estradiol and EGF in endometrial and endometriotic stroma *in vitro*. *Fertil. Steril.*, **62**, 507–13
24. Taketani, Y. and Mizuno, M. (1992). Hormonal regulation of the cell growth in an endometriotic cell culture system. *Arch. Gynecol. Obstet.*, **251**, 29–34
25. Osteen, K.G., Rodgers, W.H., Hargrove, J.T., Vasquez, J.M., Gorstein, F. and Matrisian, L.M. (1994). Steroids and growth factors can direct metalloproteinase expression in the cycling human endometrium. Abstract presented at *Society for Gynecologic Investigation*, March, Chicago
26. Gold, L., Saxena, B., Mittal, K.R., Marmor, M., Goswami, S., Nactigal, L., Korc, M. and Demopoulos, R.I. (1994). Increased expression of transforming growth factor beta isoforms and basic fibroblast growth factor in complex hyperplasia and adenocarcinoma of the endometrium: evidence for paracrine and autocrine action. *Cancer Res.*, **54**, 2347–58
27. Osteen, K.G., Bruner, K.L., Gold, L.I. and Hargrove, J.T. (1993). Steroidal regulation of TGF-β expression in normal human endometrium and endometriosis. Abstract presented at *American Fertility Society*, October, Montreal, Quebec, Canada
28. Roberts, A.B., Sporn, M.B., Assoian, R.K., Smith, J.M., Roche, N.S., Wakefield, L.M., Heine, U.I., Liotta, L.A., Falanga, V., Kehrl, J.H. and Fauci, A.S. (1986). Transforming growth factor type β: rapid induction of fibrosis and angiogenesis *in vivo* and stimulation of collagen formation *in vitro*. *Proc. Natl. Acad. Sci. USA*, **83**, 4167–71
29. Chegini, N., Gold, L.I. and Williams, R.S. (1994). Localization of TGF-β isoforms TGF-β1, TGF-β2 and TGF-β3 in surgically induced endometriosis in the rat. *Obstet. Gynecol.*, **83**, 455–61
30. Oosterlynck, D.J., Meuleman, C., Waer, M. and Koninckx, P.R. (1994). TGF-β activity is increased in the peritoneal fluid from women with endometriosis. *Obstet. Gynecol.*, **83**, 287–92
31. Spuijbroek, M.D.E.H., Dunselman, G.A.J., Menheere, P.P.C.A. and Evers, J.L.H. (1992). Early endometriosis invades the extracellular matrix. *Fertil. Steril.*, **58**, 929–33
32. Ennis, B.W. and Matrisian, L.M. (1994). Matrix degrading metalloproteinases. *J. Neuro-Oncol.*, **18**, 105–9
33. Mauviel, A. (1993). Cytokine regulation of metalloproteinase gene expression. *J. Cell. Biochem.*, **53**, 288–95
34. Osteen, K.G., Rodgers, W.H., Gaire, M., Hargrove, J.T., Gorstein, F. and Matrisian, L.M. (1994). Stromal–epithelial interaction mediates steroidal regulation of metalloproteinase expression in human endometrium. *Proc. Natl. Acad. Sci. USA*, **91**, 10129–33
35. Uria, J.A., Ferrando, A.A., Velasco, G., Freije, J.M.P. and Lopez-Otin, C. (1994). Structure and expression in breast tumors of TIMP-3, a new member of the metalloproteinase family. *Cancer Res.*, **54**, 2091–4
36. Murphy, G., Houbrechts, A., Crockett, M.I.,

Williamson, R.A., O'Shea, M. and Docherty, A.J.P. (1991). The n-terminal domain of TIMPs retains MMP inhibitory activity. *Biochemistry*, **31**, 10146–52

37. Shi, Y.E., Greene, J., Wang, M., Xiao, G. and Liu, Y.E. (1996). Loss of expression of TIMP-4, a novel human tissue inhibitor of metalloproteinase, in human breast cancer malignant progression. Presented at the *American Society for Cancer Research Special International Conference*, March, Florida
38. Rodgers, W.H., Matrisian, L.M., Giudice, L.C., Dsupin, B., Cannon, P., Svitek, C., Gorstein, F. and Osteen, K.G. (1994). Patterns of matrix metalloproteinase expression in cycling endometrium imply differential functions and regulation by steroids. *J. Clin. Invest.*, **94**, 946–53
39. Marbiax, E., Donnez, J., Courtoy, P. and Eeckout, Y. (1992). Progesterone regulates the activity of collagenase and related gelatinases A and B in human endometrial explants. *Proc. Natl. Acad. Sci. USA*, **89**, 11789–93
40. Rodgers, W.H., Osteen, K.G., Matrisian, L.M., Navre, M., Guidice, L.C. and Gorstein, F. (1994). Expression and localization of matrilysin (Pump-1, MMP-7) a matrix metalloproteinase in the human endometrium. *Am. J. Obstet. Gynecol.*, **168**, 253–60
41. Bruner, K.L., Rodgers, W.H., Korc, M., Gold, L.I., Hargrove, J.T., Matrisian, L.M. and Osteen, K.G. (1995). Transforming growth factor-β mediates the progesterone suppression of an epithelial metalloproteinase by adjacent stroma in the human endometrium. *Proc. Natl. Acad. Sci. USA*, **92**, 7362–6
42. Zamah, N.M., Dodson, M.G., Stephens, L.C., Buttram, V.C., Besch, P.K. and Kaufman, R.H. (1984). Transplantation of normal and ectopic human endometrial tissue into athymic nude mice. *Am. J. Obstet. Gynecol.*, **149**, 591–7
43. Osteen, K.G., Bruner, K.L. and Sharpe-Timms, K.L. (1996). Steroids and growth factor regulation of matrix metalloproteinase expression and endometriosis. *Semin. Reprod. Endocrinol.*, **14** (3), 247–55
44. Roberts, A.B., Anzano, M.A., Wakefield, L.M., Roche, N.S., Stern, D.S. and Sporn, M.B. (1985). Type b transforming growth factor: a bifunctional regulator of cell growth. *Proc. Natl. Acad. Sci. USA*, **82**, 119–23
45. Theodorescu, D., Sheehan, C. and Kerbel, R.S. (1993). TGF-β gene expression depends on tissue architecture. *In vitro Cell Dev.*, **29A**, 105–8
46. Saito, T., Mizumoto, H., Kuroki, K., Fujii, M., Mori, S. and Kudo, R. (1995). Expression of MMP-3 and TIMP-1 in endometriosis and the influence of danazol. *Acta Obstet. Gynecol. Jpn*, **47**, 495–6

The role of matrix metalloproteinases in the development of adenomyosis in humans and pituitary-grafted mice

M. Fujii, S. Mori, Y. Liao, T. Suzuki, M. Koizumi, T. Saito, T. Endo, S. Sagae and R. Kudo

Introduction

Adenomyosis is a benign invasive growth of functioning endometrial tissue (consisting of endometrial glands and stroma) into the myometrium, causing its derangement and disintegration[1]. Matrix metalloproteinases, enzymes whose substrates are extracellular matrix components, have been reported to be involved in several physiological and pathological processes in which tissue remodeling is implicated, such as embryonic development[2], wound healing[3] and tumor invasion[4,5].

The present study was designed to investigate the involvement of matrix metalloproteinases, particularly Pump-1, in the invasion of aberrant endometrial tissue into the myometrium, in humans as well as in a mouse model of adenomyosis induced by intrauterine pituitary grafting.

Materials and methods

Mice of the SHN strain were used in this study. They were housed in plastic cages with wood shavings in a temperature-monitored and light-controlled room (12 h light/day) and were fed with a commercial diet and tap water *ad libitum*. Induction of adenomyosis was performed according to a previously described method[6,7]. Briefly, a single pituitary obtained from an age-matched male mouse of the SHN strain was transplanted into the right uterine horn of a female mouse of the SHN strain at the age of 5–6 weeks. Three months after transplantation, each recipient mouse was sacrificed and the uterus was obtained. A part of the right horn of the bicornuate uterus was used for histological study, and the remaining uterus horn was kept at −80 °C for measurement of matrix metalloproteinase activity and RNA preparation. Human samples, obtained at surgical procedures, were kept at −80 °C for RNA preparation.

Gelatin zymography

Gelatinase activity was measured by zymography as previously described[8]. Briefly, uterine extracts (20–40 mg protein) were subjected to electrophoresis in 10% polyacrylamide gels containing 1 mg/ml gelatin. In order to confirm the activity of metalloproteinases, the gels were incubated in the presence of EDTA. Samples were diluted in non-reducing sample buffer (final concentration 1% sodium dodecyl sulfate and 5% glycerol) and electrophoresed for 3 h at a constant current of 10 mA. The gels were washed for 2 h in 2.5% Triton X-100 to remove sodium dodecyl sulfate, rinsed three times with distilled water, and then incubated for 20 h in 50 mmol/l TRIS-HCl at pH 8.0 with 5 mmol/l $CaCl_2$. After Coomassie blue staining, the density of the digested band was measured with a scanning densitometer.

RNA preparation and RT-PCR

Uterine tissue was immediately frozen in liquid nitrogen and stored at −80 °C before RNA isolation by acid guanidinium thiocyanate-phenol-chloroform extraction. mRNA was purified from total RNA by an mRNA purification kit (Biomag, Cambridge). Pump-1 primers were prepared with the Pump-1 cDNA. The reaction mixture containing pump-1 primers was subjected to 38 cycles of amplification. Each cycle included 2 min denaturation at 92 °C, 1 min annealing at 52 °C and 1 min elongation at 72 °C. A final extension time of 10 min was used in all cases. Following amplification the products were analyzed on a 1.3% agarose gel with appropriate DNA markers. Bands were visualized after staining with ethidium bromide.

Polyclonal antibody production and Western blot analysis

In order to obtain anti-Pump-1 polyclonal antibody, rabbits were immunized by standard procedures with a peptide synthesized from Pump-1 cDNA. The blot was incubated for 1 h with a 1:200 dilution of the anti-Pump-1 polyclonal antibody. A goat anti-rabbit immunoglobulin was used as the secondary antibody. Reagents for immunogold silver staining in dot and blot immune overlay assays (Amersham, Buckinghamshire, UK) were used for the detection of the immunoreactive Pump-1.

Immunohistochemical staining

Tissues were fixed with 20% formaldehyde and embedded in paraffin blocks. Paraffin sections (5 μm) were reacted with a 1:300 dilution of the anti-Pump-1 polyclonal antibody for 2 h. A goat anti-rabbit immunoglobulin was used as the secondary antibody. Avidin-biotin-horseradish peroxidase (HRP) complex solution was used for the detection of the immunoreactive Pump-1.

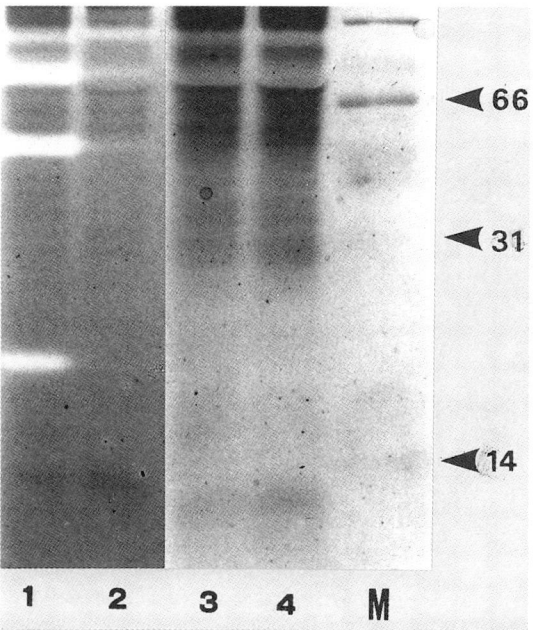

Figure 1 Gelatinase activity in mouse adenomyosis. Without EDTA, digested bands with relative masses 20 000–30 000, 50 000 and 70 000 are identified in extracts from uterus with mouse adenomyosis (lane 1), whereas no such bands are present in extracts from normal uterus (lane 2). With EDTA, the digested bands are not identified in extracts from uterus with mouse adenomyosis (lane 3) or from normal uterus (lane 4). M, marker of molecular weight

Results

Gelatin zymography was used to identify matrix metalloproteinase activity in extracts obtained from the left uterine horn of the mice that had received the intrauterine pituitary grafting (Figure 1). In the absence of EDTA, gelatinase activity was identified in three bands with relative masses 20 000–30 000, 50 000 and 70 000, in extracts obtained from the uterus with advanced adenomyosis (lane 1), whereas no gelatinase activity was identified in extracts obtained from the normal uterus (lane 2). The gelatinase activities disappeared in the presence of EDTA, suggesting that the gelatinase activities are identical to metalloproteinases.

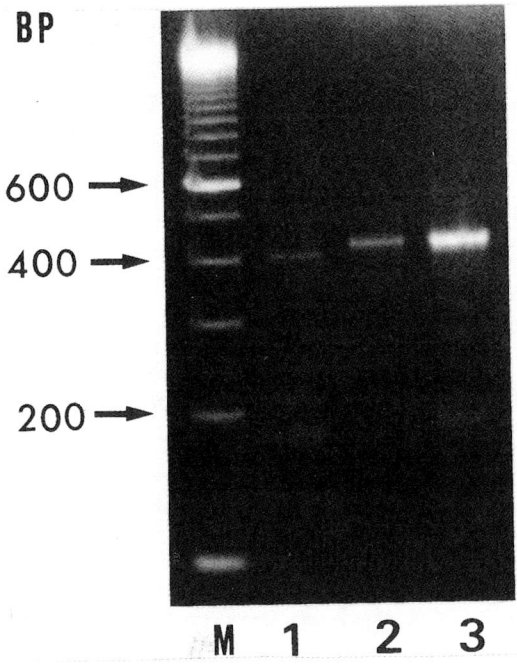

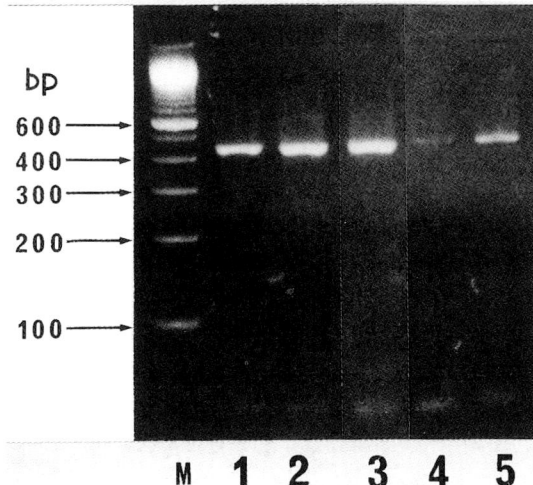

Figure 2 RT-PCR with human Pump-1 cDNA as primer in mouse adenomyosis. A band of 440 bp PCR product is identified in mouse kidney (lane 1), normal mouse uterus (lane 2), and mouse adenomyosis (lane 3)

Figure 3 RT-PCR with human Pump-1 cDNA as primer in human samples. A band of 440 bp PCR product is identified in normal uterine endometrium (lane 1), uterine adenomyosis (lanes 2 and 3), uterine adenocarcinoma (lane 4) and colon cancer (lane 5)

RT-PCR using human Pump-1 cDNA as primer in mouse adenomyosis

Th matrix metalloproteinase identified in a band of relative mass 20 000–30 000 is likely to be identical with the reported lower molecular mass matrix metalloproteinase Pump-1 (relative mass 19 000 for active form and 28 000–29 000 for latent form). Accordingly we investigated a possible involvement of Pump-1 in the development of the mouse adenomyosis. With this aim, RT-PCR was performed using human Pump-1 cDNA, the results of which are shown in Figure 2. The result showed the presence of a band of 440 bp PCR product in normal mouse uterus (lane 2) and mouse adenomyosis (lane 3), as well as in normal mouse kidney (lane 1), suggesting the involvement of Pump-1 in the development of mouse adenomyosis.

RT-PCR using human Pump-1 cDNA as primer in human samples

The data suggesting Pump-1 involvement in the development of adenomyosis in the mouse model led us to investigate a possible association of Pump-1 expression with the development of human uterine adenomyosis. RT-PCR using Pump-1 cDNA as primer was performed, the results of which are shown in Figure 3. The result showed the presence of a band of 440 bp PCR product in normal uterine endometrium (lane 1), uterine adenomyosis (lanes 2 and 3), uterine adenocarcinoma (lane 4) and colon cancer (lane 5).

Western blot analysis of human samples

Following the RT-PCR study on the expression of Pump-1 mRNA in human uterine adenomyosis, we next studied the synthesis of Pump-1 in uterine adenomyosis by Western blot analysis using anti-Pump-1 polyclonal

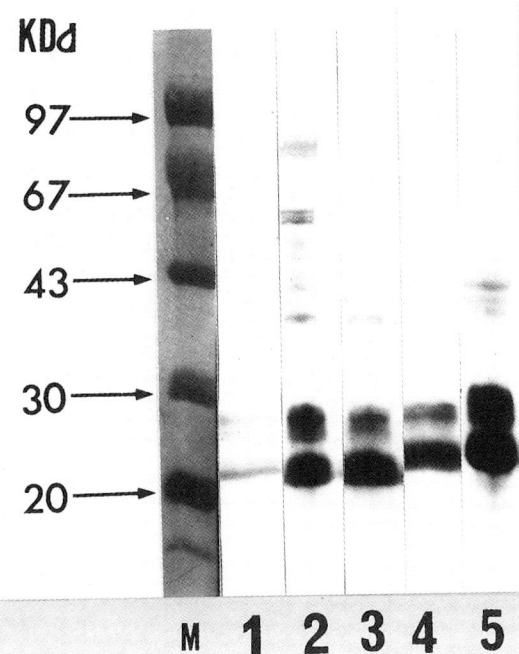

Figure 4 Western blot analysis of human samples. Samples used are the same as those giving the results in Figure 3. Normal uterine endometrium (lane 1), uterine adenomyosis (lanes 2 and 3), uterine adenocarcinoma (lane 4) and colon cancer (lane 5)

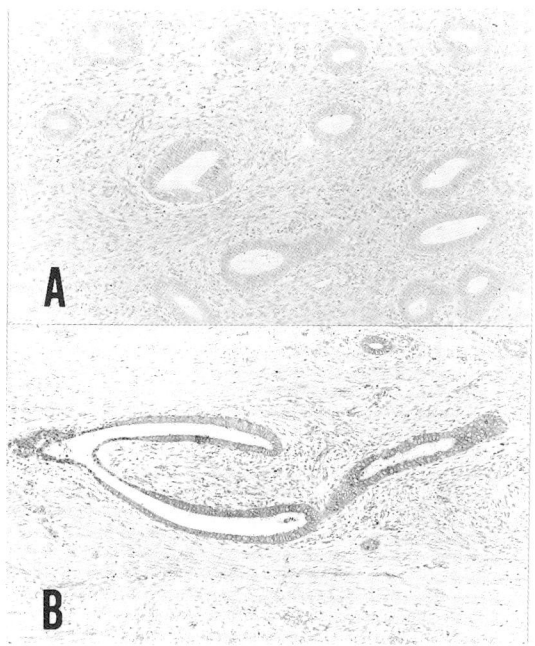

Figure 5 Immunohistochemical localization of Pump-1 in human uterine adenomyosis. Immunoreactive Pump-1 is localized in epithelial cells of human uterine adenomyosis (lower panel), whereas immunoreactive Pump-1 is not detected in normal uterine epithelial cells (upper panel)

antibody. The results are shown in Figure 4. The anti-Pump-1 polyclonal antibody was prepared by immunizing rabbits with a peptide synthesized from Pump-1 cDNA. The samples used were the same as in the previous experiment. The results showed greatly enhanced amounts of immunoreactive Pump-1 (relative mass 28 000 and 20 000 bands) in human uterine adenomyosis (lanes 2 and 3) compared with normal uterine endometrium (lane 1). The bands with relative masses 28 000 and 20 000 were also found in colon cancer (lane 5). The data, taken together, indicate the involvement of the post-transcriptional modification in the cellular Pump-1 synthesis. The results thus suggest the involvement of Pump-1 in the development of uterine adenomyosis.

Immunohistochemical localization of Pump-1 in human uterine adenomyosis

In order to localize Pump-1 in human uterine adenomyosis, immunohistochemical evaluation of human uterine adenomyosis was performed using the anti-Pump-1 antibody. The results are shown in Figure 5. Although normal human uterine epithelial cells do not contain detectable amounts of the immunoreactive Pump-1 (Figure 5a), the expression of this protein was greatly enhanced in epithelial cells of human uterine adenomyosis (Figure 5b). The data therefore indicate the localization of Pump-1 on the epithelial cells of uterine adenomyosis.

Discussion

Although adenomyosis is a benign disease, its invasiveness into the myometrium may resemble that of neoplastic cells, causing the derangement and disintegration of the myometrium. In fact, the expression of proliferating cell nuclear antigen (PCNA) has been reported to be enhanced in the tissues of endometriosis compared with normal uterine endometrium[9].

The present study showed an enhanced synthesis of Pump-1 in the tissues of uterine adenomyosis compared with normal uterine endometrium. The data suggest that an enhanced expression of Pump-1 may play an important role in the invasion of adenomyosis into the myometrium. The expression of Pump-1 in normal tissues has been limited to a few cell types such as glomerular mesangeal cells and endometrial cells. The Pump-1 expression in human endometrium changes during the reproductive cycle, and is enhanced only in the proliferative phase[10,11]. In this respect, the invasion of adenomyosis may resemble that of neoplastic cells, involving a continuous synthesis of matrix metalloproteinases such as Pump-1, which can activate collagenases.

The results of the study of Pump-1 mRNA by RT-PCR (Figure 3) and of that of immunoreactive Pump-1 (Figure 4), taken together, indicate the presence of a post-transcriptional modification in cellular Pump-1 synthesis. Furthermore, Pump-1 has been reported to undergo structural change from an inactive form to an active form before functioning as an activator of collagenases[10]. The control of Pump-1 expression is thus operated in multi-steps.

The immunohistochemical study showed the epithelial synthesis of Pump-1 in uterine adenomyosis (Figure 5). Histological studies using the mouse model for endometriosis have indicated that the invasion of endometrial parenchyma into the myometrium is preceded by the invasion of endometrial stroma through loose connective tissue in the myometrium[6,7]. We therefore speculate that the continuous epithelial synthesis of Pump-1 might be triggered by endometrial stroma, possibly in association with the function of other matrix metalloproteinases. We are currently studying the intercellular communication between endometrial parenchyma and stroma in an effort to analyze the mechanisms responsible for the continuous expression of epithelial Pump-1 in uterine adenomyosis.

In conclusion, the present data are consistent with the idea that epithelial synthesis of Pump-1 in uterine adenomyosis contributes to invasion of the adenomyosis into the myometrium.

Acknowledgements

We would like to thank Dr Yoshihiro Fujii for many helpful discussions and comments on preparing the manuscript.

References

1. Haney, A.F. (1987). *Endometriosis*, pp. 23–51. (New York: Alan R. Liss Inc.).
2. Tienari, J., Pertovaara, L., Saksela, O., Lehtonen, E. and Vartio, T. (1994). Increased expression of the matrix metalloproteinase 2 in differentiating Tera 2 human embryonal carcinoma cells. *Int. J. Cancer*, **56**, 219–23
3. Salo, T., Makela, M., Kylmaniemi, M., Harmainen, A.H. and Larjava, H. (1994). Expression of matrix metalloproteinase-2 and -9 during early human wound healing. *Lab. Invest.*, **70**, 176–82
4. Goldberg, G.I. and Eisen, A.Z. (1991). Extracellular matrix metalloproteinases in tumor invasion and metastasis. *Cancer Treat. Res.*, **53**, 421–40

5. Mori, S., Fujii, M. and Kudo, R. (1996). Expression of the small molecular weight matrix metalloproteinase in adenomyosis of the mouse uterus. *Acta Obstet. Gynaecol. Jpn*, **48**, 386–92
6. Mori, T. and Nagasawa, H. (1983). Mechanisms of development of prolactin-induced adenomyosis in mice. *Acta Anat.*, **116**, 46–54
7. Ohta, Y., Mori, T. and Nagasawa, H. (1985). Ultrastructural changes of endometrium and myometrium during development of adenomyosis in mice with ectopic pituitary transplants. *Zool. Sci.*, **2**, 239–47
8. Endo, T., Aten, R.F., Wang, F. and Behrman, H.R. (1993). Coordinate induction and activation of metalloproteinase and ascorbate depletion in structural luteolysis. *Endocrinology*, **133**, 690–8
9. Li, S.F., Nakajima, K., Masuzaka, H. and Fujii, S. (1993). The number of proliferating cell nuclear antigen positive cells in endometriotic lesions differs from that in the endometrium. *Virchow's Arch. Path. Anat.*, **423**, 257–63
10. Osteen, K.G., Rodgers, W.H., Gaire, M., Hargrove, J.T., Gorstein, F. and Matrisian, L.M. (1994). Stromal–epithelial interaction mediates steroidal regulation of metalloproteinase expression in human endometrium. *Proc. Natl. Acad. Sci. USA*, **91**, 10129–33
11. Rodgers, W.H., Osteen, K.G., Matrisian, L.M., Navre, M., Giudice, L.C. and Gorstein, F. (1993). Expression and localization of matrilysin, a matrix metalloproteinase, in human endometrium during the reproductive cycle. *Am. J. Obstet. Gynecol.*, **168**, 253–60

Endometriosis and infertility: insights with integrins used as markers of uterine receptivity

B.A. Lessey, J. Sun and J.E. Harris

Introduction

Endometriosis is defined as the presence and proliferation of endometrium outside the uterine cavity[1]. Although endometriosis is a common cause of pain and infertility in women, the mechanisms responsible for its pathogenesis and progression, and the associated infertility, remain poorly understood. This seems especially true for minimal or mild endometriosis in that the link to infertility and the effect of treatment is still in question[2]. Endometriosis, even in mild forms, may alter folliculogenesis[3,4] or ovulation[5-7], or adversely affect luteal phase function[8-10], ovum transport[11,12], sperm quality[13] and function[14], fertilization[15] and embryo quality[16,17]. Implantation defects have recently been suggested as a potential focus of investigation[18]. Peritoneal fluid factors and/or the activation of peritoneal macrophages[19,20] may contribute to alterations in endometrial function noted in human[18] and animal models[21].

We have followed a line of investigation which holds promise for understanding the etiology of endometriosis and the potential mechanisms of infertility associated with this disorder. Integrins are cell adhesion molecules (CAMs) that serve as receptors for the extracellular matrix[22]. This family of CAMs are present on virtually all cells and appear to be critical for the maintenance of normal cellular phenotype. Since endometriotic cells subsist in an environment very different from that of eutopic endometrium, we postulate that the differences in the extracellular matrix and CAMs account for many of the alterations in cellular behavior previously noted in this disorder. In addition, the presence of ectopic endometrium may alter the behavior of the eutopic endometrium, leading to defects in endometrial receptivity. In this review, we summarize what is known regarding endometrial integrins as markers of uterine receptivity in women with endometriosis.

Integrins

Integrins are heterodimeric glycoproteins consisting of an α and a β subunit that comprise a family of CAMs involved in such diverse processes as immune functions, wound healing, embryogenesis and development, and the spread of cancer cells[22]. As receptors for the extracellular matrix, these molecules are present on virtually all cells and participate in cell–cell and cell–substratum attachment, signal transduction and interaction with the cytoskeleton. Maintenance of cell shape and polarity may be a primary function of these important molecules and forms the basis for hormone receptivity and gene transcription.

As shown in Table 1, the various integrin subunits pair in limited configurations to form integrins with specific ligand preferences. While some of these 20 integrins bind only one molecule from the extracellular matrix, others, such as α3β1 or αvβ3 are quite promiscuous in their ability to recognize and bind to various extracellular matrix proteins. Regulation of integrin expression may define when

Table 1 Pairing of individual α and β subunits and ligand preference

	β1	β2	β3	β4	β5	β6	β7	β8
α1	Collagen, LM							
α2	Collagen, LM							
α3	Collagen, LM, FN†							
α4	FN						Peyer's patch, FN, VCAM-1, addressin	
α5	FN†							
α6	LM			LM				
α7	LM							
α8	?							
α9	Tenascin							
αv	FN, VN†		VN,FN,FB,vWF, TSP, OP,BSP-1†		VN†	FN		?
αx		FB, C3bi						
αm		FX,FB,C3bi, ICAM-1						
αL		ICAM-1, -2						
αIIb			FB, vWF, FN†					

LM, laminin; FN, fibronectin; VCAM, vascular cell adhesion molecule; VN, vitronectin; FB, fibrinogen; vWF, von Willebrand factor; TSP, thrombospondin; OP, osteopontin; BSP, bone sialoprotein; ICAM 1 and 2, intercellular adhesion molecules; FX, factor X; C3bi, complement component C3bi
†Recognizes RGD

and where each integrin is expressed and certain cells express integrins that must first be activated (such as platelets). On balance, these multifaceted molecules are well suited for the diverse functions they appear to have within the body. The complex patterns of integrin expression in the endometrium and early embryo and trophoblast at the time of implantation are consistent with versatility displayed by this important family of proteins.

Integrins and the endometrium

In 1992 we published the initial observation of integrin expression in the human endometrium[23]. On the basis of this and subsequent reports[24–26], it was immediately apparent that these cell adhesion molecules would be of interest in the study of implantation-related events. Based on morphological studies, the opinion is that the time of embryo attachment probably begins around cycle day 19 or 20[27]. Several integrins were constitutively expressed on either epithelia or stroma (Figure 1), but it was also noted that the α1, α4, and β3 subunits were dynamically regulated during the menstrual cycle[28]. The α1β1 collagen/laminin receptor and the α4β1 fibronectin receptor appear at the time of ovulation, but the latter 'turns off' at the close of the window of implantation around cycle days 24–25. The αvβ3 vitronectin receptor appears on the endometrial epithelium around cycle day 20 (6 days after the surge of luteinizing hormone (LH)). Of interest, however, is the finding that all three integrins are co-expressed only during the narrow window of implantation, thought to occur on cycle days 20–24. Therefore, these integrins may provide one of the first immunohistochemical markers of the time of maximal uterine receptivity. These patterns of cycle-specific integrin changes are summarized in Figure 2. Studies have recently been expanded to include

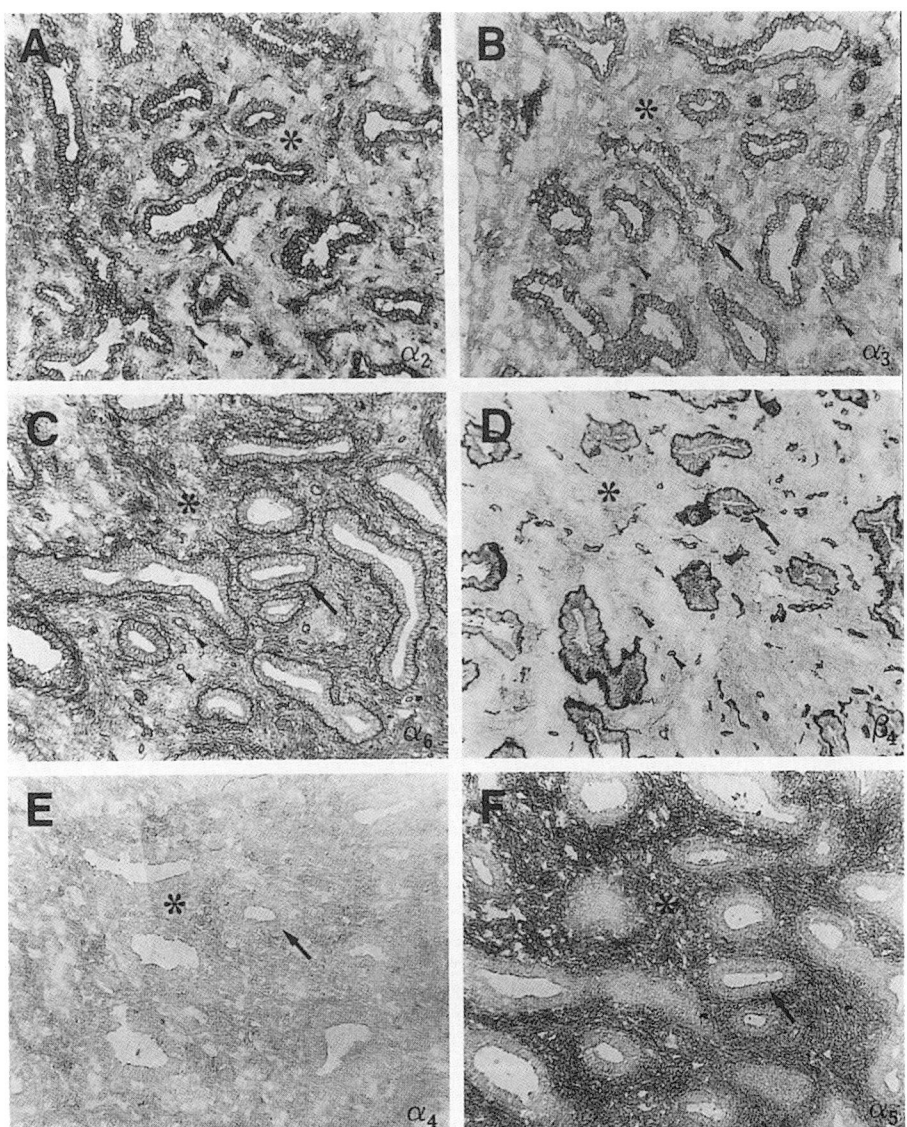

Figure 1 The profile of integrins in normal endometrium in frozen sections. Immunohistochemical staining of the collagen/laminin receptor subunits: $\alpha 2$ (A), $\alpha 3$ (B), $\alpha 6$ (C) and $\beta 4$ (D) show prominent staining of epithelium (arrows) and microvessels (arrowheads) without significant stromal staining (asterisks) for $\alpha 2$, $\alpha 3$ and $\beta 4$. Note basolateral staining for $\alpha 3$ and $\alpha 6$, and basal staining for $\beta 4$. The immunoreactions (areas of dark staining) were developed by the avidin–biotin–peroxidase complex using diaminobenzidine as a chromagen. For greater sensitivity, no counterstain was applied. Magnification: ×80. Used with permission from the publisher, Rockefeller Press, NY, from reference 23

glandular and luminal epithelium[29] and the decidualized stroma of pregnancy[28,30].

Based on what is presently known, the regulation of integrin expression in the endometrium appears to be quite complex. While the cells of normal endometrium in the fertile cycling woman appear to be tightly regulated, endometrial cancer[31] and endometriosis[32,33]

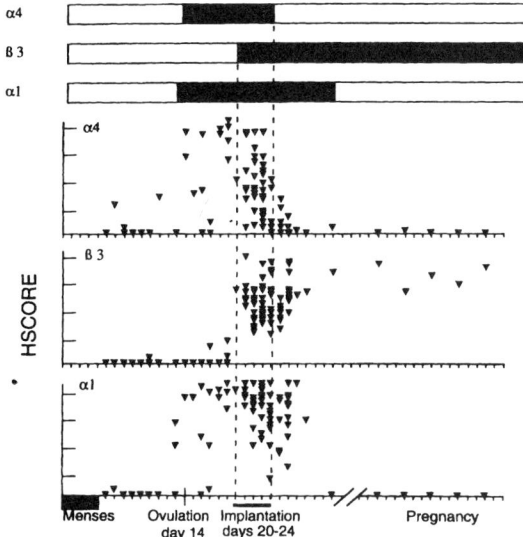

Figure 2 Relative intensity of staining for the epithelial α4, β3 and α1 integrin subunits throughout the menstrual cycle and in early pregnancy. Immunohistochemical staining was assessed by a blinded observer using the semi-quantitative HSCORE (ranging from 0 to 4), and correlated with the estimate of histological dating based on pathological criteria or on the last menstrual period in patients undergoing therapeutic pregnancy termination. The negative staining (open bars) was shown for immunostaining of an average HSCORE of ≤ 0.7 for each of the three integrin subunits. Positive staining for all three integrin subunits was seen only during a 4-day interval corresponding to cycle days 20–24, based on the histological dating criteria of Noyes and co-workers[61]. This interval of integrin co-expression corresponds to the putative window of implant-ation. Of the three, only the αvβ3 integrin was seen in the epithelium of the pregnant endometrium. Reproduced with permission of the American Society for Reproductive Medicine, from reference 28

lose the ability to express certain integrins, or express inappropriate integrins. Evidence for hormonal regulation of integrin expression was first demonstrated in 1990 by Tabibzadeh and Satyaswaroop, who showed that progesterone would induce the α1 integrin subunit in explant cultures of human, proliferative phase endometrium[34]. This phenomenon has also been demonstrated in a well-differentiated endometrial adenocarcinoma cell line (Ishikawa), provided progesterone receptors are first induced by estradiol priming[35]. The appearance of the αvβ3 vitronectin receptor appears to be tied to the down-regulation of progesterone receptors in endometrial glandular epithelium, which occurs normally by cycle days 19–20[36]; this suggests that the αvβ3 integrin, unlike α1β1, is a progesterone-*suppressed* protein. In patients with luteal phase defect, the histological delay found in this disorder is associated with a persistence of epithelial progesterone receptors and an absence of αvβ3[37]. Cytokines and growth factors are also potent inducers/inhibitors of integrins. It is not surprising to find that both stromal and epithelial cells in the endometrium respond with either induction or down-regulation of integrin expression in response to growth factors and cytokines[38,39]. As discussed below, such complexities in integrin regulation may lead to defects in endometrial receptivity, associated with endometriosis and subtle alterations in the biomolecular paracrine milieu.

Endometriosis and occult defects in uterine receptivity

Although moderate or severe endometriosis may cause infertility on the basis of mechanical disruption of ovulation or gamete transport, the effect of minimal or mild disease on cycle fecundity remains controversial[2]. Evidence that endometriosis in its milder forms contributes to infertility is based on several lines of evidence. In prospective studies normal fertile women have a significantly lower rate of endometriosis than women with infertility[40,41]. Animal models of surgically induced endometriosis have also been associated with a lower pregnancy rate[42,43]. Hahn and colleagues[21] demonstrated impaired implantation in rabbits with surgically induced endometriosis, independent of adhesion formation. This impaired implantation was transferred to normal rabbits by transfer of peritoneal

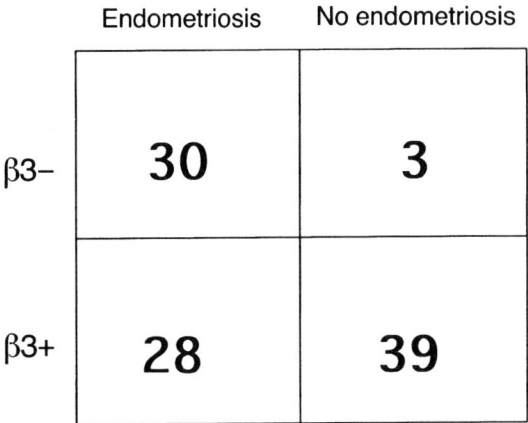

Figure 3 Prospective assessment of 100 'in-phase' endometrial biopsies in an infertile population. One hundred 'in phase' endometrial biopsies were obtained during the window of implantation (cycle days 21–23) based on the urinary luteinizing hormone surge. Immunohistochemical assessment for the αvβ3 integrin was performed as previously described[28]. Subsequent diagnostic laparoscopy was performed and the presence or absence of epithelial αvβ3 was determined. As noted, of 33 women who failed to express αvβ3, 30 were found to have endometriosis (all minimal or mild stages). Surprisingly, 28 other women were found to have endometriosis despite normal αvβ3 expression. One interpretation of these results is that women with endometriosis are a heterogeneous population comprising those with and those without uterine receptivity defects

fluid[21]. Similar studies have been carried out with human peritoneal fluid transferred into mice[44]. The third line of evidence is derived from studies of women entering a donor insemination program[45]. Cycle fecundity is significantly reduced in women with minimal endometriosis compared to women without this disorder. A fourth line of evidence comes from assisted reproductive technologies (ART). Some studies have found differences in pregnancy outcome in women with endometriosis[46], but other studies have shown no difference in the outcome between patients with endometriosis or tubal disease[47]. This may not in fact be a legitimate comparison. As hydrosalpinx may also lead to defects in implantation[48–50], the diagnosis of minimal and mild endometriosis can be shown to be associated with lower cycle fecundity rates when patients with tubal factor or hydrosalpinx are removed from the comparison[51]. Finally, women with milder forms of endometriosis prior to gamete intra-Fallopian transfer (GIFT)[52] or *in vitro* fertilization (IVF)[53] have significant improvement in pregnancy rates following medical treatment for their disease.

The pattern of cycle-dependent endometrial integrin expression is disrupted in women with endometriosis[18] and unexplained infertility[54]. The αvβ3 integrin is missing during the window of implantation in about half of all women with minimal or mild endometriosis. Further, in prospective studies, the lack of this integrin in otherwise normal endometrium had a 91% positive predictive value for the presence of endometriosis in a subsequent laparoscopy. As shown in Figure 3, in 100 prospective 'in phase' biopsies we found that 33 were missing the αvβ3 integrin. Of these, 30 were prospectively found to have endometriosis at laparoscopy (all minimal or mild disease). Interestingly, 28 women were also found to have endometriosis, but were normal with respect to this marker. Prospective follow-up of each group revealed dramatic differences in pregnancy outcome. Only four of 40 patients (10%) without normal αvβ3 expression successfully conceived, whereas over 80% of the αvβ3-positive endometriosis patients successfully achieved pregnancy. This would suggest that the long known phenomenon of pregnancy with expectant management alone, which occurs in about 50% of patients[55], might be understood in these terms. If markers could be used to identify that 50% that will not conceive due to implantation defects, inroads could be made into better diagnostic and treatment options in this unfortunate group of patients that ultimately are labeled with the diagnosis of 'unexplained' infertility.

Endometriosis and treatment options: sorting out the meta-confusion

A study to provide an adequate answer to the question of whether treatment is beneficial for the purposes of infertility in minimal or mild endometriosis has not yet been performed. To compare the effect of any treatment with expectant management alone, a prospective, randomized and blinded study design should be adopted. If the population of endometriosis patients is in fact heterogeneous, as we now believe, with half of all patients being unaffected by their disease while the remainder are profoundly infertile, it would take a surprisingly large study population to settle the issue. With the primary objective of determining the effect of therapy on pregnancy outcome and fertility in women with endometriosis, assuming a clinically meaningful difference of 20%, and assuming the alpha (type I) error to be 0.05 and the type II error to be 20% (i.e. power of 80%), over 300 endometriosis patients would be needed to randomize two treatment groups. Clearly, none of the studies to date have achieved these criteria and meta-analyses alone offer little reassurance that the issue has been settled[56,57]. One of the few studies that has demonstrated a difference in treatment outcome utilized a study design that required inclusion only after 6 months of expectant management[58], effectively selecting for women who were less likely to conceive on their own. Evidence from IVF[59] and natural cycles[60] suggests that gonadotropin-releasing hormone (GnRH) analog treatment may significantly improve clinical outcome in women with endometriosis. A large prospective, randomized and blinded study to compare the diagnostic potential of integrin testing and the role of medical management is currently being planned.

Summary

Endometriosis is an enigmatic disease that is associated with pelvic pain and infertility. New avenues of research into markers of uterine receptivity suggest that occult endometrial defects may be associated with endometriosis in some patients. The use of such markers may be useful in a non-surgical diagnostic test for endometriosis and identify women who will respond to medical therapy with improved cycle fecundity. Studies are in progress to discover the basis for such defects, but early evidence suggests that peritoneal fluid is a reservoir for biomolecular factors that may alter endometrial function. Identification of such factors may lead to better strategies for the treatment of such patients and to novel methods of contraception, targeting the endometrium and embryo implantation.

Acknowledgements

This work was supported by NIH grants HD 29448 and HD 30476. We would like to thank the many investigators for their generous donation of antibodies and reagents necessary to complete these studies.

References

1. Haney, A.F. (1990). Etiology and histogenesis of endometriosis. *Prog. Clin. Biol. Res.*, **323**, 1–14
2. Bancroft, K., Vaughan Williams, C.A. and Elstein, M. (1989). Minimal/mild endometriosis and infertility. A review. *Br. J. Obstet. Gynaecol.*, **96**, 454–60
3. Doody, M.C., Gibbons, W.E. and Buttram, V.C. Jr (1988). Linear regression analysis of ultrasound follicular growth series: evidence for an abnormality of follicular growth in endometriosis patients. *Fertil. Steril.*, **49**, 47–51
4. Wardle, P.G., McLauglin, E.A., McDermott, A.,

4. Mitchell, J.D., Ray, B.D. and Hull, M.G.R. (1985). Endometriosis and ovulatory disorder: reduced fertilization *in vitro* compared with tubal and unexplained infertility. *Lancet*, **2**, 236–9
5. Soules, M.R., Malinak, L.R., Bury, R. and Poindexter, A. (1976). Endometriosis and anovulation: a coexisting problem in the infertile female. *Am. J. Obstet. Gynecol.*, **125**, 412–17
6. Schenken, R.S., Asch, R.H., Williams, R.F. and Hodgen, G.D. (1984). Etiology of infertility in monkeys with endometriosis: luteinized unruptured follicles, luteal phase defects, pelvic adhesions, and spontaneous abortions. *Fertil. Steril.*, **41**, 122–30
7. Brosens, I.A., Koninckx, P.R. and Corveleyn, P.A. (1978). A study of plasma progesterone, oestradiol-17β, prolactin and LH levels, and of the luteal phase appearance of the ovaries in patients with endometriosis and infertility. *Br. J. Obstet. Gynaecol.*, **85**, 246–50
8. Grant, A. (1966). Additional sterility factors in endometriosis. *Fertil. Steril.*, **17**, 514–19
9. Cheesman, K.L., Ben-Nun, I., Chatterton, R.T. Jr and Cohen, M.R. (1982). Relationship of luteinizing hormone, pregnanediol-3-glucuronide and estriol-16-glucuronide in urine of infertile women with endometriosis. *Fertil. Steril.*, **38**, 542–8
10. Ayers, J.W., Birenbaum, D.L. and Menon, K.M. (1987). Luteal phase dysfunction in endometriosis: elevated progesterone levels in peripheral and ovarian veins during the follicular phase. *Fertil. Steril.*, **47**, 925–9
11. Drake, T.S., O'Brien, W.F., Ramwell, P.W. and Metz, S.A. (1981). Peritoneal fluid thromboxane B_2 and 6-keto-prostaglandin F_2 alpha in endometriosis. *Am. J. Obstet. Gynecol.*, **140**, 401–4
12. Suginami, H., Yano, K., Nakahashi, N. and Takeda, Y. (1990). Fallopian tube and fimbrial function in endometriosis: with a special reference to an ovum capture inhibitor. *Prog. Clin. Biol. Res.*, **323**, 81–97.
13. Soldati, G., Piffaretti-Yanez, A., Campana, A., Marchini, M., Luerti, M. and Balerna, M. (1989). Effect of peritoneal fluid on sperm motility and velocity distribution using objective measurements. *Fertil. Steril.*, **52**, 113–19
14. Chacho, K.J., Chacho, M.S., Andresen, P.J. and Scommegna, A. (1986). Peritoneal fluid in patients with and without endometriosis: prostanoids and macrophages and their effect on the spermatozoa penetration assay. *Am. J. Obstet. Gynecol.*, **154**, 1290–9
15. Sueldo, C.E., Lambert, H., Steinleitner, A., Rathwick, G. and Swanson, J. (1987). The effect of peritoneal fluid from patients with endometriosis on murine sperm–oocyte interaction. *Fertil. Steril.*, **48**, 697–9
16. Morcos, R.N., Gibbons, W.E. and Findley, W.E. (1985). Effect of peritoneal fluid on *in vitro* cleavage of 2-cell mouse embryos: possible role in infertility associated with endometriosis. *Fertil. Steril.*, **44**, 678–83
17. Damewood, M.D., Hesla, J.S., Schlaff, W.D., Hubbard, M., Gearhart, J.D. and Rock, J.A. (1990). Effect of serum from patients with minimal to mild endometriosis on mouse embryo development *in vitro*. *Fertil. Steril.*, **54**, 917–20
18. Lessey, B.A., Castelbaum, A.J., Sawin, S.J., Buck, C.A., Schinnar, R., Wilkins, B. and Strom, B.L. (1994). Aberrant integrin expression in the endometrium of women with endometriosis. *J. Clin. Endocrinol. Metab.*, **79**, 643–9
19. Haney, A.F., Muscata, J.J. and Weinberg, J.B. (1981). Peritoneal fluid cell populations in infertility patients. *Fertil. Steril.*, **35**, 696–8
20. Halme, J., Becker, S., Hammond, M.G., Raj, M.H.G. and Raj, S. (1983). Increased activation of pelvic macrophages in infertile women with mild endometriosis. *Am. J. Obstet. Gynecol.*, **145**, 333–7
21. Hahn, D.W., Carraher, R.P., Foldesy, R.G. and McGuire, J.L. (1986). Experimental evidence for failure to implant as a mechanism of infertility associated with endometriosis. *Am. J. Obstet. Gynecol.*, **155**, 1109–13
22. Albelda, S.M. and Buck, C.A. (1990). Integrins and other cell adhesion molecules. *FASEB J.*, **4**, 2868–80
23. Lessey, B.A., Damjanovich, L., Coutifaris, C., Castelbaum, A., Albelda, S.M. and Buck, C.A. (1992). Integrin adhesion molecules in the human endometrium. Correlation with the normal and abnormal menstrual cycle. *J. Clin. Invest.*, **90**, 188–95
24. Tabibzadeh, S. (1992). Patterns of expression of integrin molecules in human endometrium throughout the menstrual cycle. *Hum. Reprod.*, **7**, 876–82
25. Bischof, P., Redard, M., Gindre, P., Vassilakos, P. and Campana, A. (1993). Localization of alpha 2, alpha 5 and alpha 6 integrin subunits in human endometrium, decidua and tropho-

blast. *Eur. J. Obstet. Gynecol. Reprod. Biol.*, **51**, 217–26.
26. Klentzeris, L.D., Bulmer, J.N., Trejdosiewicz, L.K., Morrison, L. and Cooke, I.D. (1993). Beta-1 integrin cell adhesion molecules in the endometrium of fertile and infertile women. *Hum. Reprod.*, **8**, 1223–30
27. Hertig, A.T., Rock, J. and Adams, E.C. (1956). A description of 34 human ova within the first 17 days of development. *Am. J. Anat.*, **98**, 435–93
28. Lessey, B.A., Castelbaum, A.J., Buck, C.A., Lei, Y., Yowell, C.W. and Sun, J. (1994). Further characterization of endometrial integrins during the menstrual cycle and in pregnancy. *Fertil. Steril.*, **62**, 497–506
29. Lessey, B.A., Ilesanmi, A.O., Sun, J., Lessey, M.A., Harris, J. and Chwalisz, K. (1996). Luminal and glandular endometrial epithelium express integrins differentially throughout the menstrual cycle: implications for implantation, contraception, and infertility. *Am. J. Reprod. Immunol.*, **35**, 195–204
30. Ruck, P., Marzusch, K., Kaiserling, E., Horny, H.-P., Dietl, J., Geiselhart, A., Handgretinger, R. and Redman, C.W.G. (1994). Distribution of cell adhesion molecules in decidua of early human pregnancy: an immunohistochemical study. *Lab. Invest.*, **71**, 94–101
31. Lessey, B.A., Albelda, S., Buck, C.A., Castelbaum, A.J., Yeh, I., Kohler, M. and Berchuck, A. (1995). Distribution of integrin cell adhesion molecules in endometrial cancer. *Am. J. Pathol.*, **146**, 717–26
32. Bridges, J.E., Prentice, A., Roche, W., Englefield, P. and Thomas, E.J. (1994). Expression of integrin adhesion molecules in endometrium and endometriosis. *Br. J. Obstet. Gynaecol.*, **101**, 696–700
33. van der Linden, P.J., de Goeij, A.F., Dunselman, G.A., van der Linden, E.P., Ramaekers, F.C. and Evers, J.L. (1994). Expression of integrins and E-cadherin in cells from menstrual effluent, endometrium, peritoneal fluid, peritoneum, and endometriosis. *Fertil. Steril.*, **61**, 85–90
34. Tabibzadeh, S.S. and Satyaswaroop, P.G. (1990). Progestin-mediated induction of VLA-1 in glandular epithelium of human endometrium *in vitro*. *72nd Annual Meeting of the Endocrine Society*, no. 700
35. Lessey, B.A., Ilesanmi, A., Castelbaum, A.J., Yuan, L.-W., Somkuti, S., Chwalisz, K. and Satyaswaroop, P.G. (1996). Characterization of the functional progesterone receptor in an endometrial adenocarcinoma cell line (Ishikawa): progesterone-induced expression of the α1β1 integrin. *J. Steroid Biochem. Mol. Biol.*, **59**, 31–9
36. Lessey, B.A., Killam, A.P., Metzger, D.A., Haney, A.F., Greene, G.L. and McCarty, K.S. Jr (1988). Immunohistochemical analysis of human uterine estrogen and progesterone receptors throughout the menstrual cycle. *J. Clin. Endocrinol. Metab.*, **67**, 334–40
37. Lessey, B.A., Yeh, I.T., Castelbaum, A.J., Fritz, M.A., Ilesanmi, A.O., Korzeniowski, P., Sun, J.H. and Chwalisz, K. (1996). Endometrial progesterone receptors and markers of uterine receptivity in the window of implantation. *Fertil. Steril.*, **65**, 477–83
38. Grosskinsky, C.M., Yowell, C.W., Sun, J.H., Parise, L.V. and Lessey, B.A. (1996). Modulation of integrin expression in endometrial stroma cells *in vitro*. *J. Clin. Endocrinol. Metab.*, **81**, 2047–54
39. Somkuti, S.G., Yuan, L., Fritz, M.A. and Lessey, B.A. (1997). Epidermal growth factor and sex steroids dynamically regulate a marker of endometrial receptivity in Ishikawa cells. *J. Clin. Endo. Metab.*, in press
40. Strathy, J.H., Molgaard, C.A., Coulam, C.B. and Melton, L.J. (1982). Endometriosis and infertility: a laparoscopic study of endometriosis among fertile and infertile women. *Fertil. Steril.*, **38**, 667–75
41. Verkauf, B.S. (1987). Incidence, symptoms, and signs of endometriosis in infertile and infertile women. *J. Fla Med. Assoc.*, **74**, 671–5
42. Schenken, R.S. and Asch, R.H. (1980). Surgical induction of endometriosis in the rabbit: effects on fertility and concentration of peritoneal fluid prostaglandins. *Fertil. Steril.*, **34**, 581–7
43. Vernon, M.W. and Wilson, E.A. (1985). Studies on the surgical induction of endometriosis in the rat. *Fertil. Steril.*, **44**, 684–94
44. Illera, M.J., Rumen, J., Yuan, L.-W. and Lessey, B.A. (1995). Peritoneal fluid from infertile women with endometriosis and aberrant endometrial integrin expression blocks embryo implantation in a mouse model. *Endocrine Society 77th Annual Meeting*, P2-98, p.315
45. Jansen, R.P. (1986). Minimal endometriosis and reduced fecundability: prospective evidence

from an artificial insemination by donor program. *Fertil. Steril.*, **46**, 141–3

46. Arici, A., Oral, E., Bukulmez, O., Duleba, A., Olive, D.L. and Jones, E.E. (1996). The effect of endometriosis on implantation: results from the Yale University *in vitro* fertilization and embryo transfer program. *Fertil. Steril.*, **65**, 603–7

47. Olivennes, F., Feldberg, D., Liu, H.-C., Cohen, J., Moy, F. and Rosenwaks, Z. (1995). Endometriosis: a stage by stage analysis – the role of *in vitro* fertilization. *Fertil. Steril.*, **64**, 392–8

48. Vandromme, J., Chasse, E., Lejeune, B., Van Rysselberge, M., Delvigne, A. and Leroy, F. (1995). Hydrosalpinges in *in-vitro* fertilization: an unfavourable prognostic feature. *Hum. Reprod.*, **10**, 576–9

49. Shelton, K.E., Butler, L., Toner, J.P., Oehninger, S., and Muasher, S.J. (1996). Salpingectomy improves the pregnancy rate in *in-vitro* fertilization patients with hydrosalpinx. *Hum. Reprod.*, **11**, 523–5

50. Lessey, B.A., Castelbaum, A.J., Riben, M., Howarth, J., Tureck, R. and Meyer, W.R. (1994). Effect of hydrosalpinges on markers of uterine receptivity and success in IVF (abstr.). *American Fertility Society Annual Meeting*

51. Castelbaum, A.J., Riben, M., Howarth, J., Tureck, R. and Lessey, B.A. (1994). Minimal endometriosis impairs endometrial $\alpha v\beta 3$ integrin expression and cycle fecundity compared to tubal factor patients in an IVF program. *American Fertility Society Annual Meeting*, **P7**, S89

52. Remorgida, V., Anserini, P., Croce, S., Costa, M., Ferraiolo, A. and Capitanio, G.L. (1990). Comparison of different ovarian stimulation protocols for gamete intrafallopian transfer in patients with minimal and mild endometriosis. *Fertil. Steril.*, **53**, 1060–3

53. Chedid, S., Camus, M., Smitz, J., Van Steirteghem, A.C. and Devroey, P. (1995). Comparison among different ovarian stimulation regimens for assisted procreation procedures in patients with endometriosis. *Hum. Reprod.*, **10**, 2406–11

54. Lessey, B.A., Castelbaum, A.J., Sawin, S.J. and Sun, J. (1995). Integrins as markers of uterine receptivity in women with primary unexplained infertility. *Fertil. Steril.*, **63**, 535–42

55. Evers, J.L. (1989). The pregnancy rate of the no-treatment group in randomized clinical trials of endometriosis therapy. *Fertil. Steril.*, **52**, 906–7

56. Hughes, E.G., Fedorkow, D.M. and Collins, J.A. (1993). A quantitative overview of controlled trials in endometriosis-associated infertility. *Fertil. Steril.*, **59**, 963–70

57. Adamson, G.D. and Pasta, D.J. (1994). Surgical treatment of endometriosis-associated infertility: meta-analysis compared with survival analysis. *Am. J. Obstet. Gynecol.*, **171**, 1488–505

58. Nowroozi, K., Chase, J.S., Check, J.H. and Wu, C.H. (1987). The importance of laparoscopic coagulation of mild endometriosis in infertile women. *Int. J. Fertil.*, **32**, 442–4

59. Marcus, S.F. and Edwards, R.G. (1994). High rates of pregnancy after long-term down-regulation of women with severe endometriosis. *Am. J. Obstet. Gynecol.*, **171**, 812–17

60. Lessey, B.A., Castelbaum, A.J., Somkuti, S.G., Young, S.L. and Wolf, L. (1996). Improvement in pregnancy rates with GnRH agonist in women with infertility, minimal or mild endometriosis and aberrant $\alpha v\beta 3$ expression (abstr.). *American Society of Reproductive Medicine Annual Meeting*

61. Noyes, R.W., Hertig, A.I. and Rock, J. (1950). Dating the endometrial biopsy. *Fertil. Steril.*, **1**, 3–25

Expression of ICAM-1 in eutopic and ectopic endometrial cells

P. Viganò, B. Gaffuri, E. Somigliana, E. Iurlaro, A.M. Di Blasio and M. Vignali

Introduction

Lymphocyte adhesion to a wide array of different cells and tissue types is required for the induction and maintenance of immune responses, and is mediated by specific cell surface molecules. Although immunological specificity is regulated via antigen receptors, additional accessory molecules play an important role in cell–cell contact-mediated immune reactions[1]. One of these molecules is the intercellular adhesion molecule-1 (ICAM-1) (CD54)[2]. ICAM-1 is expressed in various lineages of hemopoietic and non-hemopoietic origin including leukocytes, fibroblasts, endothelial and epithelial cells[3,4]. It is a ligand of at least two members of the CD18 family of leukocyte adhesion molecules: LFA-1 (CD11a/CD18) and Mac-1 (CD11b/CD18)[5–8]. Structurally, ICAM-1 is a glycoprotein with relative mass 90 000, a member of the immunoglobulin supergene family with five extracellular immunoglobulin-like domains, a single transmembrane region and a short cytoplasmic tail[9,10]. The interaction of LFA-1 and ICAM-1 is essential for cell-mediated cytotoxicity[11], the interaction of T and B cells[12], homotypic adhesion of monocytes[13] and B-cell–B-cell homotypic adhesion[14]. Furthermore, ICAM-1 is necessary for lymphocyte–endothelial cell adhesion and is thought to facilitate lymphocyte migration to sites of inflammation along endothelial cells[15].

In contrast to LFA-1, which is expressed in leukocytes in a constitutive manner, ICAM-1 is up-regulated on various lineages *in vivo* and *in vitro* by proinflammatory cytokines, such as interferon-γ, interleukin 1β and tumor necrosis factor-α (TNF-α)[1,3]. In the absence of an inflammatory response, ICAM-1 can be detected only on very few cell types[5]. ICAM-1 expression depends on protein and mRNA synthesis and is at least partly regulated at the mRNA level[4,10].

Recently, a shedding form of this adhesion molecule, soluble intercellular adhesion molecule-1 (sICAM-1), has been identified and characterized in at least three identifiable molecular forms with relative molecular masses of about 240, 430 and > 500 kDa[16,17]. Soluble ICAM-1 has been detected in supernatants obtained from endothelial cells, melanoma and ovarian carcinoma cells[17]. Elevated levels of the circulating protein have been observed in inflammation, infection and cancers. In particular, sICAM-1 has been detected in the cerebrospinal fluid of patients with inflammatory neurological diseases, in synovial fluids from patients with rheumatoid arthritis, in malignant ascites of patients with ovarian carcinoma and in the broncho alveolar lavage (BAL) fluid of patients with interstitial lung disease[17]. The biological function of sICAM-1 has been studied in detail in the development and progression of cancer[18–23]. Soluble ICAM-1 has been demonstrated to be shed from tumor cells and to be still able to bind LFA-1. It can therefore disturb adhesion between immune cells (T-lymphocytes and natural killer cells) and their targets. Due to competition between sICAM-1 and (still) cell-bound ICAM-1 molecules for binding to the same receptor (LFA-1), an effective immunological reaction against the tumor is prevented[18–23].

The recent demonstration of a significantly decreased peripheral blood lymphocyte

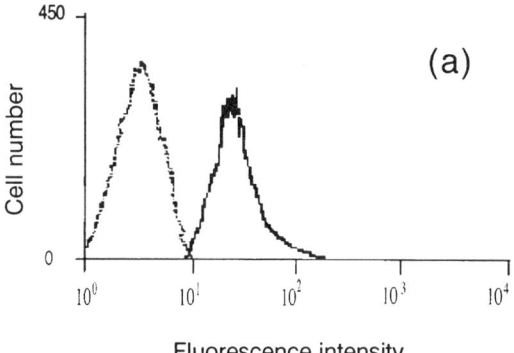
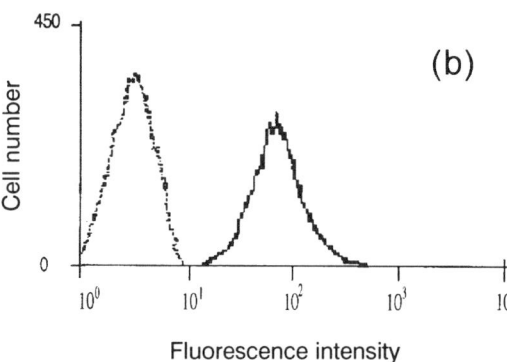

Figure 1 Representative flow cytometric profiles of intercellular adhesion molecule-1 (ICAM-1) expression on eutopic and ectopic endometrial stromal cells. Eutopic cells (a) and ectopic cells (b) were stained for ICAM-1 (solid line) and are compared with control cells (dotted line) stained only with the second fluorescent antibody (see text for details)

(PBL)-mediated cytotoxicity to autologous endometrial antigens in endometriosis patients has highlighted the importance of adhesive interaction between leukocytes and endometrial cells in the etiopathogenesis of this disease[24,25]. In particular, some indications have suggested that natural killer cells might be the specific lymphoid subpopulation responsible for this phenomenon[24–27]. However, the specific molecules involved in the natural killer cell–endometrium interaction have not yet been extensively investigated.

In the present study, we first evaluated whether surface ICAM-1 is expressed on eutopic and ectopic endometrial stromal cells. Secondly, we examined the role of this surface molecule and of its soluble form in the process of lymphocyte-mediated lysis of endometrium.

Methods and results

The expression of ICAM-1 on cultured endometrial and endometriosis stromal cells was assessed by flow cytometry. In previous studies, we successfully established and employed stromal cell monolayer cultures from normal endometrial samples and from ovarian endometrioma cyst linings[28]. For flow cytometric analysis, cells were detached from monolayers and incubated with an anti-ICAM-1 monoclonal antibody for 30 min at 4°C, followed by a fluorescein isothiocyanate–conjugate secondary IgG for 30 min at 4°C. Samples were washed twice and analyzed on a FACScan (Becton Dickinson, Mountain View, CA, USA).

Representative flow cytometric analysis of the surface expression of the ICAM-1 adhesion molecule on eutopic and ectopic endometrial stromal cells is shown in Figure 1. Visual appraisal of the profiles revealed a normal distribution of the molecule on the surface of both types of cultures. It was notable that even after long periods in culture, both types of cells retained surface ICAM-1 expression.

The functional activity of ICAM-1 on natural killer cell–endometrium interaction was tested by ^{51}Cr binding and cytotoxicity assays. Human peripheral blood mononuclear cells were isolated from heparinized blood samples and separated using a Ficoll-Isopaque discontinuous density gradient centrifugation as previously described[29]. Lymphocytes were enriched by incubating mononuclear cells in tissue culture-treated dishes for 1 h twice and saving the non-adherent cells. A fraction enriched in CD3-CD56+ cells (natural killer cells) were further purified by negative selection using a two-step panning technique with anti-CD3 and anti-CD5 monoclonal antibodies, and labeled by incubation for 60 min at 37°C with radioactive sodium chromate (^{51}Cr). Cultured

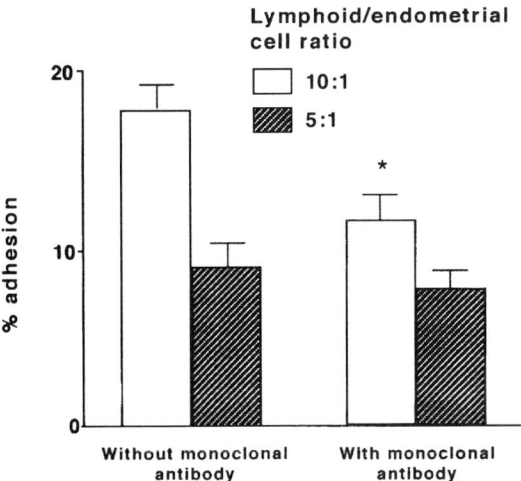

Figure 2 Natural killer cell binding to endometrial stromal cells in the presence and absence of an anti-intercellular adhesion molecule-1 (ICAM-1) monoclonal antibody. Endometrial targets were incubated with and without an anti-ICAM-1 monoclonal antibody for 1 h and then tested in a ^{51}Cr-release binding assay at the indicated lymphoid/endometrial cell ratios. Results represent the mean percentage binding ± SEM for five experiments; *represents a p value of < 0.05 compared with the control

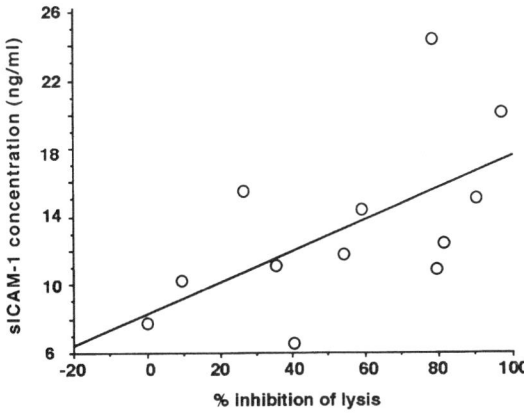

Figure 3 Correlation between levels of soluble intercellular adhesion molecule-1 (sICAM-1) in endometrial stromal cell supernatants and the percentage of inhibition of natural killer cell-mediated activity exerted by the same supernatants. Natural killer cells were incubated overnight in medium alone or in the presence of 12 different endometrial stromal supernatants. Correlation coefficient $(r) = 0.6$; $p < 0.05$

stromal cells were pretreated with and without an anti-ICAM-1 monoclonal antibody. Thereafter, natural killer cell cytotoxicity and binding to the endometrium were evaluated using previously published techniques[30,31]. As shown in Figure 2, adhesion of natural killer cells to endometrial stromal cells was inhibited by 53% by ICAM-1 monoclonal antibody. The mean binding percentage ± SEM was 17.4 ± 3.6 and 8.2 ± 2.0 in the control and ICAM-1 monoclonal antibody pretreated cells, respectively. These results therefore demonstrate that surface ICAM-1 is involved in the binding of natural killer cells to the endometrium, although it is noteworthy that the antibody could not completely abolish natural killer cell adhesion. In contrast, pretreatment of endometrial cells with ICAM-1 monoclonal antibody did not result in any consistent alteration of natural killer cell cytotoxicity (data not shown).

Finally, to evaluate whether, as observed in the tumor system, sICAM-1 might interfere with the adhesion between natural killer cells and endometrium, sICAM-1 was quantified in supernatants from endometrial stromal cultures and these concentrations were correlated with the ability of such supernatants to suppress natural killer cell-mediated cytotoxicity towards endometrial targets. The quantitative detection of sICAM-1 in endometrial supernatants was performed using a commercially available enzyme-linked immunosorbent kit provided by Bender MedSystem, Vienna, Austria. A dose of standard culture medium was also evaluated in order to exclude the presence of sICAM-1 in the culture medium. A significant correlation ($r = 0.6$, $p < 0.05$) was found between sICAM-1 levels in endometrial supernatants and the percentage of inhibition of natural killer cell-mediated lysis exerted by the same supernatant samples (Figure 3). Moreover, the results of sICAM-1 determinations in endometrial supernatants revealed that, while levels were similar for endometrial

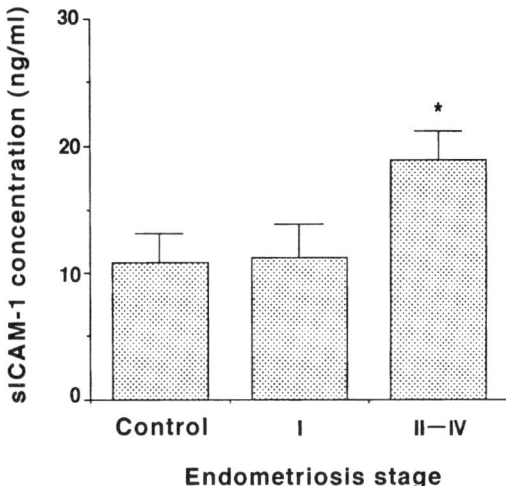

Figure 4 Endometrial stromal cell shedding of soluble intercellular adhesion molecule-1 (sICAM-1) according to the presence ($n = 13$) or absence ($n = 18$) of endometriosis. Data are expressed as mean ± SEM; *$p < 0.05$ compared with controls

samples obtained from women without evidence of endometriosis and patients with stage I disease (10.89 ± 2.2 ng/ml and 11.23 ± 2.62 ng/ml, respectively), endometrial supernatants obtained from the group of patients with advanced stage (II, III and IV) disease produced significantly higher levels of the soluble protein (18.97 ± 2.2 ng/ml) when compared to the group of control women ($p < 0.05$) (Figure 4).

Discussion

The data presented above support the following observations: (1) the adhesion molecule ICAM-1 is constitutively expressed on both eutopic and ectopic endometrial stromal cells; (2) the natural killer cell-mediated immunological recognition of endometrial targets is LFA-1/ICAM-1 pathway dependent; (3) cultured human endometrial cells are constitutively able to release sICAM-1 and this shedding is significantly higher in endometrial samples obtained from patients with advanced stage endometriosis when compared to women without the disease; and (4) sICAM-1 is endowed with the ability to influence natural killer cell function towards the endometrial target.

According to these observations, it is tempting to speculate that surface ICAM-1 may be one of the major adhesion structures through which the innate immune system ensures the elimination of ectopic cells that regularly reach the peritoneum. In contrast, its shedding may be one of the mechanisms by which refluxed endometrial cells escape immunosurveillance. An excessive release of sICAM-1 could influence the capability of endometrial cells to implant outside the uterus and thus contribute to the development of endometriosis.

It should be noted that an anti-ICAM-1 monoclonal antibody did not affect natural killer cell cytotoxic activity and did not completely abolish natural killer cell binding. It therefore seems likely that the adhesion and lytic mechanisms involved in natural killer–endometrial cell interaction comprise a heterogeneous group of molecules. This is in agreement with some immunological evidence concerning lymphocyte-mediated cytotoxic events towards a variety of targets[31]; natural killer cell-mediated cytotoxicity has been suggested to be divided into different morphologically distinguishable stages that require an elaborate set of structures. In particular, it has been suggested that the adhesion structures would serve as initial recognition molecules. This adhesion step would then lead to the activation of killer structures[31].

The release or shedding of cell surface adhesion proteins has also been described for other cell types: L-selectin from neutrophils and lymphocytes[32,33], ICAM-1, vascular cell adhesion molecule-1 (VCAM-1) and E-selectin from the surface of endothelial cells following cytokine stimulation[17], and LFA-3 from a number of different human cell lines[34]. It is at present not known how or by which mechanism(s) ICAM-1 is released into the culture media by endometrial cells. ICAM-1 has no alternative spliced form lacking the transmembrane domain and, consequently, it is likely that this ligand is proteolytically clipped at the cell surface. *In vitro* data suggest that, at least in endothelial cells, the soluble form of ICAM-1 is indeed generated by proteolytic cleavage at or near the extracellular face of the membrane[17].

Further studies are needed to clarify whether sICAM-1 has a specific role as a mediator of immune processes in the uterine cavity and to what extent such shedding contributes to the circulating plasma levels of this adhesion molecule in endometriosis.

The data reported in this study give strong evidence for a physiological role of the adhesion molecule ICAM-1 in regulating the specific leukocyte function which underlies the peritoneal immune surveillance towards endometrial cells refluxed with menstrual debris in ectopic sites. Moreover, they suggest that a disregulation of ICAM-1 expression and release might be associated with a defect of this immunological clearance, and thus contribute to the development of endometriosis.

References

1. Springer, T.A., Dustin, M.L., Kishimoto, T.K. and Marlin, S.D. (1987). The lymphocyte function associated LFA-1, CD2 and LFA-3 molecules: cell adhesion receptors of the immune system. *Annu. Rev. Immunol.*, **5**, 223–8
2. Boyd, A.W., Wawryk, S.O., Burns, G.F. and Fecondo, F.J.V. (1988). Intercellular adhesion molecule-1 (ICAM-1) has a central role in cell–cell contact mediated immune mechanism. *Proc. Natl. Acad. Sci. USA*, **85**, 3095–102
3. Dustin, M.L., Rothlein, R., Bhan, A.K., Dinarello, C.A. and Springer, T.A. (1986). A natural adherence molecule (ICAM-1): induction by IL-1 and interferon-γ, tissue distribution, biochemistry and function. *J. Immunol.*, **137**, 245–51
4. Dustin, M.L., Singer, K.H., Tuck, D.T. and Springer, T.A. (1988). Adhesion of T lymphoblasts to epidermal keratinocytes is regulated by interferon gamma and is mediated by intercellular adhesion molecule-1 (ICAM-1). *J. Exp. Med.*, **167**, 1323–9
5. Rothlein, R., Dustin, M.L., Marlin, S.D. and Springer, T.A. (1986). A human intercellular adhesion molecule (ICAM-1) distinct from LFA-1. *J. Immunol.*, **137**, 1270–8
6. Marlin, S.D. and Springer, T.A. (1987). Purified intercellular adhesion molecule-1 (ICAM-1) is a ligand for lymphocyte function-associated antigen 1 (LFA-1). *Cell*, **51**, 813–18
7. Makgoba, M.W., Sanders, M.E., Luce, G.E.G., Dustin, T.A., Springer, T.A., Clark, E.A., Mannoni, P. and Shaw, S. (1988). ICAM-1: definition by multiple antibodies of a ligand for LFA-1 dependent adhesion of B, T and myeloid cells. *Nature (London)*, **331**, 86–92
8. Diamond, M.S., Staunton, D.E., DeFourgerolles, A.R., Stacker, S.A., Garcia-Aguillar, J., Hibbs, M.L. and Springer, T.A. (1990). ICAM-1 (CD54): a counter-receptor for Mac-1 (CD11b/CD18). *J. Cell Biol.*, **111**, 3129–34
9. Staunton, D.E., Marlin, S.D., Stratowa, C., Dustin, M.L. and Springer, T.A. (1988). Primary structure of intercellular adhesion molecule-1 (ICAM-1) demonstrates interaction between members of the immunoglobulin and integrin supergene families. *Cell*, **52**, 925–36
10. Simmons, D., Makgoba, M.W. and Seed, B. (1988). ICAM-1, an adhesion ligand for LFA-1, is homologous to the neural cell adhesion molecule NCAM. *Nature*, **331**, 624–31
11. Schmidt, R.E., Bartley, G., Levine, H., Schlossman, S.F. and Ritz, J. (1985). Functional characterization of LFA-1 antigens in the interaction of human NK clones and target cells. *J. Immunol.*, **135**, 1020–7
12. Sanders, V., Snyder, J., Uhr, J. and Vitetta, E. (1986). Characterization of the physical interaction between antigen-specific B and T cells. *J. Immunol.*, **137**, 2395–402
13. Mentzer, S., Faller, D. and Burakoff, S. (1986). Interferon-induction of LFA-1 mediated homotypic adhesion of human monocytes. *J. Immunol.*, **137**, 108–13
14. Mentzer, S., Gromkowski, S., Kernsky, A., Burakoff, S. and Martz, E. (1985). LFA-1

membrane molecule in the regulation of homeotypic adhesion of human monocytes. *J. Immunol.*, **135**, 9–14

15. Dustin, M.L. and Springer, T.A. (1988). Lymphocyte function-associated antigen-1 (LFA-1) interaction with intercellular adhesion molecule-1 (ICAM-1) is one of at least three mechanisms for lymphocyte adhesion to cultured endothelial cells. *J. Cell Biol.*, **107**, 321–8

16. Seth, R., Raymond, I.D. and Makgoba, M.W. (1991). Circulating ICAM-1 isoforms: diagnostic prospects for inflammatory and immune disorders. *Lancet*, **338**, 83–4

17. Gearing, A.J.H. and Newman, W. (1993). Circulating adhesion molecules in disease. *Immunol. Today*, **14**, 506–12

18. Becker, J.C., Dummer, R., Hartmann, A.A., Burg, G. and Schmidt, R.E. (1991). Shedding of ICAM-1 from human melanoma cell lines induced by IFN-γ and tumor necrosis factor-α. *J. Immunol.*, **147**, 4398–401

19. Giavazzi, R., Chirivi, R.G.S., Garofalo, A., Rambaldi, A., Hemingway, I., Pigott, R. and Gearing, A.J.H. (1992). Soluble intercellular adhesion molecule-1 is released by human melanoma cells and is associated with tumor growth in nude mice. *Cancer Res.*, **52**, 2628–30

20. Harning, R., Mainolfi, E., Bystryn, J.C., Henn, M., Merluzzi, V.J. and Rothlein, R. (1991). Serum levels of circulating intercellular adhesion molecule-1 in human malignant melanoma. *Cancer Res.*, **51**, 5003–5

21. Johnson, J.P., Stade, B.G., Holzmann, B., Schwable, W. and Riethmuller, G. (1989). De novo expression of intercellular-adhesion molecule-1 in melanoma correlates with increased risk of metastasis. *Proc. Natl. Acad. Sci. USA*, **86**, 641–4

22. Johnson, J.P. (1991). Cell adhesion molecules of the immunoglobulin supergene family and their role in malignant transformation and progression to metastatic disease. *Cancer Metastat. Rev.*, **10**, 11–22

23. Tsujisaki, M., Imai, K., Hirata, H., Hanzawa, Y., Masuya, J., Nakano, T., Sugiyama, T., Matsui, M., Hinoda, Y. and Yachi, A. (1991). Detection of circulating intercellular adhesion molecule-1 antigen in malignant disease. *Clin. Exp. Immunol.*, **85**, 3–8

24. Viganò, P., Vercellini, P., Di Blasio, A.M., Colombo, A., Candiani, G.B. and Vignali, M. (1991). Deficient anti-endometrium lymphocyte-mediated cytotoxicity in patients with endometriosis. *Fertil. Steril.*, **56**, 894–9

25. Oosterlynck, D.J., Cornillie, F.J., Waer, M., Vanderputte, M. and Koninckx, P.R. (1991). Women with endometriosis show a defect in natural killer activity resulting in a decreased cytotoxicity to autologous endometrium. *Fertil. Steril.*, **56**, 45–51

26. Oosterlynck, D.J., Meuleman, C., Waer, M., Vanderputte, M. and Koninckx, P.R. (1992). The natural killer cell activity of peritoneal fluid is decreased in women with endometriosis. *Fertil. Steril.*, **58**, 290–5

27. Hirata, J., Kikuchi, Y., Imaizumi, E., Tode, T. and Nagata, I. (1994). Endometriotic tissues produce immunosuppressive factors. *Gynecol. Obstet. Invest.*, **37**, 43–7

28. Di Blasio, A.M., Centinaio, G., Carniti, C., Somigliana, E., Viganò, P. and Vignali, M. (1995). Basic fibroblast growth factor messenger ribonucleic acid levels in eutopic and ectopic human endometrial stromal cells as assessed by competitive polymerase chain reaction amplification. *Mol. Cell. Endocrinol.*, **115**, 169–75

29. Boyum, A. (1968). Isolation on mononuclear cells and granulocytes from human blood. *Scand. J. Clin. Lab. Invest.*, **21**, 77–81

30. Rees, R.C., Vallely, P., Clegg, A. and Potter, C.W. (1986). Suppression of natural and activated antitumour cytotoxicity by human seminal plasma. *Clin. Exp. Immunol.*, **63**, 687–91

31. Timonen, T., Patarroyo, M. and Gahmberg, C.G. (1988). CD11 a–c/CD18 and GP84 (LB-2) adhesion molecules on human large granular lymphocytes and their participation in natural killing. *J. Immunol.*, **141**, 1041–6

32. Smith, C.W., Kishimoto, T.K., Abbassi, O., Hughes, B., Rothlein, R., McIntire, L.V., Butcher, E. and Anderson, D.C. (1991). Chemotactic factors regulate lectin adhesion molecule-1 (LECAM-1)-dependent neutrophil adhesion to cytokine stimulated endothelial cells *in vitro*. *J. Clin. Invest.*, **87**, 609–18

33. Jung, T.M. and Dailey, M.O. (1990). Rapid modulation of homing receptors (p90 MEL-14) induced by activators of protein kinase C: receptor shedding due to accelerated proteolytic cleavage at the cell surface. *J. Immunol.*, **144**, 3130–6

34. Hoffman, J.C., Dengler, T.J., Knolle, P.A., Albert-Wolf, M., Roux, M., Wallich, R. and Meuer, S.C. (1993). A soluble form of the adhesion receptor CD58 (LFA-3) is present in human body fluids. *Eur. J. Immunol.*, **23**, 3003–10

The role of cell adhesion molecules in the pathogenesis of endometriosis

G.A.J. Dunselman, P.J.Q. van der Linden, A.F.P.M. de Goeij and J.L.H. Evers

Introduction

In 1921 Sampson reported on 23 cases of endometrial cysts of the ovary[1]. He considered this report to be the starting point of the development of his implantation theory for the origin of peritoneal endometriosis. In 1940 he writes: 'The material obtained from this group of cases not only furnished the first step in the development of the implantation theory but also both the incentive for and the key to its completion'[2]. According to this theory retrograde menstruation, peritoneal implantation of shed endometrial tissue and outgrowth of these endometrial cells, glands and stroma are essential elements in the development of the disease. The reflux implantation theory of Sampson is supported by the distribution of the lesions in the abdominal cavity[3], the demonstration of the viability of shed menstrual endometrium in tissue culture[4], the high prevalence of pelvic endometriosis in girls with congenital menstrual outflow obstruction[5] and animal experiments in which endometriosis was induced by the creation of uteropelvic fistulas[6].

Seventy-five years after the initial observations of Sampson, not all of the basic problems regarding his theory are solved. Retrograde menstruation is seen in the majority of women, with and without endometriotic lesions[7]. Endometrial cells can be found in the peritoneal fluid in patients with and without endometriosis in a high percentage of cases[8-11]. What happens, however, between the arrival of endometrial tissue in the abdominal cavity and the occurrence of active endometriotic lesions? In other words, how does endometrial tissue attach to the peritoneal lining? Which cell type, be it endometrial epithelial glandular tissue or stromal tissue, is making the first contact with the peritoneum? Or, alternatively, does endometrium surpass the peritoneal lining to make direct contact with the subperitoneal extracellular matrix?

Attachment

A hitherto rather neglected part of the story is the exact nature of the attachment of the endometrial tissue to the peritoneal lining. What is the 'glue' that brings the two tissue types together? Two explanations have been brought forward for the process of implantation: properties of the fibrin/fibrinolytic system and cell adhesion molecules.

Fibrin/fibrinolytic system

Sampson[12] had already postulated that the regurgitated menstrual blood acts as an irritant to the peritoneal surfaces and thus facilitates implantation. Ohtsuka[13] and Malick[14] hypothesized that a change in intra-abdominal fibrinolytic activity could play an etiological role in the development of endometriosis and the adhesions seen in this disease. They observed a decreased fibrinolytic activity of the mesothelial cells lining the peritoneal cavity in patients with endometriosis.

The fibrin exudate developing as a consequence of peritoneal damage by retrograde menstruation, combined with the decreased fibrinolytic activity, might lead to adhesion formation. In these adhesions endometrial cells might easily get caught and implant. The role of an altered fibrinolytic activity has been questioned by others. Peritoneal fluid fibrinolytic activity was shown to be the same in patients with and without endometriosis[15,16]. These authors concluded that if altered fibrinolysis plays a role in the etiology of endometriosis, these differences can possibly be found at the tissue level rather than in the peritoneal fluid.

Cell adhesion molecules

In a series of experiments we have recently shown that cell adhesion molecules potentially play a role in the development of the disease. In general, two major types of adhesion can be distinguished: cell–cell and cell–extracellular matrix adhesion[17]. Cell adhesion molecules are cell surface glycoproteins that are crucial in morphogenesis, histogenesis and in defining discrete borders between cell populations[18]. A number of cell surface glycoproteins have been identified as intercellular adhesion molecules. These cell adhesion molecules are classified into several classes: cadherins, integrins and the lectin-like glycoproteins including the immunoglobulin superfamily and selectins[19]. We focused our attention on cadherins, governing cell–cell adhesion, and integrins, governing mainly cell–extracellular matrix adhesion.

Cadherins belong to a group of calcium-dependent transmembrane glycoproteins[20]. Adhering processes which involve cadherins are homophylic: cells adhere preferentially to cells which express the same cadherin. The cytoplasmic domain regulates the cell–cell binding of the extracellular domain. The cell binding activity of cadherins depends on their association with some specific proteins and actin-based cytoskeletons (catenins). Three of these cadherins share a basic structure and are well characterized at the molecular level: E-cadherin (epithelial), N-cadherin (neural) and P-cadherin (placental). E-cadherin is expressed in all proliferating epithelial cells derived from the ectoderm and entoderm. It is widely detected in epithelial cells from all genital organs at cell–cell borders. P-cadherin is detected in basal layers of stratified epithelia only, and not in simple epithelia. It contributes to the maintenance of the proliferative compartment of epithelia, whereas E-cadherin presumably plays a major role in the formation and maintenance of epithelial tissues.

Integrins are a family of cell membrane glycoproteins consisting of an α and a β subunit that mediate cell–cell and cell–matrix interaction[21]. Currently more than 20 integrin heterodimers are known, which are composed of one of at least 14 different α and one of 8 different β chains. The majority of integrins currently known bind to various extracellular matrix components. The largest number of integrins belong to the $\beta 1$ or very late-activation antigen (VLA) subfamily. The $\beta 1$-integrins, with α chains $\alpha 1$ to $\alpha 6$, serve as receptors for matrix proteins laminin ($\alpha 1$–3, $\alpha 6$), fibronectin ($\alpha 3$–5), and type IV collagen ($\alpha 1$–3). Functionally, integrins have been found to be involved in thrombosis, inflammation, tissue repair and cancer.

Integrins have been detected in human endometrium[22-27]. Integrins could be functionally involved in implantation, trophoblast invasion and invasiveness of endometrial carcinoma cells. Integrins of the $\beta 1$ family have been studied in most detail. There is a discrepancy in the literature about the expression of some of the integrins and about the cycle dependency of their expression[18].

Cell adhesion molecules and endometriosis

The first step in characterizing the role of cell adhesion molecules in the development of endometriosis was to study the expression of the $\beta 1$-integrins and E-cadherin in cells that potentially play a role in the pathogenesis of the disease[25]. An immunohistochemical study was performed on cells from antegrade menstrual effluent, endometrium, endometrial cells in peritoneal fluid, peritoneum and endometriotic lesions in the menstrual phase and the early follicular phase of the cycle (day 2 to 5) in sixteen patients undergoing a laparoscopy in the course of an infertility work-up. All integrins tested could be detected in the endometrium samples and in endometriotic tissues. Cells in menstrual effluent and in peritoneal fluid did show expression of integrins but to a lesser extent, i.e. not in all samples studied. The same was documented for peritoneum tissue samples. E-cadherin expression was detected in all endometrial samples, while endometriotic samples, menstrual effluent samples and epithelial cells in peritoneal fluid showed E-cadherin expression to a lesser extent.

From these findings we concluded that cell adhesion molecules potentially play a role in the development of the disease. The loss of integrin and E-cadherin expression in some samples of endometrial cells in menstruum and in retrograde shed endometrium could be the result of the proteolytic activity accompanying menstruation.

To detect a possible cycle dependency we documented cadherin and integrin expression in four well-defined phases of the cycle[27]. Endometrium samples were obtained in sixteen women with regular ovulatory cycles. Expression of five β1-integrins, E-cadherin and P-cadherin was measured. E-cadherin and P-cadherin were detected in all tissue samples and did not vary throughout the menstrual cycle. Of the β1-integrins, only α2β1 integrin was modulated during the menstrual cycle and found to be absent in the midluteal phase. The cycle-dependent differences in expression of cell adhesion molecules reported could be attributed to the use of different monoclonal antibodies against integrin subunits. We compared the monoclonal dependent antibody-specific staining of integrins in endometrium samples from well-defined cycle phases with antibodies used by Lessey and co-workers[23] and those that were used in our own studies[18].

This confirmed a monoclonal antibody-specific staining pattern for the integrins α4β1 and α2β1. Since the cadherins and the β1-integrins could be detected in the late luteal phase of the cycle we hypothesized that they could be involved in the attachment of endometrial tissue to the peritoneal lining.

The next step was to test this hypothesis in an *in vitro* model. We developed an *in vitro* model to study the interaction between endometrial tissue and the extracellular matrix. As a source of endometrium tissue we used endometrial biopsies of women in the early follicular phase of the cycle. Part of the tissue was mechanically dissected. Part of the tissue was digested using collagenase to obtain single epithelial and stromal cells. Cell adhesion molecules were determined immunohistochemically in these tissue fragments and in the single cells. Adhesion to stripped amniotic membrane, i.e. devoid of epithelial lining as a model of extracellular matrix[28], was studied. We showed that endometrial, epithelial and stromal cells, after collagenase digestion, had lost their cell adhesion molecules and at the same time did not adhere to the extracellular matrix. On the contrary, mechanically dissected endometrial tissue fragments had retained their cell adhesion molecules and did adhere to the extracellular matrix. We concluded from the results of these experiments that only intact tissue fragments consisting of endometrial glandular tissue and stromal tissue do adhere to the extracellular matrix. This finding supports the contention that stromal–epithelial interactions are a prerequisite for normal functioning tissues[29]. In contrast, most studies report on collagenase-digested endometrial tissue and use the stromal cell fraction to investigate adhesion[30] or the effects of hormones and growth factors on proliferation of stromal cells[31–33]. Recently, however, others reported on the use of whole endometrial tissue fragments in an *in vitro* model to study the pathogenesis of endometriosis[34].

As we have mentioned above we could demonstrate that epithelial cells in menstrual effluent and in the peritoneal fluid did show expression of integrins but to a lesser extent than intrauterine endometrium. Menstruation has been shown to be accompanied by or even to be a result of endometrial protease activity[35].

We postulate that endometrial tissue after arrival in the peritoneal cavity is degraded by the active intra-abdominal proteolytic activity and the inherent proteolytic activity that coincides with menstruation. This degradation of tissue results in single cells and loss of cell adhesion molecules, being one of the lines of defense against the development of endometriosis. It has to be emphasized that we detected single endometrial and stromal cells rather than tissue fragments in the majority of peritoneal fluid samples studied in women with and without endometriosis[11]. Only if large tissue fragments, in a large amount, arrive in the abdominal cavity the proteolytic activity may be insufficient and more endometrial tissue fragments can adhere.

To get more insight into the problem of whether endometrial tissue adheres to the peritoneal lining or to the extracellular matrix we used the amniotic membrane model, with and without the epithelial lining[36]. Amniotic membranes allow study of adhesion to the intact epithelial side and to the other extracellular matrix side, respectively. Firstly, peritoneum and amniotic membrane were compared using light microscopy and immunohistochemistry for both epithelial and subepithelial structures. A marked resemblance was shown for the epithelial markers cytokeratin 18 and 19 and for markers for the extracellular matrix, fibronectin, collagen type IV and laminin. In view of the above-mentioned experiment only endometrial tissue fragments were used for these experiments. The endometrial fragments showed adherence to the non-epithelial side, i.e. the extracellular matrix, in all cases. Both the epithelial as well as the stromal components appeared to adhere. In contrast, adhesion to the intact epithelial side of the amniotic membrane was not observed in any case. From these results we concluded that an intact epithelial lining prevents the adherence of endometrial tissue fragments. This may be one more line of defense against the development of the disease.

The finding that an intact epithelial lining in the amniotic membrane model prevents adhesion of endometrial tissue fragments *in vitro* is endorsed by observations in women. In the first place, endometrial tissue growing on top of the peritoneal surface has not been described[37]. Secondly, Vasquez and co-workers[38], combining scanning electron microscopy and histology, have shown the presence of intraepithelial endometriosis, the surface endometriotic epithelium being in continuity with the peritoneal epithelium, and the stroma of the endometriotic lesion in continuity with subperitoneal stroma. Thirdly, for an endometrial tissue fragment to adhere to the subperitoneal extracellular matrix in cases of intact epithelial lining, the endometrium should possess invading properties and be able to destroy the epithelial lining. Interestingly, we have shown in the same amniotic membrane model that two endometrial carcinoma cell lines do adhere to either side of the amniotic membrane, indicating that the adhesion behavior of endometrial carcinoma cells is different from that of normal endometrial tissue.

Summary

Going back to the initial questions on the nature of attachment of endometrial tissue to the peritoneum we come to the following conclusions. Cell adhesion molecules are expressed in all tissues potentially involved in the pathogenesis of endometriosis. We have demonstrated a minor cycle dependency of the expression of integrins in endometrium. Late luteal endometrium shows all tested β1-integrins and E-cadherin. Endometrial cells in menstrual effluent and in the peritoneal fluid show expression of cell adhesion molecules but to a lesser extent than intrauterine endometrium. Tissue fragments and not single cells do adhere to the subperitoneal extracellular matrix. Menstruation has been shown to be accompanied by or to be even a result of endometrial protease activity. We postulate that endometrial tissue after arrival in the peritoneal cavity is degraded by the active intra-abdominal proteolytic activity and the inherent proteolytic activity that coincides with menstruation. This degradation of tissue results in single cells, that can be easily disposed of by intra-abdominal activated macrophages. Moreover it results in loss of cell adhesion molecules on these single cells. Only if large tissue fragments, in a large amount, arrive in the abdominal cavity the proteolytic activity may be insufficient and more endometrial tissue fragments are left to adhere.

References

1. Sampson, J.A. (1921). Perforating hemorrhagic (chocolate) cysts of the ovary; their importance and especially their relation to pelvic adenomas of endometrial type (adenomyoma of the uterus, rectovaginal septum, sigmoid, etc.). *Arch. Surg.*, **3**, 245–323
2. Sampson, J.A. (1940). The development of the implantation theory for the origin of peritoneal endometriosis. *Am. J. Obstet. Gynecol.*, **40**, 549–57
3. Jenkins, S., Olive, D.L. and Haney, A.F. (1986). Endometriosis: pathogenetic implications of the anatomic distribution. *Obstet. Gynecol.*, **67**, 335–8
4. Keettel, W.C. and Stein, R.J. (1951). The viability of the cast-off menstrual endometrium. *Am. J. Obstet. Gynecol.*, **61**, 440–2
5. Sanfilippo, J.S., Wakin, N.G., Schikler, K.N. and Yussman, M.A. (1986). Endometriosis in association with uterine anomaly. *Am. J. Obstet. Gynecol.*, **154**, 39–43
6. Te Linde, R.W. and Scott, R.B. (1950). Experimental endometriosis. *Am. J. Obstet. Gynecol.*, **60**, 852–8
7. Halme, J., Hammond, M.G., Hulka, J.F., Raj, S.G. and Talbert, L.M. (1984). Retrograde menstruation in healthy women and in patients with endometriosis. *Obstet. Gynecol.*, **64**, 151–4
8. Willemsen, W.N.P., Mungyer, G., Smets, H., Rolland, R., Vemer, H. and Jap, P.H.K. (1985). Behavior of cultured glandular cells obtained by flushing of the uterine cavity. *Fertil. Steril.*, **44**, 92–5
9. Bartosik, D., Jacobs, S.L. and Kelly, L.J. (1986). Endometrial tissue in peritoneal fluid. *Fertil. Steril.*, **46**, 796–800
10. Kruitwagen, R.F.P.M., Poels, L.G., Willemsen, W.N.P., de Ronde, I.J.Y., Jap, P.H.K. and Rolland, R. (1991). Endometrial epithelial cells in peritoneal fluid during the early follicular phase. *Fertil. Steril.*, **55**, 297–303
11. van der Linden, P.J.Q., Dunselman, G.A.J., de Goeij, A.F.P.M., van der Linden, E.P.M., Evers, J.L.H. and Ramaekers, F.C.S. (1995). Epithelial cells in peritoneal fluid: of endometrial origin? *Am. J. Obstet. Gynecol.*, **173**, 566–70
12. Sampson, J.A. (1927). Peritoneal endometriosis due to menstrual dissemination of endometrial tissue into the peritoneal cavity. *Am. J. Obstet. Gynecol.*, **14**, 422–69
13. Ohtsuka, N. (1980). Study on pathogenesis of adhesions in endometriosis. *Acta Obstet. Gynaecol. Jpn*, **32**, 1758–66
14. Malick, J.E. (1982). The etiology of endometriosis. *J. Am. Osteo. Assoc.*, **81**, 407–12
15. Batzofin, J.H., Holmes, S.D., Gibbons, W.E. and Buttram, V.C. Jr (1985). Peritoneal fluid plasminogen activator in endometriosis and pelvic adhesive disease. *Fertil. Steril.*, **44**, 277–9
16. Dunselman, G.A.J., Bouckaert, P.X.J.M., van Wersch, J.W.J., Brommer, E.J.P. and Evers, J.L.H. (1988). Fibrinolytic properties of peritoneal fluid in endometriosis of women. *Gynecol. Obstet. Invest.*, **26**, 302–7
17. Geiger, B., Ginsberg, D., Salomon, D. and Volberg, T. (1990). The molecular basis for the assembly and modulation of adherens-type junctions. *Cell Differ. Dev.*, **32**, 343–54
18. van der Linden, P.J.Q. (1996). Cell adhesion, cell adhesion molecules and their functional role in the human endometrium. *Early Pregnancy Biol. Med.*, **2**, 5–14
19. Katz, A.M., Rosenthal, D. and Sauder, D.M. (1991). Cell adhesion molecules. Structure, function and implication in a variety of cutaneous and other pathologic conditions. *Int. J. Dermatol.*, **30**, 153–60

20. Takeichi, M. (1988). The cadherins: cell–cell adhesion molecules controlling animal morphogenesis. *Development*, **102**, 639–55
21. Ruoshlathi, E. (1991). Integrins. *J. Clin. Invest.*, **87**, 1–5
22. Tabibzadeh, S. (1992). Patterns of expression of integrin molecules in human endometrium throughout the menstrual cycle. *Hum. Reprod.*, **7**, 639–55
23. Lessey, B.A., Damjanovich, L., Coutifaris, C., Castelbaum, A., Albelda, S.M. and Buck, C.A. (1992). Integrin adhesion molecules in the human endometrium. Correlation with the normal and abnormal menstrual cycle. *J. Clin. Invest.*, **90**, 188–95
24. Klentzeris, L.D., Bulmer, J.N., Trejdosiewicz, L.K., Morisson, L. and Cooke, I.D. (1993). Beta-1 integrin cell adhesion molecules in the endometrium of fertile and infertile women. *Hum. Reprod.*, **8**, 1223–30
25. van der Linden, P.J.Q., de Goeij, A.F.P.M., Dunselman, G.A.J., van der Linden, E.P.M., Ramaekers, F.C.S. and Evers, J.L.H. (1994). Expression of integrins and E-cadherin in cells from menstrual effluent, endometrium, peritoneal fluid, peritoneum, and endometriosis. *Fertil. Steril.*, **61**, 85–90
26. Lessey, B.A., Castelbaum, A.J., Sawin, S.W. and Sun, J. (1995). Integrins as markers of integrin receptivity in women with primary unexplained infertility. *Fertil. Steril.*, **63**, 535–42
27. van der Linden, P.J.Q., de Goeij, A.F.P.M., Dunselman, G.A.J., Erkens, H.W.H. and Evers, J.L.H. (1995). Expression of cadherins and integrins in human endometrium throughout the menstrual cycle. *Fertil. Steril.*, **63**, 1210–16
28. Liotta, L.A., Lee, C.W. and Morakis, D.J. (1980). New method for preparing large surfaces of intact human basement membrane for tumor invasion studies. *Cancer Lett.*, **11**, 141–52
29. Cunha, G.R., Bigsby, R.M., Cooke, P.S. and Sugimura, Y. (1985). Stromal–epithelial interactions in adult organs. *Cell. Diff.*, **17**, 137–48
30. Zhang, R., Wild, R.A. and Ojago, J.M. (1993). Effect of tumor necrosis factor-alpha on adhesion of human endometrial stromal cells to peritoneal mesothelial cells: an *in vitro* system. *Fertil. Steril.*, **59**, 1196–201
31. Surrey, E.S. and Halme, J. (1991). Effect of platelet-derived growth factor on endometrial stromal cell proliferation *in vitro*: a model for endometriosis? *Fertil. Steril.*, **56**, 672–9
32. Taketani, Y. and Mizuno, M. (1992). Hormonal regulation of endometriotic cell growth in primary cell culture system. *Arch. Gynecol. Obstet.*, **251**, 127–32
33. Hammond, M.G., Oh, S.T., Anners, J., Surrey, E.S. and Halme, J. (1993). The effect of growth factors on the proliferation of human endometrial stromal cells in culture. *Am. J. Obstet. Gynecol.*, **168**, 1131–8
34. Wild, R.A., Zhang, R. and Medders, D. (1994). Whole endometrial fragments form characteristics of *in vivo* endometriosis in a mesothelial cell co-culture system: an *in vitro* model for the study of the histogenesis of endometriosis. *J. Soc. Gynecol. Invest.*, **1**, 65–8
35. Rodgers, W.H., Matrisian, L.M., Giudice, L.C., Dsupin, B., Cannon, P., Svitek, C., Gorstein, F. and Osteen, K.G. (1994). Patterns of matrix metalloproteinase expression in cycling endometrium imply differential functions and regulation by steroid hormones. *J. Clin. Invest.*, **94**, 946–53
36. van der Linden, P.J.Q., de Goeij, A.F.P.M., Dunselman, G.A.J., Erkens, H.W.H. and Evers, J.L.H. (1996). Endometrial cell adhesion in an *in vitro* model using intact amniotic membranes. *Fertil. Steril.*, **65**, 76–80
37. Brosens, I.A., Puttemans, P.J. and Deprest, J. (1993). Appearances of endometriosis. *Baill. Clin. Obstet. Gynecol.*, **7**, 741–57
38. Vasquez, G., Cornillie, F. and Brosens, I.A. (1984). Peritoneal endometriosis: scanning electron microscopy and histology of minimal pelvic endometriotic lesions. *Fertil. Steril.*, **42**, 696–703

Section 5

Classification

Do we need a classification for endometriosis?

M. Canis, A. Wattiez, J.L. Pouly, G. Mage and M.A. Bruhat

Introduction

As there is no correlation between the anatomical lesions and the clinical findings in patients with endometriosis, the term pelvic endometriosis has to be illustrated using an adjective and/or a score to provide some information about the extent of the disease. Because it included a complete and simple description of surgical findings and easily comprehensible adjectives to describe each stage, the American Fertility Society (AFS) endometriosis classification system became the international language of endometriosis[1].

However, endometriosis is still an 'enigmatic' disease and we have yet to find the perfect classification system, which would provide a correct prognosis for post-treatment fertility, relief of pelvic pain and the risk of recurrence. This major difficulty should be kept in mind when proposing new systems or changes to the current classification. A change in the language can only be introduced prospectively, implying that within a few years part of the results provided by clinical studies will be lost as comparison with previous reports becomes difficult or impossible. Therefore although our current language, the revised American Fertility Society classification[2], needs to be improved and adapted to new treatments, the changes should be prospectively evaluated by some groups particularly interested in endometriosis, so as to avoid unnecessary and/or detrimental modifications.

Historical review: is there something new?

In 1949 Wicks and Larson stated: 'It is left to the individual surgeon to practice what he thinks best without a road being opened to correct his decision for future reference'[3]. They proposed the first classification of endometriosis, which included histological criteria. Cyst walls lined by phagocytic cells containing blood pigments and cellular debris were classified as grade I, whereas lesions with endometrium resembling normal endometrium and supported by an abundant endometrial stroma were described as grade IV. Sixty-one per cent of their patients were found to have grade I or II disease, which can be described as non- or low 'active'. Making a plea for more conservative surgical treatment of endometriosis, they proposed a conservative treatment for patients with low active disease. As the grading can be accomplished accurately from frozen section, the surgical management may be decided intraoperatively. Their histological criteria may need to be reconsidered to improve the surgical management and the postoperative indications of the medical treatment.

In 1951, Huffman first emphasized the need for a common language. He proposed a surgical system similar to that used when staging cervical cancer[4].

The pregnancy rates reported before 1973 ranged between 13 and 94%[5], suggesting that the populations studied were dissimilar. Because of this problem, a classification scheme, which became widely used as the Acosta classification, was designed by several investigators on a flight returning from a medical conference[6,7]. It included the size of the lesions, scarring and retraction around the implants, as well as adnexal adhesions. However this classification had several disadvantages. It did not distinguish between unilateral and bilateral adnexal disease, and some lesions were insufficiently described, resulting in doubts when staging.

In 1977, the Kistner classification emphasized the importance of tubo-ovarian adhesions and classified them according to their amenability to laparoscopic adhesiolysis[8]. This system was more complex than the Acosta classification, and did not allow the distinction between unilateral and bilateral adnexal involvement. In order to allow the distinction between unilateral and bilateral disease, Buttram proposed an 'expanded classification of endometriosis'[9], which was not better than the Acosta classification in predicting postoperative fertility[10].

In 1978 the American Fertility Society appointed a committee which published the first AFS classification[1] which became widely accepted. Each location is scored using a weighted point system to distinguish endometriotic lesions of different size. The patients are then classified in four stages: mild, moderate, severe and extensive. The AFS classification has several advantages. The scoring system is flexible enough to describe each case including those which do not follow the usual progression of the disease. This is a major improvement as compared to previous systems which tried to follow the natural history of the disease. When filling out the form, the physician has to describe all the pelvic areas, thus avoiding incomplete or vague operative reports. In addition, a scoring system is suitable for computerized analysis of data. Unfortunately the scores and cut-off points were chosen arbitrarily.

As expected, numerous criticisms have been published. The 1979 AFS classification was reliable for postoperative fertility only if comparing combined stages (stages I and II versus stage III and IV)[10]. Andrews suggested that more points should be given to bilaterality[11]. Hasson emphasized that uterosacral ligament endometriotic implants should be differentiated from other peritoneal lesions in patients with chronic pelvic pain[12] and that a three-dimensional assessment would allow an easier differentiation of superficial and deep lesions than a two-dimensional description. Too much importance was given to tubal lesions, which are rare[5]. The scores attributed to 3-cm endometriomas or to complete cul-de-sac obliteration were too low[13]. Guzick and colleagues[14], studying 214 patients treated surgically, found no significant relation between the stages and subsequent fertility.

Following all these comments, the committee was convened again and elaborated the revised AFS 1985 endometriosis classification system which is still used for infertile patients[2]. The committee decided to separate patients with minimal and mild disease, whose fertility prognosis is similar, and to group patients with severe and extensive disease. Consequently patients with bilateral and unilateral severe adnexal involvement were included in the same stage[15]. However, this new scheme included major improvements: tubal endometriosis was excluded from the score and described under additional endometriosis; peritoneal implants are described using a two- and a three-dimensional assessment; patients with complete posterior cul-de-sac obliteration are classified as severe; 16 points are attributed to dense adhesions enclosing the fimbria; high scores are attributed to dense adnexal adhesions; points attributed to a solitary adnexa are multiplied by two.

Rationale for a classification

A classification should be a common language allowing us to communicate easily, and an expert system which provides guidelines for treatment, prognosis for post-treatment fertility, for relief of pelvic pain and prevention of recurrences.

A common language

Knowledge of the extent of the disease is essential when discussing patient files or treatments. To avoid a time-consuming description, the lesions should be summarized using one word or a score, thus providing a much better description than the word endometriosis alone. This description is essential when there is no correlation between the clinical symptoms and the anatomical lesions. The operative reports are improved when using the revised AFS classification since a complete description of the pelvis is required. As improved operative reports are written with the same words all around the world, a valuable comparison of the results obtained with various treatments is possible.

This language should satisfy some requirements. The translation from anatomical lesions to 'words' should be simple, fast, easy, clear and simple, thus minimizing the surgeon's interpretation. The language should be flexible enough to allow an easy description of any case. This language needs a dictionary including accurate and simple description of each word. This dictionary, which is not yet available, is essential, as when discussing with foreign colleagues, we have often noticed that words very commonly used in clinical practice do not have the same meaning in different countries. For instance deep peritoneal implants are not clearly described in the current system. Should we consider all the typical black puckered lesions as deep lesions, or should this term be reserved for deeply infiltrating implants of more than 3 mm or 5 mm[16,17]. Similarly, the term complete cul-de-sac obliteration may be confusing for those who do not know the initial description from Sampson[18].

As one picture is worth a thousand words, color pictures are necessary in this dictionary to illustrate the words used to describe the lesions. This is particularly important when describing all the atypical peritoneal and ovarian implants. Finally, this language which should be established in English will have to be translated into other languages such as Japanese, Spanish and French.

The concept of a common language is so simple, but so difficult to establish and to accept. Indeed many experts will have to accept that the word that they are using may not become the word used in the international endometriosis language. For example, if the word 'strawberry' is chosen to describe a red peritoneal implant, many other very accurate words such as 'red flame-like lesions' may have to be abandoned. Moreover, the description used will probably be simpler than that used initially to describe all the atypical peritoneal implants. But this is necessary to make this language acceptable to everyone.

An expert system

A perfect classification should allow an accurate prognosis for post-treatment fertility, relief of pelvic pain and indicate the risk of recurrence[13]. Such an expert system is much more difficult to define. It would be obtained attributing a score to each lesion and deciding the cut-off points between the stages. Until now these scores and breakpoints have been empirically decided. The present classification is not an expert system.

When attributing a score to a lesion, one is trying to assess the effect of this lesion on postoperative outcome. This depends on several factors:

(1) The incidence of the lesion itself on the outcome, something that is rarely known, as demonstrated by numerous studies on the treatment of minimal disease;

(2) The usefulness, the effectiveness, the difficulties, the failures and the complications of the treatment;

(3) The various treatments which may be proposed, according to the patient's age and previous medical history;

(4) The delay necessary to obtain the desired outcome;

(5) The frequency and the consequences of the lesions often associated with the considered lesion.

Except for patients with mechanical infertility, our understanding of the disease is too poor to design a true expert system, which will probably not be established solely using data obtained at laparoscopy or laparotomy. As lesions found at surgery represent only one day in the spontaneous evolution of the disease, a marker for the disease 'activity' would be essential to decide the management.

Obviously, we are not able to propose a valuable expert system, and we have to accept this limit. We have to accept that the breakpoint between the stages cannot be decided using statistical or clinical results. However, we do know that these stages are useful, as the clinical problem is not the same in patients with minimal or severe disease.

The answer to the question of whether we need a common language is that we definitely do need one. But should we change everything in the current language? No we should not, because it is difficult to spread a new system and much information would be lost without any reason, as we do not have major arguments to suggest that one system would be much better than another one. Should we change the name of the language? The first consistent system was proposed by the AFS, and the pioneer should not be forgotten. However, the current language can be improved. First we can improve the way to use it, by providing guidelines for the staging technique of a patient.

Staging

Although surgical staging is now considered as the gold standard, no statement has been made concerning the best surgical approach, laparoscopy or laparotomy, and what surgical procedures are required to accurately stage a patient. When evaluating patients retrospectively from videotapes, we found that a patient with severe endometriosis cannot be staged only from laparoscopic inspection. For example, a complete examination of the pelvic peritoneum and of the posterior cul-de-sac is impossible unless large endometriomas have been punctured and emptied.

Operative laparoscopy is the best surgical staging technique. However, guidelines for laparoscopic staging are required and it is necessary to report on the form whether or not a complete pelvic examination has been achieved and which parts of the pelvis have not been fully inspected.

As ovarian punctures and adhesiolysis are often required, prerequisites to laparoscopic staging are very similar to those for laparoscopic treatment of endometriosis[19]. The following conditions are required: patients informed of a possible laparotomy; a bowel preparation administered on the day before surgery; and adequate laparoscopic retractors are required (10–15° Trendelenbourg position, efficient uterine cannulation, a good pneumoperitoneum, two or three ancillary trocars inserted in the suprapubic area). The laparoscopic staging includes the following steps:

(1) By means of the Trendelenbourg position and atraumatic forceps, the bowel and the omentum are pushed over the superior pelvic brim;

(2) The magnification provided by the laparoscope is used to inspect the anterior and posterior cul-de-sac looking for small and atypical peritoneal implants;

(3) Peritoneal cytology and/or peritoneal washing are sampled as in any patient with an ovarian cystic mass;

(4) The tubes and the ovaries are mobilized looking for tubal and ovarian adhesions;

(5) To diagnose ovarian endometriomas a complete ovariolysis is required;

(6) The broad ligaments and the anterior ovarian surface are inspected;

(7) Enlarged ovaries and/or starlike ovarian scars are routinely punctured looking for small endometriomas[20];

(8) The posterior cul-de-sac and the rectum are assessed using vaginal examination and/or vaginal and rectal probes[21];

(9) If an ovarian endometrioma has been opened, the pelvis is copiously irrigated; the internal cyst wall is inspected and biopsied in order to rule out malignancy and to differentiate endometriomas from functional chocolate cysts[22,23];

(10) The upper part of the abdomen is carefully inspected looking for bowel, appendicular or diaphragmatic endometriosis.

Expertise in operative laparoscopy is a prerequisiste to accurate staging of patients with severe disease. Similarly, awareness of the various visual appearances of peritoneal and ovarian endometriotic implants is required[24]. Moreover a recommended cycle day for diagnostic laparoscopy would be interesting, to find out whether the appearance of atypical implants is always the same.

As the laparoscope is a lens, subjective assessment of the size is obviously unreliable. The size of an implant on the videoscreen depends on the distance between the lens and the lesion. Therefore the diameter of the lesion should be measured by comparing it with laparoscopic instruments of known dimensions.

Approaching the 'activity' of endometriosis

Endometriosis 'activity' has not yet been clearly defined, but this term is often used in comments and discussions as most authors are convinced that the clinical consequences of endometriosis are more related to the 'activity' than to the extent of the disease. Studies of the implants and the peritoneal environment have been proposed for evaluation of endometriosis activity.

The implants have been studied using prostaglandin *in vitro* synthesis[25] and pathological examination[26–28]. Vernon and colleagues[25] demonstrated that *in vitro* reddish implants produce twice the amount of prostaglandin F (PGF) than brown implants, whereas black implants did not have the *in vitro* capacity to produce PGF. More recently, Nisolle and colleagues[27,28] and Donnez and associates[26] confirmed, using a usual and a three-dimensional pathological examination, that red implants are more active than black puckered lesions and have a higher vascularization and increased mitotic activity.

The peritoneal environment has been studied using peritoneal fluid volume, peritoneal cell number, concentration, activation, or production of cytokine or growth factors, and aminoterminal propeptide of type III procollagen and endometrial stromal cell proliferation[29–33]. Syrop and Halme demonstrated that postoperative fertility was related to peritoneal fluid volume[33]. Spujbroek correlated for the first time the results obtained studying the peritoneal fluid and the laparoscopic appearance of peritoneal implants[31]. He suggested that early peritoneal endometriosis is an invasive disease since the peritoneal fluid concentration of aminoterminal propeptide type III collagen was significantly increased in patients with subtle lesions[31], whereas it was not different from controls in patients without early implants.

As already suggested by Weitzmann and Buttram[7], physiological parameters will have to be incorporated into new classification systems. In our opinion, after a careful scientific evaluation, the good marker for endometriosis 'activity' will have to be cost-effective, simple and easy to assess during or just before the surgical diagnosis in every hospital. Before it can be proposed for clinical practice the marker will have to be carefully related to anatomical data and postoperative results using prospective clinical studies. Surprisingly, the peritoneal fluid volume on a recommended cycle day, which appeared very attractive as a marker, has never been re-evaluated.

Description of peritoneal endometriosis

Since 1986, several authors have emphasized the importance of atypical and subtle peritoneal implants[24–26,34]. These descriptions are essential when the evaluation of the implants is the main approach to the 'activity' of endometriosis. The relationships between laparoscopic appearances and clinical data are unclear since atypical and typical lesions are often associated in the same patient. To perform prospective studies of this essential problem, a classification of implant appearances is required. This classification of atypical lesions should include simple descriptions and carefully selected color pictures[19]. This description of peritoneal implants is now included in the management of endometriosis in the presence of pelvic pain[35–36]. The words used to describe the implants are similar to those used in the reports about subtle and atypical lesions. However, these words may not have the same meaning for all experts. Unfortunately, color pictures to document each appearance have not been published with this form. The pictures which are being prepared by the AFS committee are urgently required as the distinction between clear implants and vesicles or between white lesions and peritoneal fibrosis is not obvious and easy.

Three types of peritoneal implants will probably be distinguished: red, black and white lesions. Again, color pictures will be necessary to help everyone to classify the implants according to this classification. Similarly, a simple description and examples of what should be considered as superficial and deep peritoneal endometriosis, and guidelines on the way to assess the depth of an implant are necessary.

Over the last few years, many authors have stressed that the term minimal endometriosis is too vague. Indeed this word may be used to describe 10-cm^2 red peritoneal implants as well as a 0.3-mm diameter black peritoneal implant. To improve this description, we could add to the word minimal the estimated surface of the abnormal peritoneum and the color of the implants which are the most common in the considered patient. So the extent of the disease would be summarized as 'minimal 3 red' if the implants have a diameter of 3 cm and most of them are red, or 'minimal 0.1 black' if there is only a very small black implant.

Deep disease should be better described

Better description of deep disease is obviously necessary. As deep disease may be associated with minimal or extensive disease, it is difficult to propose a specific stage for deep disease using the scoring system used until now for infertile patients. From our clinical practice we think that deep disease is generally well described, by using the diameter and the organs involved. For instance, if a patient is treated for a 4-cm rectal nodule, everyone will anticipate that a bowel resection will probably be necessary, but this operation may be more or less difficult, depending on the extent of the associated peritoneal disease.

So that it would be easy to summarize the clinical problem of a patient with a short description including the rAFS stage and the size and organ involved by the nodule; for example severe endometriosis with a 2cm rectovaginal nodule.

A simplified revised AFS classification?

Based on the unexplained strong association of endometriomas and adhesions, Koninckx and colleagues proposed an attractive simplified classification[37]. They suggested that by increasing the points for endometriomas,

Table 1 Immediate anatomical results of laparoscopic treatment (79 patients)

	Adhesion score > 50		Adhesion score ≤ 50		Total	
	n	%	n	%	n	%
Adhesiolysis						
Complete	11*	33.3	33*	71.7	44	55.6
Partial	22	66.6	13	28.3	35	44.3
Total	33		46		79	
Treatment of ovarian endometriomas						
Complete	31†	77.5	51†	96.2	82	88.2
Drainage	9	22.5	2	3.8	11	11.8
Total	40		53		93	

*$p < 0.001$; †$p < 0.01$

Table 2 Incidence of bilateral lesions according to the AFS score

	Group 1 (AFS ≤ 70) (N = 46)		Group 2 (AFS > 70) (N = 43)	
Bilateral lesions	n	%*	n	%*
Adnexal score ≥ 20	16†	34.8	35†	81.4
Adhesion score ≥ 16	9†	19.6	28†	65.1
Ovarian score ≥ 16	13‡	28.3	24‡	55.8
Ovarian score ≥ 20	11‡	23.9	22‡	51.2

*n = number of patients who had the considered anatomical lesion on both adnexae, N = total number of patients in the group studied; †$p < 0.001$; ‡$p < 0.02$

adhesions could be omitted whereas > 95% of the patients would be staged identically. However, the following arguments should be considered: first, adhesions need to be fully described in infertile patients. Second, the association between endometriomas and adhesions may be absent in patients who underwent previous treatment. The main advantage of the AFS classification is that it is flexible enough to describe lesions which did not follow the usual progression of the disease. The adhesion scoring system is also easy to use, and the simplification would be more apparent than real. Lastly, a complete description is essential in clinical and research studies.

Should a stage V be included?

We recently proposed that a stage V needs to be considered in the next AFS classification scheme[16]. This modification is supported by the following arguments:

(1) When studying fertility after laparoscopic treatment of endometriosis, we found an intrauterine pregnancy rate of 37.5%[38]; however, we obtained no pregnancy when the AFS score was > 70, whereas 52.9% of the patients who had a score of 70 or less conceived.

(2) As shown in Table 1, this significant difference was explained by the difficulties encountered when treating patients with extensive dense adhesions; complete treatment of ovarian endometriomas was achieved significantly less often when the adhesions score including posterior cul-de-sac obliteration was > 50.

(3) As presented in Table 2, we also found that bilateral endometriomas and bilateral severe adhesions were significantly more common in patients with a score > 70[16].

(4) The prognosis is better in patients with a normal adnexa[5].

(5) We and others recently demonstrated that adhesion reformation is an all too frequent occurrence after laparoscopic treatment of dense adhesions[39,40]. Therefore, in patients with bilateral dense adhesions, conservative surgery is not an efficient treatment of infertility. This conclusion is confirmed by the results obtained at routine second-look laparoscopy performed in 53 patients with revised AFS stage IV endometriosis. At second-look laparoscopy the AFS score of patients who had an initial score

Table 3 Comparison of AFS and of adhesion score at laparoscopic treatment and at second-look laparoscopy

	Treatment	Second look	p
AFS score ≤ 70, n = 53			
AFS score	55.3 ± 7.8	21.6 ± 18.4	< 0.001
Implant score	27.2 ± 14.7	5.4 ± 6.3	< 0.001
Adhesion score	16.1 ± 11.4	12.2 ± 12.6	< 0.04
AFS score > 70, n = 22			
AFS score	96.8 ± 14.1	56.6 ± 33.6	< 0.001
Implant score	34.1 ± 13.4	8.9 ± 13.1	< 0.001
Adhesion score	39.6 ± 15.4	33.4 ± 16.8	> 0.2

Table 4 Comparison of adnexal adhesion scores at laparoscopic treatment and at second-look laparoscopy

Group	n	Laparoscopic treatment	Second-look laparoscopy	p
All adnexae	180	9.7 ± 9.8	7.9 ± 9.8	> 0.05
Severe	106	12.9 ± 10.5	10.5 ± 10.9	< 0.05
Moderate	74	4.0 ± 5.5	4.2 ± 6.3	> 0.6
40 < AFS < 71	62	8.0 ± 8.1	6.1 ± 8.1	< 0.02
AFS > 70	44	19.8 ± 9.6	16.7 ± 11.6	> 0.2
Cyst > 3 cm	72	12.6 ± 10.6	11.1 ± 11.3	> 0.3
Cyst none	108	7.1 ± 9.3	5.9 ± 8.7	> 0.05
Adhesions ≤ 4	50	1.1 ± 1.6	3.3 ± 5.9	< 0.01
Adhesions ≥ 16	45	23.4 ± 6.3	16.8 ± 11.2	< 0.01
AFS < 71	14	21.0 ± 5.6	13.4 ± 9.5	< 0.02
AFS > 70	31	24.9 ± 6.1	19.5 ± 11.6	> 0.05

> 70 is 56.6 ± 33.6, which is still very high (Table 3). This poor result is mainly explained by adhesion reformation since the adhesion score (cul-de-sac obliteration excluded) is not improved by the laparoscopic procedure ($p > 0.2$).

(6) Studying the adnexal adhesion score at laparoscopic treatment and at second-look laparoscopy in 180 adnexa, we confirmed that adhesion reformation is an essential problem and that in contrast postoperative adhesion formation is uncommon after laparoscopic treatment (Table 4).

(7) Endometriosis appears as a good indication for *in vitro* fertilization (IVF) and embryo transfer; IVF is probably the best treatment for infertile patients with extensive adhesions.

(8) An extensive stage was included in the 1979 AFS classification scheme[1].

(9) This stage is not uncommon; in our current experience stage V endometriosis is as common as stage IV and stage II and represents about 14% of our patients.

As the surgeon's interpretation is important when assessing the extent of the disease, breakpoints should be established from multicentric prospective studies, using carefully recorded videotapes so that the lesions can be staged by several investigators. A score of 70 is probably not a correct breakpoint, since a patient with this score and a complete cul-de-sac obliteration may have a normal adnexa.

Chronic pelvic pain

The AFS committee was convened again in October 1992. As the current AFS classification was designed for women with infertility and the incidence of deep infiltrating disease and pelvic adhesions is different in chronic pelvic pain patients, it was decided to propose a new system for the management of chronic pelvic pain[36]. The system proposed in December 1993 is not a classification but a form designed to standardize data collection[36]. It includes clinical and surgical data so as to study the relationship between endometriotic lesions and clinical signs and to permit the construction of a true classification for chronic pelvic pain patients.

This approach is reasonable as our knowledge of endometriosis is too poor to propose a true classification. This first and preliminary step will soon appear as essential progress in the difficult management of chronic pain associated with pelvic endometriosis. To fill in this form the surgeon has to document the appearances of peritoneal endometriotic implants. Unfortunately the system used to describe pelvic adhesion is slightly different from that used in infertile patients; this difference may appear confusing for most gynecologists used to staging their patients with the 1985 revised AFS classification. The previous adhesion scoring system was easy to use and more precise. The advantages and potential disadvantages of this new adhesion scoring system have to be carefully evaluated. In our clinic we will use both systems so as to have all the information about the extent of adnexal adhesions and to find out which system is the best one in our hands.

This pain system is mainly a research tool, but we do need such tools to improve our knowledge of the disease.

The word stage is not appropriate, since there is no correlation between the stage of the disease and the prognosis of a patient. So we have to accept that the words used are in fact a summary of the anatomical data rather than a stage. To improve this summary, one may include the description of the peritoneal implants in minimal disease and the description of the deep nodule if there is one. Operative reports would therefore be summarized as follows: extensive disease with a 3-cm rectovaginal nodule, or moderate disease with a 1-cm right utero sacral nodule.

Conclusion

A scientifically based score for each lesion would be necessary to establish a perfect expert system. We have to accept that our current knowledge is not good enough to propose such a perfect system, but we still have a lot to do to improve the language, which is used by everyone all over the world.

References

1. American Fertility Society (1979). Classification of endometriosis. *Fertil. Steril.*, **32**, 633
2. American Fertility Society (1985). Revised American Fertility Society classification of endometriosis. *Fertil. Steril.*, **43**, 351
3. Wicks, M.J. and Larson, C. P. (1949). Histologic criteria for evaluating endometriosis. *NW. Med. J.*, **48**, 611–3
4. Huffman, J.W. (1951). External endometriosis. *Am. J. Obstet. Gynecol.*, **62**, 1243–50
5. Buttram, V.C. (1985). Evolution of the revised American Fertility Society classification of endometriosis. *Fertil. Steril.*, **43**, 347–50
6. Acosta, A. A., Buttram, V. C., Besch, P. K., Malinak, L. R., Franklin, R. R. and Vanderheyden, J. D. (1973). A proposed classification of pelvic endometriosis. *Obstet. Gynecol.*, **42**, 19–23
7. Weltzman, G. A. and Buttram, V. C. (1989). Classification of endometriosis. *Obstet. Gynecol. North Am.*, **16**, 61–77
8. Kistner, R. W., Siegler, A. M. and Berhman, S. J. (1977). Suggested classification for endometriosis relationship to infertility. *Fertil. Steril.*, **28**, 1008–10
9. Buttram, V.C. (1978). An expanded classification of endometriosis. *Fertil. Steril.*, **9**, 240–2
10. Rock, J. A., Guzick, D. S., Sengos, C., Schweditsch, M., Sapp, K. and Jones, H. W. (1981). The conservative surgical treatment of endometriosis: evaluation of pregnancy success with respect to the extent of the disease as categorized using contemporary classification systems. *Fertil. Steril.*, **35**, 131–7
11. Andrews, W.C. (1981). Classification of endometriosis. *Fertil. Steril.*, **35**, 124–5
12. Hasson, H.M. (1981). Classification for endometriosis. *Fertil. Steril.*, **35**, 368–9 (letter)
13. Candiani, G.B. (1986). The classification of endometriosis: historical evolution, critical

review and present state of the art. *Acta Eur. Fertalitatis*, **17**, 85–92

14. Guzick, D.S., Bros, D.S. and Rock, J.A. (1982). Assessing the efficacy of the American Fertility Society's classification of endometriosis: application of a dose-response methodology. *Fertil. Steril.*, **38**, 171–6

15. Canis, M., Pouly, J.L., Wattiez, A., Manhes, H., Mage, G. and Bruhat, M.A. (1992). Incidence of bilateral adnexal disease in severe endometriosis (revised American Fertility Society stage IV). Should a stage V be included in the American Fertility Society classification? *Fertil. Steril.*, **57**, 691–2

16. Koninckx, P.R., Meuleman, C., Demeyere, S., Lesaffre, E. and Cornillie, F. (1991). Suggestive evidence that pelvic endometriosis is a progressive disease, whereas deeply infiltrating endometriosis is associated with pelvic pain. *Fertil. Steril.*, **55**, 759–65

17. Martin, D. C., Hubert, G. and Levy (1985). Depth of infiltration of endometriosis. *J. Gynecol. Surg.*, **5**, 55–9

18. Sampson, J. A. (1927). Peritoneal endometriomas due to the menstrual dissemination of endometrial tissue into the peritoneal cavity. *Am. J. Obstet. Gynecol.*, **14**, 422–35

19. Canis, M., Bouquet de Jolinières, J., Wattiez, A., Pouly, J.L., Mage, G. and Bruhat, M.A. (1993). Classification of endometriosis. *Baill. Clin. Obstet. Gynecol.*, **7**, 759–74

20. Candiani, G.B., Vercellini, P. and Fedele, L. (1990). Laparoscopic ovarian puncture for correct staging of endometriosis. *Fertil. Steril.*, **53**, 994–7

21. Reich, H., McGlynn, F. and Salvat, J. (1991). Laparoscopic treatment of cul-de-sac obliteration secondary to retrocervical deep endometriosis. *J. Reprod. Med.*, **36**, 516–22

22. Mage, G., Canis, M., Manhes, H., Pouly, J.L., Wattiez, A. and Bruhat, M.A. (1990). Laparoscopic management of adnexal cystic masses. *J. Gynecol. Surg.*, **6**, 71–9

23. Martin, D. C. and Demos Berry, J. (1990). Histology of chocolate cysts. *J. Gynecol. Surg.*, **6**, 43–6

24. Martin, D. C., Hubert, G. D., Vander Zwaag, R. and El-Zeky, F. (1989). Laparoscopic appearances of peritoneal endometriosis. *Fertil. Steril.*, **51**, 63–7

25. Vernon, M. W., Beard, J. S., Graves, K. and Wilson, E. A. (1986). Classification of endometriotic implants by morphologic appearance and capacity to synthesize prostaglandin F. *Fertil. Steril.*, **46**, 801–6

26. Donnez, J., Nisolle, M. and Casanas-Roux, F. (1992). Three-dimensional architectures of peritoneal endometriosis. *Fertil. Steril.*, **57**, 980–3

27. Nisolle, M., Paindaveine, B., Bourdon, A., Berliere, M., Casanas-Roux, F. and Donnez, J. (1990). Histologic study of peritoneal endometriosis. *Fertil. Steril.*, **53**, 984–8

28. Nisolle, M., Casanas-Roux, F., Anaf, V., Mine, J. M. and Donnez, J. (1993). Morphometric study of the stromal vascularization in peritoneal endometriosis. *Fertil. Steril.*, **59**, 681–4

29. Halme, J., Becker, S. and Haskill, S. (1986). Altered maturation and function of peritoneal macrophages: a possible role in pathogenesis of endometriosis. *Am. J. Obstet. Gynecol.*, **157**, 783–9

30. Olive, D. L., Montoya, I., Riehl, R. M. and Schenken, R. S. (1991). Macrophage-conditioned media enhance endometrial stromal cell proliferation *in vitro*. *Am. J. Obstet. Gynecol.*, **164**, 953–8

31. Spujbroek, M. D. E. H., Dunselman, G. A. J., Menheere, P. P. C. A. and Evers, J. L. H. (1992). Early endometriosis invades the extracellular matrix. *Fertil. Steril.*, **58**, 929–33

32. Surey, E. S. and Halme, J. (1991). Effect of platelet-derived growth factor on endometrial stromal cell proliferation *in vitro*. A model for endometriosis? *Fertil. Steril.*, **56**, 672–9

33. Syrop, C. H. and Halme, J. A. (1986). Comparison of peritoneal fluid parameters of infertile patients and the subsequent occurrence of pregnancy. *Fertil. Steril.*, **46**, 631–5

34. Jansen, R.P.S. and Russell, P. (1986). Nonpigmented endometriosis: clinical laparoscopic and pathological definition. *Am. J. Obstet. Gynecol.*, **155**, 1154–8

35. American Fertility Society (1992). Classification Plenary Session VII. *Third World Congress on Endometriosis*, Brussels, June 1–3

36. American Fertility Society (1993). Management of endometriosis in the presence of pelvic pain. *Fertil. Steril.*, **60**, 952–5

37. Koninckx, P. R., Meuleman, C., Demeyere, S., Lesaffre, E. and Cornillie, F. (1991). Suggestive evidence that pelvic endometriosis is a progressive disease, whereas deeply infiltrating endometriosis is associated with pelvic pain. *Fertil. Steril.*, **55**, 759–65

38. Canis, M., Mage, G., Manhes, H., Pouly, J.L., Wattiez, A. and Bruhat, M.A. (1989). Laparoscopic treatment of endometriosis. *Acta Obstet.*

Gynecol. Scand., Suppl. 150, 15–20
39. Canis, M., Mage, G., Wattiez, A., Chapron, C., Pouly, J.L. and Bassil, S. (1992). Second-look laparoscopy after laparoscopic cystectomy of large ovarian endometriomas. *Fertil. Steril.*, **58**, 617–19

40. Operative Laparoscopy Study Group (1991). Postoperative adhesion development after operative laparoscopy: evaluation at early second-look procedures. *Fertil. Steril.*, **55**, 700–4

Anatomic and functional considerations in the development of a classification for endometriosis for pelvic pain and infertility

B.S. Hurst and J.A. Rock

Introduction

Endometriosis has perplexed physicians since the first characterization by Sampson in 1922[1]. Even as the 21st century draws near, the causes of endometriosis-related subfertility and pelvic pain remain open to speculation. Although a wide array of palliative measures have been developed to reduce the size of lesions and symptoms, no direct treatment for endometriosis destroys implants, restores fertility and resolves pain. Sadly, since endometriosis has been so difficult to understand, leaders in our field have been unable to devise a useful classification system to direct therapy or establish a prognosis for individuals with pain or infertility. In order to establish effective treatment, a universally accepted classification system based on newly published insights must replace the currently accepted but often criticized revised-American Fertility Society (r-AFS) staging method[2]. Our modest but important goal should be to study and implement a new international staging system for endometriosis before the close of the 20th century.

Before devising a new classification scheme, the principles of simplicity, reproducibility, relevance and predictive value should be considered. Simplicity is important, since practitioners will be reluctant to use a new system if it is too difficult to understand. Simplicity does not imply that the operating physician may be lazy in establishing a proper stage. Extensive dissection may be necessary to establish a prognosis in those with pelvic pain[3].

Simplicity in the classification system should be an achievable goal if intuitively obvious aspects of endometriosis are listed. A physician should be able to use a system recalled by memory, not by the use of a scoring sheet and a calculator.

A new staging system for endometriosis must be reproducible. A physician who performs a laparoscopy, reads an operative description or reviews photographs or a videotape should be able to stage the findings with a high degree of accuracy. Intra- and interobserver variability should be minimal. Of course, classification will not be possible if an incomplete diagnostic evaluation or operative description is provided, as is occasionally seen. However, if the new system proves to be useful in determining a prognosis and treatment, accurate staging will become a clinical necessity.

The staging system must be clinically relevant to those with pain, infertility, or both. An ideal classification would provide a strong correlation between the extent of disease and subjective pain scores before or after surgery. A complete system must also show a powerful relationship between the stage and fertility, with or without surgery. The achievement of all of these goals may not be possible in a single, unified scheme. At a minimum, a new system should be useful in the prediction of treatment outcome for pain and infertility. Unfortunately, the r-AFS classification system has not been a useful predictor for endometriosis-related symptoms.

Revised American Fertility Society classification

The r-AFS classification of endometriosis was derived from a series of earlier attempts to establish a reproducible, clinically relevant scheme for staging of the extent of disease. The popularity and usefulness of gynecological cancer staging was one of the driving forces to establish a comparable system for endometriosis. The first classification of endometriosis was introduced in 1949, and the proliferation of proposed systems peaked by the 1970s[4]. In 1966, a classification for endometriosis was introduced by Beecham[5]. Staging was based entirely on speculation rather than outcome data. A new system was devised by Acosta and co-authors in 1973[6]. Endometriosis was classified as mild, moderate or severe, on the basis of a well-defined set of characteristics. This system showed a good correlation between stage and pregnancy rates after surgery[7]. However, the classification did not differentiate between unilateral and bilateral disease, and failed to gain international support[8]. Ingersoll proposed a system and correlated the success of medical therapies and pregnancy rates for each stage[9]. Another influential paper was published by Kistner and co-workers[10], who attempted to correlate the extent of endometriosis with infertility, by using a speculative system with four stages and additional subcategories. This scheme, too, was criticized as vague and occasionally misleading, and failed to account for the presence of unilateral disease[8]. None of the early systems were universally accepted, and it took the authority of the American Fertility Society to implement a viable classification, published in 1979[11]. This strategy was strongly influenced by the work of the committee members, and strongly paralleled the system suggested by Buttram in 1978[8]. The AFS 1979 classification system was widely accepted, and became the standard measure of endometriosis[12].

Flaws were evident despite a nearly universal incorporation of the AFS 1979 classification of endometriosis in the published literature. There was a poor relationship between the arbitrarily derived, point score stages of endometriosis and pregnancy outcome after therapy[7,13]. Critics noted that the AFS 1979 system was erroneously based on surgical findings instead of on pathophysiological considerations, and warned against misuse of the scoring system to evaluate the efficacy of medical therapy[14]. Supporters defended the AFS 1979 classification of endometriosis, but recognized the need for refinements[15]. By 1985, leaders in the AFS admitted the shortcomings of the old system and hailed the new, revised AFS classification of endometriosis in 1985[16]. The 1985 scheme was described as 'A more comprehensive point system...to differentiate between peritoneal and ovarian disease'[16]. The revised classification differentiated between superficial and deep endometriosis, and placed a much higher emphasis on cul-de-sac obliteration and adnexal adhesions. The system was designed to be used for infertile patients, and not intended for endometriosis-related pain. Despite the call from many to replace the AFS 1979 system with an empirically derived weighted score, the revised classification retained the arbitrary point score staging strategy[11] (Figure 1).

The goals of the r-AFS classification were to provide an objective, universal method to describe disease severity, to aid in determining therapy, to predict success, and to stratify similar patients[17]. There is no question that the first of these goals was accomplished. Nearly all data published today regarding endometriosis are reported in the r-AFS format. The other goals have not been realized, however, and we now risk chaos with implementation of numerous staging schemes if a new international classification cannot be devised. Before devising a replacement system, the strengths and weaknesses of the current system must be considered.

The major strength of the r-AFS classification is the universal acceptance as the international standard. Clinicians may compare

ENDOMETRIOSIS TODAY: ADVANCES IN RESEARCH AND PRACTICE

Patient's name _____ Date _____
Stage I (minimal)   1–5   Laparoscopy _____ Laparotomy _____ Photography _____
Stage II (mild)   6–15   Recommended treatment _____
Stage III (moderate) 16–40   _____
Stage IV (severe)   >40   _____
Total _____   Prognosis _____

	ENDOMETRIOSIS		<1 cm	1–3 cm	>3 cm
PERITONEUM	Superficial		1	2	4
	Deep		2	4	6
OVARY	R	Superficial	1	2	4
		Deep	4	16	20
	L	Superficial	1	2	4
		Deep	4	16	20
	POSTERIOR CUL-DE-SAC OBLITERATION			Partial	Complete
				4	40
	ADHESIONS		<1/3 enclosure	1/2–2/3 enclosure	>2/3 enclosure
OVARY	R	Filmy	1	2	4
		Dense	4	8	16
	L	Filmy	1	2	4
		Dense	4	8	16
TUBE	R	Filmy	1	2	4
		Dense	4*	8*	16
	L	Filmy	1	2	4
		Dense	4*	8*	16

*If the fimbriated end of the fallopian tube is completely enclosed, change the point assignment to 16

Additional endometriosis: _____   Associated pathology _____
_____   _____
_____   _____

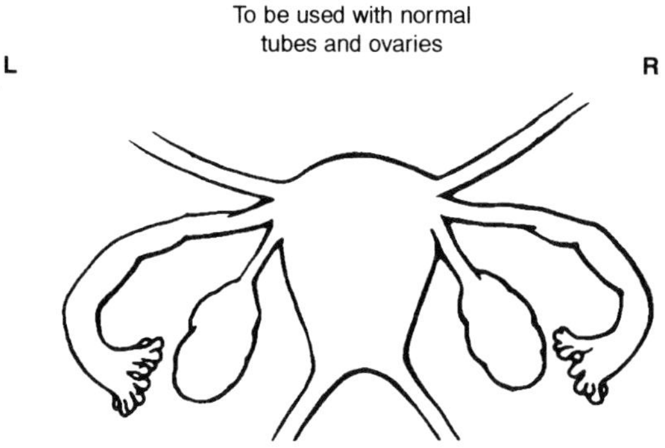

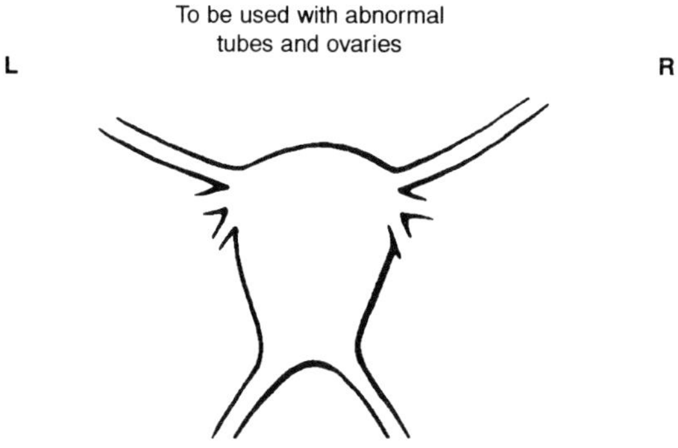

To be used with normal tubes and ovaries   To be used with abnormal tubes and ovaries

Figure 1 Revised American Fertility Classification, 1985[2]. Reproduced with permission from The American Fertility Society for Reproductive Medicine

publications describing stage-based results with a high degree of confidence. An enormous database has accumulated using r-AFS scores, and implementation of an updated system would necessitate a new start. Before abandoning the old system, we must be assured that the r-AFS classification is irreparably flawed and be sure that a new proposal will prove to be worthwhile.

Shortcomings of the r-AFS system are numerous. The 1985 r-AFS classification is neither simple to use nor highly reproducible. The complexity of the point scoring system has long been a burden, but the reproducibility has only recently been evaluated. In one study, videotapes of laparoscopies in 20 women with endometriosis were scored twice by five board-certified reproductive endocrinologists[18]. Intra- and interobserver variability caused concern, since 38% and 52% of patients, respectively, were reclassified by stage. In a large multicenter series, Rock[19] compared r-AFS laparoscopy scores in 315 women produced by study investigators and a blinded reviewer. Good to fair agreement between the investigators and the blinded reviewer was noted in this study. On the basis of these two reports, a high correlation cannot be expected among physicians who evaluate endometriosis. Whether the variation in staging is clinically significant depends on the predictive value of the r-AFS score for pain and infertility.

Many researchers have been frustrated by the lack of correlation of the r-AFS classification and pelvic pain. Marana and co-investigators[20] studied 206 women with endometriosis-related pain and found that the r-AFS classification did not reflect the intensity of symptoms. The same conclusion was reached by Stout and colleagues[21]. The extent of endometriosis was not correlated with pain levels in 102 women who were evaluated by laparoscopy. Nor does the response to treatment seem to correlate with the clinical stage. In a prospective study of 164 women, the symptomatic response with danazol and gestrinone did not differ when r-AFS scores were compared[22]. It is clearly evident that the r-AFS system is a poor measurement of endometriosis-related pain.

Recent findings provide hope for a clinically relevant staging system for pain. Koninckx and colleagues[3] described the depth and volume of endometriosis implants in a series of 643 laparoscopies performed for infertility, pelvic pain, or both. In this landmark study, deeply infiltrating endometriosis was strongly associated with pelvic pain. Women with pain tended to have larger and deeper endometriotic implants than those with isolated infertility. Based on these findings, a new emphasis on deep implants was suggested for the r-AFS system. An example is demonstrated in Figure 2. Simple laparoscopic visualization cannot determine the depth of peritoneal implants in women with pelvic pain. Complete dissection of implants should be considered as essential to the adequate surgical evaluation of endometriosis-related pain.

New insights allow a further understanding of the relationship between pain and the extent of visible disease. It appears that the frequency and severity of deep dyspareunia and dysmenorrhea is less in women with isolated ovarian endometriosis[23]. Interestingly, the severity of deep dyspareunia is inversely related to the r-AFS endometriosis score. On the other hand, histologically proven vaginal endometriosis is strongly associated with deep dyspareunia[23]. The findings in this study and the report by Koninckx and co-investigators emphasize the importance of deep endometriosis for pain[3,23]. Results from these reports should be incorporated in any new classification of endometriosis to be used for both pain and infertility.

Despite establishing the r-AFS classification for infertility, this system has not been a good predictor of pregnancy before or after treatment. For example, there appears to be little difference in pregnancy rates between those with stage I or stage II endometriosis treated expectantly, with medical therapy, after laparoscopic cautery or laser therapy, or after conservative surgery[24]. No difference was evident

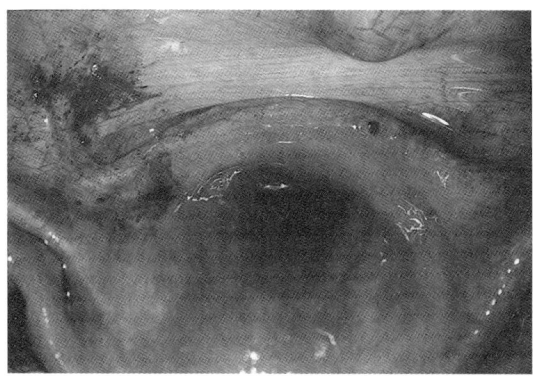

Figure 2 Peritoneal implants in patient with pelvic pain

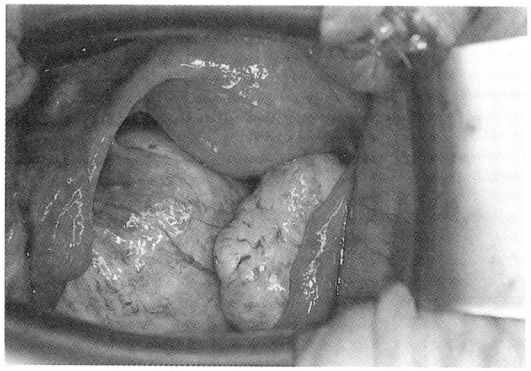

Figure 3 Large left endometrioma and smaller right endometriomas in a patient with infertility

between r-AFS stage and pregnancy rates in a small series described by Rubessa and co-authors[25], although there was a trend towards reduced rates with stage IV disease. In another report, little difference in delivery rates was evident between surgically treated stage I or stage II endometriosis: 68% vs. 53%, respectively, although success was reduced to 38% with advanced disease[26]. The similarity of pregnancy rates for surgical therapy with stage I or II disease vs. outcomes for stage III and IV endometriosis was noted with the AFS 1979 classification[7]. Since similar outcomes may be expected after surgery for those with stage I and II disease and those with III and IV stages, an argument could be made for simplification of, rather than for adding to, the complexity of the current system.

The r-AFS classification is hindered by assignment of the point score with arbitrary cut-off points for staging[13]. Figures 3 and 4 demonstrate two individuals with stage IV endometriosis and infertility. The patient in Figure 3 was assigned to stage IV, because of the presence of superficial peritoneal implants and endometriomas in both ovaries, each measuring over 3 cm. There were no adhesions and the tubal architecture was preserved. Minimal adhesive disease, easily lysed, was seen at the time of early second-look laparoscopy. The woman in Figure 4 was also assigned to stage IV. Her normal anatomic landmarks were

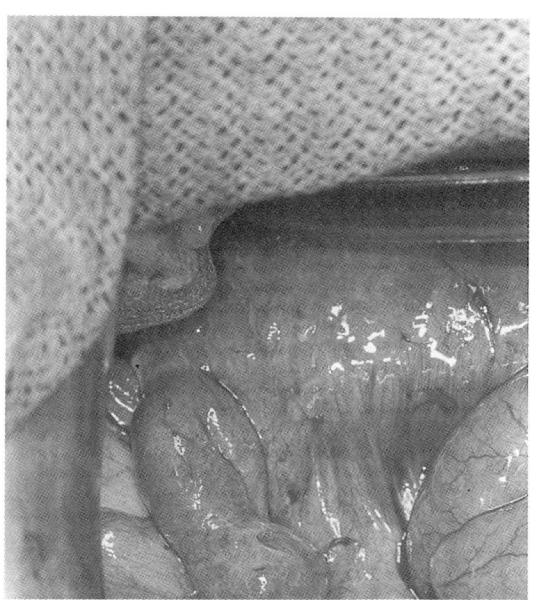

Figure 4 Massive adhesions and complete obliteration of the posterior cul-de-sac in a patient with infertility

completely distorted. Complete obliteration of the posterior cul-de-sac was seen. Both ovaries and the right Fallopian tube were buried in the cohesive adhesions binding the bowel to the posterior aspect of the uterus. The left Fallopian tube was seen, but distal occlusion was evident. Extensive superficial and deep endometriosis implants were encountered on the sidewalls and in the cul-de-sac. Early second-look laparoscopy demonstrated an improved picture, but extensive cohesive bilateral adnexal adhesions were again encountered. Despite comparable r-AFS staging, the prognosis and recommended treatments for these two patients are dramatically different. Expectant management may be appropriate in the first situation. *In vitro* fertilization would be recommended for the woman in Figure 4 by most authorities. Such discrepant approaches for two individuals with the same stage of endometriosis indicates a serious, if not fatal, flaw in the r-AFS classification system.

Unfortunately, advances in infertility therapies may hinder the scientific study needed to implement a new system. Superovulation therapy provides a significant increase in cycle fecundity, especially for those with stage I and II disease[27]. Furthermore, *in vitro* fertilization and embryo transfer (IVF-ET) has been established as a successful therapy for endometriosis, although there is some evidence that pregnancy rates may be compromised in some with advanced disease[28].

Classification for pain and infertility

The r-AFS classification was intended for those with infertility, not pain[16]. The emphasis on infertility is evident in most of the previously proposed systems[5,6,9,10]. Few investigators have attempted to devise a system for classification of both pain and infertility. Factors that correlate with pain have only recently been identified, and deep endometriosis does not seem to be an important predictor of fertility. A useful classification system for both pain and infertility may be difficult or impossible to devise. For example, if peritoneal endometriosis continues to represent the lowest stage, the relevance of deep endometriosis implants to pain will be lost. A new scheme must allow notation of the extent of superficial and deep peritoneal and serosal implants. However, if such a scheme can be formulated, it will almost certainly require a radical departure from the currently used r-AFS classification scheme.

Ovarian endometrioma influence therapy and the prognosis for fertility, but may not have a strong relationship to pain[23]. It is well established that medical therapy is not effective for endometriomas larger than 1 cm, and that surgical removal is necessary[29-31]. In addition, pregnancy success is reduced when ovarian endometriomas are larger than 3 cm or have ruptured[7]. On the other hand, pain does not appear to be related to the size of an endometrioma[23]. However, it may be a mistake to assign ovarian endometriomas a higher score than peritoneal disease, since doing so would minimize the usefulness of this classification for pain.

Adnexal adhesions and tubal compromise have a profound effect on fertility, but may not be important in pain[23]. A strong association has established and confirmed the detrimental impact of adhesions and tubal obstruction on fertility, and the decision to perform reconstructive surgery or IVF-ET is based on the nature and extent of adhesions[32]. Extensive adhesions may not require operation for restoration of fertility if IVF-ET is chosen. If the new classification is to be used for treatment based on stage, extensive adhesions should not represent a higher stage than an endometrioma, since surgery to remove an endometrioma is generally considered to be necessary for pain or infertility. If a treatment-directed classification system is the goal, a parallel site-specific scoring system rather than a progressive staging system may be useful.

Kurata and colleagues[33] have proposed a site-specific scoring system for endometriosis, called the 'TOP' classification. This system evaluates the severity of endometriosis by sites including the Fallopian tube (T), ovary (O), and peritoneum (P). Pregnancy rates were reduced with progressive tubal and peritoneal endometriosis scores, but not when the ovaries were involved. High pregnancy rates were achieved when at least one tube was normal, even when endometriomas or cul-de-sac obliteration were observed. The TOP

Table 1 Peritoneum, ovarian, adhesion classification of endometriosis

Peritoneum (P)
Superficial (s), deep (d)
   measure and record total area of superficial implant. 0 = none
Example: Ps-2, d-1 (superficial implants measure a total of 2 cm; deep implants measure a total of 1 cm)

Ovarian (O)
Right (r), left (l)
   measure and record size of endometrioma. 0 = none; s = superficial only
Example: Or-s, l-3 (right superficial, left endometrioma 3 cm diameter)

Adhesions (A) – based on least involved adnexa
Filmy (f), cohesive (c)
   0 none
   1 involving tube *or* ovary
   2 involving tube *and* ovary
   3 complete encasement of tube and ovary
Example: Ac-2 (cohesive adhesions involving least involved tube *and* ovary)

---

classification overcomes many of the limitations seen in earlier schemes, and further study to determine reproducibility and confirm clinical relevance is necessary. The TOP system may be limited as a classification predominantly of infertility, but it may serve as a template for devising a site-specific scoring system that can be applied for pain and infertility.

A new site-specific endometriosis staging system may allow clinical decisions to be made on the basis of the extent of disease and symptoms. The depth and volume of peritoneal implants are staged independently of ovarian or adhesive disease (Table 1). A separate peritoneal score including the measurement of total superficial and deep lesions should provide a clinically relevant staging for women with endometriosis-related pain without overlooking the impact of ovarian and adhesive disease in infertility patients. Ovarian endometriosis is reported as superficial implants or deep endometriomas involving the right or left ovary, with a measurement of the endometrioma included. Measurements of cysts could be based upon ultrasound findings, but surgical confirmation is required. Presence of a unilateral endometrioma would require surgical removal in most circumstances of pain or infertility. Adnexal adhesions are reported on the basis of the least involved side with subclassification describing the type and extent of tubal and ovarian involvement. The prognosis for fertility with surgical therapy should be easily established for the site-specific stage, to aid in the decision between surgical reconstruction vs. IVF-ET.

Examples of the site-specific scoring system are established for the patients shown in Figures 2, 3 and 4. Surgery for the woman in Figure 2 was performed for pain. Findings after dissection included 5-cm^2 superficial implants and 3-cm^3 deep peritoneal disease. The left ovary was normal, and a 1-cm right endometrioma was identified. A few filmy adhesions were seen between the right ovary and sidewall, but no adhesions affected the left adnexa. The site-specific stage in this example would be Ps-5, d-3; Or-1; A-0. The infertile woman in Figure 3 had no deep endometriosis, 2-cm superficial disease, a 10-cm left endometrioma, two 2-cm right endometriomas and no adnexal adhesions. Her stage would be Ps-2; Or-4, l-10; A-0. The infertile patient in Figure 4 had 7-cm superficial and 10-cm deep peritoneal implants, bilateral superficial ovarian endometriosis and cohesive adhesions with complete encasement of both tubes and ovaries. In this example, the score would be Ps-7, d-10; Or-s, l-s; Ac-3.

The peritoneal, ovarian, adhesion classification system for pain and infertility is proposed for speculation. On the basis of published reports, it is expected to be clinically relevant. However, prospective clinical studies will be necessary to establish the relevance and reproducibility of any system.

Conclusion

Despite achieving a nearly universal acceptance, the r-AFS classification of endometriosis has not been proven to be clinically relevant for establishing a prognosis or directing therapy in women with endometriosis-related pain or infertility. A linear scoring system may never be relevant for pain and infertility, since the prognostic factors are distinctly different for each. A new method of classification is necessary to incorporate both pain and infertility, and site-specific schemes may provide the greatest promise. Before any new classification system is incorporated for endometriosis, it is imperative that the system be tested and proven to be reliable. Once a staging system has been validated, co-operation among all of the international fertility and gynecology societies will be essential to avoid chaos seen in the days before the AFS classification was adopted in 1979.

References

1. Sampson, J.A. (1922). Perforating hemorrhagic (chocolate) cysts of ovary. *Arch. Surg.*, **3**, 245–323
2. The American Fertility Society (1985). Revised American Fertility Society classification of endometriosis. *Fertil. Steril.*, **43**, 351–2
3. Koninckx, P.R., Meuleman, C., Demeyers, S., Lesaffre, E. and Cornillie, F.J. (1991). Suggestive evidence that pelvic endometriosis is a progressive disease, whereas deeply infiltrating endometriosis is associated with pelvic pain. *Fertil. Steril.*, **55**, 759–65
4. Wicks, M.J. and Larson, C.P. (1949). Histologic criteria for evaluating endometriosis. *Northwest Med.*, **48**, 611
5. Beecham, C.T. (1966). Classification of endometriosis. *Obstet. Gynecol.*, **28**, 437
6. Acosta, A.A., Buttram, V.C. Jr, Besch, P.K., Malinak, L.R., Franklin, R.R. and Vanderheyden, J.D. (1973). A proposed classification of pelvic endometriosis. *Obstet. Gynecol.*, **42**, 19–25
7. Rock, J.A., Guzick, D.S., Sengos, C., Schweditsch, M., Sapp, K.C. and Jones, H.W. Jr. (1981). The conservative surgical treatment of endometriosis: evaluation of pregnancy success with respect to the extent of disease as categorized using contemporary classification systems. *Fertil. Steril.*, **35**, 131–7
8. Buttram, V.C. Jr (1978). An expanded classification of endometriosis. *Fertil. Steril.*, **30**, 240–2
9. Ingersoll, F.M. (1977). Selection of medical or surgical treatment of endometriosis. *Clin. Obstet. Gynecol.*, **20**, 849–64
10. Kistner, R.W., Siegler, A.M. and Behrman, S.J. (1977). Suggested classification for endometriosis: relationship to infertility. *Fertil. Steril.*, **28**, 1008–10
11. The American Fertility Society (1979). Classification of endometriosis. The American Fertility Society. *Fertil. Steril.*, **32**, 633–4
12. O'Shea, R.T. and Jones, W.R. (1985). Danazol: objective assessment in the treatment of endometriosis. *Clin. Reprod. Fertil.*, **3**, 205–6
13. Guzick, D.S., Bross, D.S. and Rock, J.A. (1982). Assessing the efficacy of The American Fertility Society's classification of endometriosis: application of a dose–response methodology. *Fertil. Steril.*, **38**, 171–6
14. Brosens, I.A., Cornillie, F., Koninckx, P. and Vasquez, G. (1985). Evolution of the Revised American Fertility Society Classification of Endometriosis. *Fertil. Steril.*, **44**, 714–16
15. Andrews, W.C. (1981). Classification of endometriosis. *Fertil. Steril.*, **35**, 124–5
16. Buttram, V.C. Jr (1985). Evolution of the revised American Fertility Society classification

of endometriosis. *Fertil. Steril.*, **43**, 347–50

17. Weitzman, G.A. and Buttram, V.C. Jr (1989). Classification of endometriosis. *Obstet. Gynecol. Clin. North Am.*, **16**, 61–77

18. Hornstein, M.D., Gleason, R.E., Orav, J., Haas, S.T., Friedman, A.J., Rein, M.S., Hill, J.A. and Barbieri, R.L. (1993). The reproducibility of the revised American Fertility Society classification of endometriosis. *Fertil. Steril.*, **59**, 1015–21

19. Rock, J.A. (1995). The revised American Fertility Society classification of endometriosis: reproducibility of scoring. ZOLADEX Endometriosis Study Group. *Fertil. Steril.*, **63**, 1108–10

20. Marana, R., Muzii, L., Caruana, P., Dell'Acqua, S. and Mancuso, S. (1991). Evaluation of the correlation between endometriosis extent, age of the patients and associated symptomatology. *Acta Eur. Fertil.*, **22**, 209–12

21. Stout, A.L., Steege, J.F., Dodson, W.C. and Hughes, C.L. (1991). Relationship of laparoscopic findings to self-report of pelvic pain. *Am. J. Obstet. Gynecol.*, **164**, 73–9

22. Halbe, H.W., Nakamura, M.S., Da Silveira, G.P. and Carvalho, W.P. (1995). Updating the clinical experience in endometriosis – the Brazilian perspective. *Br. J. Obstet. Gynaecol.*, **102** (Suppl. 12), 17–21

23. Vercellini, P., Trespidi, L., De Giorgi, O., Cortesi, I., Parazzini, F. and Crosignani, P.G. (1996). Endometriosis and pelvic pain: relation to disease stage and localization. *Fertil. Steril.*, **65**, 299–304

24. Paulson, J.D., Asmar, P. and Saffan, D.S. (1991). Mild and moderate endometriosis. Comparison of treatment modalities for infertile couples. *J. Reprod. Med.*, **36**, 151–5

25. Rubessa, S., Falsetti, L., Viani, A., Corazza, M. and Gastaldi, A. (1990). Conservative surgical treatment in infertile patients with endometriosis. *Acta Eur. Fertil.*, **21**, 277–80

26. Candiani, G.B., Fedele, L. and Vercellini, P. (1986). Conservative surgical treatment of endometriosis. *Acta Eur. Fertil.*, **17**, 173–80

27. Fedele, L., Bianchi, S., Marchini, M., Villa, L., Brioschi, D. and Parazzini, F. (1992). Superovulation with human menopausal gonadotropins in the treatment of infertility associated with minimal or mild endometriosis: a controlled randomized study. *Fertil. Steril.*, **58**, 28–31

28. Oehninger, S., Acosta, A.A., Kreiner, D., Muasher, S.J., Jones, H.W. Jr and Rosenwaks, Z. (1988). *In vitro* fertilization and embryo transfer (IVF/ET): an established and successful therapy for endometriosis. *J. In Vitro Fert. Embryo Transf.*, **5**, 249–56

29. Buttram, V.C. Jr, Reiter, R.C. and Ward, S. (1985). Treatment of endometriosis with danazol: report of a 6-year prospective study. *Fertil. Steril.*, **43**, 353–60

30. Biberoglu, K.O. and Behrman, S.J. (1981). Dosage aspects of danazol therapy in endometriosis: short-term and long-term effectiveness. *Am. J. Obstet. Gynecol.*, **139**, 645–54

31. Salat-Baroux, J., Giacomini, P. and Antoine, J.M. (1988). Laparoscopic control of danazol therapy on pelvic endometriosis. *Hum. Reprod.*, **3**, 197–200

32. Hurst, B.S. and Schlaff, W.D. (1966). A surgeon's perspective on ART vs microsurgery for infertility: where do we draw the line? In Rock, J.A. and Murphy, A.A. (eds.). *Advances in Obstetrics and Gynecology*, vol. 3, pp. 291–319. (St Louis: Mosby)

33. Kurata, S., Ishimaru, T., Masuzaki, H. and Yamabe, T. (1993). Relationship between the prognosis of conception and the location of pelvic involvement in endometriosis: significance of the TOP (tube, ovary, peritoneum) classification. *Asia–Oceania J. Obstet. Gynaecol.*, **19**, 391–9

Classification of endometriosis

D.K. Tran, J. Belaisch, J. Berthet, Y. Darbois, J.L. Leroy, M. Mintz, D. Querleu, C. Racinet and R. Trevoux (Endometriosis Study Group, France)

Introduction

Prerequisites for any adequate comparison of various therapeutic regimens for patients with endometriosis include the establishment of an accurate diagnosis and the use of an accepted classification system[1]. This opinion is shared by many authors[2-4]. As Brosens and colleagues[5] emphasize, a classification system 'should meet the theoretical criteria for an ideal system: have not only good descriptive potential but also be simple and practical to use'. As added by Dubuisson and Chapron it should allow 'comparisons to be made between series and multicenter study'[6].

The classification presented by the Endometriosis Study Group is not original. It employs the principles of the Tumor, Node, Metastasis (TNM) tumor classification. It also agrees with the 1978 proposals of Buttram[7], and takes into account the description criteria of other classifications[8] and the physiological data on tubo–ovarian fixity considered by Kistner and colleagues[9]. It is also partly based on the point system of the revised American Fertility Society classification[10].

The characteristics of endometriosis

Two major facts should be considered in the establishment of a classification of endometriosis. First, this disease is expressed by multiple involvements of different localizations, and second, the patients suffering from it consult their gynecologist either for infertility or for pain, and often for both of these reasons. Therefore the classification must make evident the diversity of the involvements and be useful for both groups of patients.

Other characteristics of endometriosis must also be considered. Today, the evolution of this disease is impossible to foresee. Also, the adhesions it generates are not treatable by drugs but require surgery. Lastly, the disease which is called endometriosis is perhaps of multiple nature, as suggested by Donnez and associates[11]. The score for endometriosis of different organs should therefore be kept separate. Indeed, the score should be considered within each organ, as there can be no alleviation of severity by changes occurring in the opposite direction[5].

The aim of a classification is therefore to offer the possibility of grouping together lesions of the same nature according to the criteria which are acknowledged at present. The need for a precise, 'uniform' and comprehensive classification that allows meaningful interpretation of results[7], and which can be easily used by all gynecologists, is universally admitted. We feel the FOATI classification fulfils these needs.

The FOATI classification

The basis of the FOATI classification is described here. Four types of involvement have been considered:

(1) Peritoneal involvement (foci) (**F**);

(2) Ovarian involvement (**O**);

(3) Adhesions (**A**);

(4) Tubal involvement (**T**).

As Buttram suggested[7], and due to the consequences of tubal function for fertility, we reserve a special place for tubal lesions in our classification. The inflammatory aspect of the lesions (**I**) is also taken into account, even if all gynecologists do not assign the same meaning to this characteristic. Inflammatory lesions are red and hypervascularized and the peritoneum no longer has its normal polished surface. As believed by the majority of authors, the histopathological confirmation of the endometriosis must be obtained. This examination also gives an idea of the activity and differentiation of the lesions.

Annex considerations

In most cases endometriotic involvements are bilateral. When they are not or when they are very asymmetrical, the letters R or L are associated with the FOATI formula in order to indicate the affected side for one or multiple involvements of the endometriosis.

The depth of the lesion, if easy to measure, is indicated by the letter D.

The anomaly of the cul-de-sac raises unsolved questions because of uncertainties about the physiopathology and nature of the obliteration of the cul-de-sac[11,12]. Donnez and colleagues[11] and Koninckx and associates[12] think that the obliteration might have different causes. This form of endometriosis is separately defined by the letters CDS.

Lastly, in the case where extragenital lesions of endometriosis are associated with pelvic endometriosis, they are expressed by the letter E for digestive, U for urinary, PP for pleuropulmonary and N for nervous.

The choice of the coefficients

Choosing a weighted numbering system is the most delicate part in the establishment of a classification. Along this line the objectives of the Endometriosis Study Group are very modest. One cannot require a classification system to say more than is known about a disease. It is especially impossible, today, to know how an endometriosis is going to evolve, given the large number of factors which might influence it, as we shall discuss later.

We have therefore chosen three goals. These are: to be as simple as possible; to make clear the severity of the disease; and to make evident the possibility of the occurrence of a pregnancy or the hindrances to a satisfactory tubal transport of the egg. We have designated the following coefficients to stage the disease: one point for minimal involvement; two points for moderate involvement; and three points for severe involvement. The letters and coefficients used in the FOATI system are summarized in Table 1.

The points designated for tubes and adhesions have a clear prognostic significance. Three points are given when both tubes are totally occluded or when dense adhesions completely fix the tubes. Two points are given when tubal patency is limited but a pregnancy seems possible, and one point for moderate alterations of tubes. The same criteria are applied for adhesions.

The points given for implants are based on the extent of the foci: one point for < 1 cm; two points for 1–5 cm; and three points for > 5 cm.

Like Brosens and colleagues[5], for the ovarian endometriomas we take into account only their size: small (< 1 cm), one point; medium (1–5 cm), two points; large (> 5 cm), three points. The nature of the cyst is also defined by the inflammatory aspect of the ovarian involvement. The impossibility of establishing a satisfactory categorization will appear obvious when the views of Nezhat and colleagues[13], Brosens and associates[5] and Dubuisson and Chapron[6] are compared. Even the definition of an endometrioma is a subject of debate[13]. And, like Dubuisson and Chapron[6], we consider that 'when and only when [works on endometriomas] reach conclusions which convince everyone', will modifications be integrated in the presented classification.

Table 1 Classification of endometriosis proposed by the Endometriosis Study Group

Type of involvement	Coefficient/letter
F: peritoneal involvement (foci)	F
no lesion	0
diameter < 1 cm	1
diameter 1–5 cm	2
diameter > 5 cm	3
deep	D
O: ovarian involvement	O
no lesion	0
diameter < 1 cm	1
diameter 1–5 cm	2
diameter > 5 cm or bilateral	3
A: adhesions	A
no lesion	0
tubal and ovarian mobility preserved	1
partial tubal and ovarian mobility	2
lack of tubal and ovarian mobility	3
obliteration of posterior cul-de-sac	CDS
T: tubal involvement	T
normal	0
partial occlusion (proximal or distal, unilateral or bilateral)	1
total occlusion in one tube and partial occlusion in the other	2
bilateral permanent tubal occlusion	3
I: inflammation	I
> 50% red lesions	+
< 50% red lesions	−

We know and accept that these coefficients do not have any significance in terms of prognosis and that fertility as well as pain do not depend on the extent or volume of peritoneal or ovarian involvements. Clearly we agree with Venturini and colleagues[14], when they write: 'Unfortunately all schemes to classify stages of endometriosis have so far failed to identify manifestations of the disease that respond in a predictable way to specific treatment'. An exception is made for distal tubal occlusion and dense adhesions which will never respond to medical treatment.

We consider that inflammation is present if more than 50% of the lesions are inflammatory.

The integration of all means of investigation

We believe it is essential to take into account all the ways of examining a patient suffering from endometriosis. Laparoscopy is clearly the gold standard of investigation of endometriosis, but it is not the only way. So much progress has been made in ultrasonography that, from now on, any woman consulting a physician for pain or infertility will be explored by ultrasonography. The results of this investigation should then be integrated in the classification[15,16], as are the results of conventional hysterosalpingography.

Hysterosalpingography demonstrates proximal occlusion of one or both tubes or shows diverticular images of interstitial and isthmic portions of the tube which may be endometriotic in nature and which do not always appear through the laparoscope[17,18]. Magnetic resonance images should be considered even if their significance is not completely accepted[19,20]. The simplest information given by the bimanual pelvic examination must also enter into the establishment of a coefficient since according to Koninckx and colleagues[21], and Belaisch and Madelenat[22], endometriosis of the cul-de-sac is sometimes disclosed by pelvic examination during the menstrual period and goes unseen by laparoscopy.

Advantages of the FOATI formula

At the end a very simple formula gives a precise definition of the extent of the disease, while giving information on each involvement. This is, in our opinion, the main advantage of the FOATI classification.

Expressing the results of therapies

The FOATI formula established at two different times of evaluation of the disease allows a valuable comparison of involvements and offers the possibility of interpreting results in a meaningful way. For instance, after a laparoscopic vaporization the shift from $F_2 O_{3L} A_{2L} T_{1L} I-$ to $F_1 O_0 A_{1L} T_{1L} I-$ would represent the efficacy of the surgery on the whole disease. However, a case which has shifted after medical therapy using analogs of luteinizing hormone-releasing hormone (LH RH) from $F_3 O_1 A_2 T_2 I+$ to $F_1 O_1 A_2 T_2 I-$ would confirm the sensitivity of the peritoneal implants to the medical treatment and the disappearance of inflammation, and at the same time its ineffectiveness on the tubal involvement and on the adhesions. The formula therefore precisely indicates the involvement which has propitiously evolved after the treatment, whereas general scoring would only show a global improvement of lesions.

The advantages offered by the use of a computer

Another advantage of the FOATI representation lies in the fact that it is able to use the facilities offered by computers in all kinds of classifications, as all cases which have been studied can be input according to the selected criteria. The order of the criteria may then be changed at leisure. The data capture is very simple and yet complete. It is true that the sketches of pelvic organs advised by the American Fertility Society can perfectly depict each of the involvements, but these sketches are difficult to input in order, and would use a large proportion of the computer's memory. In return, the revised American Fertility Society (AFS) scores are very easy to classify but do not give a precise topography of the disease as does the FOATI system.

Since we are aware that the revised AFS classification has been drafted by a committee comprised of some of the gynecologists with the largest knowledge of endometriosis in the world, we shall not repeat the criticism of this classification. But the very fact that a symposium is devoted to classification shows that today it is not considered satisfactory.

To take an example, the cases submitted for analysis can be presented according to the selected involvement and according to the severity. Thus, if ovarian endometriomas are selected, the simple displacement of FOATI columns will allow their presentation according to their volume. First would come the large and pure ovarian endometriomas which are more than 5 cm in diameter: $O_3 F_1 A_0 T_0 I-$; then the cysts associated with other involvements would be depicted: $O_3 F_2 A_2 T_2 I-$, $O_3 F_2 A_2 T_1 I+$, $O_3 F_2 A_1 T_2 I-$; the smaller endometriomas would appear after these: $O_2 F_2 A_3 T_2 I+$, $O_2 F_1 A_2 T_2 I-$, O_1 etc.

The record according to severity of the endometriosis

As was recently suggested by Schweppe (personal communication), the FOATI classification allows, as do the revised AFS classification and that of Acosta and associates[8,10], one to distinguish between minimal, mild, moderate and severe cases of endometriosis. For minimal forms, a coefficient of 1 would be given only to peritoneal implants; for mild forms all coefficients should be ≤ 1; for moderate forms the highest coefficient should be 2; and for severe cases at least one coefficient should be 3.

Again we must emphasize that this classification does not pretend to have any value in putting a prognosis on the evolution of the disease, regression of pain, or occurrence of pregnancy.

According to Buttram's point of view[7], we can hope that a clear morphological classification 'will lead to more definitive studies and a clearer picture of the most effective mode of therapy'. Still, we know that pain has never obeyed strict or logical rules. It is governed by anatomical as well as psychological factors. Nevertheless a very precise description of implants can be useful, and is possible in addition to the simplified expression of FOATI: color, extent and depth, as for all other involvements.

As for fertility, it clearly depends on multiple factors unrelated to endometriosis. Male and cervical factors, and age of the patient, have the greatest influence as has been proved by a study analyzing 370 cases of endometriosis classified according to both revised AFS and FOATI classification systems[23].

The hope of discovering a simple and purely morphological classification which would give valuable prognostic information on the evolution of pain and fertility of patients suffering from endometriosis is a delusion.

Factors which are insufficiently known

Nobody ignores today the fact that insufficiently known factors govern the evolution of endometriotic lesions and their sensitivity to the different modes of treatment[24]. These factors are the presence or absence of hormone receptors, the histopathological type of lesions, their degree of vascularization, the existence of growth factors and of cell adhesion molecules and other factors such as the immune condition of the patient and, last but not least, her psychological condition and the stresses to which she is submitted.

One can hope, considering the complexity of this problem, that a more fundamental knowledge of metabolic, endocrine immunological and biomolecular factors will, in the future, achieve the necessary specificity and reproducibility to provide pertinent information in these areas and open the way to a valuable classification. However, this will not happen for many years, according to Evers[25].

One might think that a classification which does not pretend to any prognostic value does not have any usefulness. It is true that if it had prognosis abilities it would be preferable. But it is necessarily useful to have at command a classification which is able to account for the different involvements in each case according to the actual state of knowledge, as this knowledge is the basis on which the therapeutic decisions are taken[26-28].

Admittedly the FOATI classification is insufficient. However, it is better than nothing. This classification is adapted to today's needs, but once we have obtained a level of evidence in the appropriate sciences, it will be easily modified.

Retrospective validation study

The FOATI classification has been used concurrently with the revised AFS classification by a group of French gynecologists in a retrospective and partly prospective study (459 patients), the results of which are given here[29].

Using the FOATI classification

Thirty patients were scored as having minimal, 75 as having mild (all coefficients ≤ 1), 174 with moderate (highest coefficient 2) and 180 patients with severe forms (at least one factor with coefficient 3).

Minimal endometriosis Thirty patients ($F_1 O_0 A_0 T_0 I+/-$) were studied. Only two patients were considered as having inflammatory lesions ($I+$) (6.6%). Thirteen patients have been treated by medical treatment and three pregnancies with delivery (23%) occurred. This pregnancy rate can be considered as rather low for minimal forms. This poor result might be due to the fact that the infertility was not due to the endometriosis in those cases.

Mild endometriosis Of 75 patients with mild disease, 48 patients presented only with tubal involvement ($F_0 O_0 A_0 T_1$). Twenty-five have been treated by medico-surgical treatment, there were eight pregnancies (32%), four miscarriages (16%), one aggravation and 12 improvements (T_1–T_0).

For 27 patients, two or three factors were given a score of one point. Three patients treated by purely medical treatment presented an improvement limited to peritoneal implants. Twenty-four patients were treated by medico-surgical treatment, and six pregnancies with

Table 2 FOATI classification of 174 patients with moderate endometriosis, in a retrospective study

Classification		n
Unique or predominant involvement		
F_2:	$F_2 O_{0-1} A_{0-1} T_{0-1} I-$	42
	$F_2 O_{0-1} A_{0-1} T_{0-1} I+$	18
O_2:	$F_{0-1} O_2 A_{0-1} T_{0-1} I-$	14
	$F_{0-1} O_2 A_{0-1} T_{0-1} I+$	4
A_2:	$F_{0-1} O_{0-1} A_2 T_{0-1} I-$	2
T_2:	$F_{0-1} O_{0-1} A_{0-1} T_2 I-$	48
Total		128
Two predominant involvements		
$F_2 O_2$:	$F_2 O_2 A_{0-1} T_{0-1} I-$	3
	$F_2 O_2 A_{0-1} T_{0-1} I+$	3
$F_2 A_2$:	$F_2 O_{0-1} A_2 T_{0-1} I-$	9
	$F_2 O_{0-1} A_2 T_{0-1} I+$	2
$F_2 T_2$:	$F_2 O_{0-1} A_{0-1} T_2 I+$	1
$O_2 A_2$:	$F_{0-1} O_2 A_2 T_{0-1} I-$	4
$O_2 T_2$:	$F_{0-1} O_2 A_{0-1} T_2 I-$	3
Three predominant involvements		
$F_2 O_2 A_2 T_{0-1} I-$		4
$F_2 O_2 A_2 T_{0-1} I+$		5
$F_2 O_2 A_{0-1} T_2 I-$		4
$F_2 O_{0-1} A_2 T_2 I-$		2
$F_{0-1} O_2 A_2 T_2 I-$		4
Four predominant involvements		
$F_2 O_2 A_2 T_2 I-$		1
$F_2 O_2 A_2 T_2 I+$		1
Total		174

delivery (22%), five miscarriages, one ectopic pregnancy and 12 improvements were obtained.

The pregnancy rate is as low as in minimal forms. Tubal obstruction has been treated by medico-surgical treatment and the pregnancy rate (32%) can be considered as correct.

Moderate endometriosis In 174 patients with moderate disease (Table 2), when a unique or predominant involvement (128 patients) was observed, the inflammatory rate was 17.2% (22 patients with I+).

The follow-up concerned 73 patients. Purely medical treatment was applied only when the lesions affected ovaries or peritoneum, and medico-surgical treatment was usually performed in the other moderate forms.

The pregnancy rate has been better than in minimal and mild forms: 30–36% for purely peritoneal involvement (F_2) and 48.5% for purely tubal involvement (T_2).

In 46 patients, two, three or four types of lesions with coefficient 2 were observed. The inflammatory rate was 26% (12 patients). The follow-up concerned 31 patients. In most cases, a medico-surgical treatment was performed and the pregnancy rate was better than in the minimal and mild forms (50–60%). Ovarian endometriomas, adhesions and tubal occlusion were probably the cause of the infertility in these cases.

Severe endometriosis 180 patients were classified with severe disease (Table 3). In cases of unique or predominant involvement, the inflammation was seldom observed: 44 of 123 patients were classified as I+ (35.75%).

The follow-up concerned 70 patients. In cases of implants alone (F_3), or predominantly peritoneal involvements ($F_3 O_{(1-2)} A_{(1-2)}$), when medical treatment was performed improvements were obtained, but no pregnancies. When applied, medico-surgical treatment gave better results: 50% pregnancy rate when tubal involvements ($T_{(1-2)}$) or adhesions ($A_{(1-2)}$) were observed. However, when tubal lesions were severe (T_3) the pregnancy rate was very low.

In cases of two or multiple factors (43 patients with two factors and 14 with 3 or 4 factors) the inflammatory rate was much higher: 76% and 71%. Only medico-surgical treatment was performed. Favorable results were obtained with $F_3 O_3$ disease. The existence of adhesions and tubal lesions was a pejorative factor of prognosis.

It appears that, with the FOATI classification, two aspects of the disease are described: endometriosis with unique or predominant involvement (66.8% of patients) and endometriosis with multiple associated lesions (33.2% of patients) (Tables 4 and 5).

Table 3 FOATI classification of 180 patients with severe endometriosis, in a retrospective study

Classification		n
Unique or predominant involvement		
F_3:	$F_3 O_{0-2} A_{0-2} T_{0-2} I-$	32
	$F_3 O_{0-2} A_{0-2} T_{0-2} I+$	18
O_3:	$F_{0-2} O_3 A_{0-2} T_{0-2} I-$	30
	$F_{0-2} O_3 A_{0-2} T_{0-2} I+$	17
A_3:	$F_{0-2} O_{0-2} A_3 T_{0-2} I-$	16
	$F_{0-2} O_{0-2} A_3 T_{0-2} I+$	9
T_3:	$F_{0-2} O_{0-2} A_{0-2} T_3 I-$	1
Total		123
Two predominant involvements		
$F_3 O_3$:	$F_3 O_3 A_{0-2} T_{0-2} I-$	3
	$F_3 O_3 A_{0-2} T_{0-2} I+$	8
$F_3 A_3$:	$F_3 O_{0-2} A_3 T_{0-2} I-$	1
	$F_3 O_{0-2} A_3 T_{0-2} I+$	17
$O_3 A_3$:	$F_{0-2} O_3 A_3 T_{0-2} I-$	8
	$F_{0-2} O_3 A_3 T_{0-2} I+$	4
$A_3 T_3$:	$F_{0-2} O_{0-2} A_3 T_3 I-$	1
	$F_{0-2} O_{0-2} A_3 T_3 I+$	1
Total		43
Three or four predominant involvements		
$F_3 O_3 A_3 T_{0-2} I-$		3
$F_3 O_3 A_3 T_{0-2} I+$		7
$F_3 O_3 A_{1-2} T_3 I-$		1
$F_3 O_3 A_3 T_3 I+$		3
Total		14
Total		180

Table 4 Endometriosis in 302 patients with unique or predominant involvement

Involvement	n
Peritoneal involvement	128
isolated; minimal or mild	30
isolated; moderate	48
major factor; severe	50
Ovarian involvement	63
isolated; moderate	16
major factor; severe	47
Adhesions	25
major factor; severe	25
Tubal involvement	86
isolated; minimal or mild	48
isolated; moderate	37
major factor; severe	1

Table 5 Endometriosis in 150 patients with multiple associated lesions

Involvement	n
Minimal/mild endometriosis	22
Peritoneal and tubal	18
Peritoneal and ovarian	2
Peritoneal, ovarian, tubal and adhesions	2
Moderate endometriosis	71
Peritoneal and ovarian	4
Peritoneal and adhesions	4
Ovarian and adhesions	2
Peritoneal and tubal	11
Peritoneal, ovarian and adhesions	16
Peritoneal, ovarian, tubal and adhesions	34
Severe endometriosis	57
Peritoneal and ovarian	11
Peritoneal and adhesions	18
Ovarian and adhesions	12
Tubal and adhesions	2
Peritoneal, ovarian and adhesions	10
Peritoneal, ovarian and tubal	1
Peritoneal, ovarian, tubal and adhesions	3

When the involvement is unique or predominant, the peritoneal endometriosis is the most frequently observed (42.5% of unique or predominant forms) and tubal endometriosis is also frequent (28.5% of unique or predominant forms).

When multiple lesions are associated, the FOATI formula gives a detailed map of pelvic endometriosis and can possibly show the efficiency of the treatment on each involvement.

The inflammatory factor increases with the severity of the lesions and is much more frequent with associated forms of endometriosis. Medical treatment and medico-surgical treatment were efficient, especially in cases of inflammatory involvement (Table 6).

Table 6 Follow-up in patients with inflammatory involvement

Severity (n)	Treatment	Outcome
Minimal/mild (2)	medical (2)	improvement (2)
Moderate (13)	medical (4)	improvement (4)
	surgical (1)	improvement (1)
	medico-surgical (8)	improvement (6)
		no improvement (2)
Severe (50)	medical (14)	improvement (10)
	surgical (4)	improvement (1)
	medico-surgical (32)	improvement (27)
		no improvement (5)

Table 7 Comparison of FOATI system with the revised American Fertility Society (AFS) classification, in a retrospective study of 459 patients

		FOATI classification		
Revised AFS stage	n	Mild/minimal	Moderate	Severe
I	167	58	90	19
II	102	2	39	61
III	82	0	14	68
IV	31	0	0	31
Unclassified	77	77	0	0

FOATI compared with the revised AFS classification

In the 167 patients considered as stage I in the revised AFS classification, only 58 patients have been scored as minimal and mild with the FOATI classification. Ninety patients were scored as having moderate forms and 19 as having severe forms.

In the stage II revised AFS patients (102), two patients were classified as having mild endometriosis (FOATI), 39 as having moderate forms and 61 as having severe forms (60% of patients with stage III revised AFS disease were considered as affected by a severe involvement of endometriosis). In the stage III revised AFS patients (82), 14 patients were scored as having moderate forms by FOATI and 68 as having severe forms.

All the patients with stage IV revised AFS disease (31) were scored as having severe forms. It appears that the FOATI classification is able to define an undisputable form of minimal endometriosis. Severe endometriosis is also clearly described. These comparisons are summarized in Table 7.

Summary

The simultaneous use of the revised AFS and FOATI classifications has appeared easy to all gynecologists who participated in this study. The set-up of a classification combining the advantages of both methods may then be envisaged. A study assessing its benefits or possible shortcomings could then be realized.

References

1. Hammond, C.B. and Haney, A.F. (1978). Conservative treatment of endometriosis. *Fertil. Steril.*, **30**, 497–509
2. American Fertility Society (1979). Classification of endometriosis. *Fertil. Steril.*, **32**, 633–4
3. Canis, M., Bouquet de Jolinieres, J., Wattiez, A., Pouly, J.L., Mage, G., Manhes, H. and Bruhat, M.A. (1993). Classification of endometriosis. *Baill. Clin. Obstet. Gynecol.*, **7**, 758–72
4. Wilson, E.A. (1987). Classification of endometriosis. In Wilson, E.A. (ed.) *Endometriosis*, pp. 78–89. (New York: A.R. Lisse)
5. Brosens, I., Donnez, J. and Benagiano, G. (1993). Improving the classification of endometriosis. *Hum. Reprod.*, **8**, 1792–5
6. Dubuisson, J.B. and Chapron, C. (1994). Classification of endometriosis. The need for modification. *Hum. Reprod.*, **9**, 2214–6

7. Buttram, V.C. (1978). An expanded classification of endometriosis. *Fertil. Steril.*, **30**, 240–2
8. Acosta, A.A., Buttram, V.C., Besch, P.K., Malinak, L.R., Frankin, R.R. and Vanderheyden, J.D. (1973). A proposed classification of pelvic endometriosis. *Obstet. Gynecol.*, **42**, 19–23
9. Kistner, R.W., Siegler, A.M. and Behrman, S.J. (1977). Suggested classification of endometriosis: relation to infertility. *Fertil. Steril.*, **28**, 1008–10
10. American Fertility Society (1985). Revised American Fertility Society classification of endometriosis. *Fertil. Steril.*, **43**, 351–2
11. Donnez, J., Nisolle, M., Casanas-Roux, F., Bassil, S. and Anaf, V. (1995). Rectovaginal septum endometriosis or adenomyosis: laparoscopic management in a series of 231 patients. *Hum. Reprod.*, **10**, 630–5
12. Koninckx, P.R., Oosterlynck, D., d'Hooghe, T. and Meuleman, C. (1994). Deeply infiltrating endometriosis is a disease whereas mild endometriosis could be considered a non-disease. *Ann. NY Acad. Sci.*, **734**, 333–41
13. Nezhat, C., Nezhat, F., Nezhat, C. and Seidman, D.S. (1994). Improving the classification of endometriotic ovarian cysts. *Hum. Reprod.*, **9**, 2212–13
14. Venturini, P.L., Semino, A. and De Cecco, L. (1995). The biological basis of medical treatment of endometriosis. *Gynecol. Endocrinol.*, **9**, 259–66
15. Guerriero, S., Mais, V., Ajossa, S., Paoletti, A.M., Angiolucci, M. and Melis, G.B. (1996). Transvaginal ultrasonography combined with CA 125 plasma levels in the diagnosis of endometrioma. *Fertil. Steril.*, **65**, 293–8
16. Kurjak, A. and Kupesic, S. (1994). Scoring system for prediction of ovarian endometriosis based on transvaginal color and pulsed Doppler sonography. *Fertil. Steril.*, **62**, 81–8
17. Musset, R., Netter, A., Poitou, P. and Rioux, J. (1977). *Précis d'Hystérosalpingographie Société Canadienne de la Fertilité.* (Québec: Les Presses de l'Université Laval)
18. Querleu, D., Boutteville, C., Notteau, G. and Crepin, G. (1987). Indirect hysterosalpingographic findings related to endometriosis. In Bruhat, M.A. and Canis, M. (eds.) *Endometriosis, Contributions to Gynecology and Obstetrics 16*, p. 320. Québec: Les Presses de l'Université Laval
19. Takahashi, K., Okada, S., Okada, M., Kitao, M., Kaji, Y. and Sugimara, K. (1996). Magnetic resonance imaging and serum CA 125 in evaluating patients with endometriomas prior to medical therapy. *Fertil. Steril.*, **65**, 288–92
20. Arrive, L., Hirical, H. and Martine, M.C. (1989). Pelvic endometriosis magnetic resonance imaging. *Radiology*, **171**, 687–92
21. Koninckx, P.R., Meuleman, C., Oosterlynck, D. and Cornillie, F.J. (1996). Diagnosis of deep endometriosis by clinical examination during menstruation and plasma CA-125 concentration. *Fertil. Steril.*, **65**, 280–7
22. Belaisch, J. and Madelenat, P. (1985). Les deux endométrioses. *Brochure du GEE*, Paris: Laboratoires Winthrop
23. Hubert, D. (1996). Thèse Médicale Maternités de Roubaix et Lille: Endometriose et Stérilité
24. Audebert, A., Bäckström, T., Barlow, D.H., Bengiano, G., Brosens, I., Bühler, K., Donnez, J., Evers, J.L.H., Pellicer, A., Mettler, L., Rönnberg, L. Smith. S.K. and Thomas, E.J. (1992). Endometriosis 1991: a discussion document. *Hum. Reprod.*, **7**, 432–5
25. Evers, J.L. (1994). Endometriosis does not exist; all women have endometriosis. *Hum. Reprod.*, **9**, 2206–9
26. Brosens, I.A. (1994). New principles in the management of endometriosis. *Acta Obstet. Gynecol. Scand.*, **159**(Suppl.), 18–21
27. Canis, M., Pouly, J.L., Wattiez, A., Manhes, H., Mage, G. and Bruhat, M.A. (1992). Incidence of bilateral adnexal disease in severe endometriosis (revised American Fertility Society (AFS) stage IV): should a stage V be included in the AFS classification? *Fertil. Steril.*, **57**, 691–2
28. Vercellini, P. and Crosignani, P.G. (1994). New guidelines are needed for the treatment of endometriosis. *Hum. Reprod.*, **9**, 2205–6
29. Tran, D.K. (1994). Classification de l'endometriose externe par la méthode FOATI. *Contracept. Fertil. Sex.*, **22**(Suppl. 12), 817–23

Section 6

Surgical treatment

Operative endoscopy and videolaparoscopy: a 20th century surgical revolution

C. Nezhat, F. Nezhat, C.H. Nezhat and S. Tazuke

Introduction

The first attempt at endoscopy was by Philip Bozzini of Italy in 1805, using a tube and a candle. After Jacobaeus of Sweden first induced pneumoperitoneum and placed a Nitze cystoscope into the peritoneal cavity in 1910, the technique was applied to diagnostic and simple sterilization procedures by Kalk in Germany and by Ruddock and Hope in the United States in the 1930s[1]. In the late 1940s, Raoul Palmer of France was the main promoter of laparoscopy in gynecology. He reported the first human tubal fulguration in 1962[1]. Victor Gomel began reporting the merits and safety of operative laparoscopy in the early 1970s[2].

At the same time, Kurt Semm headed the German-based Kiel School's development of instruments for use in operative laparoscopy, particularly fertility-enhancing procedures[3]. Bruhat and colleagues[4] and Tadir and associates[5] were among the first to report laser laparoscopy. Unfortunately, laser laparoscopy was still subject to the following limitations and not frequently used.

The advantages of operative laparoscopy were diminished by three serious drawbacks. First, the surgeon had to work crouched over the patient and had to peer with one eye through the laparoscope. Visibility was limited, the position was uncomfortable and the surgeon's back was easily fatigued. Second, the rest of the surgical team was unable to view the procedure and, as a result, was prevented from anticipating the surgeon's needs. Third, the auxiliary instruments were not available to perform procedures more complicated than tubal ligation.

In the late 1970s, we started using a video camera attached to the eyepiece of the laparoscope in human and animal laboratories[6]. The camera magnified the image and projected it onto monitors in the operating room. The major disadvantages of the laparoscope were eliminated, but the early cameras were cumbersome and the first videolaparoscopic surgery on humans was difficult because of the weight of the camera, inadequate light source, and poor resolution. As a result, its usage was not recommended and was even criticized by some (personal references available). However, the senior author persisted in using and promulgating videolaparoscopy. In the early 1980s, equipment companies began to recognize the potential market for a miniature video camera and produced lighter versions with higher resolution and better light sources. With these final modifications, all the elements were in place by 1983–84 for a revolution in abdominal and pelvic surgery[7]. As Tadir and associates stated, 'If there was a single factor that contributed to the increased interest in laparoscopic surgery, it was undoubtedly the incorporation of video equipment as an integral part of the standard endoscopic set enthusiastically promoted by Nezhat'[8].

At the combined annual meetings of the American Fertility Society and the Canadian Fertility and Andrology Society in November 1986, the senior author presented the benefits of videolaparoscopy and the results of over 600 endometriosis surgical operations performed using this technique[7]. Using the more refined cameras combined with the CO_2 laser and laparoscope, we successfully performed laparoscopic procedures on over 1000 patients, including those with extensive endometriosis[9]. Through the publication of both case reports and results of detailed studies, as well as through national and international meetings, we have promulgated the use of videolaparoscopy in abdominal surgery (benign and malignant pathology)[10–15], gastroenterology[16,17] and urology[18]. Awareness of the technique was finally created when patients recommended the procedure to acquaintances. Media attention[19–21] and word-of-mouth made operative laparoscopy one of the first truly consumer-driven medical advances.

Operative videolaparoscopy offers several benefits over an open procedure. First, pelvic and abdominal anatomy are magnified by the video camera and laparoscope, allowing the surgeon to perform microsurgical procedures. Second, the pressure created by pneumoperitoneum decreases bleeding and provides a cleaner operating field. Third, such areas as the upper abdomen, posterior cul-de-sac and posterior aspect of the broad ligaments may be more thoroughly evaluated, and with technological advances such as the development of the CO_2 laser, disease may be treated more precisely and, possibly, with a greater margin of safety. Fourth, operative laparoscopy produces fewer *de novo* adhesions[22,23] and requires a shorter recovery period. Finally, when performed by a trained and experienced surgeon, the occurrences of intraoperative and postoperative complications and morbidity are fewer than with laparotomy. An added benefit of the addition of video may be the permanent record created by taping the procedure, which may be used for future reference. This tape can be used to demonstrate techniques to other physicians, explain a procedure to a patient, review a patient's condition should further treatment become necessary, or provide information for research.

Hysterectomy

Laparoscopic hysterectomy may be defined as the complete endoscopic excision of the uterus from its attachments. In a total hysterectomy, the vaginal cuff may be repaired laparoscopically or vaginally. In a laparoscopic supracervical hysterectomy, the cervical stump is closed laparoscopically. All other combinations are variations of laparoscopically assisted vaginal hysterectomy[6,24,25].

Gynecologists recognize that vaginal hysterectomy patients experience less postoperative morbidity and pain and require a shorter period of recuperation when compared to patients having abdominal hysterectomies. However, approximately 70% of hysterectomies are still done by laparotomy. Laparoscopic and laparoscopically assisted vaginal hysterectomies have been introduced to provide an alternative to abdominal hysterectomy. Preliminary results confirm less intraoperative blood loss and shorter recuperation, without increased risk of complications[6,14,25].

Laparoscopic inspection and management, including adhesiolysis, endometriosis vaporization or excision, and salpingo-oophorectomy when indicated, are accomplished as described previously[26]. The uterus may then be removed by a standard vaginal hysterectomy technique, retaining the laparoscope for later inspection of the surgical site, or the procedure may be continued laparoscopically.

After evaluating the ureters, the infundibulopelvic ligament (or utero-ovarian ligament if the adnexa are to be retained) and the round ligament are desiccated, suture-ligated, or clipped using an automatic stapling device, then incised. Hydrodissection is used to create a bladder flap, which is then incised with a CO_2 laser or scissors. The upper portion of the broad ligament is coagulated and incised anteriorly and posteriorly. The uterine vessels are identified, skeletonized, coagulated and divided. A blackened right-angle retractor placed in the vagina allows posterior and anterior culdotomy incisions to be accomplished with the CO_2 laser or other cutting modalities.

The uterosacral ligament and the base of the cardinal ligament are approached vaginally, clamped and incised. The uterus is removed, and the vaginal mucosa is closed using a standard vaginal hysterectomy technique.

We do not advocate converting vaginal hysterectomies to laparoscopic or laparoscopically assisted vaginal hysterectomies. Rather, the laparoscopic approach is an appropriate alternative to those procedures that otherwise would require laparotomy[6,25,27].

Myomectomy

Patients with indications for laparoscopic myomectomy may be managed with gonadotropin-releasing hormone analogs for up to 3 months preoperatively. Reducing tumor size, improving operative handling, and reducing intraoperative blood loss are theoretical advantages. Three months of amenorrhea does improve preoperative hematocrit levels. However, patients are also given the option of autologous blood donation[6,28].

Laparoscopic myomectomy has two stages. The first, removing the tumor from the uterus, is generally straightforward. The second, however, removing the tumor from the abdomen, can be long and tedious[6].

A pedunculated myoma is simply excised at the stalk and bleeding is controlled with a bipolar electrocoagulator. For intramural or subserosal myomata, 5–10 ml of dilute vasopressin (20 U in 100 ml of sterile saline) is injected under the capsule. The capsule is incised and gradually dissected using a combination of suction-irrigator probe and hydrodissection. Traction on the myomas can be produced with a small hook or claw forceps. The myometrial defect is closed with 0 or 2-0 Vicryl and the subserosa is closed using 4-0 polydioxanone endosutures (Ethicon). Intraligamentous myoma are approached by incising the anterior or posterior leaf of the broad ligament (depending on the location of the myoma) after identifying the location of large vessels, ureter and bladder. Excision is then accomplished as described for subserosal myomas.

The basic surgical principles for myomectomy are identifying and removing the tumor, permanent hemostasis and eliminating the dead space. The problem in laparoscopic removal of myoma remains its extraction from the abdominal cavity, although this has been simplified by the availability of an electric morcellator[6].

Posterior colpotomy, when feasible, is the technically acceptable route for the removal of large (>5 cm) and multiple leiomyomas. Morcellation in the posterior cul-de-sac by the assistant becomes an additional option.

The strength of the uterus after laparoscopic myomectomy is unknown and must be determined to predict the ability of the organ to withstand labor and delivery. Although uterine healing appears adequate after removal of small myomas, indentations have been noted on removal of larger lesions without suturing, which might represent structural defects. Even when endosutures are applied, the meticulous reapproximation of layers available by microsurgical laparotomy is very difficult during laparoscopy. There have been reports of uterine fistula and rupture during pregnancy[29,30]. In certain cases, such as in women who wish to reproduce in the future and have deep intramural myoma(s) >5 cm, and in patients with multiple large myomas, we have replaced laparoscopic myomectomy with a modified procedure using a combination of operative laparoscopy and minilaparotomy. It is technically less difficult than laparoscopic myomectomy, allows better closure of the uterine defect and may require less time to perform[6,30]. The procedure is performed by using laparoscopy to treat associated pathology, to identify the leiomyoma(s) and bring it to a minilaparotomy incision, and to remove blood clots and debris by irrigation at the end of the procedure. Through this incision, the leiomyoma(s) is grasped, shelled and morcellated, and the uterine defect is repaired in layers.

Oophorectomy and adnexal mass management

Although the laparoscope has been proven to be a safe and effective diagnostic and therapeutic tool in the hands of experienced laparoscopists, doubts remain about the laparoscopist's ability to diagnose and properly manage early ovarian cancer if the adnexal mass is found to be malignant[31]. One of the chief concerns is that spillage of a cancer confined to the ovary may worsen prognosis. However, when an experienced surgeon follows proper protocol, adnexal masses may be safely evaluated, and the majority may be treated laparoscopically. In premenopausal women with ovarian cysts, factors to consider besides malignancy are avoiding the resection of normal ovarian tissue, and traumatization which may result in adhesion formation.

Patients should be evaluated clinically with a pelvic examination and vaginal ultrasound study, along with a review of previous intraoperative records. Simple (unilocular) cysts in premenopausal women are suppressed initially with hormonal suppressive therapy using oral contraceptive pills containing $50\,\mu g$ of estrogen, Depo-Provera or danazol (Upjohn, Kalamazoo, MI, USA). A blood sample for the serum CA-125 level or other tumor marker, if indicated, should also be obtained and saved. CA-125 measurement and ultrasonographic examination have more value in evaluating postmenopausal women than premenopausal women[32].

Intraoperative management of all patients with masses is carefully standardized and includes inspecting the pelvis, ovaries, upper abdomen and diaphragmatic surfaces for any vegetation or other sign of malignancy. Peritoneal washings are obtained for cytology. If a strong suspicion of malignancy based on intraoperative findings exists, an attempt is made to obtain frozen section biopsies without rupturing the cyst. If that is not possible, the laparoscopic procedure is terminated, and the patient will undergo a laparotomy[6].

Management of the cystic mass itself includes aspirating the fluid, followed by opening the cyst and inspecting the wall for excrescences or irregular thickening. Frozen section biopsies are obtained if the surgeon thinks that any surfaces appear suspicious. Finally, depending on the patient's age and pertinent clinical history, an ovarian cystectomy or oophorectomy may be performed[12]. Scissors, unipolar electrocoagulation or a CO_2 laser (set at 30–80 W in the ultrapulse mode) may be used to cut, and a bipolar electrocoagulator may be used for desiccation of the infundibulopelvic ligament. After exploration of the pelvis and abdomen, oophorectomy is carried out as previously described[6]. Thorough irrigation is necessary to clean the incision. After removal of the cyst, the abdominal and pelvic cavities are washed thoroughly with copious amounts of irrigation fluid, especially in cases of endometriomas, dermoid cysts or mucinous cystadenomas[6].

Before terminating the procedure, any associated pelvic pathology, such as endometriosis or other adhesions, is treated, and hemostasis is assured. Women who have undergone ovarian cystectomy for benign ovarian neoplasms (mucinous or serous cystadenomas or cystic teratomas) are followed up by a biannual pelvic examination and an ultrasound examination to look for possible recurrence at both 6 weeks and 6 months postoperatively[33].

We believe that laparoscopic evaluation and management of a benign adnexal mass performed by experienced operative laparoscopists is safe. However, no substitute exists for sound clinical judgment. A surgeon should perform the techniques he or she is comfortable with and should conduct careful preoperative patient screenings[34].

Laparoscopic ovarian cystectomy has been performed successfully during pregnancy[35]. Proper patient selection and operator experience are critical. The patient's consent should include acknowledgement that operative laparoscopy is not the standard treatment at this time and that spontaneous abortion or premature labor is possible with any surgery during pregnancy. The 10-mm trocar placement is adjusted to 6 cm or higher above the umbilicus, and pneumoperitoneum is established at less than 10 mmHg. The remaining trocars are inserted under direct visualization, and no intracervical instruments are used. Any manipulation of the uterus is accomplished gently with intra-abdominal instruments.

We have performed a laparoscopic hysterectomy and staging for a borderline ovarian tumor, without compromising the patient's prognosis[24]. As long as the metastasis and spread of the tumor are not bulky, we believe that even stage III ovarian cancer can be treated and excised laparoscopically, and removed vaginally by an experienced surgeon. The only limit to this approach is in treating advanced stages of ovarian cancer that require extensive debulking[36-38].

During our use of operative laparoscopy to manage other gynecological malignancies, we have noted several encouraging results that lead us to believe that this technique may be used more extensively in treating malignant conditions in the future. In our opinion, the applications of this technique extend beyond ovarian cancer, to endometrial and cervical cancer as well. For example, we believe that any stage of endometrial cancer can be managed laparoscopically, and that a longer portion of the vagina can be removed than with laparotomy. Furthermore, stage IA2 cervical cancer with lymphatic channel involvement, stage IB and stage IIA (especially when the lesion extends into the vagina) can be effectively managed by operative laparoscopy. For stages IIB and higher, the technique is useful for node dissection, and can be used to change the FIGO staging to clinical staging. Finally, we believe that operative laparoscopy can be used to assist pelvic exenteration[6].

Endometrioma

Superficial endometriosis of the ovaries can be treated by vaporization. Because small endometriomas (< 2 cm) tend to be fibrotic and difficult to remove, they can be biopsied and then vaporized. However, larger endometriomas must be removed completely, including the capsule, to reduce the risk of recurrence[39]. Simple aspiration or fenestration of endometriomas can lead to an unacceptably high level of recurrence[6,39-41].

Management of endometriomas must be approached in the same way as all other adnexal masses, keeping in mind that endometrioid carcinoma can coexist with endometriosis and is indistinguishable at surgery until histological results are reported[34].

When endometriomas are suspected on the basis of ultrasound appearance or previous operative reports, hormonal suppressive therapy (danazol or gonadotropin-releasing hormone (GnRH) analogs) given for 6–8 weeks preoperatively will reduce vascularity and suppress ovarian activity[42]. Consequently, intraoperative hemorrhage will be reduced, surgical manipulation of follicular or corpus luteum cysts will be avoided, and more of the normal ovarian tissue will be preserved. Similarly, 6 weeks of postoperative suppressive therapy in cases of endometrioma removal will, in our opinion, facilitate better healing. For patients who are not interested in achieving pregnancy, we suppress ovulation with oral contraceptives indefinitely.

The laparoscopic approach to an endometrioma is as follows. The cyst is first aspirated and drained through an 18-gauge aspiration needle inserted through one of the suprapubic portals. After copious irrigation of the cyst and pelvis, the cyst wall is opened further and inspected. The capsule is stripped from the ovarian stroma using two grasping forceps or excised and submitted for histological examination. Hydrodissection can be used for easier removal of the ovarian cyst capsule[43]. The ovarian defect is left to heal without suturing. If the edges of the ovarian capsule do not approximate spontaneously, one or two 4–0 PDS endosutures (Ethicon) may be used inside the ovary to approximate the edges together. It is important to keep in mind that fewer sutures will result in fewer adhesions[6,40,44].

Ovarian remnant management

With advances in the laparoscopic technique, more complicated conditions, such as ovarian remnant, which usually involves the bowel, bladder and ureter with dense adhesions, can be treated laparoscopically. For patients who have undergone previous laparotomy, the laparoscope should be inserted following a mapping technique[6,26,45].

Adhesions involving the bowel surface are injected with lactated Ringer's solution above the serosa, creating a plane of cleavage and a safe zone for laser incision[46]. Ovarian tissue embedded in the muscularis of the bowel is removed. In cases of enterotomy, the bowel is repaired with one to three interrupted 4–0 PDS endosutures or 0 Vicryl in one layer[47,48]. All patients have reported excellent results. Depending on concomitant procedures, patients may be discharged within 24–72 h of surgery. Excellent results with few complications have been reported with this technique[6,45].

Peritoneal endometriosis

Since the CO_2 laser does not penetrate water, a fluid backstop (hydrodissection) allows the surgeon to work on selected tissue with a more comfortable margin than would otherwise be available[46].

To treat endometriosis of the bladder flap, for example, an aspiration needle is used to inject 20–30 ml of lactated Ringer's solution subperitoneally in an avascular area approximately 2 cm from the endometrial lesion. This elevates the peritoneum and backs it with a fluid bed. A 0.5-cm incision is made with the laser on this elevation, through which 100–200 ml of lactated Ringer's solution is injected subperitoneally. The lesion may then be vaporized or excised using the CO_2 laser in the ultrapulse mode. For excision, a circular line is made with a radius of 0.5 cm from the lesion. The peritoneum is grasped and pulled away with the help of the CO_2 laser and the tip of a suction-irrigator probe.

When endometriosis forms scarring to the subperitoneal connective tissue, creating openings as described and injecting fluid on the lesion's lateral sides allows water to tunnel under the lesion. This often separates scarring, and the implant can then be vaporized or removed. Irrigation and washing should follow to remove all by-products and ensure complete treatment of the disease. More extensive endometriosis may be treated after removing the peritoneum, again followed by irrigation and washing.

Proper use of hydrodissection allows experienced laparoscopic surgeons to treat mild to extensive endometriosis with the CO_2 laser not only more thoroughly but also more safely than was previously possible[49].

Manipulation of and trauma to the pelvic organs should be kept to a minimum. Any excessive resection, vaporization, coagulation or manipulation in this area may predispose the patient to adhesion formation. Rock has reported good results using electrocoagulation to treat endometriosis[50].

Presacral neurectomy

Presacral neurectomy offers a surgical alternative for the amelioration of intractable dysmenorrhea[51]. Originally introduced in 1899, it fell into disfavor as a result of poor patient selection and with the introduction of non-steroidal anti-inflammatory drugs, oral contraceptives, danazol and GnRH analogs. Despite the overall success of medical therapy, approximately 30% of patients fail to obtain relief[52]. Until recently, presacral neurectomy was performed by laparotomy, limiting its application to women who had incapacitating dysmenorrhea and central pain unresponsive to medical therapy or who were undergoing laparotomy for other pelvic pathological conditions. However, recent advances in endoscopic surgery now permit a laparoscopic approach to classical presacral neurectomy in women with primary and secondary dysmenorrhea and in endometriosis-associated dysmenorrhea and central pelvic pain, where medical therapy has failed to provide adequate relief.

The sacral promontory, ureters and iliac vessels are identified. The peritoneum overlying the sacral promontory is elevated by smooth grasping forceps, and a small opening is made in the peritoneum. A suction-irrigator probe is inserted into the incision, and the peritoneum is elevated from the underlying tissue using hydrodissection[46,51]. The peritoneum is incised vertically and horizontally and extended cephalad to just below the aortic bifurcation. Bleeding points are controlled with a bipolar electrocoagulator. The following landmarks are identified beneath the peritoneum: common iliac arteries, ureter, and inferior mesenteric, superior hemorrhoidal and midsacral arteries. The loose areolar tissue is excised to gain access to the presacral nerves. Care should be exercised in clearing the areolar tissue. Bleeding in this area is difficult to control even at laparotomy. The hypogastric nerve bundle is identified, grasped and skeletonized as necessary to isolate the superior hypogastric plexus. A 3–4-cm segment of nerve tissue is excised.

Bowel endometriosis

As with other organs, the etiology of bowel endometriosis is unknown. Its occurrence was reported as early as 1922 by Sampson[53]. Following his investigation of 19 cases, he proposed that 'implantation adenoma of endometrial type of some portion of the intestinal tract may be present in at least one half of the cases of perforated ovarian hematoma of endometrial type with peritoneal implantations'[53].

Intestinal endometriosis has been reported to affect between 3 and 37% of women with endometriosis. In a series of 1573 women treated consecutively for endometriosis, 5.4% had gastrointestinal involvement. Of these, 65% had endometriosis of the rectum and rectosigmoid colon[54]. In another series of 1000 celiotomies, Williams and Pratt found that 485 women had endometriosis of which 181 (37%) had gastrointestinal involvement. Of these, 172 (95%) had rectosigmoid involvement, nine (5%) had ileal involvement and 19 (10%) had appendiceal involvement[55]. Bowel resection with or without castration has been suggested to treat symptomatic patients[54,56]. Coronado and colleagues[57] have reported satisfactory pain relief and pregnancy rates following anterior wall resection of the colon by laparotomy for deeply infiltrating lower colorectal endometriosis.

Bowel involvement is suggested by palpable tumor in the rectovaginal septum, gastrointestinal symptoms such as rectal bleeding, constipation or diarrhea associated with menses, or pain that persists after surgical removal of all recognizable lesions.

Endometriotic nodularity of the bowel and rectovaginal septum is one of the most difficult aspects of this disease to approach surgically. Because gynecologists are uncomfortable operating on the bowel and general surgeons may not be familiar with endometriosis, these cases have at times required bowel resection or temporary colostomy. Some have shown that when full-thickness bowel resection and immediate reanastomosis are performed by a surgical team familiar with the disease, low morbidity and good long-term relief of symptoms can be expected[57].

Because colorectal endometriosis is generally superficial, bowel resection should remain the last resort. We have been able to treat nearly all cases involving the rectum, rectovaginal septum, and large or small bowel laparoscopically or laparoscopically-assisted.

Women with endometriosis of the lower colon, rectum, uterosacral ligaments or rectovaginal septum often present with chronic pelvic pain, and dysmenorrhea, dyspareunia, back pain, dyschezia, constipation or diarrhea, or infertility with pelvic pain. Most women with small bowel or appendiceal endometriosis are usually asymptomatic, but may experience symptoms such as nausea and vomiting, especially in conjunction with menstruation. They rarely experience bowel obstruction.

Surgical procedures

Operative laparoscopy of the gastrointestinal tract is performed for the treatment of endometrial implants on the intestinal wall, appendix or rectovaginal space. Surgical repair of the bowel may be necessary, even in patients whose endometriosis does not invade the lumen of the gastrointestinal tract, for the repair of incidental injuries occurring during laparoscopic treatment of endometriosis in other areas of the pelvic/abdominal cavity.

Operative videolaparoscopy of the gastrointestinal tract includes lysis of bowel adhesions, as well as the treatment of superficial, infiltrative and full thickness involvement with or without stricture of the appendix, rectosigmoid colon, rectovaginal septum or small bowel.

To prepare a patient for operative laparoscopy, the surgeon should follow a protocol similar to that for laparotomy, including preoperative mechanical and antibiotic bowel preparation, as well as thorough clinical and laboratory evaluation[6].

Treatment of appendiceal endometriosis

Because approximately 50% of appendiceal lesions are detected only by palpation and may be missed by visual inspection alone, incidental appendectomy is recommended in patients with severe endometriosis[6]. We use the following technique to remove the appendix when indicated.

Appendectomy may be a primary procedure or may be performed concomitantly with other pelvic or abdominal surgeries. The incidental finding of appendiceal endometriosis or other appendiceal pathology during routine gynecological cases, and patients' frequent desire for appendectomy at the time of gynecological surgery warrant a thorough knowledge of appendectomy technique by gynecological surgeons.

Preparation for appendectomy includes inserting grasping forceps through the lower right quadrant trocar sleeve and passing the bipolar electrocoagulator and suction-irrigator probe through the midline and lower left quadrant punctures, respectively. Next, with the video laparoscope system in the umbilical channel, the appendix is located. The appendix is mobilized and examined following lysis of periappendiceal or pericecal adhesions as necessary, proceeding carefully in case of attachment to the lateral pelvic wall or retrocecal appendix. Two chromic Endoloop sutures (Ethicon) or polydioxanone sutures (Ethicon) are passed over the base of the appendix 2–5 mm from the cecum and then tied, one on top of the other. A third Endoloop suture is applied < 1 cm distal to the other sutures and then cut long, leaving a 15-cm tail to facilitate retrieval should the appendix inadvertently fall into the pelvic well. The appendix is cut between the second and third sutures placed.

The appendix is removed from the abdomen with a long grasping forceps passed through the operating channel of the laparoscope, suprapubically with the short grasper or with an Endopouch tissue removal bag (Ethicon). If appropriate, an appendix extractor may be placed via the sleeve of a 10-mm trocar, replacing the central 5-mm one. Instruments, which may be contaminated, are removed from the surgical area. Finally, the appendiceal stump and other operative sites are inspected for hemostasis and then irrigated with lactated Ringer's solution containing antibiotic solution.

Appendectomies may last from 4 to 21 min. Postoperative instructions should include avoiding solid food for 24 h. Otherwise, instructions are routine for gynecological procedures, including an outpatient evaluation the day after surgery[6].

Endometriosis of the rectosigmoid, rectovaginal septum and cul-de-sac

Most cases of rectal and rectovaginal septum endometriosis can be managed with outpatient videolaparoscopy and do not require bowel resection[58].

Location and assessment of the ureters before proceeding with this procedure is of paramount importance, especially when they are infiltrated by endometriosis. Any alteration in the direction of the ureters should be identified prior to surgery. Because ureters are lateral to the uterosacral ligament, we try to stay between the ligaments as much as possible.

Endometriosis rarely penetrates the mucosa of the colon but it commonly involves the serosa, subserosa and muscularis. The disease can be excised or vaporized thoroughly by an experienced videolaparoscopist. When major portions of both muscularis layers have been excised or vaporized, and the mucosa is reached, the bowel wall may be reinforced by sutures. The procedure is very demanding and requires maximal co-operation between the assistant and the surgeon[40].

Bowel resection

In cases of severe endometriosis of the bowel wall, bowel resection may be necessary. The technique includes laparoscopic mobilization of the lower colon followed by transvaginal/transanal prolapse or transabdominal exteriorization, and then resection and reanastomosis[16,59–62]. When the lesion involves only the anterior rectal wall near the anal verge, as in laparotomy, the rectovaginal septum is delineated by simultaneous vaginal and rectal examinations performed by an assistant. The rectum is mobilized along the rectovaginal septum. Mobilization continues along the left and right pararectal spaces by electrodesiccating and dividing branches of the hemorrhoidal artery, and partially posteriorly as well. When the rectum is sufficiently mobilized, the tumor is prolapsed to the level of the vagina or anus, the perineal body is retracted, and an RL 30 (Ethicon) multifire stapler is applied across the segment of the anterior rectal wall containing the nodule. Two staple applications may be required to traverse the width of the involved mucosa. The tumor nodule is excised using electrosurgery, and two additional interrupted 2–0 polyglactin sutures are inserted along the staple line. The rectum is returned to the pelvis under direct visualization, and closure is confirmed by insufflating the rectum with air while the cul-de-sac is filled with lactated Ringer's.

In patients with more extensive involvement and circumferential lesions, as in laparotomy, the entire rectum is mobilized, the lateral rectal pedicles are electrodesiccated, and the presacral space is entered to the level of the levator ani muscles in order to mobilize the bowel. The branches of inferior mesenteric vessels of the bowel segment to be resected are electrodesiccated and cut. The rectum is transected proximal to the lesion and the proximal limb is prolapsed vaginally, rectally, transabdominally or into the distal limb, using Babcock clamps. A 2–0 pursestring suture is inserted to the end of the proximal bowel to secure the opposing anvil of an ILS 29 or 33 stapler (Ethicon). The anvil is then replaced transvaginally, transanally or transabdominally via minilaparotomy into the pelvis along the with the proximal bowel. The rectal stump containing the endometrial lesion and fibrosis is then resected by the stapler or prolapsed out of the vagina, anus or abdomen via minilaparotomy by grasping the transected end of the rectal stump with Babcock clamps (Baxter Mueller, Chicago, IL, USA) and pulling it through the vaginal or anal canal, or the abdominal wall. The rectum is stapled shut with an RL 60 linear stapler (Ethicon) and the rectal specimen is resected and sent for analysis of surgical pathology. The rectal stump is reduced inside the pelvis and an end-to-end double stapled anastomosis is performed using the ILS 29 or 33 stapler

(Ethicon). The laparoscope is then used to attach the opposing anvil in the proximal bowel. The bowel ends are approximated, and the stapler is fired to complete the anastomosis. Intact 'doughnut' margins should be present. A proctoscope is used to examine the anastomosis for structural integrity and bleeding. Lactated Ringer's solution is inserted into the pelvis and visualized with the laparoscope as air is insufflated into the rectum to check for leakage. Air leaks may be corrected using laparoscopically placed 2–0 or 0 Vicryl sutures. Laparoscopic bowel resection by this technique is identical with resection at laparotomy, with the bipolar electrocoagulator and laser replacing the suture and scissors. Based on the location and extent of the disease, the above technique should be modified and tailored to each patient.

A simplified method for resection of severe endometriosis of the anterior wall of the colon may be used in certain cases[60]. The extent of the lesion is evaluated visually and by palpation using the tip of the suction-irrigator probe. If the lesion is low enough, an assistant can identify it by performing a rectal examination. A sigmoidoscope is used to further delineate the lesion and guide the surgeon.

The ureters should first be identified to avoid inadvertent injury. The lower colon is then mobilized in all aspects except posteriorly. Depending on the location of the lesion, the right pararectal area, left pararectal area, or both are entered. The colon is separated from the adjacent organs. Full-thickness excision is carried out, beginning above the area of visible disease. After identifying the normal tissue, the lesion is held at its proximal end with grasping forceps. An incision is made through the bowel serosa and muscularis, and the lumen is entered. The lesion is excised from the anterior rectal wall. After complete excision of the lesion, the pelvic cavity is irrigated and suctioned. Resected pieces of bowel are extracted through the operative channel of the laparoscope using a long grasping forceps, or from the anus using polyp forceps, and submitted for pathology.

The bowel is repaired transversely in one or two layers. Two traction sutures are applied to each side of the defect, transforming it into a transverse opening. The stay sutures are brought out through the right and left lower quadrant incisions. The sleeves are removed, then replaced in the peritoneal cavity next to the stay sutures, and the sutures are secured outside the abdomen. The bowel is then repaired by placing several interrupted through-and-through sutures in 0.4–0.6-cm increments until it is completely reanastomosed. We use 0-Vicryl or PDS laparoscopic sutures with a straight or curved needle (Ethicon), with extracorporeal knot tying. When the lesion is not very extensive and the bowel defect after resection is less than 4 cm, the bowel can be repaired vertically without causing stricture. At the end of the procedure, sigmoidoscopy is performed to ensure that the closure is airtight and that there is no bowel stricture[6,40,60].

Small bowel

The small bowel has the least involvement with endometriosis. It occasionally requires resection[6,40].

The genitourinary tract

Variable ureteral and bladder involvement have been reported in 1–11% of women diagnosed with endometriosis[63]. As the disease becomes more advanced, the ureter is vulnerable to endometriotic implant involvement. Endometriosis of the urinary tract can be superficial or invasive, and in sporadic cases, may even completely obstruct the ureter. The bladder wall is one of the sites least frequently involved with endometriosis. In fact, until recently, fewer than 180 cases have been reported[64]. Management options include hormone suppressive therapy, oophorectomy, hysterectomy and/or segmental cystectomy[65,66].

Decreased bladder capacity and bladder instability unresponsive to conventional therapy may be due to endometriosis. If endometriosis of the urinary tract is suspected, a complete preoperative evaluation should be performed including an intravenous pyelogram, ultrasound scan of the kidneys, and routine blood and urine workup. In selected cases where patients present recurrent hematuria, cystoscopy may be indicated.

Treatment of genitourinary tract implants

Most superficial implants of endometriosis over the ureter and the bladder can be safely treated by operative laparoscopy, utilizing hydrodissection and the CO_2 laser (or any other cutting modality). Before the introduction of hydrodissection and the CO_2 laser to the operative laparoscopic treatment of endometriosis, sensitive areas at risk of injury, such as bowel, ureter, bladder and major blood vessels, were often excluded from surgical intervention[67,68]. This omission was serious because the patient often continued to have symptoms after surgical therapy. Hydrodissection makes treatment with the CO_2 laser in these high-risk areas safer. Because the CO_2 laser beam does not penetrate fluid, treatment can be confined to the endometriotic lesion yet leave adjacent normal tissue unharmed. By creating a bed of fluid beneath the peritoneum, the risk of laser beam penetration to underlying tissue is reduced.

Superficial implants over the ureter can generally be treated by the CO_2 laser and a variation of hydrodissection. Approximately 20–30 ml of lactated Ringer's solution is injected subperitoneally on the lateral pelvic wall, elevating the peritoneum and backing it with a bed of fluid. The CO_2 laser is then used to create a 0.5-cm opening on this elevation. The peritoneum is opened anteriorly and laterally, close to the corresponding round ligament. The hydrodissection probe is then inserted into the opening and approximately 100 ml of lactated Ringer's is injected under 300-mmHg pressure into the retroperitoneal space along the course of the ureter. The fluid surrounds the ureter, moves it posteriorly and allows superficial CO_2 laser dissection or vaporization of the area.

After creating the water bed, a superpulse or ultrapulse mode of the CO_2 laser of between 20 and 80 W is used for vaporization or excision of the lesion, which should be performed with a circumference of 1–2 cm. When the lesions are large or excision is preferred, a circular line with a 1–2-cm margin is made around the lesion. The peritoneum is then grasped with an atraumatic grasping forceps and peeled away with the help of the CO_2 laser and the tip of the suction-irrigator probe. If the endometrial implant is infiltrative and has formed scarring down to the subperitoneal connective tissue, hydrodissection should be extended. By injecting around the lesion, fluid 'tunnels' beneath the lesion, which often separates the scar tissue. The lesion can then be safely treated. After vaporization or excision of these lesions, the area must be carefully irrigated to remove all remaining carbonization and verify that all remaining endometriosis has been properly treated.

Obstructed ureter

In severe cases of endometriosis, the implants may invade periureteral tissue or the ureter muscularis and cause partial or complete obstruction. The incidence of ureteral obstruction due to endometriosis is low. Most gynecologists will never encounter this entity. However, as this complication has severe effects on the patient's quality of life, any surgeon treating endometriosis must be thoroughly acquainted with the modes of treatment available. Conventional therapy consists of laparotomy and resection of the obstructed segment of the ureter[18,69].

Superficial endometriosis and fibrosis can be vaporized or excised as previously described.

However, if the ureter is obstructed partially or completely and requires resection, a retrograde ureteral catheter is placed via cystoscopy with laparoscopic guidance. Partial wall resection is carried out over the catheter. Pinpoint entries to the lumen do not usually require repair, but do require prolonged stent placement (4–6 weeks).

When the lumen is invaded, the ureter can be repaired with one to three interrupted 4–0 PDS sutures. If the lumen is completely occluded and retrograde catheter placement is unsuccessful, the ureter may be transected at that point using the laser and excising the obstructed section. Indigo carmine is injected antegrade to verify patency of the proximal lumen[18,69]. Anastomosis is performed over the ureteral catheter with four interrupted through-and-through 4–0 PDS sutures at 3, 6, 9 and 12 o'clock to approximate the proximal and distal ureteral segments or to rejoin the ureter and bladder using intracorporeal or extracorporeal knot tying. The ureteral stents can be removed 2–8 weeks postoperatively after the integrity of the repair is confirmed by intravenous pyelogram.

Bladder endometriosis

Using hydrodissection, the peritoneum over the bladder is opened and a bladder flap is created. The bladder is entered via cystotomy and the involved areas are resected using the CO_2 laser (or any other cutting modality)[70]. Simultaneous cystoscopy is performed to improve observation of the ureteral orifices and for retrograde catheterization. The defect is closed in one layer using extracorporeal or intracorporeal knot-tying techniques with 4–0 PDS or 0 polyglactin suture[71]. Cystoscopy should be performed at the end of the procedure to ensure water-tight closure. Bladder draining is continued for 10–14 days postoperatively. A repeat cystogram should be performed prior to discontinuation of bladder drainage to confirm that the bladder has healed and that there is no leakage.

Diaphragmatic endometriosis

A cardiothoracic surgeon should be available when diaphragmatic endometriosis has been diagnosed prior to the procedure or is highly suspected due to the patient's symptoms, or if all other modalities for conservative/medical management have failed. Patients may be placed in a reverse Trendelenburg position to provide more adequate visualization of the upper abdomen. Laparoscopy is performed as previously described, but additional trocars are placed in the upper quadrant (right or left according to implant location), similar to the arrangement for laparoscopic cholecystectomy or splenectomy. A grasping forceps or suction irrigator probe can be used to push the liver from the operative field to enable better exposure of the diaphragm. If the lesion is judged to be superficial, it can be vaporized using a CO_2 laser, cavitational ultrasonographic surgical aspirator (CUSA) or any other cutting modality. Deeper endometriotic lesions infiltrating the diaphragm are removed using hydrodissection and sharp dissection with the aid of a CO_2 laser set at 20–25 W. Great care must be taken to avoid injuring the phrenic nerve and surrounding organs[72,73].

Complications

Regardless of the degree of care and caution exercised, complications can occur. Timely recognition of a complication is essential to proper management. As laparoscopic surgery becomes more complex, the ability to handle an increasing number of complications endoscopically is essential.

Although it is generally agreed that diagnostic laparoscopy and laparoscopic tubal sterilization involve little risk, the potential for complication increases with the complexity of the procedures, the relative inexperience of some surgeons, and deviation from standard technique. The known rate of intraoperative and postoperative complications is less than 1%, but the risk of complications for the average gynecological surgeon probably is not reflected. Most reports are from large practices with experienced gynecologists[74], surveys of members of the American Association of Gynecologic Laparoscopists (AAGL)[75,76] and reports from tertiary referral clinics[77].

From July 1982 to December 1993 at the Center for Special Pelvic Surgery in Atlanta and Stanford University in Palo Alto[74], 6949 advanced operative laparoscopies were performed with a complication rate of 3.08%, significantly lower than that expected from laparotomy. The most common complication was abdominal wall vascular injury (inferior epigastric vessels); none required laparotomy. Intestinal and urinary tract injuries were the second most common complication. Severe adhesions and endometriosis were the main contributing factors for these injuries; most injuries were intentional during the excision and treatment of urinary tract and rectosigmoid colon endometriosis. The incidence of laparotomy to manage the complications was only 0.23%; most occurred early in experiences with operative laparoscopy. For example, in the last 5000 operations performed, only one laparotomy was necessary to control bleeding. To date, no fatalities have occurred.

Complications associated with operative laparoscopy appear to be low when procedures are performed by an experienced laparoscopist. The incidence of complications is related directly to the severity of pelvic and abdominal pathology. Adhesions and endometriosis are contributing factors to urinary tract and intestinal injury. Certain complications are unavoidable, and surgeons must be prepared to manage them by laparotomy or laparoscopy. The incidence of conversion to laparotomy to manage complications or complete a procedure tends to be higher early in one's experience[78].

In a study encompassing 17 521 diagnostic and operative procedures performed at seven centers, an overall complication rate of 3.2/1000 was found[79]. The rate for diagnostic and minor procedures was 1.1/1000 and 5.2/1000 for major and advanced operations. Laparotomies were performed for hemorrhage (17) or visceral complications (40), and injury was most common following extensive adhesiolysis and advanced laparoscopic surgery; one fatality was reported.

Limitations

Limitations of laparoscopy include the difficulty in manipulating solid masses > 20 cm, such as myomas, the possible dissemination of advanced intraperitoneal cancer resulting from laparoscopic manipulation, severe abdominal and pelvic adhesions associated with acute inflammatory bowel disease, and the current limited availability of proper instrumentation, surgical teams and skilled surgeons.

Discussion

The minimal invasiveness of videolaparoscopy remains its most prominent benefit, playing the central role in its popularization. Operative videolaparoscopy offers several other benefits over an open procedure. The video magnification of anatomy allows the most tedious procedures to be performed microsurgically. The superior visualization of the posterior cul-de-sac, posterior broad ligament and upper abdomen using this technique cannot be disputed. Further, the surgeon's eyes are within millimeters or centimeters from the tissue, via the videoscope.

The hemostasis achieved with the pressure from the pneumoperitoneum significantly adds to intraoperative exposure. In addition, *de novo* adhesion formation is at least markedly decreased with the use of laparoscopy[22,23].

While operative laparoscopy has been shown to be an excellent alternative to laparotomy for many procedures, some have called for randomized studies of the two methods[80]. Studies of this nature would provide useful statistics. However, in order for the results to be valid, the surgeon must be proficient with both laparotomy and operative laparoscopy, and must actively use both on his or her patients. We suggest that in a number of instances this is unethical. For procedures that require delicate dissection, laparoscopy is a better approach[81]. Once a surgeon is competent in operative laparoscopy, why perform laparotomy for the sake of statistical analysis, subjecting the patient to longer hospitalization, recuperation, more pain, more expense and possibly more complications?

The lightning-fast development of laparoscopy and its increasing popularity have created new dilemmas. At the same time, the old obstacles have not been overcome. Responding to popular demand, an increasing number of physicians are actively acquiring laparoscopic skills. Public pressure frequently results in inadequately trained surgeons attempting difficult laparoscopic procedures. In turn, this leads to an unacceptable increase in operative laparoscopic complications[81]. Video endoscopic procedures lack the three-dimensional perspective present with laparotomy. Successful utilization of videolaparoscopy requires that the previously trained surgeon relearn his or her operating skills. The time necessary to acquire the ability to perform advanced operative laparoscopy is typically at least as long as that for laparotomy.

Cost effectiveness has been presumed a significant benefit. However, at the present time, hospital costs associated with most operative laparoscopies, despite decreased postoperative hospitalization, continue to be higher than the costs associated with laparotomy. To compensate for the drop in revenue from a decrease in inpatient room utilization, many hospitals have increased the fees for their outpatient facilities. Also, the hospitals have increased their profit margins on the already expensive instrumentation and technology. Specifically, the use of disposable instruments adds significantly to the total cost of a procedure[82]. As an example, automatic stapling devices have emerged as a convenient time-saver, but as they are disposable, they increase cost. The expense associated with disposable stapling devices may not be justifiable, when the same results can be accomplished with bipolar electrocoagulation, or with sutures combined with widely available cutting instruments. Reusable instruments should be included in the procedure whenever possible[83].

Another reason for unrealized cost savings is the increased operative time associated with laparoscopy. The problem of prolonged operative time is exacerbated by the frequently inadequate skills of the surgeons. Although some extension in operative time is to be expected, it may be reduced by the development of new instrumentation and by the surgeon's acquisition of advanced operative skills.

Conclusion

In experienced hands, the laparoscopic approach provides an adequate route for diagnosis and treatment of endometriosis of the bowel, bladder, ureter and diaphragm. Endoscopic magnification of surgical planes, coupled with hemostasis facilitated by pneumoperitoneum and CO_2 laser, allows excellent identification of anatomic structures with this laparoscopic technique. Bipolar electrocoagulation and laser replace conventional dissection techniques and sharp instruments. Adequate laparoscopic treatment of endometriosis requires surgical skill, and of paramount importance is the operator's knowledge of this disease and its natural history.

When it comes to the treatment of extensive pelvic endometriosis, which is one of the most challenging surgical procedures (especially when it extends to the parametrium and involves the ureter and rectovaginal septum), we have rarely performed laparotomy, even for the most severe cases. Treatment of this disease often requires the expertise of a gastrointestinal, genitourinary and gynecological surgeon (pelvic surgeon), and we have been managing these types of cases for years by laparoscopy. We believe that as the years go by and the experience of surgeons increases, laparotomy will be performed less and less, and future generations of surgeons will not have to learn laparotomy first and then laparoscopy. Due to the potential benefits of laparoscopy, mainly better exposure and magnification, time will prove that learning operative laparoscopy is preferable to laparotomy and the complications of operative videolaparoscopy are less than those of laparotomy. Most of the complications of operative videolaparoscopy will be managed by this method and not by laparotomy. As acknowledged above, only a few exceptional operations, such as extensive tumor debulking, removal of giant tumors and organ transplants, still demand resorting to a large laparotomy incision. However, even portions of these procedures can be assisted by the laparoscope. Extending the many benefits of minimal access surgery to an ever growing number of patients is greatly dependent on our ability to provide proper training in advanced operative laparoscopy. However, it will probably take 20 years from now to achieve this level of expertise worldwide.

The future of operative laparoscopy rests on its widespread acceptance by the academic centers responsible for resident education. The upcoming generation of surgeons can be taught endoscopic techniques earlier in their training, allowing better assimilation of the hand–eye co-ordination necessary for videolaparoscopy. Likewise, the laparoscopic frontier will be extended with the development of instrumentation that is easier to manipulate and which will shorten operative time.

Operative endoscopy can be modified for application to almost any existing cavity in the body as instruments and technique continue to improve. Currently, the frontier areas for laparoscopy include cardiac arterial bypass surgery, heart valve replacement, and selective cerebral neuronal ablation. We reported successful endoscopic coronary bypass in a porcine model in 1992[84]. These procedures take advantage of the superior visualization of the magnified operative field and the ability to perform precise and delicate procedures using operative endoscopy.

In experienced hands, there is a significant number of personal and social benefits to patients who undergo minimal access surgery. For this reason, as time passes, more and more laparotomies will be replaced by operative videolaparoscopy. The transition from laparotomy to operative laparoscopy will happen slowly. More and more attending surgeons, especially recent graduates, will perform an increasing number of operative laparoscopies. Gradually, the postgraduate trainees will have the opportunity to be exposed to more laparoscopies than laparotomies. The trend will continue until video-assisted operative laparoscopy replaces laparotomy in almost all cases. In this country, it will most likely happen by the year 2020.

References

1. Gomel, V. (1989). Operative laparoscopy: time for acceptance. *Fertil. Steril.*, **52**, 1–11
2. Gomel, V. (1977). Salpingostomy by laparoscopy. *J. Reprod. Med.*, **18**, 265–8
3. Mettler, L., Giesel, H. and Semm, K. (1979). Treatment of female infertility due to tubal obstruction by operative laparoscopy. *Fertil. Steril.*, **32**, 384–8
4. Bruhat, M., Mage, G. and Manhes, M. (1979). Use of the CO_2 laser via laparoscopy. In Kaplan, I. (ed.) *Laser Surgery III, Proceedings of the 3rd International Society for Laser Surgery*, p. 175. (Tel Aviv: International Society for Laser Surgery)
5. Tadir, Y., Kaplain, I., Zuckerman, Z., Edelstein, T. and Ovadia, J. (1984). New instrumentation and technique for laparoscopic carbon dioxide laser operations: a preliminary report. *Obstet. Gynecol.*, **63**, 582–5
6. Nezhat, C.R., Nezhat, F.R., Luciano, A.A.,

Siegler, A.M., Metzger, D.A. and Nezhat, C.H. (eds.) (1995). *Operative Gynecologic Laparoscopy: Principles and Techniques*. (New York: McGraw-Hill)

7. Anonymous (1986). Videolaseroscopy for endometriosis care. *Obstet. Gynecol. News*, November 15–30, 41

8. Tadir, Y. and Fisch, B. (1993). Operative laparoscopy. *Am. J. Obstet. Gynecol.*, **169**, 7–12

9. Nezhat, C., Crowgey, S.R. and Garrison, C.P. (1986). Surgical treatment of endometriosis via laser laparoscopy. *Fertil. Steril.*, **45**, 778–83

10. Nezhat, C., Crowgey, S. and Nezhat, F. (1989). Videolaseroscopy for the treatment of endometriosis associated with infertility. *Fertil. Steril.*, **51**, 237–40

11. Nezhat, C. and Nezhat, F. (1991). Incidental appendectomy during videolaseroscopy. *Am. J. Obstet. Gynecol.*, **165**, 559–64

12. Nezhat, F., Nezhat, C. and Silfen, S.L. (1991). Videolaseroscopy for oophorectomy. *Am. J. Obstet. Gynecol.*, **165**, 1323–30

13. Nezhat, C., Nezhat, F. and Winer, W. (1991). Salpingectomy via laparoscopy: a new surgical approach. *J. Laparosc. Surg.*, **1**, 91–5

14. Nezhat, C., Nezhat, F., Gordon, S. and Wilkins, E. (1992). Laparoscopic versus abdominal hysterectomy. *J. Reprod. Med.*, **37**, 247–50

15. Nezhat, C., Burrell, M.O., Nezhat, F.R., Benigno, B.B. and Welander, C.E. (1992). Laparoscopic radical hysterectomy with paraaortic and pelvic node dissection. *Am. J. Obstet. Gynecol.*, **166**, 864–5

16. Nezhat, C., Pennington, E., Nezhat, F. and Silfen, S.L. (1991). Laparoscopically assisted anterior rectal wall resection and reanastomosis for deeply infiltrating endometriosis. *Surg. Laparosc. Endosc.*, **1**, 106–8

17. Nezhat, F., Nezhat, C. and Pennington, E. (1992). Laparoscopic proctectomy for infiltrating endometriosis of the rectum. *Fertil. Steril.*, **57**, 1129–32

18. Nezhat, C., Nezhat, F., and Green, B., (1992). Laparoscopic treatment of obstructed ureter due to endometriosis by resection and ureteroureterostomy. A case report. *J. Urol.*, **148**, 865–8

19. Wallis, C. (1986). The career woman's disease? *Time*, April 28, 62

20. Clark, M. and Carroll, G. (1986). Conquering endometriosis. *Newsweek*, October 13, 95

21. Cowley, G. (1990). Hanging up the knife. *Newsweek*, February 12, 58–9

22. Nezhat, C., Nezhat, F., Metzger, D.A. and Luciano, A.A. (1990). Adhesion reformation after reproductive surgery by videolaseroscopy. *Fertil. Steril.*, **53** (6), 1008–11

23. Operative Laparoscopy Study Group (1991). Postoperative adhesion development after operative laparoscopy: evaluation at early second-look procedures. *Fertil. Steril.*, **55**, 700–4

24. Nezhat, C., Nezhat, F. and Burrell, M. (1992). Laparoscopically assisted hysterectomy for the management of a borderline ovarian tumor: a case report. *J. Laparoendosc. Surg.*, **2**, 167–9

25. Nezhat, F., Nezhat, C.H., Admon, D., Gordon, S. and Nezhat, C. (1995). Complications and results of 361 hysterectomies performed at laparoscopy. *J. Am. Coll. Surg.*, **180**, 307–16

26. Nezhat, C., Nezhat, F. and Silfen, S.L. (1991). Videolaseroscopy: the CO_2 laser for advanced operative laparoscopy. *Obstet. Gynecol. Clin. North Am.*, **18** (3), 585–603

27. Summit, R.L., Stovall, T.G., Lipscomb, G.H. and Ling, F.W. (1992). Randomized comparison of laparoscopy-assisted vaginal hysterectomy in an out-patient setting. *Obstet. Gynecol.*, **80**, 895–901

28. Nezhat, C., Nezhat, F., Silfen, S., Schaffer, N. and Evans, D. (1991). Laparoscopic myomectomy. *Int. J. Fertil.*, **36**, 275–80

29. Nezhat, C. (1992). Laparoscopic myomectomy complications [letter]. *Int. J. Fertil.*, **37**, 64

30. Nezhat, C., Nezhat, F., Bess, O., Nezhat, C.H. and Mashlach, R. (1994). Laparoscopically assisted myomectomy: a report of a new technique in 57 cases. *Int. J. Fertil.*, **39** (1), 39–44

31. Maimon, M., Seltzer, V. and Boyce, J. (1991). Laparoscopic excision of ovarian neoplasms subsequently found to be malignant. *Obstet. Gynecol.*, **77**, 563–5

32. Parker, W.H. and Berek, J.S. (1990). Management of selected cystic adnexal masses in postmenopausal women by operative laparoscopy: a pilot study. *Am. J. Obstet. Gynecol.*, **163**, 1574–7

33. Nezhat, C., Winer, W. and Nezhat, F. (1989). Laparoscopic removal of dermoid cysts. *Obstet. Gynecol.*, **73**, 278–81

34. Nezhat, C., Nezhat, F., Welander, C.E. and Benigno, B. (1992). Four ovarian cancers diagnosed during laparoscopic management of 1011 adnexal masses. *Am. J. Obstet. Gynecol.*, **167**, 790–6

35. Nezhat, F., Nezhat, C., Silfen, S. and Fehnel, S. (1991). Laparoscopic ovarian cystectomy during pregnancy. *J. Laparoendosc. Surg.*, **1**, 161–4
36. Childers, J.M., Hatch, K.D., Tran, A. and Surwit, E.A. (1993). Laparoscopic para-aortic lymphadenectomy in gynecologic malignancies. *Obstet. Gynecol.*, **82** (5), 741–7
37. Querleu, D. (1993). Laparoscopic para-aortic node sampling in gynecologic oncology: a preliminary experience. *Gynecol. Oncol.*, **49**, 24–9
38. Amara, D.P., Nezhat, C., Teng, N.N.H. *et al.* (1996). Operative laparoscopy in the management of ovarian cancer. *Surg. Laparosc. Endosc.*, **1**, 38–45
39. Nezhat, C., Winer, W.K. and Nezhat, F. (1988). Is endoscopic treatment of endometriosis and endometrioma associated with better results than laparotomy? *Am. J. Gynecol. Health*, **2** (3), 10–16
40. Nezhat, C.R., Berger, G.S., Nezhat, F.R., Buttram, V.C. Jr, and Nezhat, C.H. (eds.) (1995). *Endometriosis: Advanced Management and Surgical Techniques*. (New York: Springer-Verlag)
41. Hasson, H.M. (1990). Laparoscopic management of ovarian cysts. *J. Reprod. Med.*, **25**, 863–7
42. Buttram, V.C. (1990). Use of danazol in conservative surgery. *J. Reprod. Med.*, **35**, 82–6
43. Nezhat, C., Winer, W.K., Cooper, J.D., Nezhat, F. and Nezhat, C. (1989). Endoscopic infertility surgery. *J. Reprod. Med.*, **34** (2), 127–34
44. Nezhat, C. and Nezhat, F. (1991). Postoperative adhesion formation after ovarian cystectomy with and without ovarian reconstruction. Presented at the *75th Annual Meeting of the American Fertility Society*, Orlando, October 19–24
45. Nezhat, C. and Nezhat, F. (1992). Operative laparoscopy for the management of ovarian remnant syndrome. *Fertil. Steril.*, **57**, 1003–7
46. Nezhat, C. and Nezhat, F. (1989). Safe laser excision or vaporization of peritoneal endometriosis. *Fertil. Steril.*, **52** (1), 149–51
47. Nezhat, C., Silfen, S.L., Nezhat, F. and Martin, D. (1991). Surgery for endometriosis. *Curr. Opin. Obstet. Gynecol.*, **3**, 385–93
48. Nezhat, C., Nezhat, F., Ambroze, W. and Pennington, E. (1993). Laparoscopic repair of small bowel, colon, and rectal endometriosis: a report of 26 cases. *Surg. Endosc.*, **7**, 88–9
49. Nezhat, C. (1989). Videolaseroscopy for the treatment of endometriosis. In Studd, J. (ed.) *Progress in Obstetrics and Gynecology*, 7th edn., p. 293. (Edinburgh: Churchill Livingstone)
50. Rock, J.A. (1991). Laparoscopic cautery in the treatment of endometriosis-related infertility. *Fertil. Steril.*, **55**, 246–51
51. Nezhat, C. and Nezhat, F. (1992). A simplified method of laparoscopic presacral neurectomy for the treatment of central pelvic pain due to endometriosis. *Br. J. Obstet. Gynaecol.*, **99**, 659–63
52. Tjaden, B., Schlaff, W.D., Kimball, A. and Rock, J.A. (1990). The efficacy of presacral neurectomy for the relief of midline dysmenorrhea. *Obstet. Gynecol.*, **76**, 89–91
53. Sampson, J.A. (1922). Intestinal adenomas of endometrial type. *Arch. Surg.*, **5**, 217–80
54. Prystowsky, J.B., Stryker, S.J., Ujiki, G.T. *et al.* (1988). Gastrointestinal endometriosis. *Arch. Surg.*, **123**, 855–8
55. Williams, T.J. and Pratt, J.H. (1977). Endometriosis in 1000 consecutive celiotomies: incidence and management. *Am. J. Obstet. Gynecol.*, **129**, 245–50
56. Meyers, W.C., Kelvin, F.M. and Jones, R.S. (1979). Diagnosis and surgical treatment of colonic endometriosis. *Arch. Surg.*, **114**, 169–75
57. Coronado, C., Franklin, R.R., Lotze, E.C., Bailey, H.R. and Valdes, C.T. (1990). Surgical treatment of symptomatic colorectal endometriosis. *Fertil. Steril.*, **53**, 411–6
58. Nezhat, C., Nezhat, F. and Pennington, E. (1992). Laparoscopic treatment of infiltrative rectosigmoid colon and rectovaginal septum endometriosis by the technique of videolaparoscopy and the CO_2 laser. *Br. J. Obstet. Gynaecol.*, **99**, 664–7
59. Nezhat, F., Nezhat, C., Pennington, E. and Ambroze, W. (1992). Laparoscopic segmental resection for infiltrating endometriosis of the rectosigmoid colon: a preliminary report. *Surg. Laparosc. Endosc.*, **2** (3), 212–6
60. Nezhat, C., Nezhat, F., Pennington, E. *et al.* (1994). Laparoscopic disk excision and primary repair of the anterior rectal wall for the treatment of full-thickness bowel endometriosis. *Surg. Endosc.*, **8**, 682–5
61. Redwine, D.B. and Sharpe, D.R. (1991). Laparoscopic segmental resection of the sigmoid colon. *J. Laparoendosc. Surg.*, **1**, 217–20
62. Redwine, D.B., Koning, M. and Sharpe, D.R. (1996). Laparoscopically assisted transvaginal segmental resection of the rectosigmoid colon for endometriosis. *Fertil. Steril.*, **65** (1), 193–7

63. Stanley, K.E., Utz, D.C. and Dockerty, M.B. (1965). Clinically significant endometriosis of the urinary tract. *Surg. Gynecol. Obstet.*, **120**, 491
64. Fianu, S., Ingelman-Sundberg, A., Nasiell, K., Rosen, J. and Vaclavinkova, V. (1980). Surgical treatment of post abortum endometriosis of the bladder and postoperative bladder function. *Scand. J. Urol. Nephrol.*, **14**, 151–5
65. Anderson, W.C. and Larsen, G.D. (1975). Endometriosis: treatment with hormonal pseudopregnancy and/or operation. *Am. J. Obstet. Gynecol.*, **118**, 643–51
66. Neto, W.A., Lopes, R.N., Cury, M. *et al.* (1984). Vesical endometriosis. *Urology*, **24**, 271–4
67. Davis, G.D. and Brooks, R.A. (1988). Excision of pelvic endometriosis with the carbon dioxide laser laparoscope. *Obstet. Gynecol.*, **72**, 816–9
68. Martin, D.C. and Vander Zwaag, R. (1987). Excisional techniques for endometriosis with the laser laparoscope. *J. Reprod. Med.*, **32**, 754–8
69. Nezhat, C., Nezhat, F., Nezhat, C.H., Nasserbakht, F., Rosati, M. and Seidman, D.S. (1996). Urinary tract endometriosis treated by laparoscopy. *Fertil. Steril.*, **66** (6), 920–4
70. Nezhat, C. and Nezhat, F. (1993). Laparoscopic segmental bladder resection for endometriosis. *Obstet. Gynecol.*, **81**, 882–4
71. Nezhat, C.H., Seidman, D.S., Nezhat, F., Rottenberg, H. and Nezhat, C. (1996). Laparoscopic management of intentional and unintentional cystotomy. *J. Urol.*, **156**, 1400–2
72. Nezhat, F., Nezhat, C. and Levy, J.S. (1992). Laparoscopic treatment of symptomatic diaphragmatic endometriosis: a case report. *Fertil. Steril.*, **58**, 614–16
73. Mangal, R., Taskin, O., Nezhat, C. and Franklin, R. (1996). Laparoscopic vaporization of diaphragmatic endometriosis in a woman with epigastric pain: a case report. *J. Reprod. Med.*, **41**, 64–6
74. Nezhat, F., Nezhat, C. and Nezhat, C.H. (1994). Complications of gynecologic operative laparoscopy in 6949 patients. Presented at the *Society of Laparoendoscopic Surgeons Meeting*, Seattle, WA, June
75. Phillips, J.M., Hulka, J.F., Hulka, B. *et al.* (1981). 1979 AAGL membership survey. *J. Reprod. Med.*, **26**, 529–33
76. Peterson, H.B., Hulka, J.F. and Phillips, J.M. (1990). American Association of Gynecologic Laparoscopists' 1988 membership survey on operative laparoscopy. *J. Reprod. Med.*, **35**, 587–9
77. Lehmann-Willenbrock, E., Riedel, H.H., Mecke, H. *et al.* (1992). Pelviscopy/laparoscopy and its complications in Germany 1949–1988. *J. Reprod. Med.*, **37**, 671–7
78. Levinson, C.J., Hulka, J.F. and Richardson, D.C. (1981). Laparoscopy. In Schaefer, G. and Graber, E.A. (eds.) *Complications in Obstetric and Gynecologic Surgery*, p. 281. (Philadelphia: Harper & Row)
79. Querleu, D., Chapron, C., Chevallier, L. *et al.* (1993). Complications of gynecologic laparoscopic surgery – a French multicenter collaborative study [letter]. *N. Engl. J. Med.*, **328**, 1355
80. Gant, N.F. (1992). Infertility and endometriosis: comparison of pregnancy outcomes with laparotomy versus laparoscopic techniques. *Am. J. Obstet. Gynecol.*, **166**, 1072–81
81. Garry, R. (1992). Laparoscopic alternatives to laparotomy: a new approach to gynaecological surgery. *Br. J. Obstet. Gynaecol.*, **99**, 629–32
82. Baggish, M. (1992). The most expensive hysterectomy. *J. Gynecol. Surg.*, **8**, 57
83. Baggish, M. and Nezhat, C. (1992). The medical industrial complex. *J. Gynecol. Surg.*, **8**, v–vi
84. Nezhat, C., Nezhat, F. and Nezhat, C.H. (1992). Operative laparoscopy (minimally invasive surgery): state of the art. *J. Gynecol. Surg.*, **8** (3), 111–41

Radical laparoscopic surgery for treatment of endometriosis

38

C. Wood

Peritoneal excision of endometriosis

One of the major reasons for failure in the treatment of endometriosis may be the use of inadequate surgical techniques and the reliance on drug therapy which shrinks rather than removes endometriosis[1–3]. Histological studies have demonstrated the persistence of endometriotic epithelium in a quiescent form, not easily seen at laparoscopy, after medical treatment. While diffuse multiple lesions may be more difficult to remove surgically, the highest concentrations of lesions are usually in areas of peritoneum which can be excised, the lateral pelvic wall, pouch of Douglas and the bladder. The wide expanse covered by multiple endometriotic lesions may deter the extensive use of laser or electrosurgical ablation, particularly the need to protect underlying anatomical structures from thermal damage. Bipolar electrosurgery and laser have caused injuries to the ureter and the uterine artery when used on the lateral pelvic wall[4,5]. There have been numerous anecdotal reports of ureteric trauma using laser or electrosurgery on the lateral pelvic wall, which are not reported. Spot laser or diathermy, even if targeted to all visible lesions, makes no allowance for the microscopic foci which occur in 13% of women with peritoneal endometriosis[6]. Another difficulty in providing adequate surgical treatment of endometriosis is that laparoscopic removal of endometriosis is often regarded as a minor procedure performed by trainee surgeons, whereas diffuse peritoneal endometriosis requires a variety of advanced skills including dissection of the ureter, recto-vaginal and bladder surfaces. Patients presenting to our endometriosis clinic with persistent or poorly-controlled disease most often have endometriotic lesions over the ureter or undiagnosed or neglected lesions in the pouch of Douglas.

There were no controlled trials showing that laser or electrosurgical ablation were better than excision of peritoneal endometriotic lesions when these techniques were introduced. A recurrence or persistence rate of 19% at 5 years was obtained by Redwine using laparoscopic excision[7] and was identical to that obtained by Wheeler and Malinak, 3 years after laparotomy combined with excision[8]. Excision using laser or electrosurgical techniques would be expected to produce similar results with respect to recurrence or persistence rates. Long-term recurrence after electrocoagulation or fulguration has not been satisfactorily studied, but neither is equivalent to excision, and neither would be expected to produce results similar to excision, particularly with respect to eradication of invasive disease. Success rates reported for laparoscopic laser or electrosurgical ablation have been restricted to success rates for cure of infertility ranging from 40–60% over 6–12 months[9]. Laser or electrosurgical ablation of peritoneum may be associated with significant disadvantages, the risk of thermal complications, increased costs, distortion of anatomy and pathology, difficulty in dealing with widespread disease and special training programs for surgeons.

The author's experience with severe endometriosis involves 198 patients referred to an endometriosis clinic with recurrent disease. The average number of previous drug treatments is three and the average number of

Table 1 Peritoneal resection for recurrent endometriosis in 1995 ($n = 198$)

Most extensive infiltrating lesion	Bladder	Lateral wall	Pouch of Douglas
Superficial	25	41	73
Infiltrating > 5 mm	6	5	32
Bladder/rectal lumen	4	—	12

Table 2 Ureteric dissection in patients with recurrent endometriosis ($n = 137$)

Ureter exposed by peritoneal reflection alone	75
Ureter exposure required and dissected by scissors	45
Ureteric catheters required to identify	17

Table 3 Recurrent endometriosis (average 5.7 previous treatments)

Symptoms	n	Control or cure at 6/12 months
Bladder	31	26 (84%)
Menstrual	142	129 (91%)
Coital	92	85 (92%)
Bowel	87	76 (87%)

previous surgical treatments is 2.7. The study involves patients treated over the last 3 years. Most lesions are superficial, less than 5 mm, the majority of lesions infiltrating beyond 5 mm being more common in the pouch of Douglas than the bladder and the lateral pelvic walls (Table 1). Infiltration into the rectal wall occurred in 12 patients and into the bladder wall in four patients. Ureteric dissection was required in 137 of the 198 patients, the ureter being exposed by peritoneal reflection in 75, by close ureteric dissection in 45 and in association with the use of ureteric catheters in 17 (Table 2).

Occult lesions were common. One patient with white thickening of the peritoneum on the lateral pelvic wall had five previous surgical treatments with negative histological biopsies taken from this area. Resection of the whole of the peritoneum on the lateral pelvic wall revealed an endometriotic nodule of 2×3 cm under the left ureter. One patient had two previous laser ablations of lesions on the surface of the bladder. A small white scarred area of peritoneum was excised and a 1×3 cm nodule found in the bladder muscle required excision into the bladder lumen. Another two patients with no visible lesion in the pouch of Douglas at laparoscopy had dissection of the rectovaginal septum because a nodule could be felt rectovaginally. To detect occult endometriosis excision may require removal of the peritoneum in the pouch of Douglas over the vagina and rectum or removal of the peritoneum over one or both lateral pelvic walls including the uterosacral ligament.

Adhesion formation was uncommon following extensive surgery. Further laparoscopy in 22 patients showed moderate adhesions in only one patient. In the other 21 patients new peritoneum was visible with normal color and glistening appearance.

Symptom relief at 6–12 months follow-up ranged from 84–92% for bladder, menstrual, coital and bowel pain (Table 3). In the seven patients who had persistent coital pain reoperation in three and sexual therapy in two relieved symptoms.

Adenomyosis

The diagnosis of adenomyosis using vaginal ultrasound, magnetic resonance and uterine biopsy has enabled preoperative diagnosis and the planning of conservative surgery. This has been explored by: performing endomyometrial resection when menorrhagia is a predominant symptom; myometrial electrocoagulation for infertility in the presence of localized myometrial disease; myometrial excision if uterine conservation is preferred but the patient does not wish to conceive; and partial or total hysterectomy if certain cure is required.

Electrocoagulation can be done with a mono- or bipolar needle using a vasoconstricting agent to reduce blood loss. Although postoperative adhesions are uncommon, the risk may be further reduced by placing Interceed (Johnson & Johnson) or Goretex membrane on the coagulated area. If coagulation is made in the deeper part of the adenomyotic area, avoiding the uterine surface, the area of superficial scar may be further reduced.

Adenomyomata or localized adenomyosis may be removed by excision using laparoscopic or minilaparotomy techniques. The borderline between the normal and abnormal tissue may be difficult to define but is aided by ultrasound, magnetic resonance, and the appearance, consistency and vascularity of the abnormal area. Because of the lack of the demarcation between adenomyosis and normal tissue, scissor or thermal dissection may be slow and difficult. A scalpel may be used through a 2–3-cm low abdominal incision using an abdominal elevator. This speeds dissection and reduces blood loss. Closure of the cavity may require the use of an abdominal elevator and a minilaparotomy incision of 2–4 cm to enable a sufficiently strong apposition by suture. Interceed is used if there is no superficial bleeding, or otherwise a Goretex membrane is placed over the suture line. Adenomyoma or adenomyosis in the pouch of Douglas may also involve the rectovaginal septum and disease may require removal with the uterine portion of the disease.

In 40 patients treated by conservative surgery and followed up for 3 years, 29 avoided hysterectomy. Laparoscopic excision of adenomyosis or adenomyoma was most successful curing 13 of 15 patients, laparoscopic electrosurgical coagulation cured six of nine and hysteroscopic endomyometrial loop rollerball cured 10 of 16 (Table 4). Experience of conservative surgery over 5 years shows that: hysterectomy may be avoided in the majority of patients; the improved localization of disease by color Doppler ultrasound, magnetic resonance imaging, uterine biopsy and laparoscopic uterine needling are effective; and better localization of the disease may further improve the use of conservative surgery.

Table 4 Conclusions concerning conservative surgery in adenomyosis

Conservative surgery avoided hysterectomy in 29 of 40 patients
Laparoscopic excision of adenomyosis/ adenomyoma was most successful, curing 13 of 15
Laparoscopic electrosurgical reduction cured six of nine
Hysteroscopic endomyometrial loop/rollerball cured 10 of 16

Laparoscopic oophorectomy

Oophorectomy is required if ovarian endometriosis involves 80–100% of the ovary. Ovarian adhesive entrapment with previous failed attempts at surgical mobilization and the use of anti-adhesive regimens may also require ovarian removal because of persistent pain. Following hysterectomy and resection of extrauterine endometriosis, endometriosis may recur and in these circumstances oophorectomy may assist cure. Partial oophorectomy has also been used to freeze and store a healthy portion of the ovary in order to preserve fertility.

The technique of laparoscopic oophorectomy varies markedly and there is no significant particular advantage of one technique. The ureter is first identified by visualization, dissection or the use of a ureteric catheter. The vascular pedicles may be dealt with by suture, endoloop, bipolar coagulation or staples. The ovary may be removed with the assistance of a bag or morcellation, and delivered from the abdomen through the umbilicus, the vagina after culdotomy or through a lateral abdominal incision. For the majority of patients laparoscopic oophorectomy is a simple operation.

Table 5 Comparison of laparoscopic and laparotomy oophorectomy (from reference 10)

	Laparoscopy (n = 61)	Laparotomy (n = 79)
Costs ($)	1615	3525
Time in hospital (days)	1.6	6.9
Complications	2	10
Length of operation (min)	88	—

Table 6 Pouch of Douglas endometriosis involving rectal dissection (last 100 cases)

Anterior rectal resection for circumferential lesions	9
Partial or complete thickness excision of rectal nodule for localized lesions	9
Perirectal excision of nodule or cicatrix	82

Oophorectomy may be difficult and require greater skill if the bowel is adherent to the ovary, the ureter is adherent to the ovarian mass or the ovary is adherent to the lateral pelvic wall. The surgical skills required are that of bowel dissection, ureteric dissection and internal iliac vessel identification and dissection. In difficult cases minilaparotomy or laparotomy may be preferred.

Comparison of laparoscopic and laparotomy oophorectomy have shown a reduced cost and a shorter stay in hospital with laparoscopy, and no difference in complication rates (Table 5).

Ovarian cryopreservation has been used to preserve small pieces of ovary in women who are likely to lose the ovary as a result of recurrent cyst formation, endometriosis or intending chemotherapy for cancer. A small piece of ovary, less than 1 mm^3, contains several hundred follicles, ovulation may occur with only 100 eggs remaining in the ovary and a small piece of ovary can be obtained incidentally at laparoscopic surgery or during an *in vitro* fertilization procedure. Live young have been obtained in both mice and sheep from cryopreserved pieces of ovarian tissue. In the human we have freeze-thawed small pieces of ovary and implanted the ovary into the kidney of immune deficient mice (SCID). Normal follicles have developed over 4 weeks following transplantation. Revascularization of small ovarian tissue is enhanced by the observation that ovarian remnants left inside the abdomen have grown on the surface of the bladder with histological demonstration of normal follicle survival.

Laparovaginal surgery in the pouch of Douglas

Combined laparovaginal surgery has been utilized in stage III–IV endometriosis to assist and speed surgery deep in the pelvis. A Maher abdominal wall elevator is used and the pouch of Douglas is opened to allow both laparoscopic and vaginal visualization, palpation and dissection. Finger palpation can be used to mobilize adherent ovaries or define pouch of Douglas endometriosis on the rectum or vagina. The precise definition of the lesion is then made after dissection of the rectovaginal septum and mobilization of the rectum and upper vagina. Combined laparovaginal removal of these lesions is facilitated by combining laparoscopic or vaginal surgery, whichever is most appropriate.

The most common symptoms of rectal endometriosis were constipation, diarrhea, painful defecation and deep dyspareunia. In the last 100 patients with endometriosis in the pouch of Douglas involving the rectum, most of the lesions have been removed by excision of the peritoneum, uterosacral ligaments or nodules attached to the rectum but not penetrating the rectal wall (Table 6). Nine patients required a complete or partial thickness excision of rectal disease and nine required an anterior rectal resection for circumferential lesions reaching the rectal mucosa. Most lesions on the rectum (82%) are superficial and can be removed without involving the rectal wall. Rectal bleeding occurs in only 20% of cases. The bleeding is rarely associated with ulceration through the rectal mucosa. The mechanism of the rectal bleeding

Table 7 Avoidance of hysterectomy for endometriosis

	Pouch of Douglas*	Large ovarian endometrioma	Adenomyosis
Total number in series	26	51	30
Advised to have hysterectomy	13	8	12
Cured surgically without hysterectomy	12 (93%)	8 (100%)	6 (50%)

*Previous failed medical and surgical therapy

Table 8 Hysterectomy for endometriosis ($n = 59$)

Type of hysterectomy	Associated surgery	n
Laparovaginal ($n = 52$)	Rectovaginal dissection	12
	Lateral pelvic wall	9
	Bladder	5
	Adhesiolysis	15
Abdominal ($n = 3$)	Rectal resection	2
	Sigmoid resection	1
Vaginal (adenomyosis) ($n = 4$)	—	—

is more often related to venous congestion or recurrent petechial hemorrhage at the time of menstruation. The 2-year cure rate for rectal endometriosis was 78% for the last 100 patients.

Hysterectomy

There is a declining role for hysterectomy in treating endometriosis. Long-term drug therapy such as the oral contraceptive on a 3-monthly cycle, low dose Provera or danazol, the facility of repeated laparoscopic surgery, the ability to treat the majority of endometriotic lesions by surgery localized to the area involved, the infrequency of direct uterine involvement and the development of conservative surgery for adenomyosis reduce the need for hysterectomy. Many of the patients who have been recommended to have a hysterectomy can avoid this by having conservative surgery in the pouch of Douglas, or in the ovary or uterus (Table 7).

The indications for hysterectomy are not clear-cut and are continually changing. Factors involved in the decision are the patient's ability to continue with more conservative treatment, the presence of central pain which most likely involves the uterus, pouch of Douglas disease involving the cervix and vagina, diffuse adenomyosis, failed medical and surgical therapy and rarely adhesive disease involving the uterus and ovaries. Hysterectomy in the author's practice is performed by a laparovaginal technique, with a small number having an abdominal or vaginal hysterectomy (Table 8). Vaginal hysterectomy is preferred for adenomyosis. Abdominal hysterectomy may be required when rectal or sigmoid resection is performed. The laparovaginal technique is used for all other cases when endometriosis is present in the rectum or vagina, the lateral pelvic wall or the bladder, or if there are extensive adhesions. Reasons for preferring laparovaginal hysterectomy include the improved detection of endometriosis by magnification and proximity of the laparoscope to the abnormal tissue, particularly deep in the pelvis, and improved access to remove endometriotic tissue on the rectum, vagina and lateral pelvic walls. Abdominal hysterectomy provides a reduced view of the lateral pelvic wall and reduced access to the deep pelvis. Vaginal hysterectomy does not allow inspection of the upper pelvis or easy surgical access to the lateral pelvic walls. Subtotal hysterectomy has the disadvantage of possibly leaving endometriotic tissue deep in the pelvis on the rectum, vagina or cervix.

The use of laparoscopic hysterectomy requires justification in terms of safety. Controlled trials concerning abdominal and laparoscopic hysterectomy have shown that the laparoscopic procedure has an advantage of

Table 9 Controlled trials comparing abdominal and laparoscopic hysterectomy

Trial	n	Laparoscopic operating time (min)	Laparoscopic hospital stay (days)	Laparoscopic return to normal activity (days)
Carter (1994)[13]	50	↑ 60	↓ 1	↓ 21
Langebrekke (1995)[14]	100	↑ 40	↓ 3	↓ 17
Haklin (1995)[15]	230	↑	↓	↓
Ellstrom (1994)[16]	100	↑	↓	↓
Yi Ping Yout (1995)[17]	180	↑ 73	↓ 2	?
Nezhat (1992)[18]	20	↑ 60	↓ 2	↓ 14
Phipps (1993)[19]	53	↑ 35	↓ 4	↓ 28
Total	733	↑ 35–73	↓ 1–4	↓ 14–28

↑, Increase compared to abdominal hysterectomy; ↓, decrease compared to abdominal hysterectomy

Table 10 Unintended major surgical procedures (from reference 11)

Hysterectomy	Abdominal (%)	Vaginal (%)	Laparoscopic (%)
Bladder	1–2	0.5–1.5	1.1
Bowel	0.1–0.5	0.1–0.8	0.5
Ureter	0.1–0.5	0.05–0.1	0.3

Table 11 Postoperative fever (from reference 11)

Hysterectomy	Abdominal (%)	Vaginal (%)	Laparoscopic (%)
Unexplained fever	10–20	5–8	1–4
Operative site infection	13.8–42	7.8–20	43
Urinary tract infection	1.1–5	1.7–5	< 1

Table 12 Hemorrhage (from reference 11)

Hysterectomy	Intra-operative	Post-operative	Transfusion
Abdominal			
all reports (%)	0.2–3.7	0.2–2.3	2.2–7.5
most common (%)	1–2	1–2	2–12
Vaginal			
all reports (%)	0.5–3.5	0.4–5.7	0.7–13
most common (%)	1–3	1–5	2–8
Laparoscopic			
all reports (%)	?	0.8	1.2

reduced time in hospital and early return to normal activities (Table 9). A review of complications of various types of hysterectomy reported in over 70 articles published between 1985 and 1996 has shown that major surgical complications are no different with laparoscopic, vaginal and abdominal hysterectomy (Table 10)[11]. The incidence of postoperative fever and hemorrhage, defined by the need for blood transfusion, is lower following laparoscopic than abdominal and vaginal hysterectomy (Tables 11 and 12)[11]. Results from an Australian study by the Royal Australian College of Gynaecologists, of laparoscopic hysterectomy involving 546 patients performed by 120 surgeons, have shown no increased risk of major complications associated with the laparoscopic procedure (Table 13)[12]. The major techniques for laparoscopic hysterectomy are total, subtotal or laparovaginal. The most popular is the laparovaginal technique as it allows a variable mixture of laparoscopic or vaginal surgery depending on the anatomy and pathology. The laparovaginal method using staples and stents is rapid and simple, although costs are increased by the use of disposable equipment. The Doderlein technique

Table 13 Results of Australian study of laparoscopic hysterectomy[12] ($n = 546$)

Complication	% (n)
Bladder injury	1.1 (7)
Bladder fistula	0.2 (1)
Ureteric fistula	0.2 (1)
Bowel injury	0.9 (5)
Hemorrhage	4.3 (24)
Blood transfusion	3.4 (19)
Fever	6.5 (36)
Thromboembolism	0.9 (5)
Re-admission	3.2 (18)

Table 14 Use of laparoscopic hysterectomy in three countries (from reference 12)

Country	n	Laparoscopic (%)	Vaginal (%)	Abdominal (%)
USA (1991)	731 000	4	24	72
Kaiser Hospitals, N California (1993)	11 420	5	29	66
UK (1995)	34 700	5	21	74
Australia (1994–5)	19 702	8	35	57

involves delivery of the uterus through the anterior fornix into the vagina and ligation of the major uterine vessels from the upper to lower border of the uterus. The technique is simple but may not be suitable for an enlarged uterus. The combined laparovaginal procedure using an abdominal elevator does speed and simplify surgery because two surgeons can operate, one laparoscopically and one vaginally, and surgeons have an improved view including combining a laparoscopic and vaginal panorama. A minilaparotomy may further speed the laparovaginal hysterectomy because the technique is similar to that of abdominal hysterectomy and uses similar instruments. The minilaparotomy incision is only required to be 3–4 cm. This technique is easy to learn and may be particularly helpful for training surgeons in the laparoscopy technique. Despite the advantage of laparoscopic hysterectomy, its use in three countries has been small (Table 14) – only 4–8% of hysterectomies being performed laparoscopically[12]. This may relate to the extra skills and time required to perform the operation.

References

1. Nissole-Pochet, M., Casanas-Roux, F. and Donnez, J. (1988). Histological study of ovarian endometriosis after hormonal therapy. *Fertil. Steril.*, **49**, 423–6
2. Evers, J.L.H. (1987). The second look laparoscopy for evaluation of the results of medical treatment of endometriosis should not be performed during ovarian suppression. *Fertil. Steril.*, **47**, 502–4
3. Nissole, M., Casanas-Roux, F. and Donnez, J. (1988). Histologic study of ovarian endometriosis after hormonal therapy. *Fertil. Steril.*, **51**, 237–40
4. Liu, Y.C. (1994). *Complications of Laparoscopic Surgery*. Videotape, AGES Meeting, Brisbane, October
5. Albini, S.M., Karalicki, B., Chere, M. and Polke, D.R. (1995). Delayed ureteral injury after laparoscopic surgery. Abstracts of the *World Congress of Gynecologic Endoscopy, 24th Annual Meeting of the American Association of Gynecologic Laparoscopists*, Orlando, Florida, November, p. 811
6. Murphy, A.A., Green, W.R., Babbie, D. et al. (1986). Unsuspected endometriosis diagnosed by scanning electron microscope in visually normal peritoneum. *Fertil. Steril.*, **46**, 522–4
7. Redwine, D.B. (1991). Conservative laparoscopic excision of endometriosis by sharp dissection: life table analysis of reoperation and persistent or recurrent disease. *Fertil. Steril.*, **56** (4), 628–34

8. Wheeler, J.M. and Malinak, L.R. (1983). Recurrent endometriosis: incidence, management and prognosis. *Am. J. Obstet. Gynecol.*, **146**, 247–53
9. Haney, A.F. (1993). Endometriosis-associated infertility. In Brosens, I. (ed.) *Endometriosis, Baillières Clinical Obstetrics and Gynaecology*, Vol. 7 (4), p. 805. (London: Baillière Tindall)
10. Wood, C., Maher, P., O'Callaghan, D., Hailey, D. and Downing, B. (1996). Underutilization of laparoscopic oophorectomy. *Aust NZ J Obstet. Gynaecol.*, **36**, 198–201
11. Hill, D. (1997). Complications of hysterectomy. In Wood, C. and Maher, P. (eds) *Baillière's Clinical Obstetrics and Gynaecology* (London: Baillière Tindall), Vol 11(1), p181–97
12. Wood, C. and Maher, P. (1997). Laparoscopic hysterectomy. In Wood, C. and Maher, P. (eds) *Baillière's Clinical Obstetrics and Gynaecology* (London: Baillière Tindall), Vol 11(1), p111–36
13. Carter, J.E., Rybo, J., Katz, A. and Katz, C. (1994). LAVH: A case control study with abdominal hysterectomy. *Gynaecol. Endosc.*, **3**, 25
14. Langebrekke, A., Eraker, R., Curnes, A., Nesheim, B.I., Busund, B. and Shortland, C. (1995). Laparoscopic Hysterectomy. *4th Biennial Meeting of the International Society for Gynaecologic Endoscopy*, London, UK, 26–29 April, p17
15. Haklin, E.M. and Olsson, J.H. (1995). Subtotal and total hysterectomy – a randomized postoperative trial comparing the laparoscopic and abdominal approach. *Gynaecol. Endosc.*, **4**(Supp 1), 4
16. Ellstrom, M., Haklin, M and Olsson, J.H. (1994). Laparoscopic Hysterectomy. *Gynaecol. Endosc.*, **3**(Supp 1), 32
17. Yi Ping Yout, Li Kheng Lo, Koh Liu Wok, Slih Yao Chen and Min Ho Huang (1995). Comparison of LAVH with abdominal hysterectomy. *4th Biennial Meeting of the International Society for Gynaecologic Endoscopy*, London, UK, 26–29 April, p16
18. Nezhat, F., Nezhat, C., Gordon, S. and Wilkins, E. (1992). Laparoscopic versus abdominal hysterectomy. *J. Reprod. Med.*, **37**, 247–50
19. Phipps, J.H., John, M., Hassmaien, M. and Saced, M. (1993). Laparoscopic and laparoscopically assisted vaginal hysterectomy – a series of 114 cases. *Gynaecol. Endosc.*, **2**, 7–12

Comparison of laser laparoscopic treatment of endometriosis with no treatment at all in the management of pain and infertility

C.J.G. Sutton

Introduction

In spite of recent developments in clinical pharmacology and developments in surgical technique, endometriosis remains a difficult and often frustrating disease to treat and appears to be increasingly common because of increasing awareness of the condition and the tendency of modern women to delay child bearing, thus exposing them to the consequences of more frequent retrograde menstruation than their mothers and grandmothers. It appears that anti-endometriosis drugs often result in only temporary suppression of implants[1] and for the last two decades, gynecologists have increasingly turned to surgery as the primary treatment of peritoneal endometriosis. The widespread introduction of laparoscopic surgery has meant that endometriotic implants and ovarian endometriomas can be treated at the same time as the initial laparoscopy, which confirms the diagnosis.

During the 1980s there were many published studies in the literature of the use of laser laparoscopy for the treatment of endometriosis, which claimed a success rate in relieving pain in 60–70% of patients, with a pregnancy rate of 55–80%[2–6]. Although these studies demonstrated a very low morbidity, they were either retrospective or uncontrolled and were therefore of no true scientific value, particularly since the alleviation of pain in endometriosis is purely subjective, and symptoms are difficult to evaluate. In such a retrospective study it is too easy for the surgeon to influence the patient to provide an answer that she has benefited from his surgery, and such a doctor–patient dialog could severely alter the interpretation of the results.

We therefore realized that it was necessary to prove in much the same way as medical treatments are evaluated that laparoscopic laser surgery worked, that is by a prospective, randomized, double-blind study, comparing laser laparoscopy with diagnostic laparoscopy alone, to see whether removal of these implants did in fact result in statistically significant improvements or resolution of the pain symptoms, and also to decide whether there was an increased pregnancy rate.

The placebo effect of any treatment, especially those associated with a new high technology invention such as lasers, can be significant. It was therefore very difficult to recruit patients, particularly since in their own minds they were quite certain that the laser would help them, and we had to explain quite clearly that we really did not know in our own minds what contribution the vaporization of these implants played in the alleviation of pelvic pain. The study was approved by the Hospital Ethics Committee, but they reasonably felt that it was unethical to withhold treatment from patients in severe pain due to stage IV disease, particularly because our previous experience had shown 80% pain relief in this group and a 57% pregnancy rate,

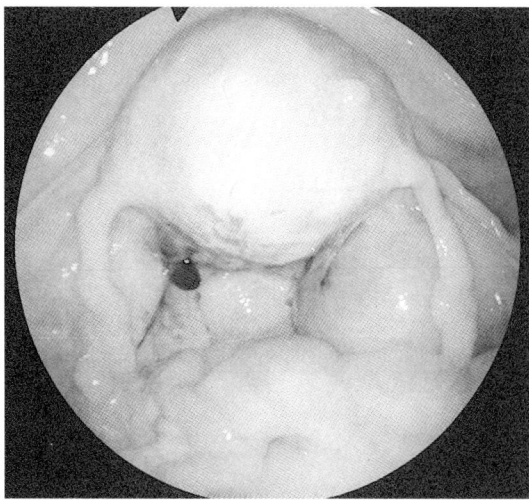

Figure 1 Severe endometriosis with large endometriomas stuck by adhesive disease to the peritoneum on the ovarian fossa. Such patients were excluded from this study

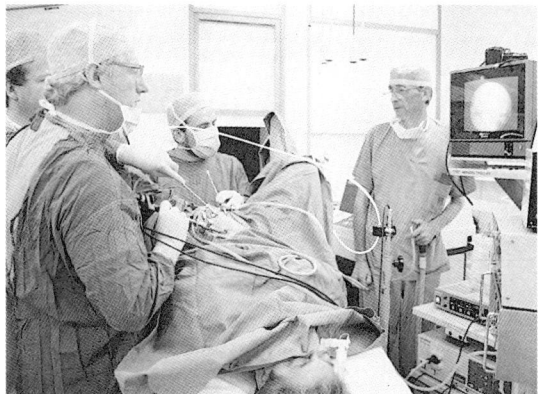

Figure 2 The KTP/532 visible light emerald green laser in use

most of whom had failed to respond to medical therapy[7] (Figure 1).

Patients and methods

The study population was recruited from women seen in the gynecological outpatient clinic with pain suggestive of endometriosis, who had been advised to undergo a diagnostic laparoscopy. To be included in the study women were neither pregnant nor lactating, were between 18 and 45 years of age, and had not received any medical or surgical treatment for endometriosis in the previous 6 months. Patients were asked to record the intensity of their pain on a linear analog scale and also to give a subjective score to their pain symptoms. Although 74 women entered the study, only 63 completed the study to the 6-month follow-up visit, since two became pregnant, five against our advice were started on hormonal contraception by their family doctor, one became severely depressed and three were lost to follow-up. At the time of laparoscopic confirmation of endometriosis a sealed envelope was opened and treatment was allocated randomly by a computer-generated randomization sequence to either laser or expectant management. The patients who had laser treatment had vaporization of all visible endometriotic implants, adhesiolysis and uterine nerve transection with either the CO_2 laser or the KTP/532 laser (Figure 2).

The patients in the no-treatment arm had only a diagnostic laparoscopy, although it was necessary to remove the sero-sanguinous fluid from the pouch of Douglas in order to perform a thorough inspection of the pelvic peritoneum. The patients were not informed whether they had received laser treatment or no treatment (expectant management) and all patients had the same three portal incisions. Patients were followed up at 3 and 6 months after surgery by an independent observer, a research nurse, who was also unaware as to which treatment had been allocated. At 6 months follow-up the randomization code was broken and if the patient had received expectant management and had no treatment and was still in pain, then laser laparoscopy was offered to them almost immediately.

Results

The results were interesting because at 3 months after surgery, 18 out of 32 (56%) in the

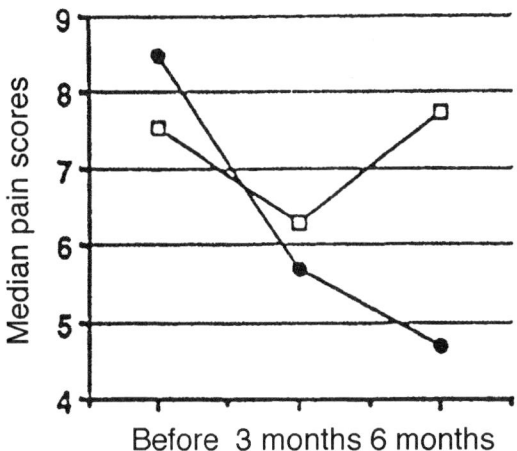

Figure 3 Median visual analog pain scores plotted against time since laser treatment (solid circles) or diagnostic laparoscopy (open squares). Taken from reference 8, with permission

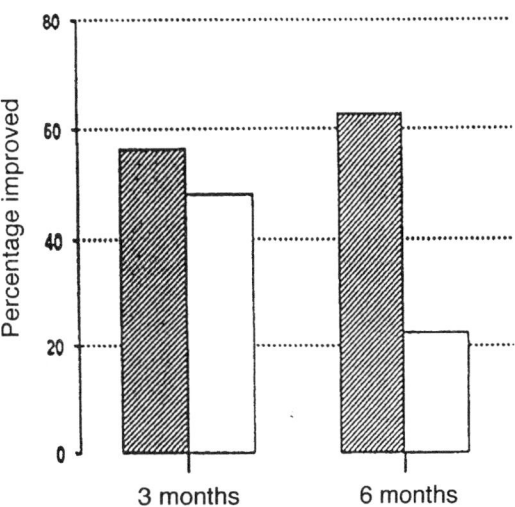

Figure 4 Proportion of patients with pain symptom alleviation according to time since laser treatment (▨) or diagnostic laparoscopy (□). Taken from reference 8, with permission

laser-treated group reported that their pain was better or improved compared with 15 of 34 (44%) in the expectant group. This difference was not statistically significant and the result of the laser surgery was much less than in our previous retrospective study[4]. We were equally very surprised to find that almost 50% of patients who had had a diagnostic laparoscopy alone appeared to be better or improved.

To our intense relief, at the 6-month follow-up, 20 of 32 (62.5%) in the laser group were better and the number in the control group had dropped down to 7 of 31 (22.6%), which was a statistically significant difference. The median value of visual analog scores related to time is shown in Figure 3. At 3 months the median decrease in pain score was 2.6 for the laser group and 1.2 for the expectant group; this was not significant ($p = 0.9$, Mann–Whitney U test). When the decrease in pain score from baseline to 6 months is analyzed, the median decrease was 2.85 for the laser group and 0.05 for the expectant group. This difference was significant ($p = 0.01$, Mann–Whitney U test) (Figures 3 and 4).

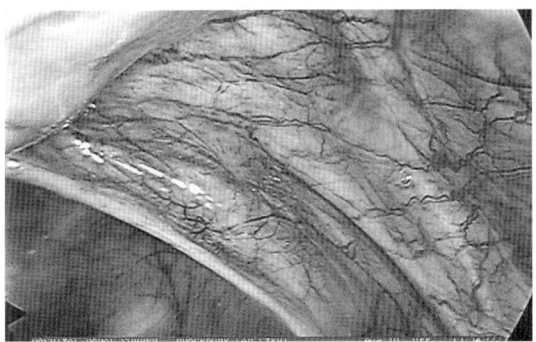

Figure 5 Small vesicles and early scarring seen in stage I disease. Since biopsy was not permitted in this study, this could be due to other inflammatory conditions

One of the problems of this study was that some of the very minimal changes in the peritoneum were interpreted as endometriosis merely by visual inspection with the laparoscope and no biopsy was permitted because that would in itself have acted as a cytoreduction of the implants. It is quite possible that some of these very subtle changes are not endometriosis at all, but merely represent post-inflammatory changes or even Walthard rests (Figure 5). If stage I patients were excluded from the evaluation, then 73.7% of patients achieved pain relief, which was extremely similar to the number that reported pain relief in our retrospective study[4,8].

Discussion

There are several interesting features of this study, which is the first one in the world to have been conducted in endoscopic laser surgery, although such randomized, prospective, double-blind studies are mandatory for the development of any new drug before it receives the approval of the statutory safety agencies. Firstly we were not entirely sure why the placebo response was so high at 3 months, and yet it dropped down at 6 months and, indeed, when patients who claimed that they were better at 6 months realized they had not had laser treatment. This placebo response has also been reported by other surgeons, notably Fedele and colleagues[9]. We are not entirely sure whether the removal of the fluid in the pelvis, which contains high concentrations of pain-mediating substances, particularly prostaglandin F, is responsible for this alleviation of pain and that it may take 3 months of retrograde menstruation before the implants re-secrete sufficient amounts of this fluid to create the same degree of pain.

Another possible explanation is a phenomenon well known among psychologists called 'pain memory', where the body anticipates pain and the mere reassurance of a laparoscopy and the expectation that one has had treatment for the disease gives relief of symptoms. Certainly such relief is relatively short-lived, and after 6 months the symptoms had not been relieved in the majority of patients and yet even then, one-fifth (22.6%) still maintained that the pain was much better than before.

The role of uterine nerve ablation

The other aspect of pain relief that this study has not addressed, was the role played by the division of the uterosacral ligaments which contain many of the afferent sensory pain fibers to the uterus[10]. At this moment in time we are doing another prospective, randomized, double-blind controlled study comparing vaporization of peritoneal implants alone with and without a uterine nerve ablation. Interestingly, the division of uterine nerves has been subject to a small study of this nature by Lichten and Bombard in 1987[11], and it will be interesting in a larger series to know what effect the uterine nerve ablation has as an additional treatment to vaporization of the endometriotic implants.

Infertility

We are also doing another study on infertility patients, but it is an extremely difficult task to recruit patients to this project because they have to wait for 1 year before the code is broken and for many patients they find that this is unacceptable. Nevertheless, we have recruited almost 50 patients to this study and already it appears that dihydrotubation and laparoscopy alone is associated with only half the number of pregnancies achieved if this is combined with laser vaporization of the endometriotic implants. It will however take another 2 or 3 years before the final results can be presented.

There is little doubt that laparoscopic laser surgery is of considerable benefit in patients with severe endometriosis, particularly with ovarian endometriomas, because the gross distortion of anatomy and adhesive disease can be dealt with by laparoscopic surgery resulting in an impressive pregnancy rate[7]. Reasonably, however, many gynecologists have been very sceptical about the role of laparoscopic surgery in improving the fertility status of women with minor degrees of endometriosis, where tubo-ovarian anatomy is usually normal and the tubes are invariably patent.

It is interesting that at the conference in Yokohama, the results of the Endocan Study were presented by Dr Maheux, and this showed clearly that regardless of the surgical modalities

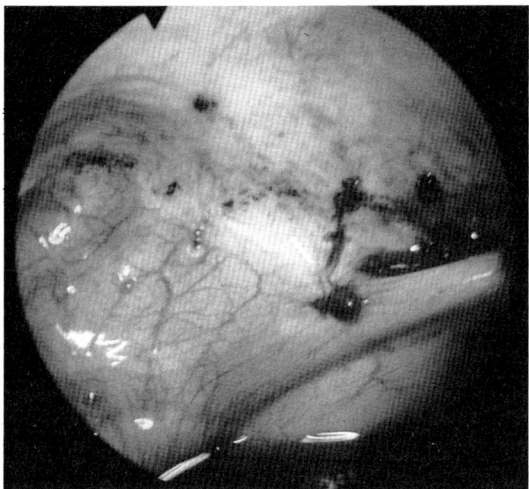

Figure 6 Peritoneal implants close to the ureter prior to precise vaporization with the CO_2 laser using a rapid rotating mirror delivery system

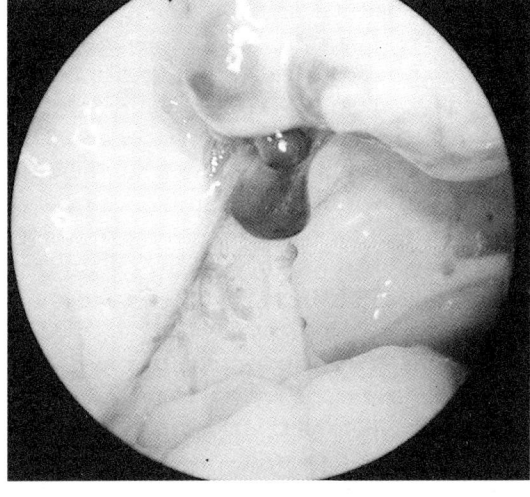

Figure 7 Hemorrhagic endometriosis with deep implants prior to removal with the KTP/532 laser

used, laparoscopic surgery for even mild forms of endometriosis can significantly increase the pregnancy rate. In an impressive study of several centers throughout Canada he has shown that 37.4% of patients treated by laparoscopic surgery conceived within a few months, whereas in those who had expectant management alone the conception rate was only 12%. Although our numbers are much smaller, they do represent the standards achieved by a single institution, and 50% of those treated in our study have so far conceived, compared with only 22% who had expectant management alone.

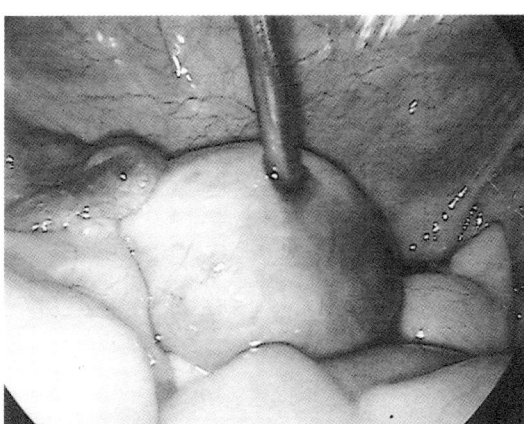

Figure 8 Ovarian endometrioma (chocolate cyst) being aspirated and irrigated prior to photocoagulation of the bleeding vessels on the internal surface of the capsule

Conclusion

At this moment in time it appears that the vaporization of peritoneal implants is associated with reasonable pain relief and increased fertility compared with no treatment at all, and the recurrence rate is much less than that associated with medical treatment[12,13].

We use the CO_2 laser for the precise vaporization of peritoneal implants (Figure 6), and if they cover a wide area or are situated on vital organs or structures, we use the Swiftlase rotating minor delivery system (Sharplan, Tel Aviv, Israel). If the endometriosis is extremely hemorrhagic (Figure 7), or is associated with ovarian endometriomas (chocolate cysts), then we remove the hemosiderin-laden fluid by irrigation and suction (Figure 8) and then use the KTP laser to photocoagulate the inside of the ovarian endometrioma. This has resulted in a pregnancy rate of 52.5%, and a pain relief rate of 80%, but has never been subjected to a randomized, double-blind, prospective, controlled study.

We feel that the laparoscope is essential for this diagnosis of this unpleasant condition in patients. In experienced hands, laser surgery can be used to remove the implants and restore the anatomy to the pelvic structures, and this should therefore be performed at the same time as the diagnostic laparoscopy, particularly since it is extremely safe. In the last 3500 cases we have had no mortality and an extremely low morbidity, and no increased time for recovery over diagnostic laparoscopy alone. We feel that in the majority of patients it avoids the need for treatment with expensive drugs, which inevitably are associated with unpleasant side-effects, are usually contraceptive and are associated with a significant recurrence rate. We admit however that the role of laser laparoscopy is less likely to be effective in minimal disease and that many of the so-called atypical lesions of endometriosis may not in fact be endometriosis at all. Nevertheless, we feel that if it is endometriosis, laser laparoscopy does at least have a role in limiting progression of the disease. Although isolated implants of endometriosis in safe areas can probably be treated by the general gynecologist, we do feel that advanced endometriosis and particularly endometriosis that is close to the ureter or the bowel should be referred to special centers where they have special experience in this type of surgery.

References

1. Evers, J.L.H. (1987). The second-look laparoscopy for evaluation of the result of medical treatment of endometriosis should not be performed during ovarian suppression. *Fertil. Steril.*, **47**, 502–4
2. Feste, J.R. (1985). Laser laparoscopy: a new modality. *J. Reprod. Med.*, **30**, 413–17
3. Nezhat, C., Winer, W., Crowgey, F. and Nezhat, F. (1989). Video laparoscopy of the treatment of endometriosis associated with infertility. *Fertil. Steril.*, **51**, 237–40
4. Sutton, C.J.G. and Hill, D. (1990). Laser laparoscopy in the treatment of endometriosis. A five year study. *Br. J. Obstet. Gynaecol.*, **97**, 181–5
5. Daniell, J.F. (1989). Fibre optic laser laparoscopy. *Baill. Clin. Obstet. Gynaecol.*, **3**, 545–62
6. Cook, A.S. and Rock, J.A. (1991). The role of laparoscopy in the treatment of endometriosis. *Fertil. Steril.*, **55**, 663–80
7. Sutton, C.J.G., Nair, S., Ewen, S.P. and Haines, P.A. (1993). A comparison between the CO_2 and KTP lasers in the treatment of large ovarian endometriomas. *Gynaecol. Endosc.*, **2**, 113
8. Sutton, C.J.G., Ewen, S.P., Whitelaw, N. and Haines, P.A. (1994). A prospective, randomised, double-blind, controlled trial of laser laparoscopy in the treatment of pelvic pain associated with minimal, mild and moderate endometriosis. *Fertil. Steril.*, **62**, 696–700
9. Fedele, L., Bianchi, S., Bocciolone, L., Nola, G.D. and Franchi, D. (1993). Buserelin acetate in the treatment of pelvic pain associated with minimal and mild endometriosis: a controlled study. *Fertil. Steril.*, **59**, 516–21
10. Sutton, C.J.G. (1994). Laser uterine nerve ablation. In Donnez, J. and Nisolle, M. (eds.) *An Atlas of Laser Operative Laparoscopy and Hysteroscopy*, pp. 47–52. (Carnforth, UK: Parthenon Publishing)
11. Lichten, E.M. and Bombard, J. (1987). Surgical treatment of dysmenorrhoea with laparoscopic uterine nerve ablation. *J. Reprod. Med.*, **32**, 37–42
12. Waller, K.G. and Shaw, R.W. (1993). Gonadotrophin-releasing hormone analogues for the treatment of endometriosis: long-term follow-up. *Fertil. Steril.*, **59**, 511–15
13. Redwine, D.B. (1991). Conservative laparoscopic excision of endometriosis by sharp dissection: life table analysis of reoperation of persistent or recurrent disease. *Fertil. Steril.*, **56**, 628–34

Laparoscopic management of infertile patients with endometriosis

K. Okuda, M. Saeki and O. Sugimoto

Introduction

Infertility has been estimated to be present in 68% of patients with endometriosis[1]. It has been reported that endometriosis in its initial stage is a consequence, rather than a cause of infertility[2]. However, most clinicians would agree that endometriosis which is associated with tubal or ovarian damage or adhesion formation will materially affect future fertility. From this perspective, it has been shown that conservative surgery by laparotomy for endometriosis is beneficial for some infertile women[3]. Recently, many gynecologists have started treating endometriosis by surgical laparoscopy[1,4,5]. Laparoscopic surgery was introduced in our hospital in 1988 as conservative surgery for endometriosis. We progressed from aspiration and alcohol fixation of chocolate cysts, to performing laparoscopic cystectomies for chocolate cysts. A number of recent studies have addressed the improved fertility rate after laparoscopic surgery using laser and a combination of gonadotropin-releasing hormone (GnRH) analogs[5]. However, there is still considerable controversy regarding the appropriate treatment for endometriosis. Based on the pregnancy outcomes of 179 patients with infertility who underwent laparoscopic surgery, we discuss laparoscopic management of infertile patients with endometriosis.

Materials and method

Between January 1988 and December 1994 in the Department of Obstetrics and Gynecology of Osaka Medical College, and between January 1993 and December 1995 in the Gynecology Department of NTT Kyoto Hospital, 510 patients were treated for endometriosis. We performed definitive surgery on 75 patients, who received hysterectomy and/or bilateral oophorectomy, 420 patients underwent conservative surgeries and 15 other procedures. The conservative surgeries can be divided into 118 laparotomies (including 32 patients who underwent diagnostic laparoscopy before surgery), 56 diagnostic laparoscopies, 195 laparoscopic surgeries and 50 vaginal alcohol fixations of chocolate cysts.

This paper retrospectively analyzes the laparoscopic surgery cases. Among 195 cases, 10 cases were complicated by male infertility (sperm quantity $< 20 \times 10^6$/ml, mobility $< 30\%$), and 43 cases lost to follow-up were excluded from this study. In the laparoscopic surgery group, there were 142 cases treated for infertility. These patients were further divided into two groups, group I (142 patients) had not previously undergone surgery for endometriosis, while group II (37 patients) had previously undergone conservative surgery.

Results

Patients who had initially undergone conservative surgery

The cumulative pregnancy rate rose rapidly to 23.8% 7 months after laparoscopic surgery, and reached 31.4% by 13 months (Figure 1). From 13 months to 44 months after surgery,

Table 1 Pregnancy rates for 105 patients who underwent initial conservative surgery by laparoscopy

Stage	No. of patients	No. of pregnancies	% pregnant	Spontaneous abortions	% abortions
Stage I	24	11	45.8	3	27.3
Stage II	17	11	64.7	2	18.2
Stage III	27	10	37.0	1	10.0
Stage IV	37	7	18.9	0	0
Total	105	39	37.1	6	15.4

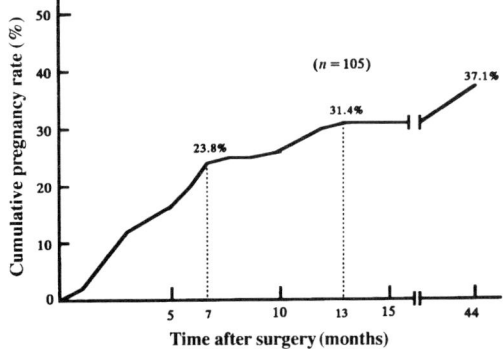

Figure 1 Cumulative pregnancy rate of the patients who underwent initial conservative surgery by laparoscopy

the pregnancy rate increased by only an additional 5.7%, to 37.1%. According to the revised classification of the American Fertility Society (AFS)[7], the highest pregnancy rate of 64.7% was achieved by patients in stage II, 45.8% by those in stage I, 37.0% by those in stage III, and the lowest pregnancy rate of 18.9% by those in stage IV (Table 1). These results show that laparoscopic surgery is more effective in patients with mild to moderate endometriosis than in patients with severe endometriosis.

Figures 2 and 3 show that the success of laparoscopic surgery in enabling pregnancy was based on the location and severity of endometrial lesions. The postoperative pregnancy rate in relation to severity of peritoneal lesions showed an inverse correlation, indicating that the severity of peritoneal lesions does not adversely affect pregnancy rates after laparoscopic surgery. However, the pregnancy rate declined as the severity of ovarian endometriosis, ovarian adhesion and tubal adhesion increased. The pregnancy rate in patients with an ovarian adhesion score greater than 4 dropped off dramatically from 49 to 20%. There was no pregnancy among 20 patients with an ovarian adhesion score over 16. The correlation between tubal adhesion severity and pregnancy rate was similar to the correlation between the ovarian adhesion severity and pregnancy rate. The pregnancy rate was reduced significantly from 44.4% when the severity was below 4, to 8.8% when the severity was 5 or above. Pregnancy rates were higher with a Douglas adhesion score of zero (45.9%), but did not appear to differ due to adhesion severity when comparing a score of 4 (24.0%) with a score of 40 (26.3%).

To confirm the significance of adnexal adhesions on the pregnancy rate after laparoscopic surgery, we examined the distribution of pregnancies among patients with adnexal adhesions. Figure 4 shows that the distribution of successful and unsuccessful pregnancies was based on coordinates which reflect the severity of both tubal adhesion and ovarian adhesions. The pregnancy rate was very low, only 10% in 30 patients with a tubal adhesion score over 4 and an ovarian adhesion score over 8 points. However, the pregnancy success rate was very high, 48% in 75 patients with a tubal adhesion score below 4 and an ovarian adhesion score of 8 points. This indicates that using laser or fibrin glue to

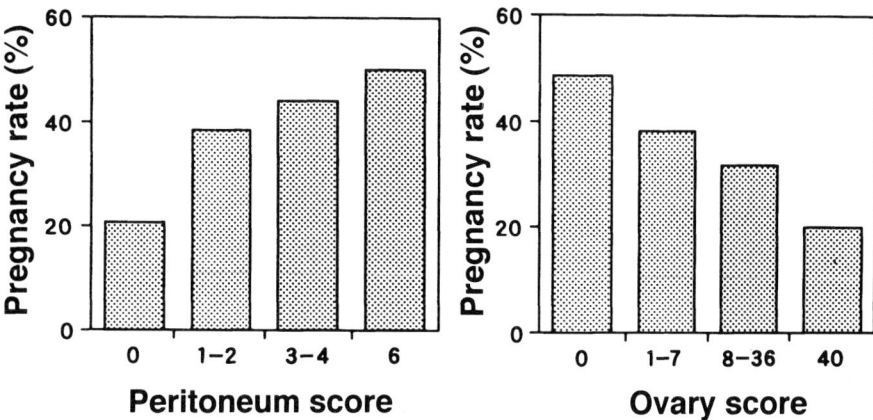

Figure 2 Postoperative pregnancy rates in relation to the severity of peritoneal and ovarian lesions

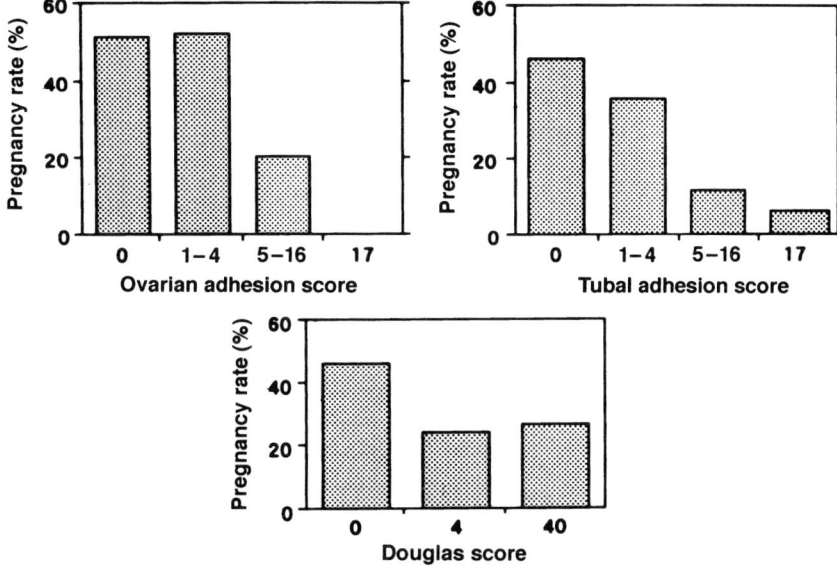

Figure 3 Postoperative pregnancy rates in relation to the severity of adnexal, ovarian and Douglas adhesion

avoid reformation of adhesion is not sufficient. Considering these findings, we recommend that patients with severe adnexal adhesions be referred to an *in vitro* fertilization/embryo transfer program.

Patients undergoing conservative surgery for the first time were classified into 35 patients receiving preoperative medical therapy (PMT), and 70 patients receiving laparoscopic surgery only. There were no significant differences in age (30.4 ± 2.1 and 31.2 ± 8.5 years), infertility duration (4.3 ± 3.5 and 4.6 ± 3.8 years), primary infertility (74.9 and 72.9%) or revised AFS score (32.2 ± 16.3 and 38.6 ± 21.9) between the two groups.

The overall pregnancy rate was significantly

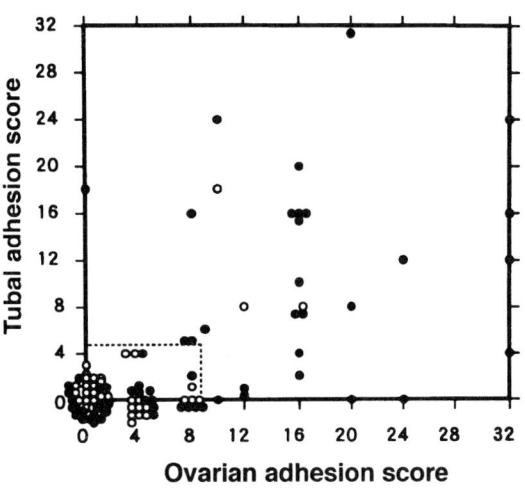

Figure 4 Distribution of pregnant (○) and non-pregnant (●) patients based on the severity of both tubal adhesion and ovarian adhesion

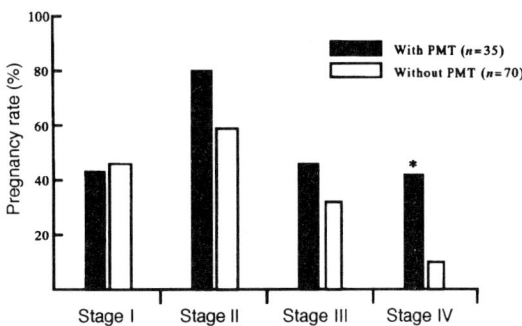

Figure 5 Comparison of pregnancy rates between patients with preoperative medical treatment (PMT) and those without PMT. *$p < 0.05$ compared with no PMT

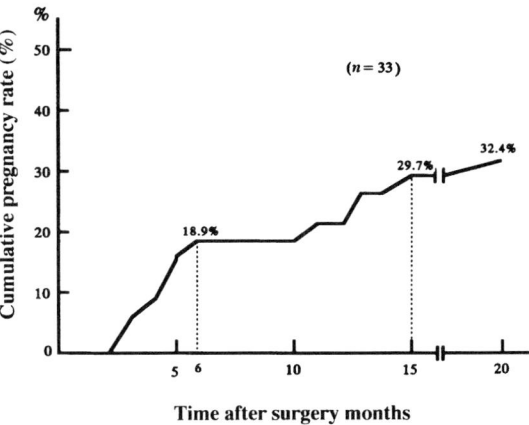

Figure 6 Cumulative pregnancy rate after laparoscopic surgery for recurrent endometriosis

increased by PMT. Pregnancy rates in patients receiving PMT were 48.6% vs. only 31.4% in patients without PMT. When patients were grouped by endometriosis staging (Figure 5), PMT did not provide a comparative advantage to the pregnancy rate in patients with stage I disease. However, PMT appeared to positively increase the pregnancy rate in patients with stage II, III or IV endometriosis, compared to the rate in patients who did not receive PMT. PMT resulted in the largest difference in pregnancy rates among patients with stage IV disease, 42% (5/12) with PMT vs. 8% (2/24) without PMT.

Patients who had previously undergone conservative surgery

There was no difference in age (31.1 ± 4.1 and 30.5 ± 3.4 years), infertility duration (5.1 ± 3.8 and 5.1 ± 3.4 years) or primary infertility (73.3 and 75.7%) between the patients who underwent initial laparoscopic surgery and those who underwent repetitive conservative surgery. Although the revised AFS score was higher in the repetitive conservative surgery group (40.8 ± 36.4) than in the initial laparoscopic surgery group (51.6 ± 31.6), the difference was not significant.

The cumulative pregnancy rate reached 18.9% by 6 months postoperatively, and continued to climb to reach 29.7% by 15 months after surgery, then peaked at 32.4%, 20 months postoperatively (Figure 6). The interval until pregnancy after repetitive conservative surgery was similar to that in patients undergoing their first laparoscopic surgery. The cumulative pregnancy rate in patients receiving repetitive laparoscopic

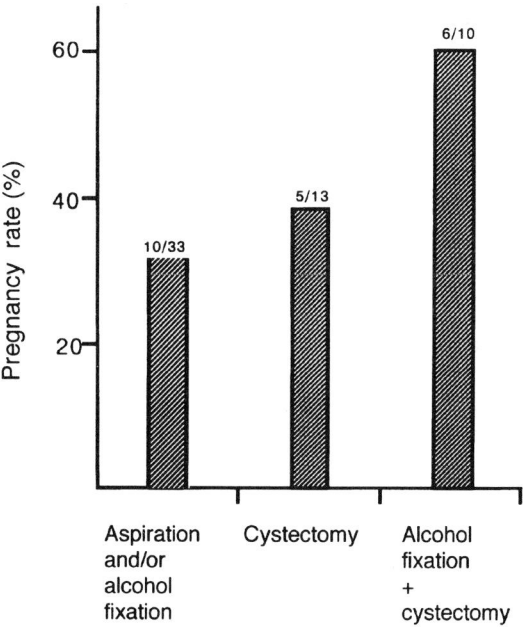

Figure 7 Comparison of the pregnancy rates after different laparoscopic procedures to treat chocolate cysts

Discussion

Conservative surgery is considered one of the possible treatments for endometriosis[3]. Recently, many gynecologists have started treating endometriosis by surgical laparoscopy[1,4,5]. A number of recent studies[4,5] have addressed improvement of the fertility rate by laparoscopic surgery. However, analyzing the fertility results in patients treated for endometriosis is difficult and uncertain, because it is difficult to study homogeneous cases without any other infertility causes. There is still considerable controversy regarding the appropriate treatment for endometriosis. In this study, preoperative medical treatment (PMT) significantly increased the pregnancy rate from 31.4 to 48.6%. In stage IV disease, there was a significant difference in pregnancy rates. However, medical treatment provided no comparative advantage to the pregnancy rate in stage I disease. Donnez and colleagues[6] reported that hormone therapy reduced the size of chocolate cysts and the inflammatory aspect of the adhesions. It was suggested that these effects of hormone therapy could be beneficial in preventing re-formation after laparoscopic surgery. So hormone therapy is recommended before surgery to improve the fertility rate, if the patient is clinically suspected of endometriosis.

The cumulative pregnancy rate was 37.4% after laparoscopic surgery in patients followed over 6 months. According to the revised AFS classification, the pregnancy rate in patients with mild to moderate endometriosis was significantly higher than that of those with severe disease. Whether pregnancy rates correlate with the revised AFS classification remains controversial. Nezhat and colleagues[4] reported that the pregnancy rate does not differ between stages of endometriosis. However, Donnez and associates[5] reported that the pregnancy rate in stage III patients was higher than that in stage IV patients. The significance of adnexal adhesions on the pregnancy rate after laparoscopic surgery was clearly shown in this study. Great efforts have

surgery was comparable to that of those receiving their first laparoscopic surgery. We conclude that repetitive surgery utilizing a laparoscopic procedure can effectively improve the fertility rate.

We advanced from aspiration and alcohol fixation of chocolate cysts, to performing laparoscopic cystectomies for chocolate cyst. However, the pregnancy rate did not significantly increase in the patients undergoing laparoscopic cystectomy (38%) compared to that in those undergoing aspiration and alcohol fixation (30%) of chocolate cysts (Figure 7). To reduce the size of chocolate cysts, we performed vaginal aspiration and alcohol fixation of the chocolate cysts prior to laparoscopic cystectomy. Six of ten patients became pregnant after this procedure. To date, only a small group has undergone this procedure, but a high pregnancy rate was achieved by this intervention.

been made to prevent re-formation of adhesions, using laser surgery or fibrin glue. However, it is difficult to avoid re-formation of adhesions after lysis of adnexal adhesions or cystectomy, even by laparoscopy. It is important to use less invasive procedures in laparoscopic surgery. We recommend reducing the size of chocolate cysts with vaginal aspiration and alcohol fixation prior to laparoscopic cystectomy. Donnez and colleagues[6] reported that GnRH agonist and drainage in patients with large chocolate cysts reduced the size of the cysts and the 'activity' of endometriotic lesions in the ovary as well as the peritoneum. In this study, a pregnancy rate of 60% was achieved using this method, vs. 38% for laparoscopic cystectomy alone, and 30% for aspiration and alcohol fixation alone. The effectiveness of this procedure should be investigated in a larger number of patients. However, vaginal aspiration is a less invasive treatment than laparoscopic aspiration for patients with chocolate cysts.

Recurrence of endometriosis is frequent in patients treated by conservative surgery and ranges from 2 to 47%. Candiani and colleagues[8] showed that repetitive conservative surgery by laparotomy for recurrence of endometriosis is an effective therapeutic option for infertile patients with recurrent endometriosis. Our data also showed that repetitive surgery utilizing a laparoscopic procedure is useful for improving the fertility rate. The cumulative pregnancy rate (32.4%) by laparoscopy is comparable to that by laparotomy (30.7%). If the patient does not conceive within 13 months after the initial laparoscopic surgery, laparoscopy is necessary to evaluate the severity of endometriosis, and repetitive laparoscopic surgery is indicated to improve the fertility rate. It is suggested that laparoscopic conservative surgery is an effective therapeutic option for infertile patients with recurrent endometriosis.

In conclusion, to improve the pregnancy rate we propose the following intervention. First, medical treatment for 3–6 months before laparoscopic surgery. Second, vaginal aspiration and alcohol fixation of chocolate cysts prior to surgery. Third, repetitive laparoscopic surgery 13 months after the first laparoscopic surgery, if necessary.

References

1. Koninckx, P.R., Lesaffre, E., Meuleman, C., Cornillie, F.J. and Demeyre, S. (1991). Suggestive evidence that pelvic endometriosis is a progressive disease, whereas deeply infiltrating endometriosis is associated with pelvic pain. *Fertil. Steril.*, **55**, 759–65
2. Shenken, R.S. and Malinak, L.R. (1982). Conservative surgery versus expectant management for the infertile patient with mild endometriosis. *Fertil. Steril.*, **37**, 183–6
3. Buttram, V.C. (1979). Surgical treatment of endometriosis in the infertile female: a modified approach. *Fertil. Steril.*, **32**, 635–40
4. Nezhat, C., Crowgey, S. and Nezhat, F. (1989). Videolaserscopy for the treatment of endometriosis associated with infertility. *Fertil. Steril.*, **51**, 237–40
5. Donnez, J. Nisolle, M., Anaf, V., Semts, M., Bassil, S. and CasanasRoux, F. (1994). Endoscopic management of peritoneal and ovarian endometriosis. In Donnez, J. and Nisolle, M. (eds.) *An Atlas of Laser Operative Laparoscopy and Hysteroscopy*, pp. 63–74. (New York: Parthenon Publishing)
6. Donnez, J., Anaf, V., Nisolle, M., Clerckx-Braun, F., Gillerot, S. and Casanas-Roux, F. (1994). Ovarian endometrial cysts: the role of gonadotropin-releasing hormone agonist and/or drainage. *Fertil. Steril.*, **62**, 63–6
7. The American Fertility Society (1989). Revised classification of endometriosis. *Fertil. Steril.*, **52**, 27–30
8. Candiani, G.B., Fedele, L., Vercellini, P., Bianchi, S. and Di Nola, G. (1991). Repetitive conservative surgery for recurrence of endometriosis. *Obstet. Gynecol.*, **77**, 421–4

Office microlaparoscopy under local anesthesia for endometriosis

S.F. Palter

Introduction

Laparoscopic surgery has been in the forefront of gynecologic surgical innovation in the past decade. Major benefits which have been realized by the utilization of laparoscopy include: a reduced size of surgical incisions; reduced length of hospital stays; increased utilization of outpatient surgery; a more rapid postoperative recovery period; reduced morbidity; and reduced total costs of treatment. Recent refinements in surgical technique and instrumentation have allowed the development of a new incarnation of laparoscopy which has the potential to further realize each of these goals. Office microlaparoscopy under local anesthesia is the most recent advance in gynecologic minimally invasive surgery.

The performance of laparoscopy without general anesthesia is not a new concept. In fact, laparoscopy was initially developed as a local anesthetic procedure[1-11]. Over the past 75 years laparoscopy has gradually shifted to a procedure primarily performed under general anesthesia. This transformation in anesthetic technique has necessitated that the procedure be performed in a traditional operating room (hospital or outpatient surgical center). Unfortunately, this degree of resource utilization, including a full operating room, anesthesiologist and general anesthesia, and full postoperative recovery room, is in excess of what is required for simple diagnostic laparoscopy. Recent focus on cost containment has led to a re-evaluation of the technique of laparoscopy under local anesthesia. This is similar to the transformation of colonoscopy and cystoscopy to procedures primarily performed in outpatient procedure rooms under local anesthesia. The overall concept is to use an appropriate level of resources for each procedure and not to over-utilize resources which are not required. The older protocols for local anesthetic laparoscopy have been further modified by the technological innovation of micro- (or sub-5-mm) laparoscopy, which has raised tolerance and lengthened the time procedures can be performed (increasing the likelihood of adequate and complete examinations).

The technique of office laparoscopy under local anesthesia is especially suited to meet the current pressures of quality vs. cost in an era of managed care. It is likely that this technique will soon become a major part of the practicing gynecologist's diagnostic and operative armamentarium. Advantages of office microlaparoscopy under local anesthesia are realized by the practitioner, the patient and the managed care-provider. Patients benefit from decreased scheduling delays, a more rapid postoperative recovery with decreased pain, decreased total procedure costs and a greater involvement in the procedure. Physicians will also benefit from a greater control over the scheduling of the procedure, the potential to perform laparoscopy in a traditional office procedure room and streamlined care delivery. All of this translates into reduced total costs, decreased disability, a more rapid return to the workforce and greater total satisfaction.

Anesthesia and its impact on technique

Traditional thought in the USA has dictated that laparoscopy is a procedure that requires general anesthesia. Many arguments are given in support of this, including the arguments that general anesthesia is required for adequate intraoperative pain control; that creation of a pneumoperitoneum compromises diaphragmatic excursion and dictates intubation and mechanical ventilation to assure adequate oxygenation; that there is a need for paralysis of the patient to prevent intra-operative movement and inadvertent injury; and that there is a need for mechanical ventilation to clear CO_2 absorbed from the pneumoperitoneum. Each of these arguments is based upon anecdote and speculation rather than actual data. In fact, there is a long history to support the safety, feasibility and advantages of laparoscopy under local anesthesia, and which refutes these arguments[7,8].

Most reports of laparoscopy under local anesthesia were performed with some degree of supplemental intravenous sedation in addition to local anesthesia[3,4,9-13]. In these reports, the term local anesthesia is used liberally to differentiate the procedures from those performed under general anesthesia, even if supplemental intravenous agents are used. The prime consideration in the use of intravenous (or 'conscious') sedation is the preservation of patient alertness and responsiveness. In doing so, the patient will independently preserve the integrity of her own airway and maintain adequate ventilation. In contrast, under general anesthesia, there is partial or complete loss of protective reflexes. Should the patient not remain responsive to verbal instructions, the line into general anesthesia has been crossed and the risk of the procedure increases dramatically.

Procedures can be performed under strict local anesthesia; however, this results in diminished operative time and tolerance, and prohibits all but the most simple procedures. Historically, laparoscopy under strict local anesthesia (using traditional-sized instrumentation) was limited to 10–15 min of operative time before patient discomfort became limiting. We have found that by using the microlaparoscopes and adding supplemental intravenous sedation we can extend operative times to 30–45 min on a regular basis, with our longest case lasting over 1 h. Current studies are ongoing to compare objectively the tolerance of traditional (5- and 10-mm) laparoscopes as compared with the newer micro- (2- and 3-mm) instrumentation under local anesthesia.

Diagnosis of endometriosis

Endometriosis is associated with a wide variety of presenting signs and symptoms. It has been well documented that there is a poor correlation between extent of disease and either type or severity of symptomatology. Pelvic endometriosis commonly presents with dysmenorrhea, chronic pelvic pain, infertility, menstrual irregularities or dyspareunia. Other patients may have extensive disease yet remain symptom-free.

Pelvic pain is one of the most common symptoms of pelvic endometriosis. A wide variety of manifestations have been associated with the disease including primary or secondary dysmenorrhea, dyspareunia, chronic pelvic pain, abdominal pain and backache. Although the exact prevalence of endometriosis in women who have pelvic pain is variable, a high percentage have been shown to have endometriosis when both cyclic pelvic pain and dysmenorrhea are present. Despite this, endometriosis remains a diagnostic dilemma. Many of the presenting signs and symptoms are of non-specific or poorly localized pain and symptoms may be highly variable throughout the menstrual cycle. Physical examination findings are related to the location and stage of disease and patients with mild to moderate stage disease often have normal examinations[14]. Available diagnostic modalities for endometriosis include laparoscopy, sonography, computerized tomographic (CT) scanning, magnetic resonance imaging (MRI) and serum protein testing (CA-125, PP-14). Among these, laparoscopy has been the 'gold standard' method of diagnosis. Unfortunately, the laparoscopic appearance of endometriosis is highly variable with the recent recognition of many atypical forms of lesions. Difficulty in recognizing these lesions often results in false-negative operations[15]. Even more common, however, is a delay in performing laparoscopy in favor of reliance on non-invasive diagnostic modalities or empiric treatment. Frequently cited reasons for this delay include an over-reliance on physical examination and symptoms, a desire to avoid operative interventions (especially in younger patients), misdiagnosis (pelvic inflammatory disease etc.) and the high cost associated with laparoscopy. Many of these presumed 'low-likelihood' patients, including teenagers, have been shown frequently to have endometriosis[16].

Physicians must then decide the 'threshold for laparoscopy' for each patient, or how severe the pain must become before it warrants an operative intervention. Instead, many will initially choose to treat with a combination of watchful waiting, oral contraceptives or progestational agents, and non-steroidal anti-inflammatory agents. Recently, there has been an increase in empiric treatments including antibiotics and gonadotropin-releasing hormone agonists (GnRHa). The net result of all of these is often a delay in obtaining definitive diagnosis and inappropriate treatment.

Unfortunately, non-invasive methods of diagnosis all suffer from poor sensitivity and specificity. Sonography is best suited for the diagnosis of ovarian endometriosis where it is fairly reliable[17]. It is a poor technique for the diagnosis of focal lesions outside of the ovary with a sensitivity as low as 11%[18]. CT scanning suffers from a similar lack of ability to discriminate focal endometriotic lesions unless a significant space occupied by lesions is present[19]. More recently, advances in MRI have made it a promising technique for the non-invasive diagnosis of endometriosis[20]. However, at present this technique is not well standardized, requires special expertise, is expensive and has not been well validated.

Use of office microlaparoscopy for endometriosis

Office microlaparoscopy has the potential to become a standard method of evaluation of the patient with suspected endometriosis. The procedure has been successfully performed on patients presenting with both chronic pelvic pain and infertility. In addition to the ability to visually identify endometriotic lesions, biopsies can be taken to obtain a tissue diagnosis. The major limitation to the technique is that it is primarily a diagnostic tool. Therapeutic options are currently limited by safety concerns (with limited emergent hemostasis options), patient tolerance and microlaparoscopy equipment limitations. In view of this, some physicians choose to perform diagnostic microlaparoscopy under local anesthesia as a preoperative adjuvant to traditional operative laparoscopy. In this situation, diagnostic laparoscopy (with conscious pain mapping, if indicated) is first performed under local anesthesia. If no pathology is encountered, the procedure is terminated. When pathology is found, and is localized, the surgeon can choose to convert to traditional operative laparoscopy under general anesthesia at the time of the same procedure.

Office microlaparoscopy for chronic pelvic pain

A prospective cohort study was conducted by Palter and Olive[12] on patients presenting with chronic pelvic pain and requiring diagnostic laparoscopy who all had office microlaparoscopy performed under local anesthesia, the results of which are presented in Table 1[12]. Patients were queried preoperatively, and 30 min and 1 week postoperatively with a specially designed questionnaire and a modification of the McGill Pain Inventory scale. A specific subset of questions evaluated the recovery period and time until return to usual activities including diet, work and sexual activity.

Table 1 Results of office microlaparoscopy under local anesthesia for chronic pelvic pain (CPP) and infertility (INF)

	All	CPP	INF
Age (years)	35.33	36.45	34.56
Gravidy	0.96	1.55	0.56*
Operative time (min)	20.85	23.91	18.75
Recovery time (min)	51.65	51.64	51.67
Fentanyl (µg)	81.48	90.91	75.00*
Versed (mg)	3.20	4.00	2.66*
Pain scale score	5.87	7.00	5.04*
30-min postoperative pain score	1.48	3.17	0.53**
Time to normal activity (days)	1.88	1.73	2.01
Time to return to work (days)	1.70	2.23	1.29*
Time to resume intercourse (days)	4.61	5.42	4.21
Postoperative medical usage (tablets ibu)	4.88	9.45	1.53**

*$p < 0.05$; **$p < 0.005$, CPP compared with INF; ibu, Ibuprofen (600 mg)

The technique of 'conscious pain mapping' was developed for use during office laparoscopy under local anesthesia in patients with chronic pelvic pain[12]. Here, the pelvis is systematically inspected and the major structures grasped or probed in a standardized fashion. Any visible areas of pathology (e.g. endometriosis, adhesions or scarring) are also probed. Patients are asked to rate the pain of this grasping with a weighted 0–10 point scale. Conscious pain mapping demonstrated distinct patterns of pain in patients with chronic pelvic pain: either no identifiable pain; or focal pain which may or may not be associated with focal lesions; or a generalized visceral hypersensitivity in all areas of the pelvis and abdominal cavity. This third pattern, generalized visceral hypersensitivity (GVH), was not found in patients undergoing diagnostic laparoscopy for infertility who did not also have chronic pelvic pain, regardless of the presence of visualized pathology (adhesions or endometriosis). GVH has been observed in patients with and without focal pathology. Pathophysiologically, GVH may represent an abnormal response to normal visceral sensations, a response to chronic focal pain (the 'kindling phenomenon'), microscopic endometriosis, or a response to secreted substances and generalized inflammation[13,21]. We believe that patients with endometriosis who exhibit GVH may respond better to medical or combination therapies than to surgical excision alone. Current studies are ongoing to address this question.

Office microlaparoscopy for the evaluation of infertility

A cohort study was performed by Palter and Olive on all patients requiring diagnostic laparoscopy as part of the general infertility work-up at the Reproductive Endocrinology Division of Yale University[13]. They investigated whether a complete infertility evaluation could be performed under local anesthesia in an office setting. All of these patients reported that they were highly satisfied with the procedure, 96% would repeat the procedure in the office under local anesthesia, and 93% preferred the office laparoscopy to a previous traditional operating room-based laparoscopy. There were no procedures that were unable to be performed due to patient or equipment failures, and no procedures required general anesthesia. All aspects of the infertility investigation were able to be performed successfully including chromopertubation, biopsy of endometriosis and inspection of all areas of the pelvis and abdomen. The average procedure length was 18 min and ranged from 8 to 50 min. Furthermore, patients were stable for discharge in less than 50 min. The average patient required minimal to no postoperative medication and returned to full usual activities within 24 h. Analysis of costs demonstrated an approximate 75% reduction in costs as compared with traditional laparoscopy. These results would suggest that the use of office microlaparoscopy may allow diagnostic laparoscopy to be considered earlier in the infertility investigation.

Conclusions

Endometriosis remains one of the most commonly encountered gynecological diseases. Despite a high prevalence and multiple diagnostic options, it remains difficult to diagnose accurately without operative intervention. Unfortunately, delay in performing diagnostic laparoscopy in favor of less accurate methods remains a major limitation in obtaining an accurate diagnosis. Office microlaparoscopy under local anesthesia enables practitioners to quickly, easily, and effectively obtain a visual and/or tissue diagnosis of endometriosis. In addition, total costs of obtaining this diagnosis are drastically reduced when compared with traditional laparoscopy.

In the future, office microlaparoscopy has the potential to become the standard method of diagnosis of endometriosis. Hopefully the ease of use will translate into a lowered threshold for laparoscopy and earlier diagnosis of disease. Conscious pain mapping represents the first technique unique to microlaparoscopy under local anesthesia and has the potential to help physicians better choose between the therapeutic options available for a given patient. As a research and monitoring tool, office microlaparoscopy under local anesthesia enables physicians to perform multiple or repeat procedures with a minimum of pain, expense and trauma. Finally, many physicians will choose to perform microlaparoscopy under local anesthesia in hospital operating rooms, procedure rooms or surgicenters. In this way, the benefits of laparoscopy under local anesthesia are realized while avoiding start-up costs and lack of back-up in office laparoscopy.

References

1. Gunning, J.E. (1974). The history of laparoscopy. *J. Reprod. Med.*, **12**, 222–6
2. Short, A.R. (1925). The use of celioscopy. *Br. Med. J.*, **2**, 254
3. Childers, J.M., Hatch, K.D. and Surwit, E.A. (1992). Office laparoscopy and biopsy for evaluation of patients with intraperitoneal carcinomatosis using a new optical catheter. *Gynecol. Oncol.*, **47**, 337–42
4. Steege, J.F. (1994). Repeated clinic laparoscopy for the treatment of pelvic adhesions: a pilot study. *Obstet. Gynecol.*, **83**, 276–9
5. Metha, P.V. (1989). A total of 250 136 laparoscopic sterilizations by single operator. *Br. J. Obstet. Gynaecol.*, **96**, 1024–34
6. Snabes, M.C. and Poindexter A.N. III, (1991). Laparoscopic tubal sterilization under local anesthesia in women with cyanotic heart disease. *Obstet. Gynecol.*, **78**, 437–40
7. Peterson, H.B., Hulka, J.F., Spielman, F.J., Lee, S. and Marchbanks, P.A. (1987). Local vs. general anesthesia for laparoscopic sterilization: randomized study. *Obstet. Gynecol.*, **70**, 903–8
8. Brown, D.R., Fishburne, J.I., Roberson, V.O. and Hulka, J.V. (1976). Ventilatory and blood gas changes during laparoscopy with local anesthesia. *Am. J. Obstet. Gynecol.*, **124**, 741–5
9. Wheeless C.R. Jr, (1972). Outpatient laparoscopic sterilization under local anesthesia. *Obstet. Gynecol.*, **39**, 767–70
10. Alexander, G.D., Goldrath, M., Brown, E.M. and Smiler, B.G. (1973). Outpatient laparoscopic sterilization under local anesthesia. *Am. J. Obstet. Gynecol.*, **116**, 1065–8
11. Fishburne, J.I., Omran, K.F., Hulka, J.F., Mercer, J.P. and Edelman, D.A. (1974). Laparoscopic tubal clip sterilization under local anesthesia. *Fertil. Steril.*, **25**, 762–6
12. Palter, S. and Olive, D. (1996). Office laparoscopy under local anesthesia for chronic pelvic pain: utility, acceptance, and cost-benefit analysis. *J. Am. Assoc. Gynecol. Laparosc.*, **3**, 359–64
13. Palter, S.F. and Olive, D.L. (1995). Office laparoscopy under local anesthesia for infertility: utility, acceptance, and cost-benefit/outcome analyses. *Fertil. Steril.*, **64**, S8–S9

14. Rawson, J.M.R. (1991). Prevalence of endometriosis in asymptomatic women. *J. Reprod. Med.*, **36**, 513–15
15. Stripling, M.C., Martin, D.C., Chatman, D.L. *et al.* (1988). Subtle appearance of pelvic endometriosis. *Fertil. Steril.*, **49**, 427
16. Huffman, J.W. (1981). Endometriosis in young teenage girls. *Pediatr. Ann.*, **10**, 44–9
17. Mais, V., Guerriero, S., Ajossa, S., Angiolucci, M., Paoletti, A.M. and Melis, G.B. (1993). The efficiency of transvaginal ultrasonography in the diagnosis of endometrioma. *Fertil. Steril.*, **5**, 776–80
18. Friedman, H., Vogelzangh, R.L., Mendelson, E.B., Neiman, H.L. and Cohen, M. (1985). Endometriosis detection by US with laparoscopic correlation. *Radiology*, **157**, 217–20
19. Fishman, E.K., Scatarige, J.C., Saksouk, F.A., Rosenheim, N.B. and Siegelmann, S.S. (1983). Computed tomography of endometriosis. *J. Comput. Assist. Tomogr.*, **7**, 257–64
20. Arrive, L., Hrick, H. and Martin, M.C. (1989). Pelvic endometriosis: MR imaging. *Radiology*, **171**, 687–92
21. Murphy, A.A., Green, W.R., Bobbi, D. *et al.* (1986). Unsuspected endometriosis documented by scanning electron microscopy in visually normal peritoneum. *Fertil. Steril.*, **46**, 522

Meta-analysis and evidence-based guidelines for treating endometriosis-associated infertility

G.D. Adamson

Introduction

This manuscript evaluates the best treatment for endometriosis-associated infertility. The options for treatment include no treatment, medical treatment and surgical treatment by laparoscopy or laparotomy. An array of studies has addressed these alternative treatments. Many reports have significant limitations because they are retrospective or lack controls. It has been difficult to determine the optimal treatment because prospective randomized trials are rarely performed. Even prospective studies done with controls have limitations because of differences among the treatment groups, but they represent the best studies to date with respect to surgical treatment for endometriosis. Although it is not possible to account for all differences among treatment groups in the absence of randomization, identified differences can be controlled using statistical methods such as survival analysis with fixed covariates. Below is a summary of data which have been collected over the past 18 years which help to provide information to develop a consensus on the appropriate treatment of endometriosis-associated infertility.

Treatment of endometriosis-associated infertility

It has become increasingly possible in the past 15 years to treat endometriosis at the time of diagnostic laparoscopy. Numerous studies have evaluated pregnancy rates following laparoscopic treatment of endometriosis. One of the earlier papers evaluating outcomes was, in fact, performed to study a method for designing a surgical staging system[1]. With no treatment, the life-table estimated 3-year pregnancy rate was 40%, with oral contraceptives 33% and with surgery 53%. These results were not statistically significantly different and showed that no treatment was a reasonable approach for many patients with minimal or mild endometriosis.

With the increasing facility of laparoscopy to treat more extensive disease, the effectiveness of laparoscopy compared to laparotomy for treating endometriomata was evaluated with prospectively collected data. This showed 1- and 3-year life-table estimated cumulative pregnancy rates of 30% and 52% for the laparoscopy group, compared to 23% and 46%, respectively, for the laparotomy group (Breslow $p = 0.48$). Monthly fecundity over 3 years was 2.4% for the laparoscopy group and 2% for the laparotomy group[2]. This controlled study using prospectively tabulated data confirmed that CO_2 laser laparoscopy was a safe and effective treatment for endometriomata. Pregnancy rates after CO_2 laser laparoscopy were equivalent to those obtained by laparotomy and were independent of size and number of endometriomata and stage of pelvic disease. It was shown that laparoscopy with the CO_2 laser allowed precise treatment of extensive pelvic disease, and the less invasive surgery provided obvious advantages to the patient. However, it was also noted that this type of surgery could be technically demanding.

A large study with prospectively recorded data was carried out to evaluate pregnancy rates following laparoscopy for endometriosis, compared with no treatment, medical treatment and laparotomy, and was published in January 1993[3]. This study of 579 patients showed that laparoscopy pregnancy rates were equal to or higher than other treatment options for the entire population of 579 patients as well as an endometriosis-only subset consisting of patients with at least one normal tube and fimbria, and normal male factor ($n = 258$) (Table 1). Laparoscopic treatment of endometriosis was found to result in equivalent or higher pregnancy rates than other treatments, whether or not disease was minimal, mild, moderate or severe. Furthermore, even when significant variables, such as years of infertility, revised American Fertility Society (AFS) total endometriosis score, ovulation treatment, fimbrial score and tubal score were controlled for, the laparoscopy crude pregnancy rates were equal to or higher than other treatments. These differences were up to 101% better than other treatment modalities and could consequently be of clinical significance to the patient. In particular, in the endometriosis-only subset, it was shown that laparoscopy for moderate and severe endometriosis was statistically significantly better with respect to subsequent pregnancy rates than laparotomy ($p = 0.03$) (Table 2).

As skill and experience with the laparoscope increased, further studies evaluated estimated life-table pregnancy rates for treatment of complete posterior cul-de-sac endometriosis obliteration. These data showed that laparoscopy and laparotomy were not statistically significantly different in terms of outcome for the patient, even when there was very extensive disease[4].

Hughes and colleagues published an excellent paper which was a quantitative overview of controlled trials in endometriosis infertility[5]. We subsequently performed a study to evaluate and expand this meta-analysis and to compare it with our prospective cohort study data, thereby hopefully increasing our understanding of the best treatment for endometriosis-associated infertility[6].

Meta-analysis is a recent popular method being utilized to evaluate evidence in clinical situations in which prospective randomized trials are difficult or impossible to perform[7]. Meta-analysis is the formal combination of evidence from a series of separate studies. Studies are selected according to predetermined criteria, and the evidence is combined across those studies using statistical techniques. Unfortunately, meta-analyses also suffer from weaknesses which can limit their utility.

The results of our analysis provided strong evidence that there was no significant difference in crude pregnancy rates between medical treatment and no treatment (Figure 1)[6]. The combined estimated risk ratio was 0.98 with a 95% confidence interval of 0.81–1.18. In the figure the central dot for each study represents the point estimate of relative risk of pregnancy for no treatment compared to medical treatment. Dots to the right of the vertical line at unity indicate studies in which medical treatment resulted in higher crude pregnancy rates. Dots to the left of the vertical line indicate studies in which no treatment resulted in higher crude pregnancy rates. The horizontal lines indicate a 95% confidence interval for the true relative risk based on that study. Longer lines indicate more uncertainty which occurs in studies with a smaller number of patients. Lines that include unity (as all do in Figure 1) mean that the study showed no statistically significant difference in crude pregnancy rates between medical treatment and no treatment. The lowest line on the figure shows the estimated relative risk and associated 95% confidence interval obtained by combining the evidence from all the studies using the Mantel–Haenszel approach[6].

A combined Mantel–Haenszel estimate from our study is summarized in Figure 2. Medical treatment alone did not produce higher pregnancy rates compared to no treatment, and therefore is not appropriate for treatment of endometriosis-associated infertility. Other

Table 1 Estimated cumulative life-table percentage pregnancy rates by treatment group for different stages of endometriosis

Stage	Treatment	Entire patient population					Endometriosis-only subset		
		n	3-year pregnancies[†]	1 year	2 years	3 years	3-year pregnancies[†]	1 year	2 years	3 years
Minimal/mild	None	20	11	48.6 ± 11.7	61.1 ± 11.8	61.1 ± 11.8	14	10	64.3 ± 12.8	71.4 ± 12.1	71.4 ± 12.1
	Medical	49	24	30.4 ± 7.1	56.1 ± 8.2	64.0 ± 8.5	34	14	27.1 ± 8.2	47.5 ± 9.8	54.1 ± 10.5
	Laparoscopy	285	144	43.0 ± 3.2	60.3 ± 3.5	67.6 ± 3.8	148	78	45.9 ± 4.5	62.1 ± 4.9	71.6 ± 5.2
	Laparotomy	87	44	38.3 ± 5.7	52.5 ± 6.2	68.8 ± 6.5	18	9	32.4 ± 12.0	47.4 ± 13.2	64.4 ± 13.4
Moderate/severe*	Laparoscopy	76	30	22.8 ± 5.2	42.9 ± 6.7	59.2 ± 7.8	34	17	25.1 ± 8.3	65.1 ± 10.7	79.1 ± 10.0
	Laparotomy	61	21	27.2 ± 5.8	37.0 ± 6.5	37.0 ± 6.5	10	2	20.0 ± 12.7	20.0 ± 12.7	20.0 ± 12.7

[†]Actual number of patients pregnant within 3 years; *One patient treated medically excluded

Table 2 Comparison of laparoscopic treatment of endometriosis for infertility with other treatment modalities

Treatment comparison	Entire patient population ($n = 579$)		Endometriosis-only subset* ($n = 258$)	
	Increased pregnancy rate when treated laparoscopically	p-value	Increased pregnancy rate when treated laparoscopically	p-value
Laparoscopy vs. no treatment**	7%	0.83	−14%	0.64
Laparoscopy vs. medical treatment**	42%	0.088	101%	0.007
Laparoscopy vs. laparotomy	29%	0.13	87%	0.031

*At least one Fallopian tube and fimbria normal, and normal male factor; **all patients receiving no treatment or medical treatments had minimal or mild disease

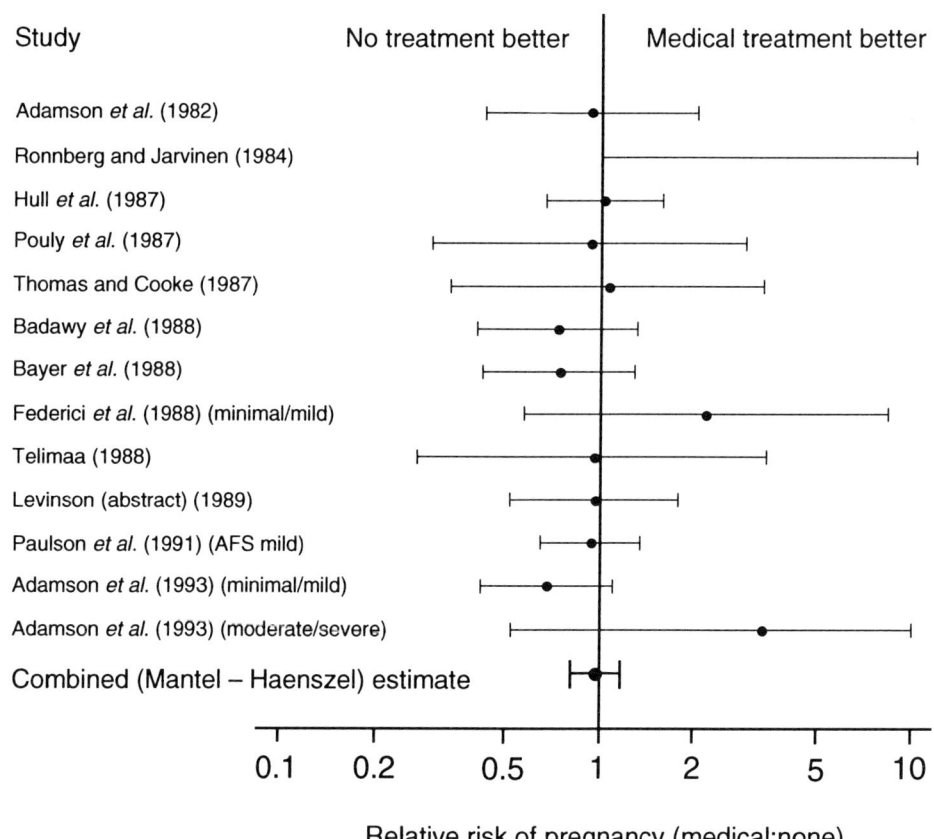

Figure 1 Results of meta-analysis of medical vs. no treatment of endometriosis-associated infertility (reproduced from reference 7). The point estimated risk ratio is shown as a dot and the 95% confidence interval by the bar. If the bar does not cross the line marked '1' there is a statistical difference between the treatments ($p < 0.05$)

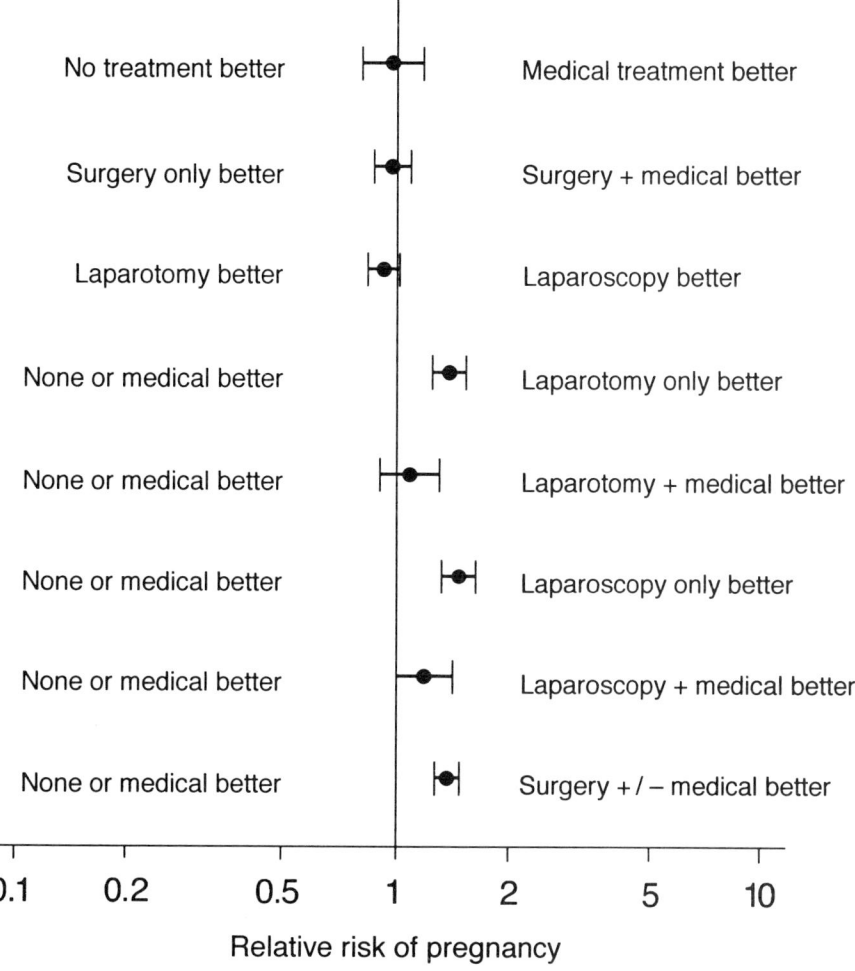

Figure 2 Summary of a combined Mantel–Haenszel estimate for each of the pairwise comparisons performed. The point estimated risk ratio is shown as a dot and the 95% confidence interval by the bar. If the bar does not cross the line marked '1' there is a statistical difference between the treatments ($p < 0.05$)

meta-analyses in our study show that surgery alone had pregnancy rates that were just as good as surgery followed by medical treatment with a relative risk of 0.97 and 95% confidence interval of 0.87–1.09. When laparoscopy was compared with laparotomy, there was no significant difference between laparoscopy and laparotomy with a relative risk of 0.93 and a 95% confidence interval of 0.84–1.02. When surgical treatment was compared to no treatment or medical treatment, the combined evidence clearly favored surgery, with surgical treatment producing crude pregnancy rates that were estimated to be 38% higher than non-surgical treatment. The 95% confidence interval was 28–48% higher.

Our study highlighted differences between meta-analysis and life-table analysis results. In the treatment comparison for no treatment vs. medical treatment, meta-analysis showed the same outcome whereas life-table analysis showed that no treatment was better. In the treatment comparison of laparoscopy vs. laparotomy the meta-analysis showed there was no difference in outcome whereas the life-table analysis showed laparoscopy was better for moderate and severe disease. The reason for these differences is that the life-table analysis took into account the amount of time to conceive, whereas the meta-analysis did not. Patients in the medical treatment group took longer to conceive, but eventually their pregnancy rate was equivalent to those in the no treatment group. Their treatment took longer because of the 6-month delay while they were taking medications. Patients in the laparotomy group had apparent equivalent pregnancy rates in the meta-analysis group because they had much longer follow-up than the laparoscopy patients.

In summary, the first set of conclusions from our study dealt with differences between types of studies. Meta-analysis requires careful and strict setting of rules to select and analyze studies formally. In addition, application of these rules can sometimes be ambiguous. Meta-analysis also cannot account for differences in length of follow-up, and also cannot account for differences among groups.

With respect to a comparison of studies, some strategies which can improve our understanding of clinical situations not amenable to prospective randomized trials include: reporting 1-, 2- and 3-year life-table pregnancy rates with 95% confidence intervals; stratifying groups by diagnosis and/or treatment; adjusting differences between groups by using survival analysis with fixed covariates and/or propensity scores; and utilizing multiple statistical approaches to analyze cohort studies.

A third, more clinically oriented set of conclusions were made. These are that medical treatment of endometriosis-associated infertility is inappropriate. Secondly, no treatment may be appropriate in selected patients with minimal or mild disease. Thirdly, surgical treatment is generally better than no treatment or medical treatment. Finally, laparoscopy pregnancy rates can be equivalent to laparotomy pregnancy rates.

In 1994 the American Society for Reproductive Medicine (ASRM) established a subcommittee to develop guidelines for assisted reproductive technologies. This committee has utilized the Agency for Health Care Policy and Research (AHCPR) methodology which involves a very systematic and ordered approach to developing practice guidelines. An evidence model was developed to clarify the clinical questions which needed to be answered (Figure 3). An exhaustive review of the English language literature since 1975 identified 1046 potentially relevant citations of papers concerning endometriosis and infertility treatment. A review of all of these papers identified 223 which had usable pregnancy rates and could be analyzed. Analysis of all these papers has just been completed. Preliminary results again confirm that surgical treatment is superior to medical or no treatment for all stages of disease (Table 3). Therefore, yet another study performed using different study design and a rigorous methodology confirms the rationale for surgical treatment of endometriosis. Further, a recently reported randomized trial has demonstrated superior pregnancy rates following laparoscopic ablation of minimal or mild endometriosis compared with no treatment[8].

Summary

Overall, it is clear that laparoscopic treatment of endometriosis can be performed safely and efficaciously. All the data support a very strong therapeutic impact of diagnostic and operative laparoscopy on endometriosis especially in its more severe forms. However, some laparoscopic surgeries for endometriosis can be extremely complex and should only be attempted by those with the requisite training, experience and skill.

EVIDENCE MODEL

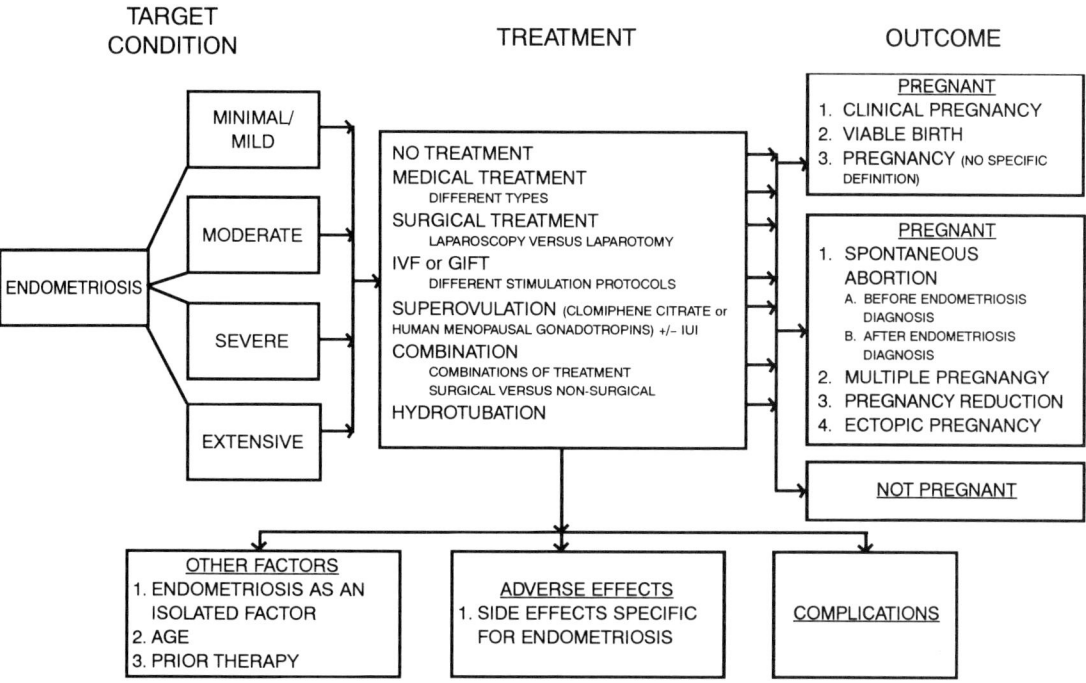

Figure 3 Evidence Model developed so that all intended linkages are identified and appropriate questions to be answered by the literature search are formulated

Table 3 Pregnancy rates for infertile patients with endometriosis in studies reporting comparison of medical and laparoscopy treatment

Stage of disease	Treatment group	n	Number pregnant	Percentage pregnant
Minimal/mild	No treatment	895	335	37.4
	Medical	987	326	33.0
	Surgical	3006	1553	51.7
Moderate	No treatment	103	23	22.3
	Medical	301	142	47.2
	Surgical	1476	764	51.8
Severe/extensive	No treatment	65	2	3.1
	Medical	67	20	29.9
	Surgical	894	369	41.3

References

1. Adamson, G.D., Frison, L. and Lamb, E. (1982). Endometriosis: studies of a method for the design of a surgical staging system. *Fertil. Steril.*, **38**, 659–66
2. Adamson, G.D., Subak, L.L., Pasta, D.J., Hurd, S.J., von Franque, O. and Rodriguez, B.D. (1992). Comparison of CO_2 laser laparoscopy with laparotomy for treatment of endometriomata. *Fertil. Steril.*, **57**, 965–73
3. Adamson, G.D., Hurd, S.J., Pasta, D.J. and Rodriguez, B.D. (1993). Laparoscopic endometriosis treatment: is it better? *Fertil. Steril.*, **59**, 35–44
4. Adamson, G.D., Rodriguez, B.D., Hurd, S.J. and Pasta, D.J. (1992). Laparoscopy vs. laparotomy for treatment of posterior cul-de-sac obliteration. *American Association of Gynecologic Laparoscopists,* Chicago, Illinois, September 24–27 (Abstract)
5. Hughes, E.G., Fedorkow, D.M. and Collins, J.A. (1993). A quantitative overview of controlled trials in endometriosis-associated infertility. *Fertil. Steril.* **59**, 963–70
6. Adamson, G.D. and Pasta. D.J. (1994). Surgical treatment of endometriosis-associated infertility: meta-analysis combined with survival analysis. *Am. J. Obstet. Gynecol.*, **171**(6), 1488–505
7. Sacks, H.S., Berrier, J. and Reitman, D. (1987). Meta-analyses of randomized controlled trials. *N. Engl. J. Med.*, **316**, 450–5
8. Maheux, R., Marcoux, S., Berube, S. and the Canadian Collaborative Group on Endometriosis (1996). Surgical laparoscopy in infertile women with minimal/mild endometriosis: a randomized controlled trial. *Vth World Congress on Endometriosis*, Yokohama, Japan, October 21–24 (Abstract)

Section 7

Medical treatment

The anticipated results from expectant management

A.F. Haney

Introduction

Endometriosis-associated infertility remains one of the most frequent yet frustrating clinical situations encountered in reproductive medicine. It had previously been widely accepted that the endometrial implants, by virtue of their very presence, were responsible for the failure to conceive, without a specific mechanism being identified. Although adnexal adhesions or endometriomas may certainly co-exist with or be caused by endometrial implants, the vast majority of infertile women having endometriosis identified today have a relatively small amount of disease without mechanical compromise of the pelvic viscera[1].

The mechanism(s) of endometriosis-associated infertility remain to be established[2]. Attention has focused on macrophage and natural killer cell function, but no single mechanism has been confirmed to be responsible for the failure to conceive in the absence of mechanical compromise of the pelvic viscera. Until a causal relationship can be established, it is just as plausible a hypothesis that infertility causes endometriosis as it is that endometriosis causes infertility. Until a mechanism is identified, the relationship between endometriosis and infertility in the absence of mechanical compromise will remain highly controversial[3].

Any consideration of how to treat endometriosis-associated infertility must take into account the nature of the observed reproductive failure encountered. These couples are clearly not sterile, but rather, have a lower monthly probability of pregnancy (cycle fecundity), and are properly termed 'subfertile' or 'infertile'. Additionally, the female partners in many of these couples are in their later reproductive years and have to contend with the natural age-related decline in cycle fecundity. As a consequence, it seems clear that any therapeutic trials involving surgical destruction/excision or suppression of the endometrial implants and claiming an improvement in fertility must include untreated controls and be age-matched for the female partner as well as for other fertility-lowering factors. Unfortunately, the vast majority of the available data regarding the treatment of endometriosis-associated infertility are predominantly anecdotal and retrospective, suffering from substantial selection bias and the absence of optimal study designs, specifically lacking untreated control groups or comparison to another unproven therapy. This discussion will focus on an exploration of the available information regarding the likelihood that pregnancy will occur in the absence of treatment or so-called 'expectant management' in couples with endometriosis-associated infertility. The goal is to allow the reader to make a better judgement of the different therapeutic interventions, assess currently available treatment options and assist in designing future treatment trials, so as to adequately test newly proposed treatment modalities.

Implications of the results of 'expectant management' in the evaluation of infertility therapy

In couples with endometriosis-associated infertility, treatment-independent conceptions have been universally observed[4-6], albeit with a low monthly fecundity, approximately 1–3%. After any therapeutic intervention, the natural tendency is to attribute all subsequent pregnancies to a beneficial effect of the treatment. The relative proportion of couples with treatment-dependent pregnancies can only be determined when randomized untreated control groups are included in clinical trials. Unfortunately, the vast majority of studies reporting treatment results do not include appropriate control groups. Until therapeutic trials uniformly include untreated controls, attractive-sounding but ineffective treatments will remain the most frequently utilized options, squandering the most precious commodity possessed by infertile couples, time.

Comparing different treatments for the infertility associated with endometriosis has also been made difficult by the lack of uniform standards by which success is measured. Most commonly, crude pregnancy rates have been employed, defined as the number of pregnancies divided by the total number of patients treated[3]. This is the easiest measure of fertility to collect when retrospectively analyzing data; however, there are two main problems with this approach. First, it does not take into account patient selection bias and secondly it is dramatically influenced by the length of follow-up. As a consequence, pregnancy rates will be positively influenced by selection of patients with the milder forms of the disease and by a longer interval of observation. The majority of available studies are not at all comparable with regard to the patient population and length of follow-up. Many authors attempt to obtain a more homogeneous group by 'correcting' or excluding patients who have other infertility factors that might influence the results. This does not, however, correct for the observation interval, and the factors being corrected for are not uniform between studies.

Another method frequently employed in retrospective studies is life-table analysis, which corrects for variable lengths of follow-up. This analytic technique calculates the theoretical probability of a pregnancy occurring at any follow-up interval. It is necessary to create a mathematical model describing the parameters for comparative purposes which is less accurate than evaluating actual outcomes. This method also does not address the issue of sample bias and, without an expectantly managed control group, the illusion of treatment-dependent success is often created by the occurrence of treatment-independent pregnancies in the absence of true efficacy.

Monthly fecundity rates have been the most recent addition to the evaluation of efficacy and can be calculated by taking the total number of pregnancies and dividing by the number of months of pregnancy exposure[7]. No couples, even those lost to follow-up, should be excluded, and these patients contribute to the total number of months of follow-up as if they did not conceive, assuming that if they conceived, they would be more likely not to be 'lost'. This is a relatively easy calculation and is not dependent upon the follow-up interval, but it cannot address the issue of selection bias. A major drawback is that there are not an infinite number of oocytes and the natural age-related fertility decline will continue to influence the results. A two-parameter model for life-table analysis has been developed utilizing a 'cure' rate and retaining the monthly probability of pregnancy[8]. Again, this method will not correct for sample bias and has the potential to assign efficacy incorrectly to an ineffective therapeutic modality.

At this point in our understanding of the treatment of endometriosis-associated infertility, the value of any type of retrospective analysis is dubious. There is simply no adequate alternative to the prospective randomized clinical trial with an untreated control group to eliminate the problem of sample bias. Although the other methods can be applied to retrospective observational data and help gain insight into which treatment modalities will be worthy of further consideration for clinical testing, the definitive conclusion of efficacy will depend upon randomized clinical trials, including expectantly managed control groups.

The risk–benefit decision for treatments of endometriosis-associated infertility

When infertile couples decide upon therapy, they are assuming that they will choose an option that has been demonstrated to increase their cycle fecundity. If a surgical option is chosen, the potential benefit must be weighed against the risks of immediate surgical complications and the likelihood of creating fertility-reducing postoperative pelvic adhesions. If a medical suppression regimen is selected, there are the problems of complications from the treatment itself and the loss of time while ovulation is suppressed, when the couple cannot even attempt pregnancy. When the proposed treatments do not have proven benefit over expectant management, it is difficult to justify any treatment focused toward the endometriotic implants. As a result, any purported treatment must be rigorously tested against expectant management before it can be offered as therapy for the infertility associated with endometriosis.

Available data on expectant management

In order to determine the efficacy of any treatment, a randomized controlled trial comparing the proposed treatment to expectant management should be performed. The available data regarding the cycle fecundity with expectant management are derived from the relatively small number of randomized trials with untreated control groups. This approach reduces the likelihood of selection bias and, at least for the population under study, allows the quantitation of the treatment-independent pregnancies against which potential treatments can be tested. Table 1 summarizes the available data from the randomized untreated control groups. The variation in the cycle fecundity between studies is likely to relate to the patient selection biases present with each investigation.

The importance of these data are that they suggest that a relatively large number of couples with endometriosis-associated infertility without mechanical compromise of the pelvic viscera will conceive following laparoscopic diagnosis, although the fecundity is substantially lower than that of the general population. A monthly fecundity rate of 2.9% has even been observed with higher stages of endometriosis[13], indicating that, despite more extensive disease, a significant number of pregnancies can be anticipated to be treatment-independent.

Table 1 Results of expectant management in randomized clinical trials

Study	n	% pregnant	Cycle fecundity
Garcia and David[9]	17	64.7	0.050*
Schenken and Malinak[10]	18	72.2	0.102*
Seibel et al.[11]	28	50.0	0.111*
Portuondo et al.[12]	31	61.2	0.083
Olive et al.[13]	34	52.9	0.057
Thomas and Cooke[14]	17	23.5	0.023*
Bayer et al.[15]	36	47.2	0.073
Telimaa[16]	5	40.0	0.042*
Overton et al.[17]	14	50.0	0.083†
Total	200	51.3	0.069

*Estimated 6-month interval averages; †estimated 12-month interval averages

Conclusions

The following facts can be established about the infertility associated with endometriosis:

(1) Endometriosis cannot be etiologically linked to the infertility experienced by these couples

(2) There is no specific mechanism identified that can account for the infertility

(3) Expectant management is associated with a definable cycle fecundity varying between 2.3% and 11.1% in published randomized clinical trials

(4) There are no studies unequivocally demonstrating the efficacy of medical or surgical treatments, and these proposed therapies are associated with potential problems such as surgical complications and a prolonged delay during medical therapy before an attempt at pregnancy is possible.

In appreciation of these facts, inclusion of expectantly managed (untreated) control groups will be required in treatment trials before efficacy can be established. It is imperative not to compare new therapies to currently available, but equally unproven, treatment modalities. These studies will need to be randomized clinical trials in order to minimize patient selection bias and to be large enough to possess sufficient statistical power for unequivocal testing of efficacy. Until such studies are carried out, the optimal treatment of endometriosis-associated infertility will remain elusive.

References

1. Olive, D.L. and Haney, A.F. (1986). Endometriosis. In DeCherney, A.H. (ed.) *Reproductive Failure*, pp. 153–201. (New York: Churchill Livingstone)
2. Metzger, D.A. and Haney, A.F. (1988). Endometriosis: etiology and pathophysiology of infertility. *Clin. Obstet. Gynecol.*, **31**, 801–12
3. Olive, D.L. and Haney, A.F. (1986). Endometriosis-associated infertility: a critical review of therapeutic approaches. *Obstet. Gynecol. Surv.*, **41**, 538–55
4. Lenton, E.A., Weston, G.A. and Cooke, I.A. (1977). Long-term follow-up of the apparently normal couple with a complaint of infertility. *Fertil. Steril.*, **28**, 913–19
5. Templeton, A.A. and Penney, G.C. (1982). The incidence, characteristics, and prognosis of patients whose infertility is unexplained. *Fertil. Steril.*, **37**, 175–82
6. Collins, J.A., Writom, W., Janes, L.B. and Wilson, E.H. (1983). Treatment independent pregnancies among infertile couples. *N. Engl. J. Med.*, **309**, 1201–6
7. Cramer, D.W., Walker, A.M. and Schiff, I. (1979). Statistical methods in evaluating the outcome of infertility therapy. *Fertil. Steril.*, **32**, 80–6
8. Guzick D.S. and Rock, J.A. (1981). Estimation of a model of cumulative pregnancy following infertility therapy. *Am. J. Obstet. Gynecol.*, **140**, 573–8
9. Garcia, C.R. and David, S.S. (1977). Pelvic endometriosis: infertility and pelvic pain. *Am. J. Obstet. Gynecol.*, **129**, 740–7
10. Schenken, R.S. and Malinak, L.R. (1982). Conservative surgery vs. expectant management for the infertile patient with mild endometriosis. *Fertil. Steril.*, **37**, 183–6
11. Seibel, M.M., Berger, M.J., Weinstein, F.G. and Taymor, M.L. (1982). The effectiveness of danazol on subsequent fertility in minimal endometriosis. *Fertil. Steril.*, **38**, 534–7
12. Portuondo, J.A., Echanojauregui, A.D., Herran, C. and Alijarte, I. (1983). Early conception in patients with untreated mild endometriosis. *Fertil. Steril.*, **39**, 22–5
13. Olive, D.L., Stohs, G.F., Metzger, D.A. and Franklin, R.R. (1985). Expectant management and hydrotubations in the treatment of endometriosis associated infertility. *Fertil. Steril.*, **44**, 35–41
14. Thomas, E.J. and Cooke, I. (1987). Successful treatment of asymptomatic endometriosis: does it benefit infertile women? *Br. Med. J.*, **294**, 1117–19
15. Bayer, S.R., Seibel, M., Saffan, D.S., Berger, M.J. and Taymor, M. (1988). Efficacy of danazol treatment for minimal endometriosis in infertile women. *J. Reprod. Med.*, **33**, 179–83
16. Telimaa, S. (1988). Danazol and medroxyprogesterone acetate are inefficacious in the treatment of infertility in endometriosis. *Fertil. Steril.*, **50**, 872–5
17. Overton, C.E., Lindsay, P.C., Johal, B., Collins, S.A., Siddle, N.C., Shaw, R.W. and Barlow, D.H. (1994). A randomized, double-blind, placebo-controlled study of luteal phase dehydrogesterone (Duphaston) in women with minimal to mild endometriosis. *Fertil. Steril.*, **62**, 701–7

Effects of medical treatment on active lesions of peritoneal endometriosis

N. Terakawa and T. Harada

Introduction

Endometriosis is the presence of functioning endometrial glands and stroma outside the uterine cavity. The prominent symptoms of the disease are chronic pelvic pain and infertility, which are significant problems in gynecology. The disease affects approximately 10% of all women of reproductive age, and the need for an effective non-surgical treatment is pressing, particularly for patients concerned about their future fertility. At present, medical treatment of endometriosis is dominated by use of danazol and gonadotropin-releasing hormone (GnRH) agonists. Both danazol and GnRH agonists are effective in the treatment of endometriosis[1]. Dramatic improvement has been noted in terms of both symptoms and signs and laparoscopic findings. The uncorrected fertility rate has been reported as approximately 40%[1].

A cause-and-effect relation between minimal or mild endometriosis and infertility is not currently known. Peritoneal fluid in women with endometriosis contains an increased number of activated macrophages that secrete a variety of local products such as cytokines[2]. Cytokines have been implicated in the control of implantation and the growth of endometrial cells outside the uterus[3,4], and are also believed to be related to infertility in women with endometriosis. Recently it has been shown that cytokines such as interleukin-6 are secreted by endometriotic cells and are present in peritoneal fluid[5]. Peritoneal endometriosis can be classified as red, black or white lesions. Red-colored and gland-like lesions are considered to be active forms of endometriosis, because vascularization and mitotic activity are shown to be most prominent in these lesions[6].

In this study, we investigated the correlations between peritoneal fluid levels of cytokines and the size and the numbers of active lesions of peritoneal endometriosis in infertile patients, and then examined the effects of medical treatment on active endometriotic lesions. The effect of interleukin-6 on the development of single-cell mouse embryos was also evaluated.

Materials and methods

Subjects

Peritoneal fluid was obtained from 45 infertile patients who underwent laparoscopy for infertility work-up or laparoscopic surgery for endometriosis. Of the 45 patients studied, 28 patients had pelvic endometriosis and 17 patients were free of endometriosis. Eight out of the 28 patients with endometriosis were treated daily for 6 months with 900 µg buserelin or with 400 mg danazol before the laparoscopic examination. Endometriosis was staged according to the criteria of the revised American Fertility Society (AFS) classification system by laparoscopic inspection of the pelvis[7]. Observations and surgical procedures were recorded on videotape. We estimated the size and the numbers of all active lesions at the laparoscopy and on the videotapes. Active lesions were identified according to the criteria of Jansen and Russell[8] and Wiegerinck and colleagues[9]. In this study, active lesions of peritoneal endometriosis were graded

Table 1 Grading of active lesions of peritoneal endometriosis

Grade 0	No active lesion
Grade 1	An active lesion < 1 cm in diameter
Grade 2	An active lesion 1–2 cm in diameter, or two separate lesions < 1 cm in diameter
Grade 3	An active lesion ≥ 2 cm in diameter, or more than one lesion other than those classified as Grade 2

according to the size and the numbers of the lesions, as shown in Table 1.

Collection and isolation of samples

Peritoneal fluid was obtained via a laparoscopic cannula immediately after the introduction of the laparoscope. Aspiration was performed under direct visualization from the posterior cul-de-sac and anterior vesico-uterine fold. We recorded the total volume of fluid obtained. Fluid samples were centrifuged at $800\,g$ for 10 min at 4 °C to separate the cell pellet and the supernatant. The cell-free supernatant was then stored at –70 °C until assay.

Assays of cytokines

The concentrations of interleukin-6 and tumor necrosis factor-α (TNF-α) were determined using specific sandwich enzyme-linked immunosorbent assays (ELISA) (R & D Systems, Minneapolis, MN, USA). The detection limit of the ELISA was 0.1 pg/ml for both interleukin-6 and TNF-α. The intra-assay variations were less than 5%.

Embryo collection and culture

Female 5–6-week-old B6C3F1 mice were superovulated by intraperitoneal injection of 7.5 IU pregnant mares serum gonadotropin (Peamex; Sankyo Zoki Co. Ltd, Tokyo, Japan) and 7.5 IU human chorionic gonadotropin (hCG, Pregnyl; N.V. Organon, Tokyo, Japan). Immediately after injection of hCG, the females were mated with males of the same strain. One-cell embryos were collected from the oviducts after 20 h and washed in (N-[2-Hydroxyethyl]piperazine-N'-[2-ethanesulfonic acid]) (HEPES)-buffered human tubal fluid (HTF) medium containing 1 mg/ml bovine serum albumin (BSA) (Fraction V; Sigma Chemical Co., St Louis, MO, USA)[10]. The embryos were cultured in HTF medium containing 50–500 pg/ml human recombinant interleukin-6 (Chinese hamster ovary (CHO)-cell derived, Genzyme, Cambridge, MA, USA).

Statistical analysis

All values were expressed as mean ± SE, and the data on concentrations of cytokines in peritoneal fluid were analyzed statistically with non-parametric analysis. The data on embryo development was analyzed by the χ^2 test.

Results

Concentrations of TNF-α in peritoneal fluid from patients with endometriosis showed a tendency to increase with the grading of active lesions, and a significantly high level of TNF-α was found in the fluid from patients with grade 3 lesions (Figure 1). Concentrations of TNF-α in the fluid of patients who were treated with either danazol or GnRH agonists were significantly low compared with those from patients with grade 3 lesions. Interleukin-6 was also found to be produced in significantly higher amounts as the size or the numbers of active lesions increased (Figure 2). Medical treatment again decreased the production of interleukin-6. Six out of eight infertile patients treated with either danazol or GnRH agonists achieved pregnancy. Three of them conceived within 6 months after finish of medical treatment.

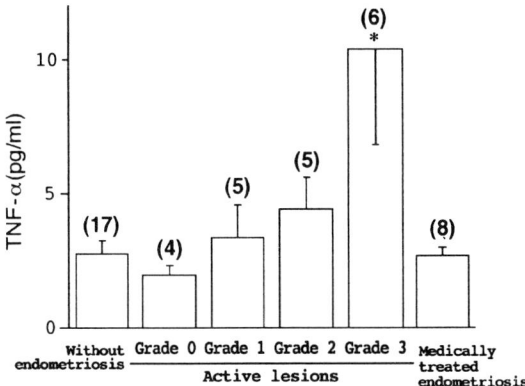

Figure 1 Concentrations of tumor necrosis factor-α (TNF-α) in peritoneal fluid of infertile patients with or without endometriosis. Numbers within parentheses indicate the numbers of patients. *$p < 0.05$ compared with patients without endometriosis and medically treated patients

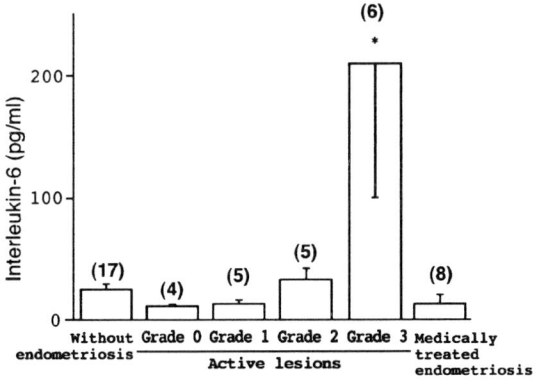

Figure 2 Concentrations of interleukin-6 in peritoneal fluid of infertile patients with or without endometriosis. *$p < 0.05$ compared with patients without endometriosis, patients with Grade 0 disease, and medically treated patients

We next examined whether the medical treatment actually improves active lesions of peritoneal endometriosis. Change in active lesions of endometriosis after medical treatment was investigated in seven individual patients. As expected, medical treatment with either buserelin or danazol caused almost complete regression of active lesions of endometriosis (Figure 3).

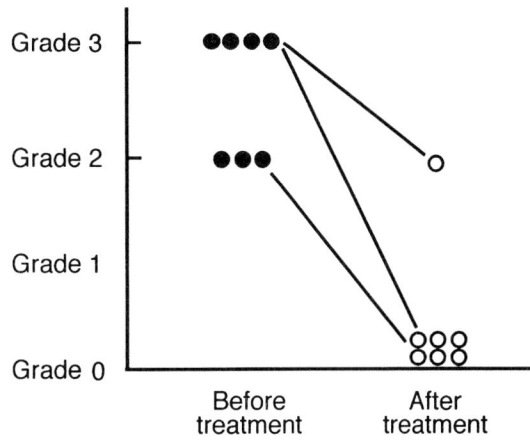

Figure 3 Changes in grade of active lesions of endometriosis after medical treatment. Laparoscopic examination was performed in seven individual patients with endometriosis before and after medical treatment

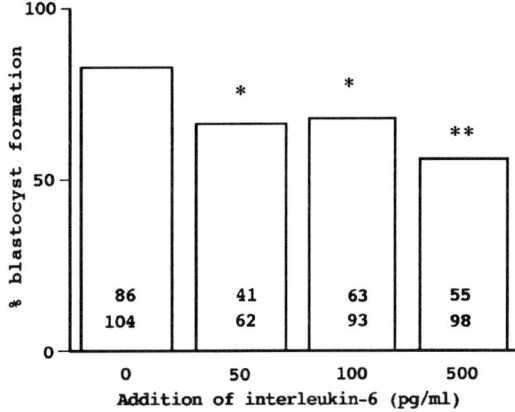

Figure 4 Effects of interleukin-6 on blastocyst formation of one-cell mouse embryos. Numbers within the bars indicate numbers of blastocysts and one-cell embryos. *$p < 0.05$ and **$p < 0.01$ compared with control

Mouse embryo development has been shown to be adversely affected by peritoneal fluid from patients with mild endometriosis[11]. In this study, addition of interleukin-6 significantly reduced the rates of development of one-cell embryos to blastocyst stage (Figure 4).

Discussion

In the present study, peritoneal fluid levels of interleukin-6 and TNF-α were increased in infertile patients with active lesions of endometriosis. Medical treatment with either danazol or GnRH agonists caused almost complete regression of the active lesions and significantly reduced the concentrations of cytokines in peritoneal fluid. After medical treatment, patients with reduced levels of cytokines became pregnant. Addition of human recombinant interleukin-6 to the culture medium suppressed the rate of blastocyst formation of mouse embryos. These results suggest that increased peritoneal fluid levels of cytokines in patients with endometriosis may reduce fertility by adversely affecting embryonic development.

Peritoneal endometriosis is classified as red, white or black lesions[6]. Vascularization[6] and metabolic activities[12] are most pronounced in red lesions. Red-colored lesions have been shown to invade the extracellular matrix[13]. Red-colored lesions are therefore considered to be active lesions in the early stages of endometriosis. The present study showed that an increased number of red-colored lesions was correlated with elevated concentrations of cytokines in peritoneal fluid. Interleukin-6 is a multifunctional cytokine involved in the regulation of immune response, hematopoiesis and inflammation. It is produced in response to infection or injury by a variety of cell types, including monocytes, lymphocytes, fibroblasts, endothelial cells and keratinocytes[14]. The peritoneal fluid level of interleukin-6 is increased in women with pelvic pathology[15]. Recent findings have shown that ectopic endometrial stromal cells present in peritoneal endometriotic implants may be another important source of interleukin-6[5,16]. The present findings also suggest that peritoneal endometriosis, particularly the so-called 'red' lesions, may be a source of interleukin-6 and TNF-α.

In the present study, it can be concluded that medical treatment improves the active lesions of endometriosis and reduces the production of cytokines such as interleukin-6 which adversely affect reproductive physiology.

References

1. Henzl, M.R., Corson, S.L., Moghissi, K., Buttram, V.C., Berqvist, C. and Jacobson, J. (1988). Administration of nasal nafarelin as compared with oral danazol for endometriosis. *N. Engl. J. Med.*, **318**, 485–9
2. Ramey, J.W. and Archer, D.F. (1993). Peritoneal fluid: its relevance to the development of endometriosis. *Fertil. Steril.*, **60**, 1–14
3. Oosterlynck, D.J., Meuleman, C., Sobis, H., Vandeputte, M. and Koninckx, P.R. (1993). Angiogenic activity of peritoneal fluid from women with endometriosis. *Fertil. Steril.*, **59**, 778–82
4. Halme, J. (1989). Release of tumor necrosis factor-alpha by human peritoneal macrophages *in vivo* and *in vitro*. *Am. J. Obstet. Gynecol.*, **161**, 1718–25
5. Tseng, J.F., Ryan, I.P., Milam, T.D., Murai, J.T., Shriock, E.D., Landers, D.V. and Taylor, R.N. (1996). Interleukin-6 secretion *in vitro* is up-regulated in ectopic and eutopic endometrial stromal cells from women with endometriosis. *J. Clin. Endocrinol. Metab.*, **81**, 1118–22
6. Nissole, M., Casanas-Roux, F., Anaf, V., Mince, J.M. and Donnez, J. (1993). Morphometric study of the stromal vascularization in peritoneal endometriosis. *Fertil. Steril.*, **59**, 681–4
7. The American Fertility Society (1985). Revised American Fertility Society classification of endometriosis: 1985. *Fertil. Steril.*, **43**, 351–2
8. Jansen, R.P. and Russell, P. (1986). Non-pigmented endometriosis: clinical, laparoscopic, and pathologic definition. *Am. J. Obstet. Gynecol.*, **155**, 1154–9
9. Wiegerinck, M.A.H.M., Van Dop, P.A. and Brosens, I.A. (1993). The staging of peritoneal

endometriosis by the type of active lesion in addition to the revised American Fertility Society classification. *Fertil. Steril.*, **60**, 461–4

10. Harada, T., Tanikawa, M., Iwabe, T., Onohara, Y., Mio, Y. and Terakawa, N. (1992). Measurement of uptake and incorporation of nucleic acid precursors by preimplantation mouse embryos after development *in vivo* and *in vitro*. *J. Assist. Reprod. Genet.*, **9**, 551–6

11. Prough, S.G., Aksel, S., Gilmore, S.M. and Yeoman, R.R. (1990). Peritoneal fluid fractions from patients with endometriosis do not promote two-cell mouse embryo growth. *Fertil. Steril.*, **54**, 927–30

12. Vernon, M.W., Beard, J.S., Graves, K. and Wilson, E.A. (1986). Classification of endometriotic implants by morphologic appearance and activity to synthesize prostaglandin F. *Fertil. Steril.*, **46**, 801–6

13. Spuijbroek, M.D.E., Dunselman, G.A.J., Menheere, P.P.C.A. and Evers, J.L.H. (1992). Early endometriosis invades the extracellular matrix. *Fertil. Steril.*, **58**, 929–33

14. Kishimoto, T. (1989). The biology of interleukin-6. *Blood*, **74**, 1–10

15. Buyalos, R.P., Funari, V.A., Azziz, R., Watson, J.M. and Martinez-Maza, O. (1992). Elevated interleukin-6 levels in peritoneal fluid of patients with pelvic pathology. *Fertil. Steril.*, **58**, 302–6

16. Rier, S.E., Zarmakoupis, P.N., Hu, X. and Becker, J.L. (1995). Dysregulation of interleukin-6 responses in ectopic endometrial stromal cells: correlation with decreased soluble receptor levels in peritoneal fluid of women with endometriosis. *J. Clin. Endocrinol. Metab.*, **80**, 1431–7

Treatment of endometriosis with mifepristone (RU486)

L.M. Kettel

Introduction

The first antiprogestin which became available for clinical use is mifepristone, popularly known by its industrial nomenclature as RU486. RU486 was developed as part of a research program headed by E.E. Baulieu, at Roussel-Uclaf, a French pharmaceutical company, to develop antiglucocorticoid compounds. RU486 is short for RU38486 and is the internal number used by Roussel-Uclaf to catalog compounds with this specific biologic activity. Early in its development, it was discovered that RU486 bound to both the glucocorticoid and progesterone receptors. As with all steroid hormone antagonists, RU486 competes with the native ligand (progesterone or cortisol) for binding sites on the steroid hormone receptor. Once RU486 has bound to the receptor, the natural ligand cannot bind and, therefore, cannot exert its biologic action. RU486 is an orally active anti-progesterone steroid analog with a long half-life.

In 1982, Herrmann and colleagues conducted the first clinical studies of RU486 in women[1]. In his initial report, 11 pregnant women (estimated gestational age range 6–8 weeks) were given RU486 200 mg four times daily for 4 days (total 3200 mg). Nine of the eleven women experienced vaginal bleeding and miscarried within 3 days of completing treatment (one required dilatation and curettage for hemorrhage). These results were so striking that RU486 became known as the 'abortion pill', despite an abundance of additional clinical applications predicted when the compound was first discovered. Many of these additional clinical applications have been explored, but only in a preliminary fashion[2]. Included on this list are endometriosis, uterine fibroids, premenstrual syndrome, ectopic pregnancy and breast cancer. The political controversy surrounding the use of this medication for pregnancy termination has severely restricted the availability of the compound to investigators for appropriate testing, and has also decreased the willingness of the parent company to invest in a drug which polarizes the worldwide community.

Background

Endometriosis is a disease associated with significant pelvic pain, dysmenorrhea and infertility. It affects as many as 1 in 15 women of reproductive age and may be identified in as many as 25% of women with infertility[3,4]. In this condition, functioning endometrial glands and stroma proliferate outside the uterine cavity. The growth of endometriosis is stimulated by the ovarian steroids, estrogen and progesterone, and in the absence of these hormones the symptoms of endometriosis improve. Both progesterone and estrogen receptors are found in endometriotic implants. However, only half of these implants are in phase with normal endometrium, indicating a non-uniformity in the hormone responsiveness of the implants[5].

Current medical treatments of endometriosis depend on suppression of ovarian function and induction of endometrial atrophy. Both danazol and the gonadotropin-releasing hormone (GnRH) agonist analogs (leuprolide, nafarelin, goserelin) have been used effectively for the treatment of endometriosis. However,

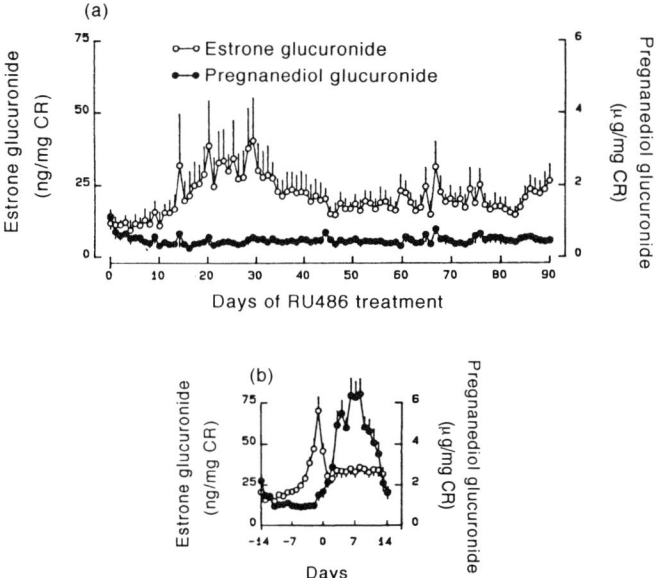

Figure 1 (a) Mean (±SE) urinary estrone glucuronide and pregnanediol glucuronide levels normalized to creatinine (CR) in six women during treatment with RU486 100 mg/day for 3 months. (b) Mean (±SE) urinary estrone glucuronide and pregnanediol glucuronide in 13 normally cycling women. Data are centered around the day after the estrone glucuronide peak. (From reference 12, with permission)

both of these compounds have significant adverse effects which limit their widespread utility. It is apparent that the development of novel, effective and long-term medical treatments with few or no side-effects would be a significant advance in the management of symptomatic endometriosis.

RU486 has been shown to inhibit ovulation[6–8] and disrupt endometrial integrity[9–11]. Based on these observations, we hypothesized that long-term RU486 administration may induce a condition of chronic anovulation associated with endometriotic disruption in patients with symptomatic endometriosis.

Clinical studies

In a pilot study we observed that the administration of RU486 100 mg daily for 3 months resulted in ovarian acyclicity and improvement in pelvic pain in six patients with symptomatic endometriosis in whom other therapies had failed[12] (Figure 1). In this preliminary report we did not observe a visible regression of endometriosis, but realized that the treatment interval (3 months) may have been inadequate. In addition, the dose selected (100 mg) increased the 24 h mean serum cortisol and adreno-corticotropic hormone (ACTH) levels.

A follow-up study was conducted in an attempt to dissociate the antiglucocorticoid side-effects of RU486 from its antiprogesterone actions and to induce a reduction in endometriosis by extending the duration of treatment (6 months) and lowering the dose of RU486 administered (50 mg daily)[13]. Eight patients were enrolled in this study. All patients became amenorrheic

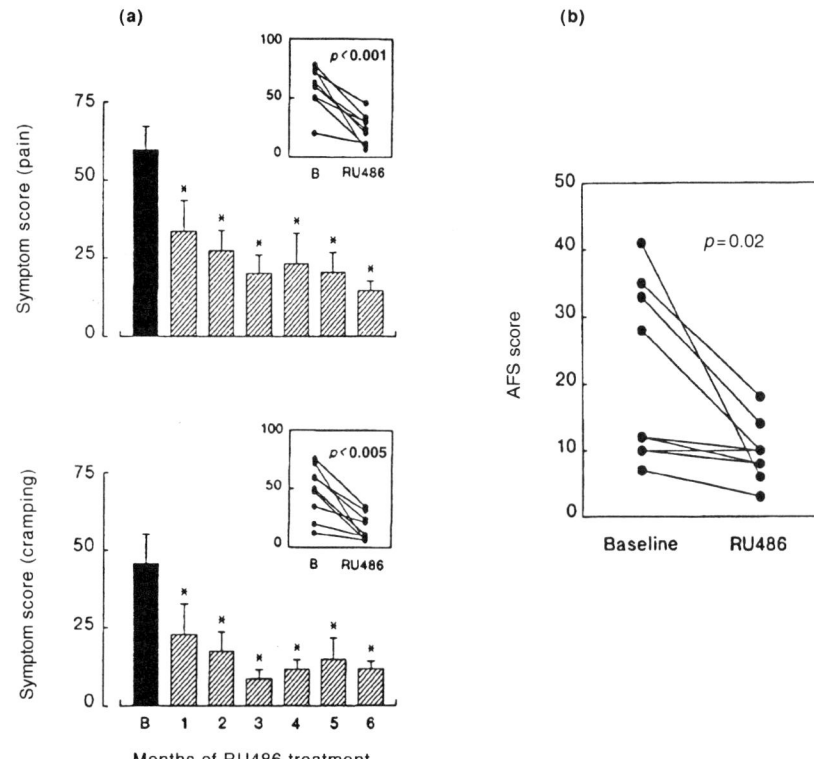

Figure 2 (a) Mean (± SE) symptom scores for pain and cramping determined by daily visual analog scale inventories completed before (B, baseline) and at monthly intervals during treatment with mifepristone (RU486) 50 mg daily. The inserts show symptom scores for each patient recorded during the baseline month (30-day mean) and the combined 6-month treatment interval (180-day mean). *$p < 0.05$ compared with baseline). (b) Endometriosis scores (American Fertility Society) for each patient before and after 6 months of treatment with mifepristone (RU486) 50 mg daily. (From reference 13, with permission)

during therapy and demonstrated anovulatory urinary steroid profiles. A significant decrease in pelvic pain ($p < 0.001$) and dysmenorrhea ($p < 0.005$) occurred in all subjects within the first 4 weeks of treatment and persisted throughout therapy (Figure 2). Endometriosis scores, as determined by the American Fertility Society classification system, decreased by approximately 50% following RU486 treatment. There was no change in 24 h mean serum cortisol with preservation of the normal circadian rhythm. One patient developed a mild increase in liver transaminases which resolved after therapy. No other significant adverse effects were noted.

The endocrine milieu created by long-term therapy with RU486 is characterized by mid-follicular levels of estradiol and progesterone. This unopposed condition of estrogen exposure to the endometrium has led to some concerns about the potential for development of endometrial hyperplasia. In primates, the long-term administration of RU486 leads to endometriotic lesion and endometrial atrophy[14]. In women, we have observed that treatment with RU486 50 mg daily for 3–6 months resulted in a mixed proliferative/secretory endometrium associated with cystic dilatation and increased stromal density without evidence of atypia[15]. These findings are consistent with observations in ovariectomized monkeys treated with RU486 1 mg/kg plus estradiol[16]. While overt endometrial hyperplasia was not identified in the doses used for these studies, careful follow-up of women receiving this medication is clearly required.

Conclusions

Both of these pilot studies point to a potentially promising use for antiprogesterones. More than 400 different antiprogesterone analogs have been synthesized by different pharmaceutical companies worldwide. These compounds differ in their antiprogesterone and antiglucocorticoid potencies and their binding to different progesterone receptors. Whether these differences prove to give advantages over RU486 remains to be seen, but they highlight the potential future for this new family of steroid analogs.

References

1. Herrmann, W., Wyss, R., Riondel, A., Philibert, D., Teutsch, G., Sakiz, E. and Baulieu, E.-E. (1982). Effet d'un stéroide anti-progestérone chez la femme: interruption du cycle menstruel et de la grossesse au début. *Compt. Rendus Acad. Sci. (Paris)*, **294**, 933–8
2. Kettel, L.M. (1995). Clinical applications of RU486. In Pitkin, R.M. and Scott, J.R. (eds.) *Clinical Obstetrics and Gynecology*, Vol. 38, pp. 921–34. (Philadelphia: Lippincott-Raven Publishers)
3. Drake, T.S. and Grunert, G.M. (1980). The unsuspected pelvic factor in the infertility investigations. *Fertil. Steril.*, **34**, 27–32
4. Peterson, E.P. and Behrman, S.J. (1970). Laparoscopy of the infertile patient. *Obstet. Gynecol.*, **36**, 363–7
5. Tamaya, T., Motoyaha, T., Ohono, Y., Ide, N., Tsurusaki, T. and Okada, H. (1979). Steroid receptor levels and histology of endometriosis and adenomyosis. *Fertil. Steril.*, **31**, 396–400
6. Liu, J.H., Garzo, G., Morris, S., Stuenkel, C.A., Ulmann, A. and Yen, S.S.C. (1987). Disruption of follicular maturation and delay of ovulation after administration of the antiprogesterone RU486. *J. Clin. Endocrinol. Metab.*, **65**, 1135–40
7. Shoupe, D., Mishell, D.J., Page, M.A., Madkour, H., Spitz, I.M. and Lobo, R.A. (1987). Effects of the antiprogesterone RU486 in normal women. II. Administration in the late follicular phase. *Am. J. Obstet. Gynecol.*, **157**, 1421–6
8. Luukkainen, T. and Heikinheimo, O. (1988). Inhibition of folliculogenesis and ovulation by the antiprogesterone RU486. *Fertil. Steril.*, **49**, 961–3
9. Swahn, M., Johannisson, E. and Daniore, V. (1988). The effect of RU486 administered during the proliferative and secretory phase of the cycle on the bleeding pattern, hormonal parameters and the endometrium. *Hum. Reprod.*, **3**, 915–21
10. Garzo, V.G., Liu, J.H., Ulmann, A., Baulieu, E. and Yen, S.S.C. (1988). Effects of an antiprogesterone (RU486) on the hypothalamic–hypophyseal–ovarian–endometrial axis during the luteal phase of the menstrual cycle. *J. Clin. Endocrinol. Metab.*, **66**, 508–17
11. Schaison, G., George, M., Lestrat, N. and Baulieu, E. (1985). Effects of the antiprogesterone steroid RU486 during midluteal phase in normal women. *J. Clin. Endocrinol. Metab.*, **61**, 484–9
12. Kettel, L.M., Murphy, A.A., Mortola, J.F., Liu, J.H., Ulmann, A. and Yen, S.S.C. (1991). Endocrine responses to long-term administration of the antiprogesterone RU486 in patients with pelvic endometriosis. *Fertil. Steril.*, **56**, 402–7
13. Kettel, L.M., Murphy, A.A., Morales, A.J., Ulmann, A., Baulieu, E.-E. and Yen, S.S.C. (1996). Treatment of endometriosis with the antiprogesterone mifepristone (RU486). *Fertil. Steril.*, **65**, 23–8

14. Grow, D.R., Williams, R.F., Hsiu, J.G. and Hodgen, G.D. (1996). Antiprogestin and/or gonadotropin-releasing hormone agonist for endometriosis treatment and bone maintenance: a 1-year primate study. *J. Clin. Endocrinol. Metab.*, **81**, 1933–9
15. Murphy, A.A., Kettel, L.M., Morales, A.J., Roberts, V., Parmley, T. and Yen, S.S.C. (1995). Endometrial effects of long term, low dose administration of RU486. *Fertil. Steril.*, **63**, 761–6
16. Slayden, O.D. and Brenner, R. (1994). RU486 action after estrogen priming in the endometrium and oviducts of Rhesus monkeys (*Macaca mulatta*). *J. Clin. Endocrinol. Metab.*, **78**, 440–8

Fundamental and phase I clinical study of YM511, a new aromatase inhibitor

H. Shigeta, H. Minaguchi, H. Kudoh, K. Noguchi, M. Ikeda and N. Nakamura

Introduction

Aromatase is the enzyme that changes androgen into estrogen by 'aromatizing' the A ring of androgen. It is one of the cytochrome P450 enzymes and is present in the gonads (ovaries and testicles), brain, fat, muscle and skin. By blocking aromatase activity, estrogen biosynthesis can be inhibited. Thus, an aromatase inhibitor could be effective in estrogen-dependent diseases such as breast cancer, endometriosis, endometrial cancer and uterine myoma.

Although several aromatase inhibitors have already been developed and examined in clinical trials, none has proved to be of value for the treatment of estrogen-dependent diseases. They inhibit the biosynthesis of other steroids because of insufficient specificity for aromatase and do not have sufficient potency in lowering serum estrogen levels for the treatment of these diseases. Their indication to date is therefore limited to breast cancer in postmenopausal women.

YM511 is a novel non-steroidal aromatase inhibitor. We found that it had a very strong and specific inhibitory effect on aromatase activity, and we therefore examined its effectiveness and toxicity in experimental animals, and followed this by clinical phase I study in post- and premenopausal women.

Fundamental study

Inhibitory effect on aromatase activity

The inhibitory effect on aromatase activity was examined by incubating $1\beta,2\beta$-[^{3}H]androstenedione with rat ovarian or human placental microsomes. The results showed that YM511 inhibited aromatase activity with an IC_{50} of 0.4 nmol/l in the rat ovary and of 0.13 nmol/l in the human placenta. Kinetic analysis showed that YM511 was a competitive inhibitor, with K_i value of 0.11 nmol/l.

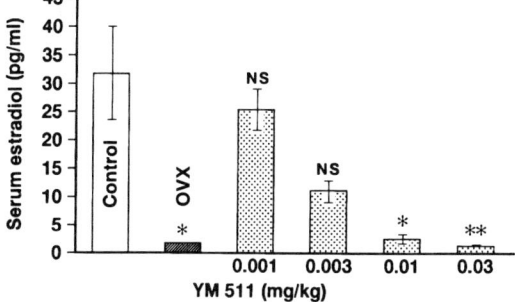

Figure 1 Effect of oral administration of YM511 on serum estradiol concentration in adult female rats (OVX, ovariectomy; NS, not significant; *$p < 0.05$ vs. control; **$p < 0.01$ vs. control)

Reduction of serum estrogen concentration

YM511 was orally administered to female rats, and blood samples were taken 3 h later. YM511 was shown to reduce the serum estradiol concentration, as measured by radioimmunoassay (RIA), dose-dependently in normal adult female rats (Figure 1). Administration of 0.01 mg/kg YM511 reduced the estradiol level to that observed in ovariectomized rats.

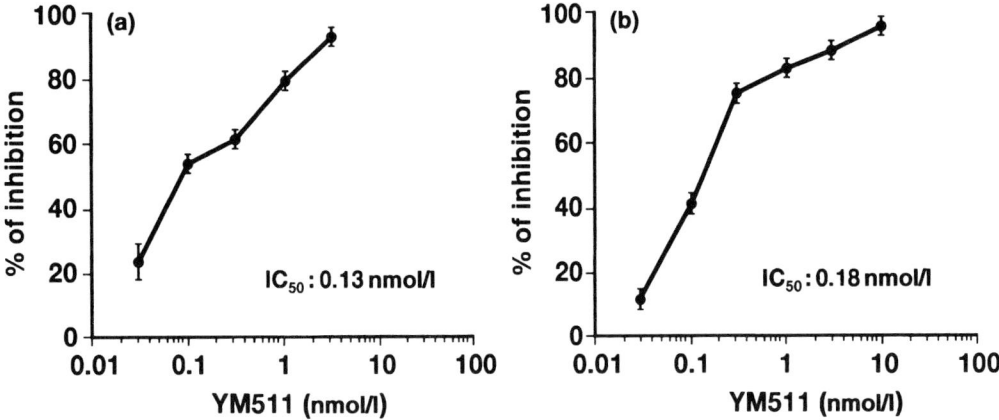

Figure 2 Inhibition by YM511 of cell growth (a) and DNA synthesis (b) in MCF-7 cells stimulated by testosterone

Effects on cell growth of MCF-7 cells

MCF-7 cells (human breast cancer cell line) were grown with testosterone and various concentrations of YM511. Both the cell growth and DNA synthesis of these cells were inhibited by YM511 in a dose-dependent manner (Figure 2). The IC_{50} was 0.13 nmol/l in cell growth and 0.18 nmol/l in DNA synthesis.

Effects on other enzymes and hormones

Effects on other P450 enzymes In vitro experiments with rat testicular microsomes or bovine adrenal mitochondria revealed that 10 µmol/l of YM511 inhibited steroid C17-20 lyase weakly (12.2%) but had no effect on 17α-hydroxylase and 11β-hydroxylase activity.

Effects on serum concentration of progesterone, LH and FSH Two weeks' administration of YM511 to 10-week-old female rats decreased the serum progesterone level, increased the luteinizing hormone (LH) level and had no effect on the follicle-stimulating hormone (FSH) level.

Effects on other steroid hormone levels YM511 weakly inhibited adrenocorticotropic hormone (ACTH)-induced aldosterone and cortisol levels, and human chorionic gonadotropin (hCG)-induced testosterone level *in vitro* in rat adrenal cells, rabbit adrenal cells and rat testicular cells, respectively. It had no effect on ACTH-induced aldosterone and cortisol levels *in vivo* in rats and guinea-pigs, respectively.

General pharmacology and toxicity studies

No remarkable findings were observed in general pharmacology and toxicity studies, including studies on dose toxicity, reproductive and developmental toxicity, antigenicity, mutagenicity and irritation.

Absorption, distribution and metabolism

YM511 was well absorbed in the intestine and colon of rats. The bioavailability of YM511 in rats and dogs was extremely high, indicating that it is almost completely absorbed on oral administration. The serum concentration reached the maximum level 1.5–3 h after oral administration in rats. YM511 was rapidly distributed to many organs, including the ovary, fat and brain. It was excreted mainly in the urine of the rat.

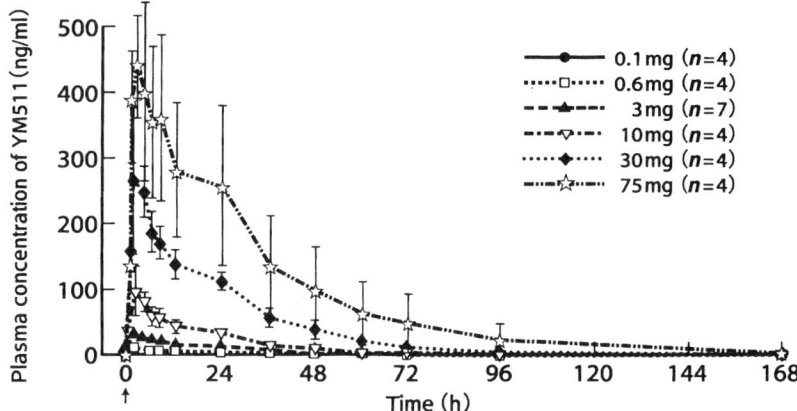

Figure 3 Plasma concentration profiles of YM511 in healthy postmenopausal women as a function of time after single oral administration (arrow) of various doses of YM511 (mean ± SD)

Phase I clinical study in healthy postmenopausal women

The tolerance, pharmacokinetics and effects of YM511 on hormonal concentration in healthy postmenopausal women have been studied after single oral administration (0.1, 0.6, 3, 10, 30 and 75 mg; $n = 28$) and repeated oral administration (20 mg once a day for 10 days, 50 mg once a day for 10 days; $n = 12$).

Tolerance

In single and repeated oral administration studies, no subjective symptoms strictly associated with the drug were observed. As for laboratory test values, deviations from normal ranges were occasionally observed, but none of these changes were clinically significant.

Drug pharmacokinetics

After single oral administration of YM511, the plasma concentration of the drug increased in a dose-dependent manner and there was a linear relationship for both C_{max} and the area under the curve (AUC) (Figure 3). In the repeated oral administration study, the plasma concentration of YM511 reached a plateau on days 5–6 (Figure 4). The pharmacokinetics of YM511 was not affected by food. The half-life of YM511 was approximately 20 h.

Effects on hormonal concentrations

Following single oral administration of the drug at doses of 0.1, 0.6, 3, 10, 30 or 75 mg, the serum concentrations of estrone and estradiol were suppressed to 15.8–44.2% and 19.7–45.9%, respectively, compared to the preadministration level (Figure 5). In the repeated administration study over 10 days, serum estrone and estradiol levels were suppressed to 38.8–56.8% and 30.3–54.9%, respectively, by administration of 20 mg/day; and to 27.2–39.3% and 21.0–36.1%, respectively, by administration of 50 mg/day, compared to the preadministration level. YM511 had no influence on serum levels of other hormones (LH, FSH, prolactin, thyroid stimulating hormone, progesterone, testosterone, cortisol, aldosterone, androstenedione and dehydroepiandrosterone).

Phase I clinical study in healthy premenopausal women

The tolerance, pharmacokinetics and effects of YM511 on hormonal concentration have

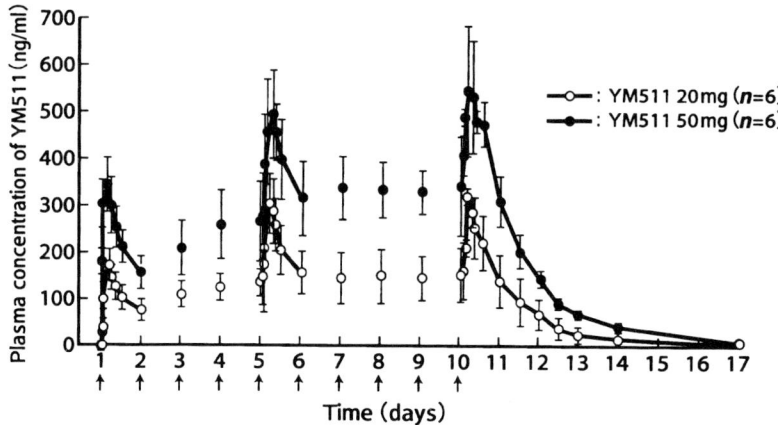

Figure 4 Plasma concentration profiles of YM511 in healthy postmenopausal women as a function of time after multiple oral administration (arrows) of 20 mg and 50 mg YM511 (mean ± SD)

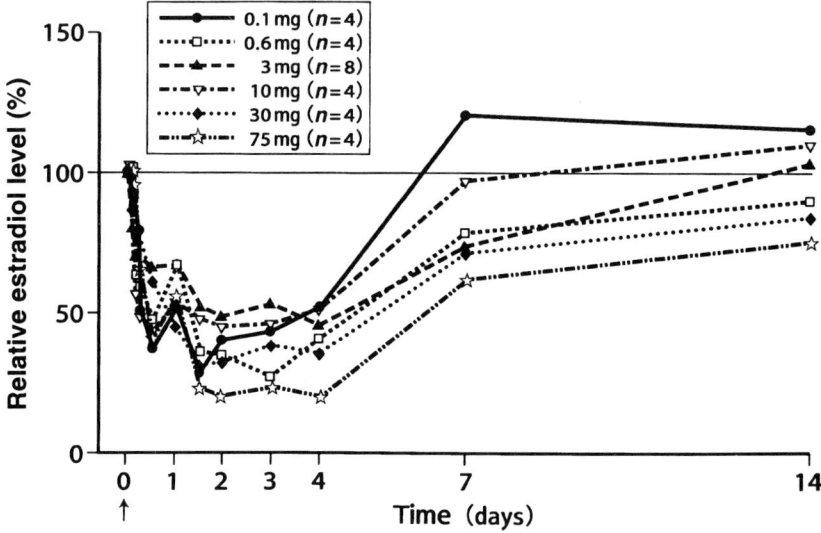

Figure 5 Serum concentration of estradiol in healthy postmenopausal women after single oral administration (arrow) of various doses of YM511 (with pre-dosage level as 100)

been studied in premenopausal women after single oral administration (1, 10, 30 and 75 mg; $n = 12$).

Tolerance

No adverse events strictly associated with YM511 and laboratory abnormalities were found.

Drug pharmacokinetics

After single oral administration of YM511, there was a linear relationship for both C_{max} and AUC over a dose range of 1–75 mg.

Effects on hormonal concentrations

The serum concentrations of estradiol were suppressed after single oral administration

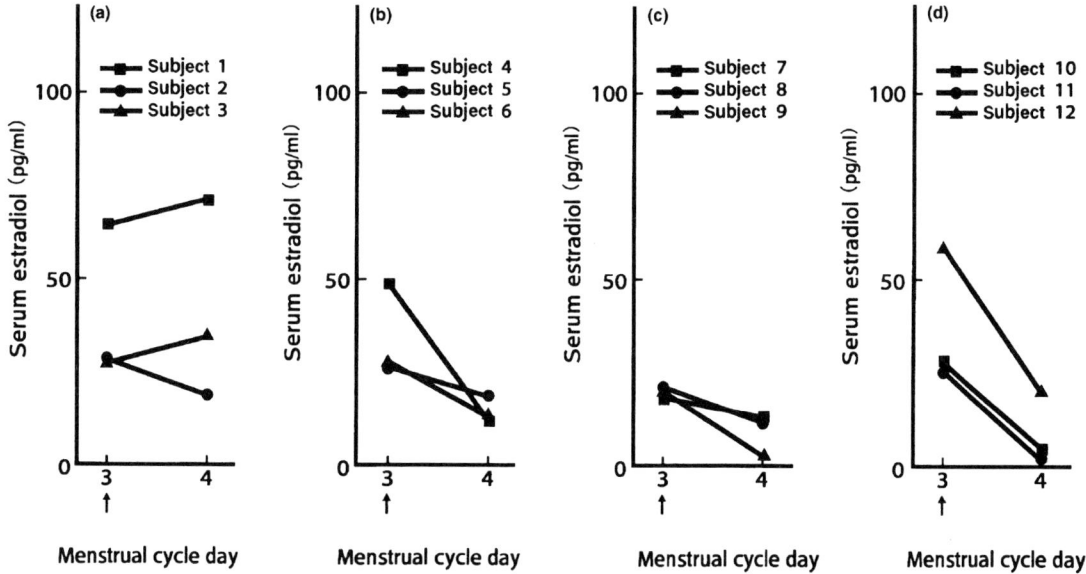

Figure 6 Serum concentration of estradiol in healthy premenopausal women after single oral administration of various doses of YM511: (a) 1 mg; (b) 10 mg; (c) 30 mg; (d) 75 mg

(third day of the menstrual cycle) of YM511 at the doses from 10 mg (Figure 6). Other hormones tended to increase from 10 mg (LH and FSH) and from 30 mg (androstenedione and testosterone).

Conclusions

YM511 is a novel non-steroidal aromatase inhibitor. It has strong and specific inhibitory effects for aromatase activity by competitive inhibition. It is well tolerated in a wide range of doses, and once-daily oral administration is enough to reduce serum estradiol levels in pre- and postmenopausal women. It is expected that YM511 will be effective in postmenopausal breast cancer, because it has no influence on other serum hormones such as LH, FSH and testosterone in postmenopausal women and it inhibits the growth of MCF-7 cells (human breast cancer cell line). Three cases of female aromatase deficiency have been reported to date[1-3]. These cases have indicated the need for vigilance regarding ovarian cysts and virilization, similar symptoms to those of polycystic ovary syndrome, at the time of administration of YM511. However, it must be remembered that aromatase deficiency does not have serious effects on health except these symptoms, and that all these abnormalities can be treated by estrogen. Furthermore, it is apparent that estrogen deficiency does not disturb psychosexual development. Because YM511 has been shown to reduce the serum estradiol level in premenopausal women, it is expected to be useful for the treatment of estrogen-dependent diseases such as endometriosis and uterine myoma. Our preliminary experiments have revealed that YM511 inhibited the growth of endometrial tissues implanted under the kidney capsule in rats. Further studies are being conducted to confirm the effectiveness of YM511 in premenopausal women.

References

1. Shozu, M., Akasofu, K., Harada, T. and Kubota, Y. (1991). A new cause of female pseudohermaphroditism: placental aromatase deficiency. *J. Clin. Endocrinol. Metab.*, **72**, 560–6
2. Conte, F.A., Grumbach, M.M., Ito, Y., Fisher, C.R. and Simpson, E.R. (1994). A syndrome of female pseudohermaphroditism, hypergonadotropic hypogonadism, and multicystic ovaries associated with missense mutations in the gene encoding aromatase (P450arom). *J. Clin. Endocrinol. Metab.*, **78**, 1287–92
3. Morishima, A., Grumbach, M.M., Simpson, E.R., Fisher, C. and Kenan, Q. (1995). Aromatase deficiency in male and female siblings caused by a novel mutation and the physiological role of estrogens. *J. Clin. Endocrinol. Metab.*, **80**, 3689–98

Section 8

GnRH agonists

Development of LHRH analogs: past, present and future

B. Lunenfeld

Ever since the isolation, identification and synthesis of gonadotropin-releasing hormone (GnRH) in 1971, the interest in the application of GnRH analogs has experienced an explosive growth rate.

The potency of GnRH and its analogs as stimulators (when administered in a precise pulsatile fashion) or GnRH agonists or antagonists as inhibitors of pituitary gonadotropin secretion (when administered chronically) permitted its exploration as a method of 'reversible medical gonadectomy' applied to the treatment of diseases dependent on gonadal steroids. It served as a basis for developing four types of treatment modalities, based on different rationales:

(1) To suppress sex steroids in diseases in which development or progress is sex steroid-dependent (metastatic prostatic cancer, hormone-dependent breast and endometrial cancer, uterine fibroids and endometrosis);

(2) To inhibit the precocious appearance of mature type GnRH pulsatility (central precocious puberty) or delay the normal onset of pubertal GnRH pulsatility, in order to postpone epididymal closure and in combination with growth hormone to permit growth to continue in slowly growing children;

(3) To control the dynamics of gonadotropin secretion in induction or ovulation or superovulation (as adjunctive treatment of anovulation, polycystic ovary disease and assisted reproduction protocols); and

(4) To exploit the possible local effects of GnRH agonists or antagonists on tissues having GnRH receptors (some types of malignancies, uterine fibroids, etc.).

Immense efforts have produced several thousand analogs and six of the most potent analogs are commercially available around the world for different clinical indications (Table 1).

Unlike the potent GnRH agonists, whose availability has allowed their widespread use during the past 10 years, the lack of production of suitable antagonists working by receptor occupancy has been disappointing. Progress in the synthesis of antagonists has been slower, since several amino acids have to be substituted in the GnRH molecule. Antagonists also require precise topological features for high binding affinity to the receptor. In the past, antagonists have had several disadvantages. Their effective dose was 1000 times that of agonists. Furthermore, the introduction of hydrophobic amino acids in positions 1, 2 and 3, as well as the addition of very basic groups in position 6, has often led to high histamine release from rat mast cells and induced cutaneous anaphylactoid reactionlike reactions. Table 2 describes the different generations of GnRH antagonists and their status. The newer generations of antagonists, particularly the latest ones, show only negligible histamine release and therefore take advantage of the remarkably acute and potent properties.

The necessary criteria for antagonist efficiency can now be defined more clearly. These are:

(1) High gonadotropin suppressive potency;
(2) Low histamine release;

ENDOMETRIOSIS TODAY: ADVANCES IN RESEARCH AND PRACTICE

Table 1 GnRH agonists available as approved drugs

Name	Structure	Route of administration
Leuprolide (Lupron, Trenantone, Enantone)	pGlu-His-Trp-Ser-Tyr-DLeu-Leu-Arg-Pro-NHEt	Subcutaneous (sc); sc 1 and 3 month depot 2 month rod implant
Buserelin (Superfact, Supercur, Superfact depot)	pGlu-His-Trp-Ser-Tyr-DSer(O^tBu)-Leu-Arg-Pro-NHEt	sc, nasal, depot, 3 months' depot
Nafarelin (Synarel)	pGlu-His-Trp-Ser-Tyr-D2Nal-Leu-Arg-Pro-GlyNH$_2$	sc, nasal
Goserelin (Zoladex)	pGlu-His-Trp-Ser-Tyr-DSer(O^tBu)-Leu-Arg-Pro-AzaglyNH$_2$	sc, depot
Histrelin (Supprelin)	pGlu-His-Trp-Ser-Tyr-DHis(Bzl)-Leu-Arg-Pro-AzaglyNH$_2$	sc
Decapeptyl	pGlu-His-Trp-Ser-Tyr-DTrp-Leu-Arg-Pro-GlyNH$_2$	sc, depot

Table 2 GnRH antagonists in clinical or preclinical studies

Name	Structure	Status
Generation 1		
4F Ant (Rivier J, Salk Inst.)	NAc$\Delta^{3,4}$Pro-D4FPhe-DTrp-Ser-Tyr-DTrp-Leu-Arg-Pro-GlyNH$_2$	Phase I
Generation 2		
NalArg (Rivier J, Salk Inst.)	NAcD2Nal-D4FPhe-DTrp-Ser-Tyr-DArg-Leu-Arg-Pro-GlyNH$_2$	Preclinical
Detirelix (Nestor J, Syntex)	NAcD2Nal-D4ClPhe-DTrp-Ser-Tyr-DHarg(Et$_2$)-Leu-Arg-Pro-DAlaNH$_2$	Phase I
Generation 3		
NalGlu (Rivier J, Salk Inst.)	NAcD2Nal-D4ClPhe-D3Pal-Ser-Arg-DGlu(AA)-Leu-Arg-Pro-DAlaNH$_2$	Phase I/II
Antide (Folkers K, Serono)	NAcD2Nal-D4ClPhe-D3Pal-Ser-Lys(Nic)-DDLys(Nic)-Leu-Lys(Isp)-Pro-DAlaNH$_2$	Phase I
Org-30850 (Organon)	NAcD4ClPhe-D4ClPhe-DBal-Ser-Tyr-DLys-Leu-Arg-Pro-DAlaNH$_2$	Phase I
Ramorelix (Sandow J, Hoechst)	NAcD2Nal-D4ClPhe-DTrp-Ser-Tyr-DSer(Rha)-Leu-Arg-Pro-AzaglyNH$_2$	Phase I
Cetrorelix (Schally AV, Asta Pharma)	NAcD2Nal-D4ClPhe-D3Pal-Ser-Tyr-DCit-Leu-Arg-Pro-DAlaNH$_2$	Phase I/II/III
Ganirelix (Nestor J, Syntex, Organon)	NAcD2Nal-D4ClPhe-D3Pal-Ser-Tyr-DHarg(Et$_2$)-Leu-Harg(Et$_2$)-Pro-DAlaNH$_2$	Phase I/II
A-75998 (Haviv F, TAP/Abbott)	NAcD2Nal-D4ClPhe-D3Pal-Ser-NMeTyr-DLys(Nic)-Leu-Lys(Isp)-Pro-DAlaNH$_2$	Phase I
Azaline B (Rivier J, Salk Inst.)	NAcD2Nal-D4ClPhe-D3Pal-Ser-Aph(atz)-DAph(atz)-Leu-Lys(Isp)-Pro-DAlaNH$_2$	Preclinical
Antarelix (Europeptides)	NAcD2Nal-D4ClPhe-D3Pal-Ser-Tyr-DHcit-Leu-Lys(Isp)-Pro-DAlaNH$_2$	Preclinical

(3) Decreased complexity and increased ease of synthesis;

(4) Easy formulation in an aqueous vehicle (solubility) with no or low gelling effects. Gelling gives rise to a subcutaneous depot effect, which may result in irritations at the site of injection and may cause random and mostly unpredictable release into the circulation; and

(5) Controllable and predictable duration of action.

Taking into account the difficulties encountered in devising effective, safe and simple to produce GnRH antagonists, the question arises whether such agents are really needed for clinical use and, if so, what are the exact indications for their application? Antagonists would seem to be required:

(1) In all clinical situations in which the flare-up has a pronounced negative effect;

(2) In situations in which the suppressing effect is required to appear immediately after administration;

(3) In situations in which the suppressive effect has to be exactly controlled; and

(4) In situations in which instant reversal of the suppressive effect (by pulsatile GnRH application) is necessary.

In order to be used for any of the above-mentioned conditions, GnRH antagonists must be extremely potent and long-acting, and exhibit negligible side-effects such as histamine release. In order to be commercially viable, these analogs also need to meet rigorous criteria, such as being easy to formulate for slow or acute release and economical to make.

It seems that third-generation GnRH antagonists are potent and well tolerated inhibitors of the pituitary gonadal axis in men and women. Preliminary studies indicate that they rapidly and reversibly suppress testicular and ovarian function in a dose-dependent manner and may be clinically effective and acceptable drugs for the treatment of gonadal hormone-dependent disorders.

Results with some of the newer antagonists in clinical situations have demonstrated that in normal women the estradiol positive feed-back is abolished by GnRH antagonist administration. During controlled ovarian hyperstimulation, antagonist administration prevented endogenous luteinizing hormone (LH) surges, thus allowing complete follicular maturation prior to the triggering of ovulation with human chorionic gonadotropin (hCG).

Future therapy consisting of a combination of a GnRH agonist and antagonist could be imagined, in which the agonist would be used initially to reduce pituitary gonadotrope receptors and would be followed by administration of a smaller amount of antagonist in order to obtain a subtle, exactly dose-dependent effect. In situations in which chronic therapy is necessary and the initial flare-up harmful, a different type of combination therapy could also be imagined, i.e. initial suppression of gonadotropin activity by antagonist, followed by continuous GnRH agonist application.

Presently available analogs of GnRH are not deliverable orally, but great progress has been made with alternatives to daily injections, first by intranasal insufflation and then by the potentially more compliance-compatible 1–3-month depot injectable formulations (Figure 1). The delivery systems could still be improved, however, to enable more convenient chronic application (oral, vaginal or possibly transdermal).

The recent cloning of the mouse and human GnRH receptors and elucidation of their sequences have elicited a great deal of scientific interest and activity, both in structural biology and in drug design. Using the published sequences, several laboratories have modeled the GnRH receptor and are trying to refine it experimentally. The model of the structure of the receptor will be utilized to design more efficient analogs as well as peptidomimetic or non-peptidic orally active antagonists.

We are finally beginning to understand the molecular biology and mechanism of action of GnRH and its analogs. GnRH binds to and

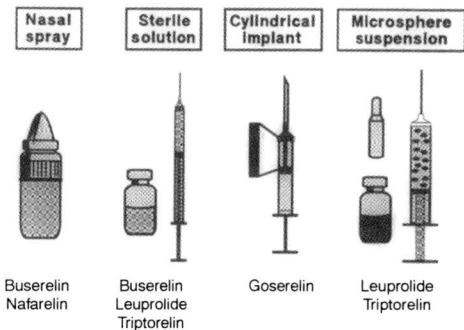

Figure 1 Various formulations of different GnRH agonists (see Table 1)

Figure 2 (below) Proposed model for GnRH receptor activation. G protein is activated following the binding of GnRH to its receptor. Thereafter, phospholipase C (PLC-PIP$_2$) and phosphatidyl-choline-specific phospholipase D (PLD-PC) are activated. The activated phospholipases elevate the second messengers diacylglycerol (DAG) and inositol trisphosphate (IP$_3$), which mobilize Ca^{2+} from internal pools stored in the endoplasmic reticulum (ER). The second messengers activate PKC subspecies, which are involved in gonado-tropin release and biosynthesis. GnRH may cause the stimulation of phospholipase A$_2$ (PLA$_2$) via PKC-independent activation of the cytosolic protein kinase cascade (MAPK). Reproduced with permission from Naor, Z. (1996). Signal transduction of the GnRH receptor. In Lunenfeld, B. and Insler, V. *GnRH Analogues: The State of the Art*, p.14. (Carnforth, UK: Parthenon Publishing)

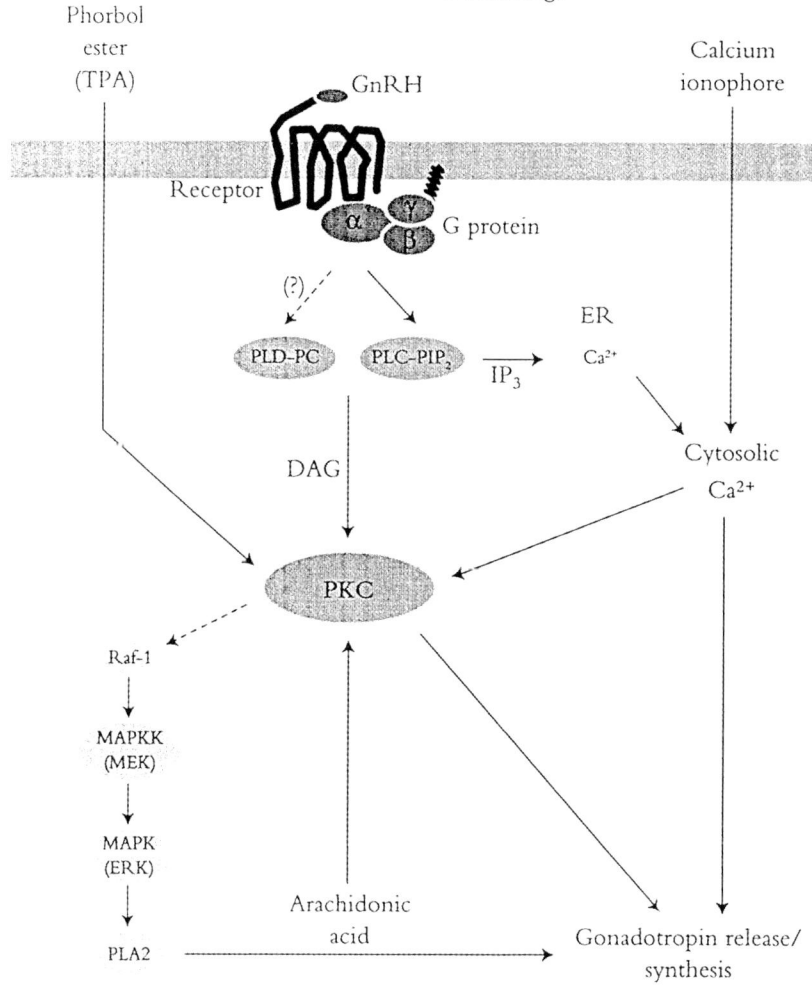

activates the gonadotropes to elicit the release and synthesis of gonadotropins. Separate mechanisms might be involved in gonadotropin release and synthesis (Figure 2).

Following the binding of GnRH to a specific receptor (cloned recently) GnRH activates several phospholipases to produce water-soluble and insoluble mediators of its action. Furthermore, there has been elucidation of the major components of the cellular basis of desensitization such as the loss of measurable GnRH receptor from the plasma membrane, the loss of functional GnRH receptor-linked calcium ion channels and the loss of the ability to transfer gonadotropin from a non-releasable to a releasable pool.

GnRH regulates gene transcription through distinct GnRH-responsive DNA sequences. Continuous exposure to GnRH desensitizes the signaling pathways that mediate transcriptional regulation. These biosynthetic effects of GnRH may account in part for the long-term effects of GnRH analogs.

Widespread clinical use of commercially available GnRH agonists has proven their efficacy in the treatment of metastatic prostatic cancer, precocious puberty and endometriosis, and as adjunctive therapy in the management of benign gynecological diseases and reproductive disorders.

We seem to arrive at a consensus that GnRH analogs in the management of leiomyomata should be restricted to the tumors producing specific symptoms such as pelvic pain, menorrhagia or infertility. GnRH analog administration in such patients with shrinkage of the uterus and fibroids and decreasing blood supply is efficient in diminishing the intraoperative blood loss and shortening of the duration of surgery for uterine fibroids. Such preoperative treatment may therefore be a useful addition to surgery in cases with symptomatic fibroid uteri, by improving the patient's preoperative status and providing concurrent symptom relief. It can allow for restoration of iron stores and hemoglobin levels, so that autodonation of blood preoperatively becomes possible.

The 30–40% reduction in size may permit laparoscopic or hysteroscopic enucleation of the fibroid. In some cases agonist or antagonist therapy may postpone or even eliminate the need for surgery, converting symptomatic into asymptomatic conditions. However, in most cases, relief is temporary, and regrowth to pretreatment size occurs within 3 months of cessation of therapy. For inoperable patients, long-term GnRH analog treatment and add-back therapy could constitute an alternative, especially during the years immediately preceding the menopause.

Studies reported also indicate that GnRH analogs offer an alternative and successful therapeutic approach and should be able to control, quite efficiently and quickly, benign gynecological disorders associated with excessive menstrual blood loss.

In the medical management of endometriosis, one can conclude that GnRH analogs are potent therapeutic agents that bring about not only suppression of endometrial lesions but also relief of symptoms. A novel aspect of treatment with GnRH agonist regimens is the addition of estrogens to alleviate hypoestrogenic symptoms. Preliminary data indicate that, in fact, the add-back regimen may accomplish these goals. An in-depth literature review revealed that the efficacies of medroxyprogesterone acetate (MPA), gestrinone, danazol and GnRH analogs in the treatment of pelvic pain for endometriosis are largely comparable. However, despite favorable results during treatment, about 50% of women experienced recurrence of pelvic pain a few months to a few years following the termination of therapy. Because of the chronic nature of endometriosis, the average symptomatic patient will probably require and receive several courses of medical therapy during her reproductive life. Some women will unquestionably exhibit side-effects to one or several of these drugs; others will be unresponsive or intolerant. Assuming equal effectiveness between progestogens, danazol and GnRH analogs, the availability of several drugs enables the physician to select the most suitable medication for the patient at any given time.

In the management of the infertile patient, when conventional treatment regimes had failed, GnRH analogs have been successfully utilized to suppress the pituitary–ovarian axis prior to stimulation of follicular growth and induction of ovulation, concomitantly with exogenous follicle-stimulating hormone (FSH). This triphasic approach has also been efficiently used for the stimulation of multiple follicular recruitment growth and development in assisted reproductive techniques (ART). It will prevent drop-outs due to an untimely LH surge, and increase live birth rate by reducing the undesirable late follicular LH levels, which have been associated with decreased fertilization potential and increased pregnancy wastage. It is estimated that in many countries more than 70% of superovulation protocols include the use of GnRH analogs, illustrating their increasing popularity.

Prostatic cancer, and more specifically the advanced forms with metastasis, were and remain a challenge for oncologists and urologists. Since GnRH analogs can replace the psychological debilitating syndrome of surgical castration with only minimal side-effects, they are being widely used in the management of prostatic cancer.

GnRH analogs are being investigated for their therapeutic advantage in hormone-dependent breast cancer and for ovarian cancer. Some tumor types, such as pancreatic acinar tumors and osteosarcomas, may need to be redefined according to their hormonal dependency. Co-administration of GnRH analogs with somatostatin analogs may also be beneficial for treatment of certain tumors.

It has become clear during the last few years that the physically, psychologically and socially debilitating syndrome of central or true isosexual precocious puberty is now treatable on more than a symptomatic level. Several large-scale studies with GnRH agonists are now of sufficient duration to suggest that a major influence on final adult height may result if treatment is commenced early enough and continued for long enough. Moreover, it has been suggested that delaying the onset of puberty in slowly growing children, and concomitantly treating them with growth hormone, may allow growth to continue and permit an increase in their final adult height. Conclusive data on this subject will probably be presented in a few years.

As always, with any new class of therapeutic agents, safety considerations must be paramount. Potent endocrine drugs such as the GnRH analogs should not be expected to be without side-effects. These unwanted effects will include sequelae of their mechanism of action and reflect the induction of a hypogonadotropic hypogonadism, such as vasomotor symptoms in both sexes and osteoporotic changes in women.

At present, it is debated whether both the symptoms of the underlying disease and the adverse effects derived from ovarian quiescence can be reliably suppressed by the combined treatment of GnRH analogs with low-dose estrogen–gestagen, with low-dose estrogen replacement therapy or with synthetic steroids. Recent data also seem to indicate that the beneficial effects of initial high-dose GnRH analog treatment can be preserved by continuing treatment with sub-threshold doses, which may result in only partial pituitary suppression, resulting in continuous low-grade estrogen production.

Relatively new data have now become available, indicating that persistence of minimal amounts of GnRH analogs during the luteal phase at the time of implantation seems to have no adverse effects on pregnancy rate and fetal well-being. Furthermore, it has been demonstrated that GnRH analogs did not exert any fetotoxicity or embryotoxicity in rabbits or monkeys. Moreover, none of the currently available data suggest that agonists exert toxic or teratogenic effects in pregnant women who received GnRH analog treatment accidentally.

The value of GnRH agonists in treatment of female infertility by using the induction of superovulation (COH) modality has proven to be impressive. By abolishing untimely LH surges the combined pituitary suppression/ovarian stimulation therapy has significantly improved the pregnancy rates. This, however, was associated with a longer duration of therapy and a higher dose requirement of gonadotropins. Recent studies have shown that a short-term application of a GnRH antagonist during a defined period of follicular development prevented the appearance of a premature LH surge, thus allowing complete follicular maturation prior to the triggering of ovulation with hCG. This type of combined therapy could obviously offset the objectionable features of GnRH agonist/gonadotropin treatment. Their immediate inhibition of gonadotropins, without the flare-up effect may have a profound influence on their use in ovulation induction and ART procedures. Three different protocols are being investigated. The German protocol with multiple applications seems effective but does not have any major advantages over the current use of GnRH agonists. The French protocol which advocates the use of a single, or sometimes double, application may have some beneficial effect on ART, since it will reduce the amount of gonadotropins as well as the number of days of application without affecting results. Recently a revival of either unstimulated cycles or clomiphene-stimulated cycles combined with a single injection of GnRH antagonist has been proposed. This protocol employs the availability of GnRH antagonists which enable the abolishment of the LH surge but also inhibits an already beginning LH surge. This principle is being investigated to revive either unstimulated or clomiphene-induced ART cycles. By the time of the next GnRH meeting in Geneva, February 1999, sufficient data should have accumulated to be able to judge these new developments. Furthermore, a sequential treatment consisting of pituitary–ovarian suppression by a GnRH antagonist followed by induction of follicular growth by pulsatile GnRH can also be envisaged.

Additional basic research concerning the biology of GnRH should be carried out. The binding and function of GnRH analogs in other organs besides the pituitary must be explored. Confirmation of recently produced experimental data could open new avenues for the management of benign prostatic hyperplasia (BPH) and control of some malignant tumors by application of specific GnRH antagonists. An effort should also be made to discriminate between the actions of agonists and antagonists with respect to the effect on FSH and free alpha-subunit secretion, tumor cell proliferation and the immune response.

Role of GnRH agonist type and formulation in the management of endometriosis

M. Filicori

Endometriosis is a classical indication for gonadotropin-releasing hormone (GnRH) agonists, and the potency, route of administration and delivery systems used for different agonists are discussed here. Assessment of differences in potency for the GnRH agonists include *in vitro* assays (luteinizing hormone (LH) and follicle-stimulating hormone (FSH) measurement from dispersed pituitary cells, receptor binding assays) and *in vivo* assays (stimulation of LH release in immature or ovariectomized rats, ovulation induction, stimulation of uterine growth). For example, results of one study[1] which assessed the potency of different GnRH agonists using an ovariectomized rat assay showed that leuprorelin had the highest activity (Figure 1). However, when making comparisons between GnRH agonists, it must be stressed that results can differ depending on which assay is used, making it important to compare agonists using the same assay and under the same experimental conditions[2-4].

In addition to the different types of agonists available, they are also marketed in different formulations, ranging from short-acting subcutaneous forms, intranasal administrations and the depot preparations, available as the microencapsulated forms or implants, in which the GnRH agonist is bound to a biodegradable matrix formed by polylactide glycolide (PLG) copolymers that provide controlled release. PLG copolymers are available as microcapsules or implants, with GnRH release dynamics profoundly influenced by the formulation of these copolymers. In general implants can accommodate greater peptide loads making them preferable for ultralong administration, although leuprorelin also has a 3-monthly microencapsulated form. Implant coating with a barrier compound such as cyanoacrylate or changing the ratio of the PLG polymer can affect and delay peptide diffusion.

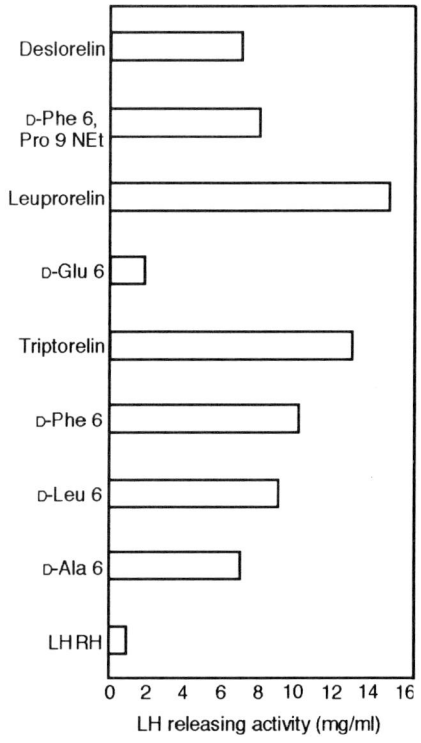

Figure 1 Potency of different GnRH agonists (ovariectomized rat assay) (reproduced from reference 1). NEt, N-ethilamide; LHRH, luteinizing hormone-releasing hormone

We conducted a comparative study which assessed the efficacy of different GnRH agonists in terms of induction of amenorrhea, pituitary suppression and ovarian suppression[5]. Forty infertile women, aged less than 36 years, were randomized to four different regimens; Group B received the very high dose of 300 µg buserelin twice daily, a dose known to cause profound pituitary and ovarian suppression; Group G, goserelin 3.6 mg depot every 28 days; Group L, leuprorelin 3.75 mg depot every 28 days; and Group T, triptorelin 3.75 mg intramuscularly every 28 days. The duration of the study was 3 months.

Evaluations included baseline measurements of LH, FSH and estradiol taken prior to starting the GnRH agonist; a second evaluation the day after the third GnRH agonist dose was administered (days 56–57) and a final measurement at the end of the trial (day 84). Aggregate data showed that LH was profoundly suppressed, FSH suppressed to a lesser degree, and estradiol well suppressed in general, although goserelin and triptorelin tended to have estradiol concentrations which were more variable. While 35 out of 40 patients achieved estradiol levels which were below castration threshold at the second evaluation (Figure 2), by the end of the study all patients except two receiving goserelin had complete suppression. Both of these two had concentrations above 70 pmol/l, and both had uterine bleeding.

While all compounds profoundly suppressed immuno-LH in the third month, FSH suppression with depot forms was less marked than with high dose short-acting agonists, and signs of incomplete ovarian function block may be present using depots, particularly with goserelin.

Translation of this information to the management of endometriosis is difficult, but most depot GnRH agonists were very effective in inducing profound amenorrhea compared

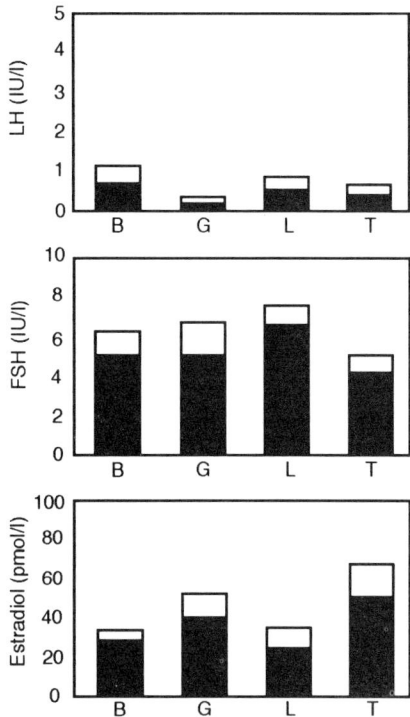

Figure 2 Gonadotropin and 17β-estradiol response to GnRH (second evaluation performed on days 56–57 of study protocol). B, buserelin; G, goserelin; L, leuprorelin; T, triptorelin

to intranasal agonists, while goserelin implants resulted in about 10% of patients having breakthrough bleeding throughout the duration of the study.

In conclusion, different pharmaceutical formulations profoundly influence GnRH agonist delivery kinetics, and the GnRH agonist release profile from depot is influenced by polymer ratio and system type. In addition, GnRH agonist depots may differ in their capacity to completely suppress estrogen secretion and induce amenorrhea. Finally, the implications of these differences for the management of endometriosis remain to be fully established.

References

1. Coy, D.H., Vilchez-Martinez, J.A. and Coy, E.J. (1976). Analogs of luteinizing hormone-releasing hormone with increased biological activity produced by D-amino acid substitutions in position 6. *J. Med. Chem.* **19**, 423–5
2. Nestor, J.J. Jr. (1987). Design of LHRH agonist drug candidates. *J. Androl.*, **8**, 4–8
3. Filicori, M. and Flamigni, C. (1988). GnRH agonists and antagonists: a review of their current status. *Drugs*, **35**, 63–82
4. Conn, P.M. and Crowley, W.F. Jr. (1991). Gonadotropin-releasing hormone and its analogues. *N. Engl. J. Med.*, **324**, 93–103
5. Filicori, M., Flamigni, C., Cognigni, G., Dellai, P., Arnone, R., Falbo, A. and Capelli, M. (1993). Comparison of the suppressive capacity of different depot gonadotropin-releasing hormone analogs in women. *J. Clin. Endocrinol. Metab.*, **77**, 130–3

GnRH analogs in the management of endometriosis

K.-W. Schweppe

Introduction

As early as 1982, Meldrun and colleagues[1] introduced the gonadotropin-releasing hormone (GnRH) analogs as a possible new approach to the treatment of endometriosis. In the 10 years following the initial report, many non-comparative studies were published confirming the significant reduction in symptoms of endometriosis during and after medical therapy with GnRH analogs. All these clinical trials confirmed the ability of the GnRH analogs to suppress estradiol serum levels after the first month of treatment to the menopausal range, to induce hypoestrogenic amenorrhea and to achieve pain relief. No relevant disturbances of metabolic processes (such as liver function, lipid metabolism) were found, except an estrogen-dependent demineralization of bone mass.

The effect on the endometriotic implants is not dependent upon the degree of suppression of ovarian estrogen synthesis. Patients with intermittent estradiol rise during intranasal application and consecutive vaginal spottings had the same degree of pelviscopic confirmed regression as patients with continuous sufficient ovarian suppression[2]. Complete suppression may therefore not be necessary for the achievement of a clinical response of endometriosis, as demonstrated in trials with different dose regimens by Shaw and Matta[3] and Minaguchi and associates[4].

Between 1986 and 1995 several randomized comparative or double-blind placebo-controlled studies were published, which have compared the efficacy of different GnRH analogs with that of the danazol regimen[5-16]. All data proved that, independent of the severity of the disease, treatment of endometriosis with GnRH agonists led to a marked regression of implants and reduction of size of ovarian endometriomas, to the same degree as danazol, the standard of the past.

In a special symposium dealing with the newest international data on the place of the GnRH analog leuprorelin in the treatment of endometriosis, Dr Filicori (Italy) covered the importance of different types and the formulation of GnRH agonists and Dr Crosignanis (Italy) compared the effects of a monthly depot injection versus an ultra long-acting preparation. Clinical results with special reference to long-term effects were presented by Dr Tuketani (Japan); Dr Winkel (USA) discussed GnRH agonist therapy in combination with surgical treatment. Finally, Dr Bouchard (France) gave practical recommendations concerning indications and criteria for medical treatment of endometriosis.

These facts will characterize the actual situation of our knowledge about GnRH analogs and hopefully improve our practical guidelines for the treatment of this enigmatic disease. During the *4th International Symposium on GnRH Analogs*, which was held in Geneva this year, the attempt during the discussion to reach a consensus about the place of GnRH analogs failed because of numerous unsolved questions on the therapeutic strategies. There was, however, agreement that:

(1) Endometriosis is a benign, proliferative, sex steroid-dependent disease of women, which mostly affects the reproductive organs; it has an unclear etiology and its

pathogenesis is not yet completely understood;

(2) After uterine fibroids endometriosis is the second most common benign condition affecting women of reproductive age. Cardinal symptoms and signs are dysmenorrhea, pelvic pain, dyspareunia, urinary and defecation disorders as well as uncharacteristic abdominal and back pain appearing cyclically or acyclically;

(3) Endometriosis has an association with infertility. In advanced stages organ damage and adhesions represent mechanical causes of infertility;

(4) The diagnosis must be verified by directed biopsy and histological evaluation;

(5) Clinical relevance should be assessed on the basis of extent, location, type and color of endometriotic lesions and cysts;

(6) Undertreatment as well as overtreatment either with medical drugs or surgery has to be avoided; and

(7) Since endometriosis is often a progressive disease that continues during the reproductive age and has a high risk of recurrence, periodical gynecological follow-ups including sonographic examinations are necessary.

There was controversy regarding the following topics:

(1) The currently most effective treatment for active and inactive lesions;

(2) The indications for symptomatic, medical or surgical treatment; and

(3) The usefulness of medical treatment prior to or after surgery.

Conclusions

Putting all the reported new findings and reviewed data together we can draw the following conclusions:

(1) GnRH agonists as depot preparations are preferable to other formulations, because they provide a profound and constant ovarian suppression (M. Filicori);

(2) Although the regression of endometriosis, the pregnancy rates and the recurrence rates are independent of the route of administration and dosage of GnRH agonists, patient compliance, amenorrhea rates and subjective improvement are better with depot preparations with high dosages, i.e. leuprorelin 3.75 mg monthly (Y. Taketani);

(3) Patient acceptability is even better with a 3-monthly depot (P.G. Crosignani);

(4) Postoperative treatment with leuprorelin acetate significantly reduces the recurrence rates of ovarian endometriomas. The most effective therapy for patients with endometriosis-induced pain is the excision of endometriotic implants and the sequelae of endometriosis. Similar results can be obtained if, after laser ablation, a 6-month course of leuprorelin depot is given to reduce the recurrence of subjective complaints (C.A. Winkel);

(5) Medical treatment of endometriosis is indicated in cases of recurrent disease and to consolidate surgery. In infertile patients, the fecundity cannot be improved by medical therapy alone; therefore assisted reproduction must be taken into consideration; and

(6) From all medical therapies available (danazol, progestins, GnRH agonists and antiprogestins), at this stage GnRH agonists are the best anti-estrogenic treatment for endometriosis (P. Bouchard).

These evidence-based guidelines should be used in gynecological practice to improve the therapeutic options for patients, to reduce side-effects of treatment and to achieve longer-lasting disease-free intervals.

References

1. Meldrun, D.R., Chang, R.J., Lu, J. et al. (1982). Medical oophorectomy using a long-acting GnRH agonist: a possible new approach to the treatment of endometriosis. *J. Clin. Endocrinol. Metab.*, **54**, 1081–3
2. Ochs, H., Cirkel, U. and Schneider, H.P.G. (1993). Correlation between ovarian suppression and regression of endometriosis: decapeptyl versus danazol. Presented at the *3rd International Symposium on GnRH Analogues in Cancer and Human Reproduction*, Geneva, (Abstr.)
3. Shaw, R.W. and Matta, W. (1986). Reversible pituitary ovarian suppression induced by an LHRH agonist in the treatment of endometriosis. Comparison of two dose regimens. *Clin. Reprod. Fertil.*, **4**, 329–36
4. Minaguchi, H., Vermura, T.L. and Shitzu, K. (1986). Clinical study on finding the optimal dose of a potent LHRH agonist (buserelin) for the treatment of endometriosis – multicentre trial in Japan. In Rolland, R., Chandha, D.R. and Wilemsen, W.P.N. (eds.) *Gonadotrophin Down Regulation in Gynaecological Practice*, pp. 211–25. (New York: Alan R. Liss)
5. Henzl, M.R., Corson, S.L. Moghissi, K. et al. (1988). Administration of nasal narfarelin as compared with oral danazol for endometriosis. *N. Engl. J. Med.*, **318**, 455–89
6. Matta, W.H. and Shaw, R.W. (1986). A comparative study between buserelin and danazol in the treatment of endometriosis. *Br. J. Clin. Pract.*, **41** (Suppl. 48), 69–73
7. Kiesel, L., Thomas, K., Tempore, A. et al. (1989). Efficacy and safety of buserelin treatment in women with endometriosis – a multicentre open-label study. *Gynaecol. Endocrinol.*, **3** (Suppl. 2), 5–19
8. Sondheimer, S.J., Klioze, S.S., Schreider, J., Setescak, L. and Spiro, T. (1990). A comparison of the efficacy and safety of buserelin vs. danazol in the treatment of endometriosis. In Chadra, D.R. and Buttram, V.C. Jr (eds.) *Current Concepts in Endometriosis*, pp. 253–67. (New York: Alan R. Liss)
9. Lemay, A. (1988). Comparison of GnRH analogues to conventional therapy in endometriosis. Presented at the *International Symposium on GnRH Analogues*, Geneva, Abstr. 020
10. The Narfarelin European Endometriosis Group (1992). A large scale danazol controlled trial of efficacy and safety with one year follow-up. *Fertil. Steril.*, **57**, 514–22
11. Shaw, R.W. (1992). An open randomised comparative study on the effect of goserelin and danazol in the treatment of endometriosis. *Fertil. Steril.*, **58**, 265–72
12. Wheeler, J.M., Knittle, J.D. and Miller, J.D. (1992). Depot leuprolide versus danazol in the treatment of women with symptomatic endometriosis. *Am. J. Obstet. Gynecol.*, **167**, 1367–71
13. Rock, J.A., Truglia, J.A., Caplan, R.J. and the Zoladex Endometriosis Study Group (1993). Zoladex (goserelin acetate implant) in the treatment of endometriosis: a randomised comparison with danazol. *Obstet. Gynecol.*, **82**, 198–205
14. Cirkel, U., Ochs, H. and Schneider, H.P.G. (1995). A randomized, comparative trial of triptorelin depot (D-Trp6-LHRH) and danazol in the treatment of endometriosis. *Eur. J. Obstet. Gynecol. Reprod. Biol.*, **59**, 61–9
15. Reichel, R.P., Schweppe, K.-W. and ZES-Group (1992). Goserelin depot in the treatment of endometriosis. *Fertil. Steril.*, **57**, 1197–202
16. Schweppe, K.-W. (1994). Stellenwert von Zoldex-Gyn in der Endometriosebehandlung. In Schweppe, K.-W., Bastert, G., Alt, D. and Klosterhalfen, B. (eds.) *GnRH-Agonisten in der Behandlung von Endometriose und Uterus myomatosus*, pp. 1–19 (München, Bern, Wien, New York: Zuckschwerdt)

Treatment of symptomatic endometriosis with leuprolide in a 3-monthly versus a monthly depot formulation

P.G. Crosignani, W. Vegetti, L. De Cecco, A. Sémino, A. Gastaldi, P. La Commare, P.L. Venturini, P. Vercellini and S. Oldani

Introduction

Gonadotropin-releasing hormone (GnRH) agonists are highly effective in the relief of pain symptoms associated with endometriosis and constitute the therapeutic reference standard among medical treatments[1-5]. It has been demonstrated that depot formulations are better tolerated and induce a more profound and stable hypo-estrogenism than intranasal sprays or daily subcutaneous or intramuscular injections[6,7]. Recently a 3-monthly depot formulation of leuprolide acetate has become available for clinical assessment in urology and gynecology[8]. We designed a pilot study to evaluate the efficacy and acceptability of one injection of a GnRH agonist every 12 weeks compared with the usual administration every 4 weeks in the treatment of symptomatic pelvic endometriosis.

Materials and methods

The main objective of this multicenter, open-label randomized pilot study was to evaluate the efficacy of 6 months of treatment with leuprolide in a 3-monthly versus a monthly intramuscular depot injection in the relief of chronic pelvic pain in women with endometriosis. Secondary aims were to assess variations in luteinizing hormone (LH), follicle-stimulating hormone (FSH) and 17β-estradiol serum levels, the effects of the two formulations on endometriotic implants at follow-up laparoscopy, the acceptability of the two treatment schedules and modifications in bone mineral density during therapy. The protocol was approved by the local ethics committees and the patients gave their written consent to the study. Premenopausal women (FSH < 30 mIU/ml) of 18–38 years of age with symptomatic endometriosis at stage I–IV of the revised American Fertility Society (rAFS) classification[9] diagnosed at laparoscopy, were considered for recruitment to the trial. Exclusion criteria were pregnancy, breast-feeding, obesity (body mass index > 26), total serum cholesterol levels > 300 mg/dl, cardiovascular, hepatic, renal and neoplastic diseases, and hormonal treatments or oral contraceptive use in the previous 2 months. Eligible patients were randomized according to a computer-generated sequence to receive an intramuscular injection of leuprolide acetate 11.25 mg every 84 days (Group 1), or 3.75 mg every 28 days (Group 2) for 6 months, beginning on the first day of menstruation. Participating subjects agreed to use barrier contraception for the entire study period and for 8 weeks thereafter. At baseline and at 3 and 6 months the patients underwent general and gynecological examination, routine biochemistry tests, and hormonal determinations (FSH, LH, 17β-estradiol and progesterone). The women were also asked to grade the degree of their pain symptoms according to the 0–3 points verbal rating scale devised by Biberoglu and Behrman[10], which defines dysmenorrhea according to loss of work efficiency and need for bed rest (some loss of work efficiency, mild, 1; in bed part of one day, occasional loss of work, moderate, 2; in bed for one or more days, incapacitation, severe, 3), non-menstrual pain according to degree of discomfort and use of analgesics (occasional pelvic discomfort, mild, 1; noticeable discomfort for most of the cycle, moderate, 2; pain persisting during the cycle or requiring strong analgesics, severe, 3) and deep dyspareunia according to limitation of sexual activity (discomfort tolerated, mild, 1; intercourse painful to the point of interruption, moderate, 2; intercourse avoided because of pain, severe, 3). We graded pelvic tenderness (minimal tenderness on palpation, mild, 1; extensive tenderness on palpation, moderate, 2; unable to palpate because of tenderness, severe, 3) and induration (uterus freely mobile, induration of the cul-de-sac, mild, 1; thickened and indurated adnexa and cul-de-sac, restricted uterine mobility, moderate, 2; nodular adnexa and cul-de-sac, frozen uterus, severe, 3) at gynecological examination at the same time points. At the end of the treatment period a follow-up laparoscopy was scheduled to monitor the effect of therapy on endometriotic lesions and revised AFS score. Bone mineral density of the lumbar spine at the L2–L4 region was measured at baseline and at the end of therapy by dual energy X-ray absorptiometry (Hologic QDR 1000, Hologic Inc., Waltham, MA, USA; or Norland XR-26, Norland Corporation, Fort Atkinson, WI, USA). The bone mineral density of each patient was monitored with the same instrument. Differences in accuracy among instruments were minimized by normalizing the data as percentage changes from baseline. Measurements and data analysis were performed using standard procedures with the original software provided by the manufacturer. At the 6-month assessment the women were requested to grade the acceptability of their treatment schedule (3-monthly versus monthly depot injections) as good, fair, or poor.

Clinical characteristics of the subjects in the two groups were compared by means of unpaired Student's t- and χ^2 tests. Within- and between-group variations in pain symptoms and pelvic findings scores at baseline and the end of treatment were evaluated with Wilcoxon's matched-pairs signed-ranks and Mann–Whitney U-tests. Variations in routine biochemistry tests, serum hormone levels, endometriosis revised AFS scores, and bone mineral density values were analyzed at the same time points by paired and unpaired Student's t-test as appropriate. The χ^2 test was used to compare the frequency of good tolerability of the treatment schedule in the two study groups. All tests were two-sided. Probability values less than 5% were considered as statistically significant.

Results

A total of 30 women were enrolled in the trial in three academic departments of northern Italy (Clinica Ostetrica e Ginecologica I, University of Milano; Clinica Ostetrica e Ginecologica, University of Genova; and Clinica Ostetrica e Ginecologica, University of Brescia), 15 of whom were allocated to the 3-monthly depot treatment and 15 to the monthly one. No significant difference in clinical characteristics was observed between the groups (Table 1). One Group 1 patient withdrew from the study because she did not want to undergo venipunctures and follow-up laparoscopy, and one Group 2 subject stopped therapy at the third month because of a desire to conceive. Non-menstrual pelvic pain was significantly reduced at both the 3- and 6-month evaluations, without between-group differences (Table 2). An appreciable reduction was also observed in both groups in deep dyspareunia scores, but the differences between the basal and 6-month values did not reach statistical significance due to the limited sample size. Dysmenorrhea obviously disappeared in concomitance with the amenorrheic status induced by the GnRH agonist in both formulations. With regard to findings at vaginal examination, pelvic tenderness was significantly reduced by both 3- and 1-monthly depot injections whereas pelvic induration was not modified by either regimen. Serum LH and 17β-estradiol levels were significantly suppressed at 12 and 24 weeks compared with baseline values, being respectively, at the above different time points, 8.0 ± 8.3, 0.7 ± 0.4 and 1.0 ± 1.1 mIU/ml and 105 ± 69, 14 ± 7 and 13 ± 6 pg/ml in Group 1 and 5.4 ± 2.8, 0.9 ± 0.7 and 1.1 ± 1.0 mIU/ml and 95 ± 61, 15 ± 11 and 16 ± 13 pg/ml in Group 2, without differences between the groups. The monthly depot caused a slightly more marked inhibition of serum FSH levels with respect to the 3-monthly preparation. In fact, FSH values at baseline, 12 and 24 weeks were, respectively, 7.2 ± 7.4, 4.9 ± 2.8 and 4.1 ± 3.0 mIU/ml in Group 1 and 6.1 ± 7.1, 3.8 ± 1.4 and 2.9 ± 1.1 mIU/ml in Group 2. Progesterone levels were always in the anovulatory range during therapy. No significant variations were observed in routine biochemistry tests. Treatment with both leuprolide depot formulations induced a significant reduction in endometriotic lesions. Mean (SD) revised AFS scores at baseline and at follow-up laparoscopy were, respectively, 32.8 (25.1) and 12.2 (9.3) in ten subjects of Group 1 and 29.0 (22.7) and 13.1 (15.3) in nine subjects of Group 2 (paired t-test, $p < 0.05$). Hot flushes were reported by 12 (80%) women in each group, vaginal dryness by three (20%) in Group 1 and two (13%) in Group 2, and abdominal pain, arthralgia and depression by three different subjects in Group 2 (7% in each case). Three-monthly injections were accepted significantly better than monthly ones. In fact, 13 women in Group 1 graded the acceptability of their treatment schedule as 'good' compared with seven in Group 2 ($\chi^2 = 5.40$, $p = 0.02$, odds ratio 7.4, 95% confidence interval, 1.2–45.0). A total of 20 patients (10 in each study group) underwent complete serial lumbar dual X-ray absorptiometry. A statistically significant variation of lumbar spine bone mineral density was observed at the end of leuprolide treatment in both study groups ($p < 0.01$), the percentage decrease from baseline being 5.2%

Table 1 Clinical characteristics of the study subjects according to treatment allocation. Data are presented as mean ± SD or number (%) of patients

	Group 1 (3-monthly depot formulation)	Group 2 (monthly depot formulation)
Age (years)	28.6 ± 6.0	31.0 ± 5.2
Weight (kg)	54.4 ± 4.8	54.7 ± 6.2
Height (cm)	164 ± 6	164 ± 5
Number parous	2 (13.3%)	4 (26.7%)
Disease stage*		
stage I	1 (6.7%)	2 (13.3%)
stage II	1 (6.7%)	2 (13.3%)
stage III	5 (33.3%)	4 (26.7%)
stage IV	8 (53.3%)	7 (46.7%)

*According to the revised American Fertility Society classification of endometriosis[9]

and 4.9% in the 3-monthly and 1-monthly depot arms, respectively.

Discussion

There is general consensus on the efficacy of GnRH agonist treatment in selected benign gynecological diseases[1–5]. Monthly depot preparations have been demonstrated to induce a deeper and more stable hypo-estrogenism with better acceptability than intranasal sprays or daily injections[6,7]. A further improvement in treatment acceptability and patient compliance should be offered by 3-monthly depot formulations but very limited data are available in the literature, especially on the efficacy of these sustained release preparations in terms of ovarian suppression and clinical results in comparison with the usual monthly injections[8,11]. As far as we know, no studies have yet been published on treatment with a 3-monthly GnRH agonist depot preparation in patients with endometriosis. In the present study we did not observe significant between-group differences in LH concentrations. The reduction in serum FSH levels was statistically

Table 2 Pain symptom scores* in patients with endometriosis before, during and after leuprolide therapy according to treatment schedule allocation. Data are presented as mean ± SD

Type of symptom and treatment schedule	Baseline	3 months	6 months
Dysmenorrhea			
3-monthly depot	2.8 ± 1.1	—	—
monthly depot	2.9 ± 1.0	—	—
Deep dyspareunia			
3-monthly depot	1.8 ± 0.9	1.3 ± 0.7	1.3 ± 0.7
monthly depot	2.1 ± 1.2	1.2 ± 0.4	1.3 ± 0.7
Non-menstrual pain			
3-monthly depot	2.1 ± 0.6	1.4 ± 0.5**	1.1 ± 0.3**
monthly depot	2.1 ± 0.8	1.2 ± 0.4**	1.2 ± 0.4**
Pelvic tenderness			
3-monthly depot	2.2 ± 0.6	1.8 ± 0.4**	1.2 ± 0.7**
monthly depot	2.4 ± 0.9	1.5 ± 0.7**	1.6 ± 0.7**
Induration			
3-monthly depot	1.7 ± 0.8	1.5 ± 0.7	1.1 ± 0.3
monthly depot	1.9 ± 0.9	1.6 ± 0.7	1.5 ± 0.5

*According to the verbal rating scale devised by Biberoglu and Behrman[10]; **$p < 0.05$, Wilcoxon's matched-pairs signed-ranks test

significant only in the monthly depot group, but this is probably related to the limited number of observations. In fact, all women were amenorrheic during treatment and 17β-estradiol levels were always suppressed in both groups. Pain symptoms assessed by the Biberoglu and Behrman scale[10] were alleviated by both leuprolide acetate preparations. Pelvic induration was not relieved by treatment, but this is not surprising due to the mainly fibrotic and cicatricial nature of this phenomenon, which may not undergo great modifications during medical therapies. Laparoscopic evaluation at the end of the study period demonstrated that both leuprolide acetate regimens induced a reduction in endometriotic lesions as assessed by the revised AFS score. However, it has been demonstrated that this effect may be temporary and limited to the hypoestrogenic period[12,13]. The percentage decreases of lumbar spine bone mineral density after 6 months of treatment were very similar in the two study groups and substantially in accordance with literature data[14,15]. The limited sample size is one of the main drawbacks of our study, which was however designed to demonstrate important differences in patient tolerance of the 3-monthly and the monthly preparations. In this regard, the acceptability of the treatment schedule was considered as 'good' by significantly more women in the 3-monthly depot group than in the monthly one.

In conclusion, the results of our multicenter, randomized pilot study demonstrated that 3-monthly and monthly depot preparations of leuprolide acetate are both efficacious in inducing ovarian suppression, lesion regression and pain relief in subjects with symptomatic endometriosis. However, due to better patient acceptability, the 3-monthly depot injections may be preferred when a 6-month treatment is indicated.

Acknowledgement

We are grateful to Takeda Italia Farmaceutici, Rome, Italy, for supplying leuprolide depot injections, preparing the randomization procedures, and giving financial support to the study.

References

1. Barbieri, R.L. (1990). Endometriosis 1990. Current treatment approaches. *Drugs*, **39**, 502–10
2. Shaw, R.W. (1991). GnRH analogues in the treatment of endometriosis – rationale and efficacy. In Thomas, E. and Rock, J. (eds.) *Modern Approaches to Endometriosis*, pp. 257–74. (Dordrecht, The Netherlands: Kluwer Academic Publishers)
3. Shaw, R.W. (1992). Treatment of endometriosis. *Lancet*, **340**, 1267–70
4. Kaupilla, A. (1993). Changing concepts of medical treatment of endometriosis. *Acta Obstet. Gynecol. Scand.*, **72**, 324–36
5. Emmi, A.M. (1993). The use of GnRH agonist in the medical therapy of endometriosis in the woman with pain. *Semin. Reprod. Endocrinol.*, **11**, 119–26
6. Donnez, J., Nisolle-Pochet, M., Clerckx-Braun, F., Sandow, J. and Casanas-Roux, F. (1989). Administration of nasal buserelin as compared with subcutaneous buserelin implant for endometriosis. *Fertil. Steril.*, **52**, 27–30
7. Shaw, R.W. (1995). Evaluation of treatment with gonadotrophin releasing hormone analogues. In Shaw, R.W. (ed.) *Endometriosis. Current Understanding and Management*, pp. 206–34. (Oxford: Blackwell Science)
8. Okada, H., Doken, Y., Ogawa, Y. and Toguchi, H. (1994). Preparation of three-month depot injectable microspheres of leuprorelin acetate using biodegradable polymers. *Pharm. Res.*, **11**, 1143–7
9. American Fertility Society (1985). Revised American Fertility Society classification of endometriosis. *Fertil. Steril.*, **43**, 351–2
10. Biberoglu, K.O. and Behrman, S.J. (1981). Dosage aspects of danazol therapy in endometriosis: short-term and long-term effectiveness. *Am. J. Obstet. Gynecol.*, **139**, 645–54
11. Dijkman, G.A., Fernandez del Moral, P., Plasman, J.W.M.H., Pull, H.C., van der Meijden, A.P.M., Debruyne, F.M.J., Hutchinson, F.G. and Furr, B.J.A. (1990). A new longer-acting LHRH analog depot: preliminary results of a Dutch open phase II clinical study on a 10.8 mg Zoladex 3-monthly depot. *Eur. Urol.*, **18** (Suppl. 3), 22–5
12. Evers, J.L.H. (1987). The second-look laparoscopy for evaluation of the results of medical treatment of endometriosis should not be performed during ovarian suppression. *Fertil. Steril.*, **47**, 502–4
13. Nisolle-Pochet, M., Casanas-Roux, F. and Donnez, J. (1988). Histological study of ovarian endometriosis after hormonal therapy. *Fertil. Steril.*, **49**, 423–6
14. Dawood, M.Y. (1993). Impact of medical treatment of endometriosis on bone mass. *Am. J. Obstet. Gynecol.*, **168**, 674–84
15. Orwoll, E.S., Yuzpe, A.A., Burry, K.A., Heinrichs, L., Buttram, V.C. and Hornstein, M.D. (1994). Nafarelin therapy in endometriosis: long-term effects on bone mineral density. *Am. J. Obstet. Gynecol.*, **171**, 1221–5

Use of leuprolide acetate in combination with surgical treatment for women with endometriosis

C.A. Winkel and M. Bray

Introduction

The first case of pelvic endometriosis was described by Rokitansky in 1860, and by 1921 the entire world's literature consisted of 20 reported cases[1]. Since then, the incidence of the disease has appeared to increase, as more and more clinicians learn to recognize the protean manifestations of this disease, as it appears at the time of diagnostic laparoscopy. Whether there has truly been an increase in the prevalence of endometriosis or whether we are simply learning to recognize it better and thus making the diagnosis more often, the gynecologist today finds himself or herself faced with the problem of providing treatment for women with complaints secondary to the presence of endometriosis who desire to retain or improve their fertility potential.

The associations between endometriosis and the ability to conceive and between endometriosis and chronic pelvic pain and dyspareunia are well recognized. A thorough discussion of the mechanisms involved is beyond the scope of this chapter. As more and more has been learned about this enigmatic disease, however, new understanding enables us to make advances in our techniques for management of women with endometriosis. For example, the depth of infiltration of endometriotic lesions has been demonstrated to correlate directly with severity of pain symptoms[2]. More than that, the pathophysiology of endometriosis seems to vary considerably, depending on whether the lesions are superficial or infiltrative. Early disease, which looks different from late disease[3,4], appears to present primarily as superficial lesions, whereas the deep lesions increase progressively with increasing age[5]. Deep lesions and superficial lesions appear to be biologically different, the former being associated with decreased natural killer cell activity[6] and the latter secreting their biochemical products towards the peritoneal cavity, thereby disrupting normal reproductive functions[7].

Perhaps more important than any of the scientific data that have appeared regarding the functional biology of endometriosis is the realization that the depth of invasion of endometriotic lesions correlates very poorly with the visible surface area of involvement. Two-dimensional visual inspection of the peritoneal surfaces of the pelvis will often fail to detect the infiltrating lesions and thus grossly underestimate the volume of disease present. Failure of the surgeon to appreciate accurately the extent of disease is likely to lead to incomplete therapy and incomplete or short-lived resolution of symptoms. Potentially even worse, however, is the creation of a situation that may allow the disease to progress. For these reasons, although endometriosis that is associated solely with infertility (typically the surface-type lesions) may be treated easily by simple cautery or laser ablation, we believe that endometriosis which is associated with a significant component of pelvic pain can be treated effectively only by excisional therapy.

The difficulty with excisional therapy for the complete surgical treatment of the women with infiltrating lesions of endometriosis lies in the fact that the surgeon may be unable to detect all of the lesions, unable by way of location to excise completely the entire infiltrative lesions, or lack the training, skill and experience to feel comfortable in undertaking that sort of surgical therapy. This may be especially true in the case of ovarian endometriomas in which the cyst cavity is large and the cyst wall is not amenable to complete resection. Under these circumstances, we have found previously that adjunctive medical therapy with a gonadotropin releasing hormone (GnRH) analog, such as leuprolide acetate, offers additional success in eradicating symptoms as well as in prolonging the symptom-free interval[8].

Materials and methods

To test the effectiveness of the use of leuprolide acetate in conjunction with surgical resection for women with ovarian endometriomas, we evaluated the outcomes with regard to recurrence of ovarian endometrioma in a group of 61 women with ovarian endometriomas that were discovered on pelvic examination and confirmed by ultrasonographic findings of an adnexal mass consistent with an endometrioma.

At the time of surgery, all women had the endometriomas opened and drained. Attempt was made to remove all endometriotic tissue that could be visualized. This was accomplished both by resection and by 'teasing' of the cyst wall away from the underlying ovarian stroma. Unless the incision in the capsule of the ovary was longer than 4 cm or significant bleeding was observed, the ovarian capsule was not sutured closed.

Forty-eight of the women with surgically documented endometriosis agreed to treatment with leuprolide acetate for a period of 3–6 months following surgical therapy. Thirteen of the women with endometriomas refused therapy with leuprolide acetate following surgical treatment. All 61 women were followed for a period of at least 18 months. During the follow-up period, all women underwent serial sonography and pelvic examinations in an attempt to document recurrence of ovarian endometrioma. The women who refused therapy with leuprolide acetate were of similar age, gravidity and parity and had ovarian endometriomas similar in size and number to those women treated with leuprolide acetate.

We have also undertaken outcome studies, with regard to recurrence of pain, of 240 women with pelvic pain and pelvic endometriosis documented at the time of diagnostic laparoscopy by histological evaluation. A total of 178 women were treated by surgical excision and 62 were treated by laser ablation of the endometriosis. Of those women treated by ablative therapy, 23 were treated postoperatively with leuprolide acetate and the other 39 were not.

The women who underwent surgical excision were treated laparoscopically. The technique employed a contact Nd-YAG laser for the excision of the endometriosis. Ablation of endometriotic lesions was accomplished with either a carbon dioxide laser or a contact Nd-YAG laser using a flat contact tip. During ablative therapy, the surgeon attempted to ablate the entire lesion.

All women were followed postoperatively for recurrence of symptoms of pain. No attempt was made to quantify pain. If patients experienced recurrent pain that persisted for 2 months or more, they were said to have recurrent pain.

Results

Of the women who presented with a preoperative diagnosis of ovarian endometrioma, all 61 were taken to the operating room at Thomas Jefferson University Hospital. Diagnostic laparoscopy confirmed the finding of ovarian endometriomas that ranged in size from 1 to 10 cm. Eight women had unilateral ovarian endometriomas and 53 had bilateral endometriomas. During the 18-month follow-up, one of the 48 women treated with post-

Table 1 Outcomes of 61 women with ovarian endometriomas treated surgically with or without adjunctive medical therapy with leuprolide acetate (LA)

Treatment	n	Endometrioma after follow-up period	
		6 months	18 months
Surgery alone	13	11	0
Surgery plus LA	48	0	1

operative leuprolide acetate developed a sonographically suggested ovarian endometrioma (Table 1). This patient, who previously had had a unilateral endometrioma, underwent reoperation and was found to have a 4-cm ovarian endometrioma that involved the same ovary previously affected.

Eleven of 13 women who refused therapy with leuprolide acetate postoperatively were found on sonographic re-evaluation to have developed a recurrent or subsequent endometrioma. All 11 women developed the repeat ovarian lesions within the first 6 months postoperatively, although the exact time of recurrence cannot be stated, since the ultrasonography was first accomplished at 6 months following the surgical treatment and all 11 women had evidence of recurrence at that time. The two women without recurrence continued to be followed for an additional 12 months and did not develop new ovarian endometriomas.

With regard to the women treated for pelvic pain, 178 were treated by surgical excision of endometriosis and 160 remained symptom free for 18 months of follow-up. Thereafter, 28 of the 160 were lost to follow-up and further outcome of those 28 remains unknown. The other 132 were followed for up to 18 more months. Twenty-nine women (22%) have remained pain free. The other 103 subsequently experienced recurrent symptoms within the last 18-month follow-up period (Table 2).

Of the women treated with ablation of endometriosis, 39 received no postoperative leuprolide acetate therapy. Twenty-three experienced recurrent symptoms of pain within 18 months of the surgery. Two experienced pain within the first 6 months, eight in the second 6 months and 13 within the last 6 months. The 15 who did not experience pain within 18 months' follow-up were able to be followed for an additional 16 months. During that time, nine experienced recurrent pain within the following 12 months. Two experienced recurrent pain in the last 2 months of follow-up. The rest (four) were then lost to subsequent follow-up.

Of the 23 women treated with leuprolide acetate postablative therapy, two were lost to follow-up by 9 months after surgery. All of these women had been treated for 6 months with leuprolide acetate. The remaining 21 women were followed for a period of up to 24 months. One experienced recurrence of symptoms in the 19th month of follow-up. Three

Table 2 Outcomes of 240 women with endometriosis and pelvic pain treated surgically with or without adjunctive medical therapy with leuprolide acetate (LA)

Treatment	n	Pain free after follow-up period				Lost to follow-up
		12 months	18 months	24 months	36 months	
Excision	178	170 (96%)*	160 (90%)**	103 (58%)**	29	28
Ablation alone	39	27 (69%)	15 (38%)	9 (23%)	5	4
Ablation plus LA	23	21 (91%)	21 (91%)**	16 (70%)**	—	2

*Excision significantly different from ablation alone and ablation plus LA, $p < 0.05$; **excision and ablation plus LA significantly different from ablation alone, $p < 0.05$

experienced recurrent symptoms in the 24th month of follow-up and the remaining 16 remained pain free.

Discussion

Endometriosis probably represents a host of physiological abnormalities represented by the finding of endometrium-like tissue in extra-uterine sites. It has been hypothesized that women with endometriosis could be categorized into one of three groups:

(1) Those who experience no change in physiology in response to endometrial cells within the peritoneal cavity. These are the women in whom endometriosis is found incidentally;

(2) Those who experience an exaggerated immunological response. Perhaps these are the women who develop intense fibrosis and infiltration; and

(3) Those who experience a blunted immunological response. Perhaps these are the women who experience large areas of surface involvement but minimal invasive disease.

It is quite clear, regardless of whether the pathophysiology is incompletely understood or not, that neither surgical therapy alone nor medical therapy alone have proven to be optimal in all patients. On the basis of the outcomes of the patients whom we have monitored after surgical management of ovarian endometriomas with and without GnRH agonist, it appears that adjunctive medical treatment offers a significant likelihood of preventing the short-term recurrence of ovarian endometrioma formation.

The manner in which we undertook to evaluate ablative vs. excisional therapy for the treatment of women with endometriosis and complaint of pelvic pain prevents us from answering several questions that need to be addressed. However, it is most important that we conclude from these data that ablative therapy, when combined with adjunctive medical treatment with leuprolide acetate, offers a greater pain-free interval than does ablative therapy alone. We did not attempt to evaluate the potential benefit of combining excisional therapy with postoperative leuprolide acetate therapy. That clearly does need to be accomplished. However, for the surgeon who does not feel comfortable undertaking excisional therapy, or when the particular situation is not amenable to complete excision, we recommend that the addition of postoperative treatment with leuprolide acetate offers the opportunity to increase the pain-free interval postoperatively.

Conclusion

On the basis of the data that we have accumulated it appears that the addition of postoperative therapy with leuprolide acetate offers a significant reduction in the incidence of recurrence of ovarian endometrioma during the first 18 months following surgical therapy for the same. Failure to utilize leuprolide acetate seems to be associated with a very high incidence of recurrence of ovarian endometrioma within the first 6 months. Excisional therapy seems to offer an advantage in terms of the pain-free interval following surgery for endometriosis. When excisional therapy cannot be accomplished and ablative therapy is the method employed, the addition of leuprolide acetate as postoperative adjunctive therapy is associated with a significant improvement in the postoperative pain-free interval.

References

1. Cattell, R.B. and Swinton, N.W. (1936). Endometriosis with reference to conservative treatment. *N. Engl. J. Med.*, **214**, 341–4
2. Cornillie, F.J., Oosterlynck, D., Lauweryns, J.M. and Koninckx, P.R. (1990). Deeply infiltrating pelvic endometriosis: histology and clinical significance. *Fertil. Steril.*, **53**, 978–83
3. Martin, D.C., Hubert, G.D., Vander Zwaag, R. and El-Keky, R.A. (1989). Laparoscopic appearances of peritoneal endometriosis. *Fertil. Steril.*, **51**, 63–7
4. Redwine, D.B. (1987). Age-related evolution in color and appearance of endometriosis. *Fertil. Steril.*, **48**, 1062–3
5. Koninckx, P.R., Meuleman, C., Demeyere, S., Lesaffre, E. and Cornillie, F.J. (1991). Suggestive evidence that pelvic endometriosis is a progressive disease, whereas deeply infiltrating endometriosis is associated with pelvic pain. *Fertil. Steril.*, **55**, 759–65
6. Oosterlynck, D.J., Cornillie, F.J., Waer, M., Vandeputte, M. and Koninckx, P.R. (1991). Women with endometriosis show a defect in natural killer activity resulting in decreased cytotoxicity to analogous endometrium. *Fertil. Steril.*, **56**, 45–51
7. Koninckx, P.R., Riittinen, L., Seppala, M. and Cornillie, F.J. (1992). CA-125 and placental protein 14 concentrations in plasma and peritoneal fluid of women with deeply infiltrating endometriosis. *Fertil. Steril.*, **57**, 523–30
8. Winkel, C.A., Miller, C., Lyons, T. and McCarus, T. (1992). Laser treatment of women with ovarian endometrioma. *International Congress of Gynecologic Endoscopy*. American Association of Gynecologic Laparoscopy, Annual Meeting, September 23–27, Chicago, Illinois

Dose-related effects of leuprorelin acetate depot on the endocrinological changes and clinical improvement in women with endometriosis

Y. Taketani, T. Uemura, H. Hoshiai and N. Terakawa

Introduction

Leuprorelin acetate is a highly potent gonadotropin-releasing hormone (GnRH) agonist which is currently available in a monthly injectable depot form[1]. Leuprorelin depot allows continuous low-dose release of the agonist over a period of at least 4 weeks.

GnRH agonists achieve a reversible and prominent suppression of gonadotropin release through a mechanism of pituitary desensitization with resultant hypoestrogenism, which makes it a useful therapeutic measure against estrogen-dependent diseases including endometriosis and fibroma.

In this study, we conducted a multicenter clinical trial to compare the effects of different doses of leuprorelin in terms of endocrinological variables and clinical utility in Japanese women affected with endometriosis.

Materials and methods

A total of 144 women with endometriosis were recruited into this study. Diagnosis of the disease was, in principle, verified based on laparoscopic examination or laparotomy. They were randomized to receive different doses of leuprorelin acetate depot once every 4 weeks, six times, for a treatment period of 24 weeks. The doses of leuprorelin were divided into five groups: 0.47 mg, 0.94 mg, 1.88 mg, 3.75 mg and 5.63 mg. Leuprorelin was injected subcutaneously, beginning within 3–5 days of menses.

We evaluated the changes in serum luteinizing hormone (LH) and follicle-stimulating hormone (FSH) levels and their responses to GnRH (100 μg intramuscularly) every 4 weeks. Serum levels of estradiol, testosterone, prolactin, growth hormone, thyroxine, cortisol and cancer antigen (CA) 125 were determined.

The clinical improvement and leuprorelin-related untoward effects were assessed. The effect of leuprorelin on the size of endometriotic cysts was also evaluated.

Results

Changes in the average LH levels produced by different doses of leuprorelin are shown in Figure 1. In general, LH levels were equally suppressed in the 0.94 mg, 1.88 μg, 3.75 mg and 5.63 mg groups. Noticeably, the average LH levels tended to decrease with time during the treatment, excluding an initial flare-up period. LH levels returned to pretreatment levels 12 weeks after the last injection, and the change in pituitary sensitivity to native GnRH was then examined (Figure 2). In the 0.47 mg group, the desensitization was incomplete. In the 0.94 μg and 1.88 mg groups, although LH release in response to

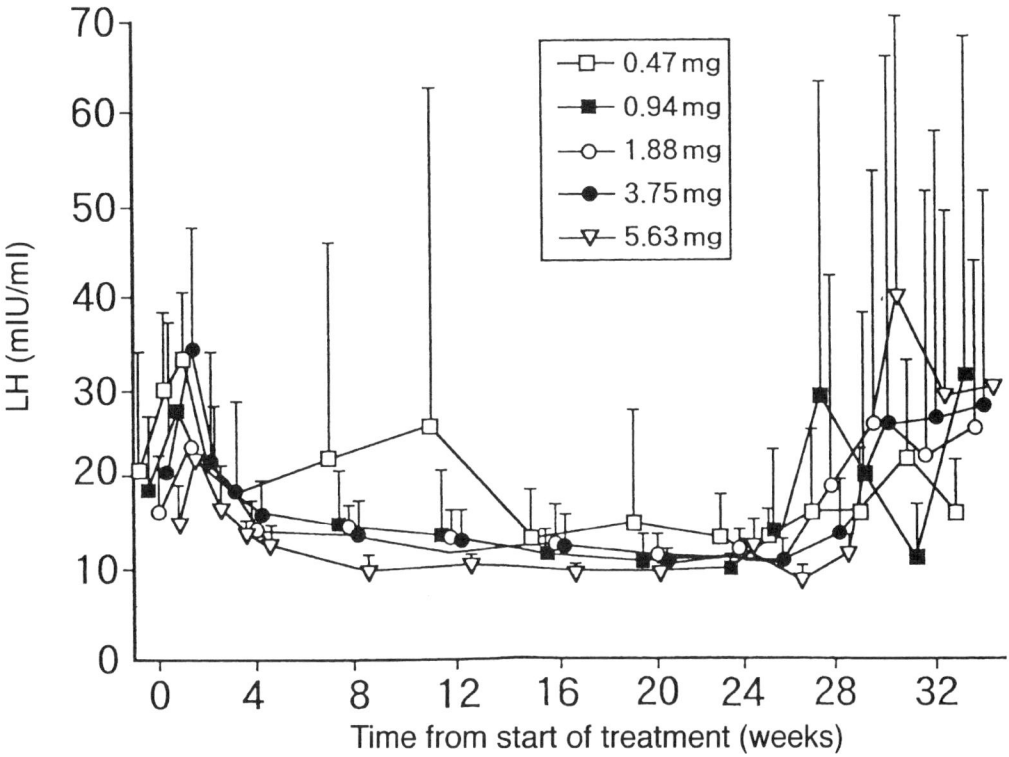

Figure 1 Changes in serum luteinizing hormone (LH) levels (mean ± SD) in cases treated with different doses of leuprorelin acetate depot

GnRH was basically blunted, sporadic LH responses were observed. LH response was completely eliminated in the 3.75 mg group.

Figure 3 illustrates the changes in serum FSH levels during leuprorelin treatment. Unlike LH, basal FSH levels were suppressed differently for the doses ranging from 0.47 to 3.75 mg. In addition, an increase in FSH levels during the flare-up period was hardly observable. FSH release in response to GnRH during leuprorelin treatment was preserved to some extent, even in the 3.75 mg group, a result which was in contrast to LH release.

Estradiol levels remained suppressed during the treatment after an initial transient increase for groups receiving 0.94 mg or more. At doses of 0.94 mg and more the average estradiol levels were equally suppressed (Figure 4). At 4 weeks and onward, 85–90% of cases exhibited estradiol levels below 30 pg/ml in both the 1.88 and 3.75 mg groups.

Testosterone levels tended to decrease marginally with leuprorelin administration. Regarding other hormones such as prolactin, growth hormone, thyroxine and cortisol, their serum levels were unaltered by leuprorelin treatment.

Due to the presence of endometriosis, serum CA 125 levels were elevated before the treatment. Leuprorelin produced a constant suppression of CA 125 levels at as early as 4 weeks of treatment and thereafter up to 24 weeks, suggesting that CA 125 levels move in parallel with estradiol levels and, therefore, do not reflect the extent of endometriotic lesions, at least during the GnRH analog treatment.

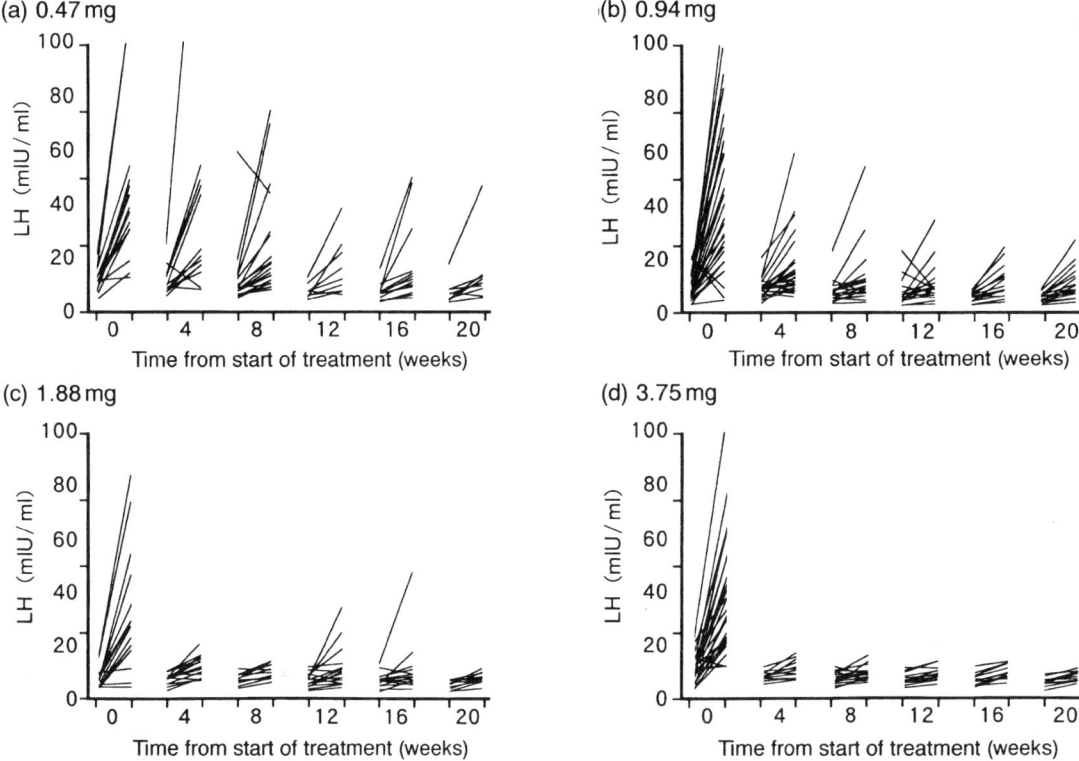

Figure 2 Effects of different doses of leuprorelin acetate depot on the release of luteinizing hormone (LH) in response to gonadotropin-releasing hormone (GnRH) agonist

We examined the incidence of escape ovulation during the treatment by analyzing basal body temperature charts. Ovulation was observed during the first 4 weeks in the majority of cases irrespective of the leuprorelin dose. The incidence of ovulation diminished with increasing doses of leuprorelin between 4 and 24 weeks and no ovulation was found in the cases given 3.75 mg during this period.

Bleeding during the treatment is a major concern for patients. During the first 4 weeks, 77% of cases experienced bleeding with 70% of them describing this as spotting or only a small amount of blood loss. From 4 weeks onward, the incidence of bleeding decreased with increasing doses of leuprorelin (Table 1).

Overall clinical efficacy of leuprorelin at 24 weeks was assessed by taking all subjective and objective findings into account. The rate of improvement was dose-dependent (Figure 5). In the 3.75 mg group, 94% of cases were considered to be markedly or considerably

Table 1 Status of uterine bleeding during leuprorelin acetate depot administration between 4 and 24 weeks

Dose (mg)	Number in group	Number with no bleeding (%)
0.47	20	7 (35.0)
0.94	38	20 (52.6)
1.88	29	18 (62.1)
3.75	35	30 (85.7)
5.63	7	6 (85.7)

Note that the total does not equal 144, as some women had no bleeding

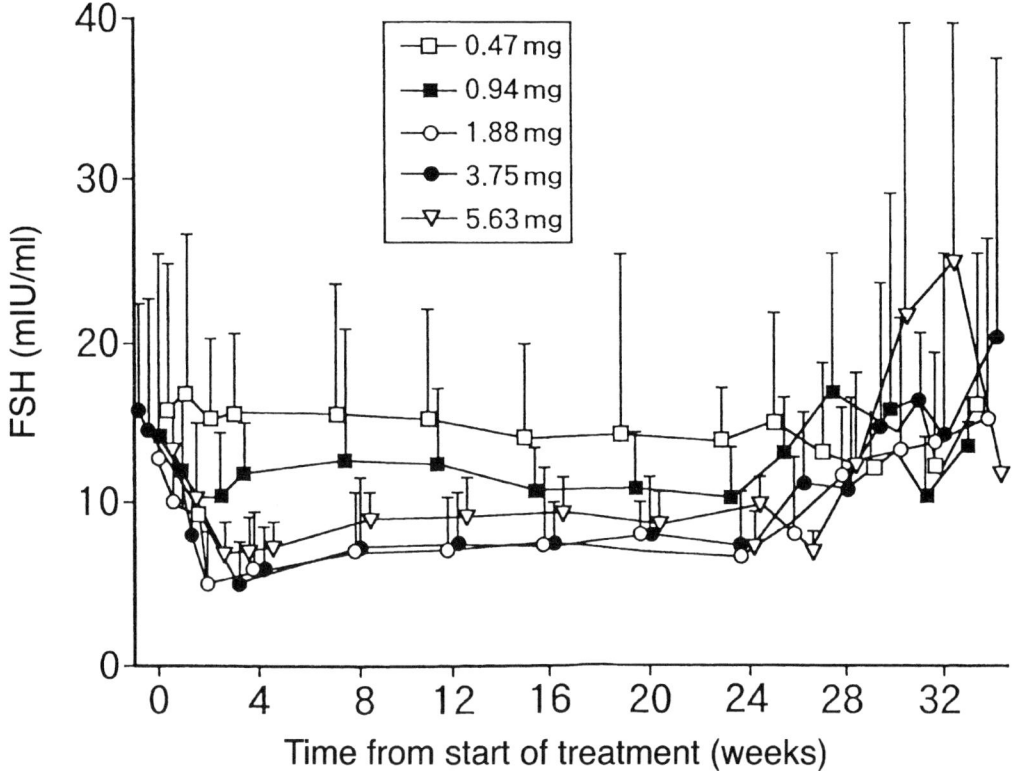

Figure 3 Changes in serum follicle-stimulating hormone (FSH) levels (mean ± SD) in cases treated with different doses of leuprorelin acetate depot

improved. Although apparent differences in the degree of estradiol suppression were not detected among the 0.94, 1.88 and 3.75 mg groups, interestingly, a dose-response clinical effect was shown in these groups.

As most patients on GnRH analog therapy are amenorrheic during the treatment, symptoms associated with menstruation cannot be evaluated. Thus, we assessed the general improvement of both subjective and objective findings related to endometriosis at the first menstruation after treatment. Although the rate of markedly improved cases was higher in the 3.75 mg group, the rate of either marked or considerable improvement was almost the same in the 0.94, 1.88 and 3.75 mg groups (Figure 6).

The effect of leuprorelin on endometriotic cysts was investigated. At 8 weeks, there was a tendency for tumor size to reduce in every treatment group. At 24 weeks, 3.75 mg leuprorelin produced a 48% marked reduction rate and an 83% marked or considerable reduction in the tumor size.

Over 80% of the cases in groups receiving 0.94 mg or more developed side-effects. However, about 70% of the side-effects were hot flushes and, therefore, most of the side-effects associated with leuprorelin were minimal and not problematic.

General usefulness of leuprorelin in the treatment of endometriosis was evaluated based on the patients' own assessments. The overall usefulness rate increased with increasing dose of leuprorelin. The usefulness at first menstruation after the cessation of the treatment is shown in Figure 7. About 70% of patients in the 1.88 and 3.75 mg groups felt

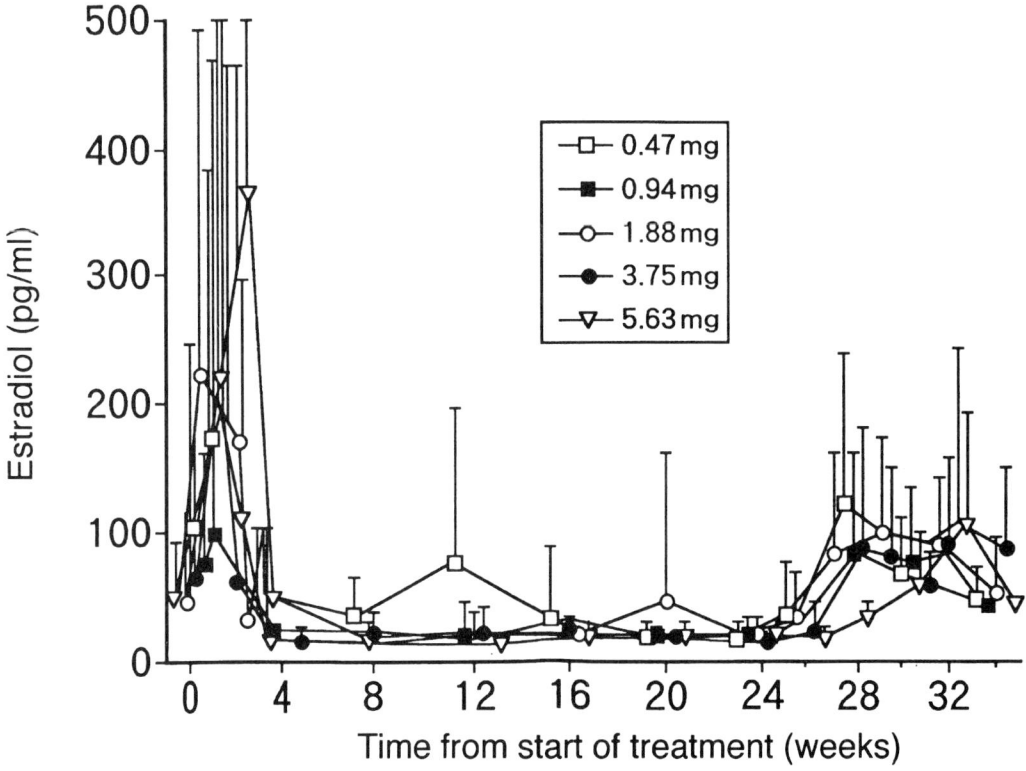

Figure 4 Effects of different doses of leuprorelin acetate depot on the serum levels (mean ± SD) of estradiol

that the treatment was markedly or moderately useful.

Patients were also followed-up for a period of 1–2 years after stopping leuprorelin therapy, allowing assessment of pregnancy and recurrence rates. In 198 patients desiring to become pregnant, 57 (28.8%) did conceive, and 48 babies were delivered. Two anomalies were found, which were inguinal hernia in one, and atrial septal defect in another. These two anomalies are relatively frequent. In addition, the patients in question conceived about 6 months after the final dose of the study drug; hence, the anomalies were hardly treatment-related. Recurrence of endometriosis was reported in 37%, based on objective findings. The period before recurrence was 326 ± 183 days. The leuprorelin dose did not correlate with either the conception or recurrence rates.

Discussion

The aim of this study was to investigate the effects of varying doses of leuprorelin on the endocrinological changes and clinical efficacy in Japanese women afflicted with endometriosis.

In regard to gonadotropin release, leuprorelin at doses of 0.94 mg or more seemed to suppress basal LH levels equally. However, if we looked into LH levels on an individual basis, the patients receiving 0.94 mg leuprorelin exhibited sporadically higher LH levels over 20 mIU/ml, whereas those on the 1.88 mg or greater dose displayed sustained suppression of LH levels. It appeared that basal LH levels tended to decrease in patients on 0.94 mg or more after 4 weeks up to 24 weeks. This finding is in keeping with clinical data obtained in Germany[2].

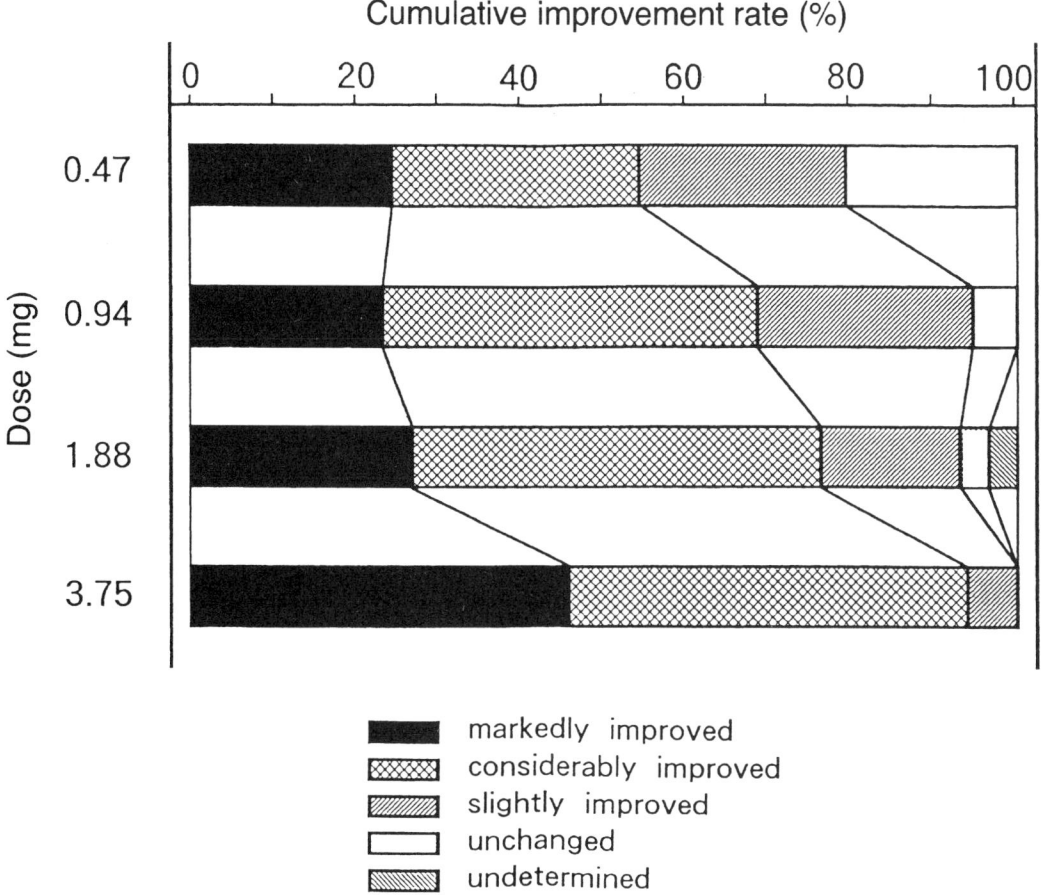

Figure 5 General improvement of subjective and objective findings of endometriosis in cases treated with different doses of leuprorelin acetate depot 24 weeks after treatment

It is noteworthy that the flare-up phase of FSH was barely recognizable, if at all. In addition, unlike LH, basal FSH levels were suppressed in a dose-dependent manner at leuprorelin doses between 0.47 and 3.75 mg, and the degree of basal FSH suppression seemed to be attenuated with time over the treatment period. An earlier report showed that leuprorelin-induced suppression of FSH levels was less marked compared with LH levels[3]. These findings suggest that release of LH and FSH are regulated by GnRH in a different way.

Leuprorelin at doses of 0.94 mg or more suppressed estradiol levels. However, the incidences of bleeding or ovulation during the treatment diminished with increasing doses of leuprorelin. Occurrence of sporadic higher estradiol levels found in patients on 0.94 mg or 1.88 mg may account for their higher incidence of bleeding and ovulation.

We have also conducted a double-blind multicenter study to compare the effects of leuprorelin at 3.75 mg versus intranasal buserelin (900 µg/day) on the endocrinological profiles and clinical efficacy (data not shown). Judging from this study, particularly based on the degree of estrogen suppression and incidences of ovulation or bleeding during the treatment, the degree of suppression

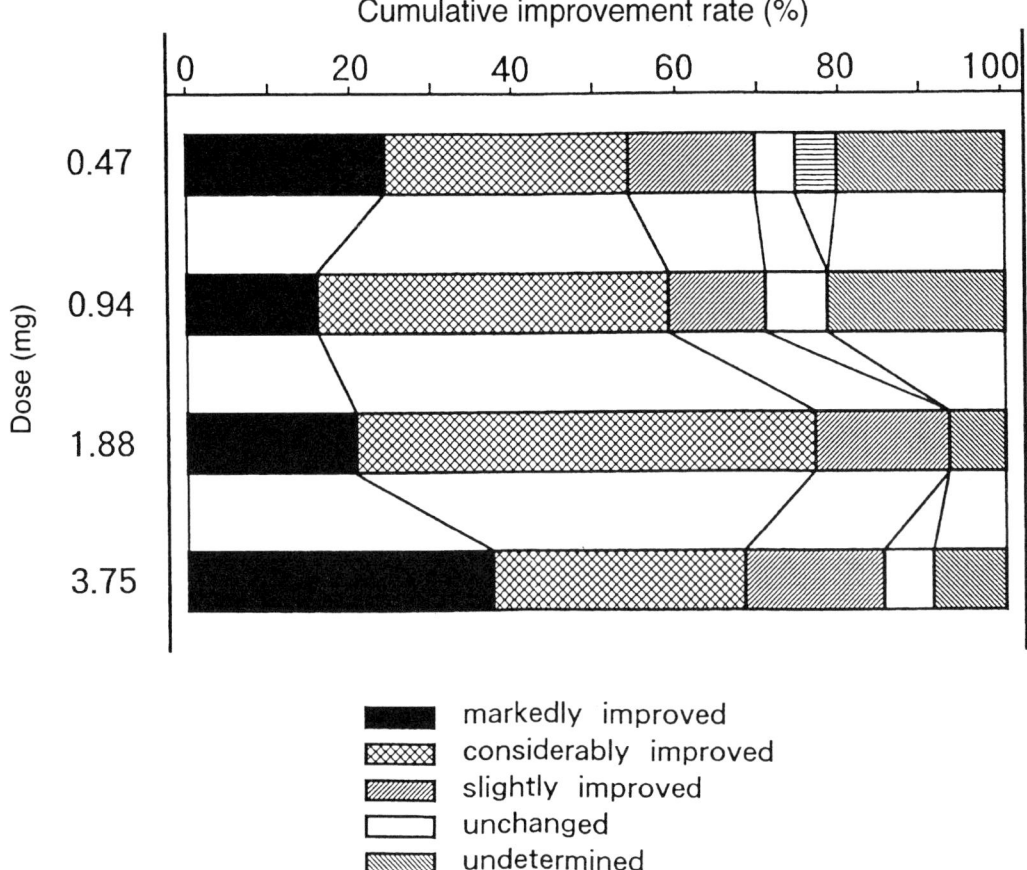

Figure 6 General improvement of subjective and objective findings of endometriosis in cases treated with different doses of leuprorelin acetate depot at first menstruation after treatment

caused by 900 μg/day intranasal buserelin seemed to match that found with 0.94 mg leuprorelin. However, it is obvious that larger doses of GnRH agonists induce more estrogen-deficient symptoms. Hence, the choice between intranasal buserelin and depot leuprorelin is not a straightforward decision.

As expected from present data demonstrating that leuprorelin suppressed ovarian functions dose-relatedly, the rate of marked and considerable improvement increased with increasing doses of leuprorelin between 0.47 and 3.75 mg. The rates of improvement at 24 weeks in patients on 1.88 mg and 3.75 mg leuprorelin were 87% and 94%, respectively. These rates are at least as effective as those reported to date on the clinical efficacy of buserelin[4]. It appears that leuprorelin at 3.75 mg is most useful and, therefore, the most desirable dose for the treatment of endometriosis. However, leuprorelin at 1.88 mg is no less effective than the earlier reported clinical efficacy of GnRH analogs, and thus could be an optimal dose in certain women.

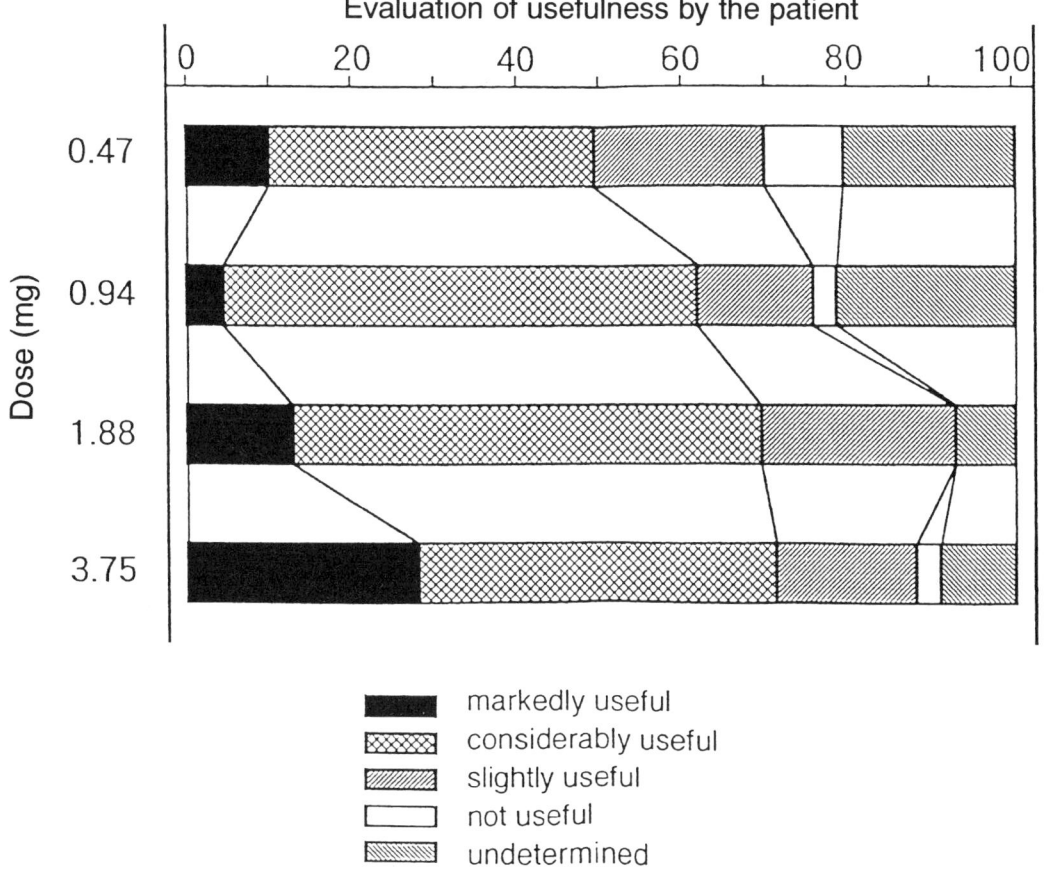

Figure 7 Usefulness of leuprorelin acetate as determined by patients at first menstruation after treatment

References

1. Okada, H., Inoue, Y., Heya, T. et al. (1991). Pharmacokinetics of once-a-month injectable microspheres of leuprolide acetate. *Pharm. Res.*, **8**, 787–91
2. Cirkel, U., Ochs, H. and Schneider, H.P.G. (1992). Experience with leuprorelin acetate depot in the treatment of fibroids: German multicenter study. *Clin. Ther.*, **14**, 37–47
3. Golan, A., Bukovsky, I., Schneider, D. et al. (1989). D-try-6-luteinizing hormone-releasing hormone microcapsules in the treatment of uterine leiomyomas. *Fertil. Steril.*, **52**, 406–11
4. Lemay, A., Malheux, R., Jean, C. et al. (1986). Efficacy of different modalities of LHRH agonist (buserelin) administration on the inhibition of the pituitary–ovarian axis for the treatment of endometriosis. In Rolland, R., Chadha, D. R. and Willemsen, W.N.P. (eds.) *Gonadotropin Down Regulation in Gynecological Practice*, p. 157. (New York: Alan Liss)

Section 9

Danazol

Analysis of danazol action

K. Kato, K. Kato and N. Wake

Introduction

It is well known that danazol, an isoxazole derivative of the synthetic steroid 17α-ethinyl/testosterone, is effective in the treatment of endometriosis. Although the pharmacological action of danazol is not fully understood, the literature describes the diverse effects of danazol. Danazol decreases the estrogen receptor level[1] and increases the progesterone receptor level[2]. Danazol suppresses aromatase and estrone sulfatase activity[3]. It has the ability to bind with steroid receptors and behaves in the same way as androgen, glucocorticoid or progestin[4]. In addition, danazol is associated with the suppression of interleukin-1β and tumor necrosis factor production by monocytes[5]. The effects of danazol seem to be multiple and complex.

Epidermal growth factor (EGF) and estrogen are able to promote the growth of endometriotic cells[6,7]. The growth promoting signal from EGF is transmitted to the Ras protein. There is considerable evidence indicating that the Ras protein acts as a critical relay switch controlling the signal pathways that connect the cell surface with the nucleus. It then triggers the activation of a cascade of serine/threonine kinases, which includes Raf-1 and MAPK (mitogen-activated protein kinase)[8–10]. Activated MAPK then translocates to the nucleus where it phosphorylates and activates transcription factors which, in turn, cause a change in the gene expression responsible for growth stimulation. The recent finding that MAPK activates the estrogen receptor functionally through ER-AF1 phosphorylation suggests that the estrogen receptor is one of the downstream targets of the Ras-mediated signal transduction pathway[11]. These results provide for the possibility that danazol has an inhibitory effect on endometriotic cell growth through its effect on the signal pathways.

In this study we examined the effects of danazol on both MAPK activity and the transcriptional activity by estrogen receptor, in order to demonstrate its interrupting action on growth factor signaling.

Results

Effect of danazol on cell growth

We used three kinds of reconstituted NIH3T3 cells that implied the NIH3T3 transfected vector alone (mock cell), that transfected activated [^{12}Val] K-ras mutant (K12V cell) and that transfected human estrogen receptor cDNA (ER cell). The activated K-ras mutant remarkably altered the morphology of NIH3T3 cell-lines but the vector alone and the human estrogen receptor cDNA left the cell-lines unchanged. K12V cells exhibited a colony-forming ability in soft agar cultures and produced massive tumors when implanted in nude mice. However, neither mock nor estrogen receptor cells exhibited any transformed phenotype.

First of all, we examined the effect of danazol on this cell growth. Cells were incubated for 10 days in the presence of danazol (10^{-7} mol/l) and the number of viable cells resulting was compared with those in the control group. An inhibitory effect on cell growth by danazol was shown in the three reconstituted cells (Figure 1). The most dominant inhibition was recognized in K12V cells. Ten days incubation in the presence of danazol decreased the viable cell numbers to 36% of that in the control

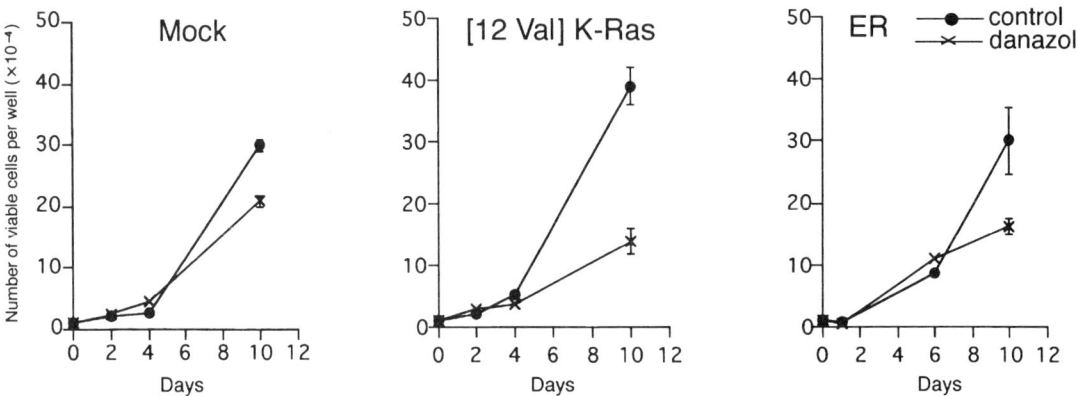

Figure 1 Effect of danazol on cell growth. Cells were plated at 1.0×10^4 cells per $2.0\,mm^2$ in 24-well plates (Falcon) in DMEM supplemented with 10% calf serum and incubated overnight. The medium was replaced in the presence or absence of danazol ($10^{-7}\,mol/l$). The number of viable cells was counted on day 1 or 2, 4 or 6 and 10. Each value was a mean of three independent experiments. Danazol inhibited cell growth in all cell-lines ($p < 0.01$), but the inhibition rate was most significant in K12V cells ($p < 0.001$)

group. However, the inhibitory effect by danazol was not so significant in mock (70%) and estrogen receptor (53%) cells. In addition to the inhibitory effect on the *in vitro* cell growth, danazol has the potential to suppress the colony-forming efficiency of K12V cells. In the presence of danazol, the colony numbers were reduced to 54% of that in the control group.

Effect of danazol on MAPK activity

MAPK is an important serine/threonine kinase in the growth factor signaling cascade. A variety of growth factors activate MAPK resulting in the alteration in gene expression associated with cell growth promotion. We demonstrated that danazol has the potential to significantly inhibit the *in vitro* growth and colony-forming efficiency of K12V cells. Thus, we investigated the association between the inhibitory effect by danazol with suppressed MAPK activity. Cells were incubated with phenol-red free DMEM containing 1% charcoal-dextran treated calf serum for 2 days, followed by a further 1 day incubation in the presence of $10^{-7}\,mol/l$ danazol. Cell lysates were resolved by SDS/PAGE. We investigated the relative ratio between phosphorylated and unphosphorylated forms of MAPK. The active and phosphorylated form of MAPK was detected in K12V cells (Figure 2). Danazol significantly reduced the ratio of the active form. In mock cells and estrogen receptor cells, the active form of MAPK was not clearly detected in the absence of danazol and thus we could not determine the effect of danazol on these cells. In contrast to the wild type K-Ras, the activated [12Val]

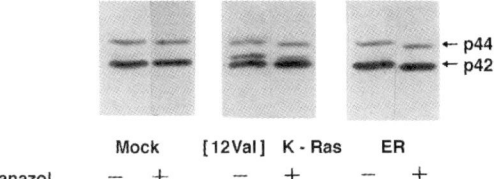

Figure 2 Effect of danazol on MAPK activation. Cells were incubated in phenol-red free DMEM containing 1% charcoal-dextran treated calf serum for 2 days and $10^{-7}\,mol/l$ danazol was added to the medium. Cells were lysed and lysates were resolved by SDS/PAGE. MAPK activation was determined by Western blot analysis to detect the phosphorylated active and non-phosphorylated inactive forms of p42MAPK/ERK2 and p44MAPK/ERK1. The phosphorylated active form was detected in K12V cells and danazol decreased MAPK activation

K-Ras mutant fails to function as a biological switch between GTP-bound and GDP-bound states, resulting in a constitutive stimulation of the downstream target such as MAPK. Detection of the active form in only K12V cells in the low serum (1%) condition would be responsible for the effect of this gain of function mutation. The reduced ratio of active form of MAPK suggested an ability of danazol to inhibit the activation of MAPK by interfering with the downstream target of Ras. These results suggest the possibility that the inhibitory effect by danazol on *in vitro* growth and the colony-forming potential of K12V cells, corresponds to the interrupted signal transduction between Ras and MAPK.

Effect of danazol on estrogen receptor-mediated transcriptional activity

MAP kinase enhances the activity of ER-AF1 by stimulating the phosphorylation of serine residue at codon 118. Based on this evidence, we considered the possibility that estrogen receptor activity is modulated by danazol through the suppression of MAPK activity. Functional activation of estrogen receptor requires activation of both AF1 and AF2, that may be modulated by independently transmitted signals[12]. The estrogen signal is transmitted to the nucleus by binding with the estrogen receptor, resulting in the putative activation of AF2. Estrogen receptor activated by dimerization between estrogen and estrogen receptor, and phosphorylation of AF1 by MAPK, tightly binds with estrogen-responsive DNA sequences and acts as a transcription factor. To investigate how danazol modulates the estrogen receptor-mediated transcription through the particular DNA sequences, we transiently transfected mock, K12V and ER cells with the pCAT-enhancer vector which contained an SV 40 enhancer element and Vit A2 ERE. In the charcoal-treated, low serum (1%) condition, estrogen stimulated the CAT activity in all three mock, K12V and ER cells. Danazol decreased the level of estrogen-

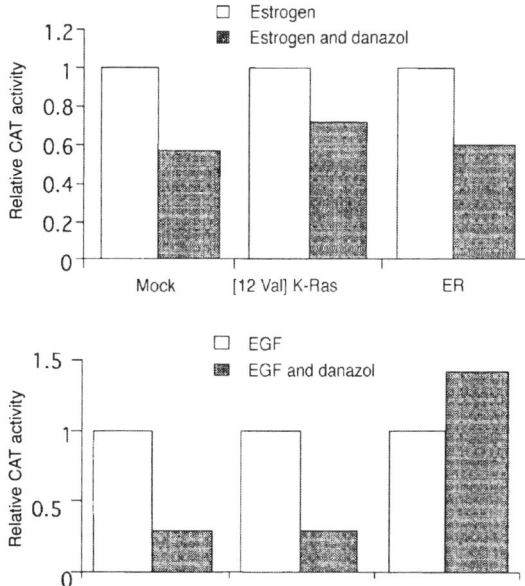

Figure 3 Effect of danazol on estrogen receptor-mediated transcriptional activity. Each cell was transfected with the pCAT vector that contained vitellogenin A2 ERE. CAT activity was investigated in both the presence and absence of danazol (10^{-7} mol/l). The results of transactivation in the presence of danazol were shown as a fold-induction comparison in relation to the control group results. Both groups contained 1% charcoal-dextran treated calf serum supplemented by 10^{-7} mol/l estrogen or 50 ng/ml epidermal growth factor (EGF), respectively

mediated CAT activation (Figure 3). The danazol treatment resulted in the suppression of estrogen-stimulated CAT activity in mock, K12V and ER cells, to 57%, 72% and 60%, respectively. These results are consistent with the idea that danazol partially blocks ligand-dependent estrogen receptor activation.

EGF is associated with the activation of estrogen receptor transcriptional activity[13] by initiating the signaling to MAPK. Thus, we examined the effect of EGF on the CAT activity. In the presence of EGF, stimulation of CAT activity was shown in K12V cells and estrogen receptor cells, although the level of stimulation was lower than that by estrogen.

Again, danazol blocked EGF stimulation (Figure 3). However, suppression of CAT activity was less remarkable in the case of estrogen receptor cells and the reason for this remains unclear. The obtained results from the CAT assay clearly demonstrate that danazol has the ability to suppress the functional activation of estrogen receptor by affecting the two independently transmitted signals necessary for estrogen receptor activation.

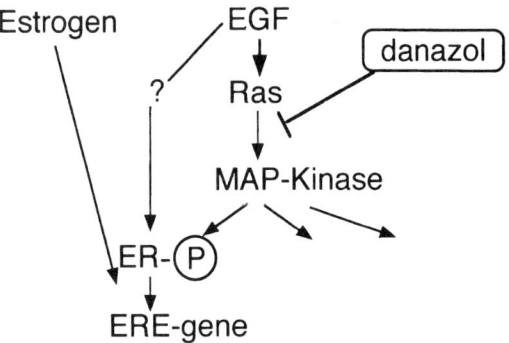

Figure 4 The model of danazol action. EGF, epidermal growth factor; ER, estrogen receptor; MAP, mitogen-activated protein; P, phosphorylation

Discussion

Estrogen receptor has two transcriptional activation domains, AF1 and AF2, which are located in the NH2-terminal A/B region and in the ligand-binding E region, respectively. Some of the signals passing through the membrane-associated receptor tyrosine kinase – Ras, Raf, MAPK – enhance the activity of ER-AF1. Heterodimer formation between estrogen and estrogen receptor is required for the activation of AF2. The present data provide for the possibility that danazol has the potential to attenuate the ER-AF1 activation by suppressing MAPK activity. In addition to this effect, danazol blocks the estrogen-mediated, functional activation of estrogen receptor. The interruption of two independently transmitted signals required for the functional activation of estrogen receptor is one of the basic pharmacological actions of danazol (Figure 4). The suppression of estrogen receptor activity by danazol could be responsible for the inhibition of *in vitro* growth and the colony-forming efficiency of K12V cells, since enhanced transcriptional activity by estrogen receptor plays a critical role in NIH3T3 cell transformation.

Acknowledgements

We are grateful to Dr Pierre Chambon (Laboratoire de Genetique Moleculaire des Eucaryotes du CNRS) for providing pSG5 estrogen receptor and we also thank Dr Channing Der (University of North Carolina) for gifts of oZIP neo SV (X)1 K-ras4B(12V)

References

1. Fujimoto, J., Hori, M., Itoh, T., Ichigo, S., Nishigaki, M. and Tamaya, T. (1995). Danazol decreases transcription of estrogen receptor gene in human monocytes. *Gen. Pharmacol.*, **26**, 507–16
2. Gledhill, J.M., Barker, S., Wanless, C., Hinson, J.P., Puddefoot, J.R. Panahy, C., Goode, A.W. and Vinson, G.P. (1992). Progesterone receptor induction by danazol in cultured cancer cells and the rat uterus. *J. Steroid Biochem. Mol. Biol.*, **43**, 289–96
3. Yamamoto, T., Noguchi, T., Tamura, T., Kitawaki, J. and Okada, H. (1993). Evidence for estrogen synthesis in adenomyotic tissues. *Am. J. Obstet. Gynecol.*, **169**, 734–8
4. Barbieri, R.L. and Ryan, K.L. (1981). Danazol: endocrine pharmacology and therapeutic application. *Am. J. Obstet. Gynecol.*, **141**, 453–63

5. Mori, H., Nakagawa, M., Itoh, N., Wada, K. and Tamaya, T. (1990). Danazol suppresses the production of interleukin-1β and tumor necrosis factor by human monocytes. *Am. J. Reprod. Immunol.*, **24**, 45–50
6. Taketani, Y. and Mizuno, M. (1992). Hormonal regulation of endometriotic cell growth in primary cell culture system. *Arch. Gynecol. Obstet.*, **251**, 127–32
7. Huang, J.C. and Yeh, J. (1994). Quantitative analysis of epidermal growth factor receptor gene expression in endometriosis. *J. Clin. Endocrinol. Metab.*, **79**, 1097–101
8. Vojek, A.B., Hollenberg, S.M. and Cooper, J.A. (1993). Mammalian *ras* interacts directly with serine/threonine kinase Raf. *Cell*, **74**, 205–14
9. Warne, P., Viciana, P. and Downward, J. (1993). Direct interaction of *ras* and the amino-terminal region of Raf-1 *in vitro*. *Nature (London)*, **364**, 352–5
10. Zhang, X.F., Settleman, J., Kyriakis, J.M., Takeuchi-Suzuki, E., Elledge, S.J., Marshall, M.S., Brude, J.T., Rapp, U.R. and Avruch, J. (1993). Normal and oncogenic p12ras proteins bind to the amino-terminal regulatory domain of c-Raf-1. *Nature (London)*, **364**, 308–13
11. Kato, S., Endoh, H., Masuhiro, Y., Kitamoto, T., Uchiyama, S., Sasaki, H., Masushige, S., Gotoh, Y., Nishida, E., Kawashima, H., Metzger, D. and Chambon, P. (1995). Activation of the estrogen receptor through phosphorylation by mitogen-activated protein kinase. *Science*, **270**, 1491–4
12. Kumar, V., Green, S., Stack, G., Berry, M., Jin, J.R. and Chambon, P. (1987). Functional domains of the human estrogen receptor. *Cell*, **51**, 941–51
13. Ignar-Trowbridge, D.M., Teng, C.T., Ross, K.A., Parker, M.G., Korach, K.S. and McLachlan, J.A. (1993). Peptide growth factors elicit estrogen receptor-dependent transcriptional activation of an estrogen-responsive element. *Mol. Endocrinol.*, **7**, 992–8

Danazol decreases estrogen receptor (ER) and ER mRNA levels in peripheral monocytes due to suppression of the transcription rate of the ER gene

J. Fujimoto, S. Ichigo, M. Hori, R. Misao, R. Hirose, Y. Nakanishi, H. Sakaguchi and T. Tamaya

Introduction

Evidence has accumulated to indicate that the functions of the monocyte/macrophage in pelvic endometriosis are partly associated with infertility. Peritoneal macrophages are activated in the peritoneal effusion of the patient. Estrogen alone and/or with progesterone, especially at the physiological level, stimulates the production of interleukin-1 (IL-1) and tumor necrosis factor (TNF) in the activated monocytes[1,2] (Figure 1) and the expression of macrophage colony-stimulating factor (M-CSF) receptor with the activation of tyrosine kinase in peripheral monocytes[3] (Figure 2). Macrophages secrete IL-1 and TNF[4,5], and exert phagocytic action mediated by activated tyrosine kinase of the M-CSF receptor in the macrophage[6–8], resulting in the damage of gametocytes, and the disturbance of fertilization and embryo development in the Fallopian tube[9,10].

With the acknowledgement that macrophages are derived from peripheral monocytes, the following evidence has been accumulated. The induction of IL-1 and TNF production in peripheral monocytes is enhanced by estradiol 17β and progesterone at the physiological level, but is constantly inhibited by danazol[2]. Peripheral monocytes express the estrogen receptor (ER) (36.3 ± 8.9 fmol/μg DNA) and progesterone receptor (0.74 ± 0.10 fmol/μg DNA), and danazol reduces the ER level in the *in vitro* culture[11].

In this study, the levels of the ER and its mRNA in peripheral monocytes (as a substitute for peritoneal macrophages) were determined during the menstrual cycle and long-term treatment with danazol. The effects of danazol on the stability of ER mRNA and the transcription of the ER gene to ER mRNA were studied, to clarify the mechanism by which danazol decreases the monocyte ER level.

Materials and methods

Our previous report[12] described the isolation of peripheral monocytes, the ER assay, the isolation of total RNA from peripheral monocytes, reverse transcription–polymerase chain reaction (RT–PCR)–Southern blot analysis to determine the ER mRNA level and analysis of the degradation rate of ER mRNA and the transcription rate of the ER gene to ER mRNA (run-on assay).

Statistical analysis was performed with Student's *t*-test; differences were considered significant if the *p*-value was less than 0.05.

Results

Expression of the ER in the monocytes

Saturation analysis and Scatchard plot analysis for the ER[13] were performed in the

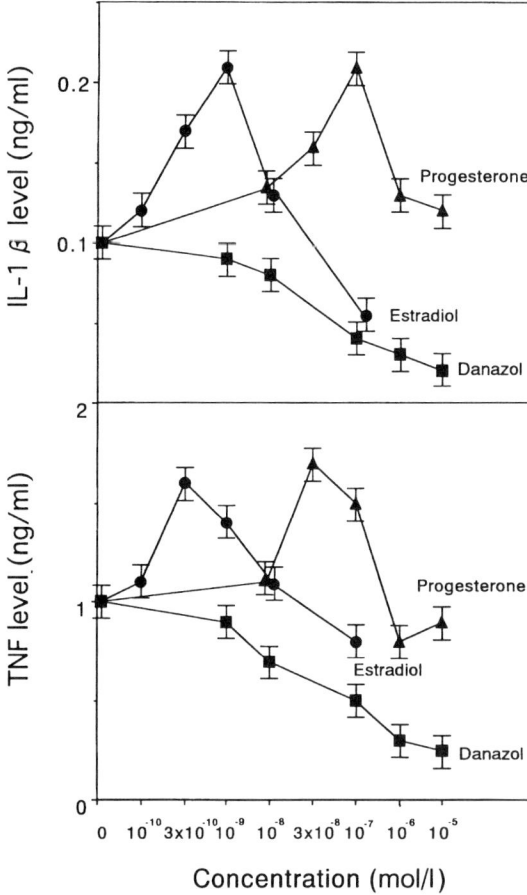

Figure 1 Effect of estradiol, progesterone and danazol on the generation of IL-1β and TNF in the monocytes. The monocytes were incubated with various concentrations of estradiol, progesterone and danazol; 6 h later OK-432 was added at a final concentration of 0.2 KE/ml, and the monocytes were incubated for 24 h. The levels of IL-1β and TNF were measured by an ^{125}I radioimmunoassay kit (Medgenix) and an enzyme-linked immunosorbent assay kit (T Cell Science), respectively. Data are the mean ± SD of five determinations in triplicate

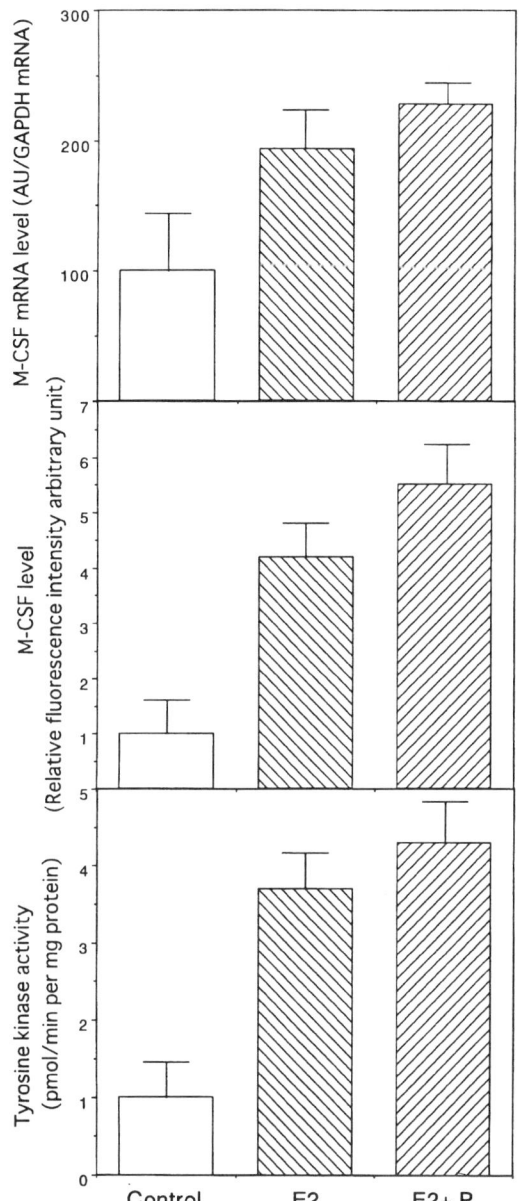

Figure 2 (Above right) Effect of estradiol and progesterone on the expression of M-CSF receptor and its mRNA with the activity of tyrosine kinase in the monocytes. The monocytes at the secretory phase of the menstrual cycle were treated with 1 μmol/l estradiol (E2) and progesterone (P) for 3 h. The level of M-CSF receptor mRNA was determined by reverse transcription–polymerase chain reaction–Southern blot analysis, and assigned as an arbitrary unit/GAPDH mRNA. The level of M-CSF receptor was determined by the intensity of fluorescence on the surface of the monocytes labeled with FITC-conjugated M-CSF. The activity of tyrosine kinase in the monocytes was measured by the Tyrosine Kinase Assay System Kit (Gibco BRL) 5 min after M-CSF was added. Data are the mean ± SD of six determinations in triplicate

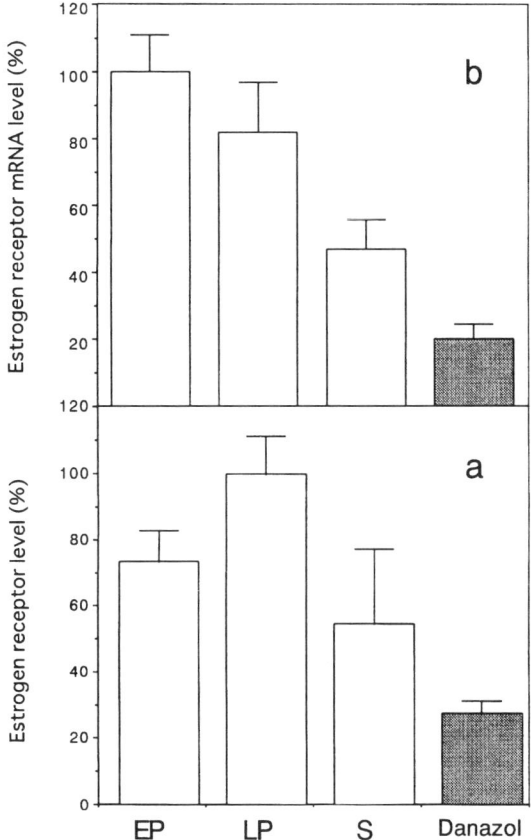

Figure 3 The estrogen receptor (ER) and its mRNA levels in the monocytes. (a) The cytosol, nuclear KCl extract and nuclear non-KCl extract fractions (100 μl) in the monocytes were incubated with 1.0 to 8.0 nmol/l [^{3}H]estradiol plus a 200-fold molar excess of dihydrotestosterone, and those with or without a 200-fold molar excess diethylstilbestrol at 20°C for 120 min. Radioactivity of the bound form was determined, and Scatchard plot analysis was carried out. Cellular expression levels of the ER were evaluated by summing the maximal estrogen binding sites of each fraction. Data are the mean ± SD of 5–10 determinations in triplicate. (b) Each value represents the mean (± SD) ER mRNA level in the monocytes in each menstrual cycle and with the treatment of danazol. The value of ER mRNA in the monocytes in the early proliferative phase (EP) was designated as 100%. Data are the mean ± SD of four determinations in triplicate. LP, late proliferative phase; S, secretory phase

monocytes. The dissociation constants (Kd) of the ER ($n = 15$) in monocytes during the menstrual cycle, early proliferative phase, late proliferative phase and secretory phase were identical at approximately 10^{-9} mol/l, and the Kd in the monocytes from the patients to whom danazol was administered for over 1 month was not affected by the treatment. There were no significant differences in Kd among the monocytes with or without danazol administration.

The mean (± SD) ER level in the monocytes in the early proliferative phase ($n = 5$), the late proliferative phase ($n = 5$) and the secretory phase ($n = 5$) was 34.7 ± 3.4, 47.5 ± 5.1 and 26.7 ± 8.3 fmol/μg DNA, respectively (Figure 3a). The ER level in the monocytes was the highest in the late proliferative phase ($p < 0.05$) of the menstrual cycle. The mean ER level in the monocytes of the danazol-treated patients was 13.0 ± 0.8 fmol/μg DNA (Figure 3a), showing that danazol *in vivo* significantly ($p < 0.05$) reduced the ER level in the monocytes to approximately 27% of that of the late proliferative phase.

Expression of ER mRNA in the monocytes

The mean (± SD) ER mRNA level in the monocytes in the early proliferative phase ($n = 4$), the late proliferative phase ($n = 4$) and the secretory phase ($n = 4$) was 40.5 ± 2.89 (100.0 ± 7.1%), 33.1 ± 6.06 (81.7 ± 14.9%) and 18.9 ± 2.51 (46.7 ± 6.2%) pg/μg total RNA, respectively (Figure 3b). The ER mRNA level in the monocytes was decreasing with the advance of the menstrual cycle. The ER mRNA level in the monocytes from the danazol-treated patients ($n = 4$) was 8.44 ± 1.22 pg/μg total RNA (Figure 3b), showing that danazol *in vivo* significantly ($p < 0.05$) reduced the ER mRNA level in monocytes to approximately 21% of that of the early proliferative phase.

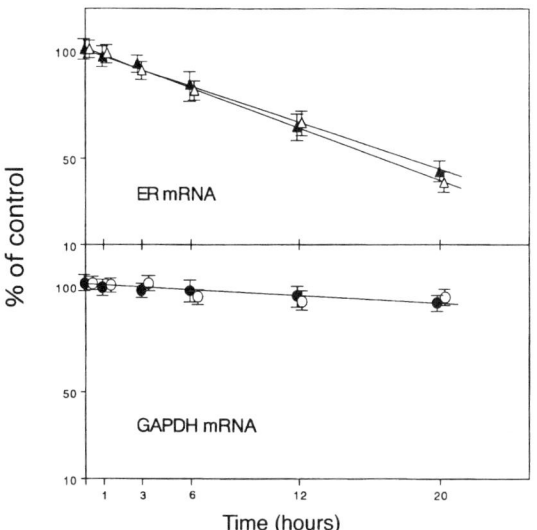
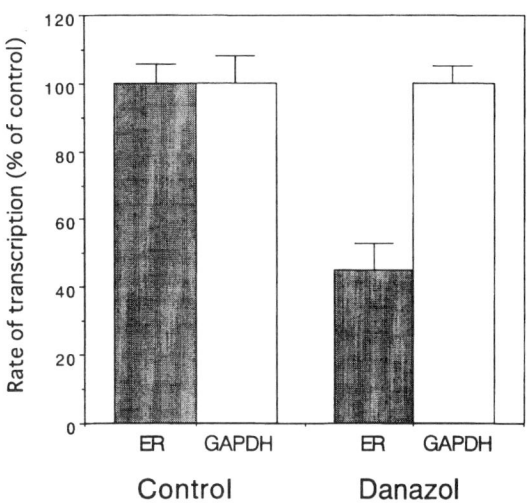

Figure 4 Effect of danazol on the rate of degradation of estrogen receptor (ER) mRNA in the monocytes. The monocytes were incubated without and with 1 µmol/l danazol for 8 h, until the addition of actinomycin-D (5 µg/ml). The monocytes were harvested at the time indicated. Total RNA was isolated and assayed by RT-PCR amplification. Each value represents the mean ± SD of duplicate determinations from three experiments

Figure 5 Effect of danazol on the rate of transcription of the estrogen receptor (ER) gene in the monocytes. The monocytes were incubated without and with 1 µmol/l danazol for 8 h, until the nuclei were isolated. The rate of ER and GAPDH gene transcription was measured by a run-on assay. Data represent the mean ± SD of triplicate determinations from two experiments

Degradation rate of ER mRNA in the monocytes

The half-life of ER mRNA in monocytes without or with exposure to danazol at 1 µmol/l for 8 h was 11.0 and 11.6 h, respectively (Figure 4). The half-life of glyceraldehyde-3-phosphate dehydrogenase (GAPDH) mRNA in monocytes with and without exposure to danazol was approximately 50 h (Figure 4). This suggests that danazol does not affect the degradation rate of ER mRNA or GAPDH mRNA, namely their stability.

Transcription rate of ER gene to ER mRNA (run-on assay) in the monocytes

The amount of generated ER or GAPDH mRNA *in vitro* was analyzed by the hybridization of ER cDNA or GAPDH DNA fragments amplified by PCR on a nylon membrane (Figure 5). Danazol did not decrease the transcription rate of the GAPDH gene to GAPDH mRNA, but decreased that of the ER gene to ER mRNA significantly ($p < 0.05$) to approximately 47% of the control (Figure 5).

Discussion

The expression level of ER mRNA in monocytes was the highest in the early proliferative phase of the menstrual cycle, and that of ER in monocytes was the highest in the late proliferative phase of the menstrual cycle. There was a time lag of the peak between the levels of ER mRNA and ER. The expressions of these two in monocytes seem to be regulated predominantly by estrogen. The time lag of those expressions may be explained as the time lag between the translation of ER mRNA and the accumulation of ER protein. The expression levels of ER mRNA and ER were decreased during the secretory phase. There is a plausible explanation that progesterone reduces the expression, as one of its biological functions, resulting in the inhibition of cellular proliferation (antiestrogenic effect). Danazol exerts an antiestrogenic effect which is known from the clinical evidence obtained in the treatment of endometriosis and from the experimental evidence[14]. Danazol *in vitro* neither modulates the Kd of ER, nor markedly inhibits the binding of [^{3}H]estradiol to the cytosol fraction of monocytes[12]. Therefore, danazol is not considered to have an effect on the quality of the ER in monocytes. Danazol *in vivo* lowers the ER level in the uterus[15]. Its mechanism remains to be clarified, and is considered to be derived partly from the interaction of danazol with the synthesis of the ER, which is related to other steroid receptors[16].

The long-term downregulation of a hormone receptor partly involves the downregulation of its mRNA, i.e. the degradation of its mRNA by the homologous[17] and/or heterologous hormone[18]. We determined the degradation rate of ER mRNA produced by danazol. The half-life (11.0 h) of ER mRNA in monocytes after the exposure to danazol at 1 μmol/l for 8 h was similar to that (11.6 h) without treatment. These findings indicate that danazol does not affect the degradation rate of ER mRNA in monocytes, but downregulates the ER level in monocytes. Danazol decreased the transcription rate of the ER gene to ER mRNA to approximately 47% of that of the control. In addition, serum estradiol, progesterone and testosterone levels before and after danazol administration were 54.1 ± 13.6 pg/ml and 47.8 ± 14.7 pg/ml; 0.82 ± 0.33 ng/ml and 0.77 ± 0.22 ng/ml; and 0.62 ± 0.35 ng/ml and 0.70 ± 0.42 ng/ml; respectively by Coat-A-Count radioimmunoassay kits (Nippon DPC Corp., Tokyo, Japan). This suggests that danazol decreases estrogen responsiveness in the monocytes, at least in part, via the reduction of transcription of the ER gene to ER mRNA, and the reduction of the ER level in monocytes, regardless of the alteration of serum steroid hormone levels. These findings suggest that danazol, in local treatment[19], is effective as an antiestrogenic drug on monocyte/macrophage-related infertility in pelvic endometriosis, concomitantly with the reduction of cytokines IL-1 and/or TNF from peritoneal macrophages, and the suppression of the phagocytic activity of the macrophages.

References

1. Polan, M.L., Daniele, A. and Kuo, A. (1988). Gonadal steroids modulate human monocyte interleukin-1 (IL-1) activity. *Fertil. Steril.*, **49**, 964–8
2. Mori, H., Nakagawa, M., Itoh, N., Wada, K. and Tamaya, T. (1990). Danazol suppresses the production of interleukin-1β and tumor necrosis factor by human monocytes. *Am. J. Reprod. Immunol.*, **24**, 45–50
3. Fujimoto, J., Hori, M., Ichigo, S., Itoh, T., Saio, M., Takami, T. and Tamaya, T. (1995). Induction of M-CSF receptor and its mRNA, and activation of tyrosine kinase in peripheral monocytes by oestradiol-17β and progesterone. *Ann. Clin. Biochem.*, **32**, 399–404
4. Fakih, H., Baggett, B., Holtz, G., Tsang, K., Lee, J.C. and Williamson, H.O. (1987). Interleukin-1: a possible role in the infertility associated with endometriosis. *Fertil. Steril.*, **47**, 213–17
5. Eisermann, J., Odem, R.R., Gast, M.J., Collins, J.L. and Pineda, J. (1988). Tumor necrosis factor in peritoneal fluid of women undergoing laparoscopic surgery. *Fertil. Steril.*, **50**, 573–9
6. Yeung, Y.G., Jubinsky, P.T., Sengupta, A., Yeung, D.C.Y. and Stanley, E.R. (1987). Purification of the colony-stimulating factor 1 receptor and demonstration of its tyrosine kinase activity. *Proc. Natl. Acad. Sci. USA*, **84**, 1268–71

7. Sherr, C., Rettenmier, C.W., Sacca, R., Roussel, M.F., Look, A.T. and Stanley, E.R. (1985). The c-*fms* proto-oncogene product is related to the receptor for the molecular phagocyte colony-stimulating factor, CSF-1. *Cell*, **41**, 665–76
8. Stanley, E.R., Guilbert, L.J., Tushinski, R.J. and Bartelmez, S.H. (1983). A mononuclear phagocyte lineage-specific hemopoietic growth factor. *J. Cell Biochem.*, **21**, 151–9
9. Hill, J.A., Cohen, J. and Anderson, D.J. (1989). The effect of lymphokines and monokines on human sperm fertilizing ability in the zona-free hamster egg penetration test. *Am. J. Obstet. Gynecol.*, **160**, 1154–9
10. Hill, J.A., Haimovici, F. and Anderson, D.J. (1987). Products of activated lymphocytes and macrophages inhibit mouse embryo development *in vitro*. *J. Immunol.*, **139**, 2250–4
11. Wada, K., Itoh, T., Nakagawa, M., Misao, R., Mori, H. and Tamaya, T. (1992). Estrogen binding sites in peripheral blood monocytes and effects of danazol on their sites *in vitro*. *Gen. Pharmacol.*, **23**, 693–700
12. Fujimoto, J., Hori, M., Itoh, T., Ichigo, S., Nishigaki, M. and Tamaya, T. (1995). Danazol decreases transcription of estrogen receptor gene in human monocytes. *Gen. Pharmacol.*, **26**, 507–16
13. Scatchard, G. (1979). The attraction of proteins for small molecules and ions. *Ann. NY Acad. Sci.*, **51**, 660–72
14. Dmowski, W.P. (1979). Endocrine properties and clinical application of danazol. *Fertil. Steril.*, **31**, 237–51
15. Tamaya, T., Wada, K., Mori, H. and Imai, A. (1991). Different effects on oestrogen binding sites and anti-oestrogenic action of danazol and progesterone. *Ann. Clin. Biochem.*, **28**, 250–2
16. Tamaya, T., Wada, K., Fujimoto, J., Yamada, T. and Okada, H. (1984). Danazol binding to steroid receptors in human uterine endometrium. *Fertil. Steril.*, **41**, 732–5
17. Fujimoto, J., Straub, R.E. and Gershengorn, M.C. (1991). Thyrotropin-releasing hormone (TRH) and phorbol myristate acetate decrease TRH receptor messenger RNA in rat pituitary GH_3 cells: evidence that protein kinase-C mediates the TRH effect. *Mol. Endocrinol.*, **5**, 1527–32
18. Fujimoto, J. and Gershengorn, M.C. (1991). Evidence for dual regulation of protein kinase A and C thyrotropin-releasing hormone receptor mRNA in GH_3 cells. *Endocrinology*, **129**, 3430–2
19. Igarashi, M. (1990). A new therapy for pelvic endometriosis and uterine adenomyosis: local effect of vaginal and intrauterine danazol application. *Asia–Oceania J. Obstet. Gynaecol.*, **16**, 1–12

Effects of danazol pretreatment for patients with endometriosis on their *in vitro* fertilization and embryo transfer outcomes

N. Suganuma, T. Moriwaki, T. Ando, O. Narita, M. Osawa, T. Tanaka, H. Saito, M. Seki, O. Tsutsumi, H. Kanzaki, A. Hoshiai, S. Yamano, Y. Nagata, K. Matsuura and H. Okamura (EMART group)

Introduction

Recently, for the treatment of infertile patients, assisted reproductive technology has been well developed, and applied in the clinical gynecological field. Treatment using *in vitro* fertilization and embryo transfer (IVF–ET) was first used successfully in England, and the first test-tube baby was born in 1978. This technique has spread quickly all over the world, and been applied clinically for the treatment of infertile couples. In Japan, the first baby was born by IVF–ET in 1983. After that, the number of clinics performing IVF increased rapidly. In 1988, the number of IVF clinics was only 54, and the number of cycles of oocyte-retrieval per year was 1700. However, in 1994, the number of clinics performing IVF reached 236, and the number of retrievals per year was about 30 000. Now, more than 5000 IVF babies are born per year in Japan. This means that the IVF–ET method has been established as a clinical therapeutic procedure for infertility.

For IVF-ET, the first indication was tubal factor infertility, because the method is summarized as induction of conception omitting the Fallopian tubes. Oocytes are retrieved directly from mature follicles before ovulation, and insemination is performed in the laboratory *in vitro*. Fertilized oocytes are cultured and the subsequent embryos are transferred into the uterine cavity with an embryo transfer tube. Thus, patients whose Fallopian tubes are obstructed can conceive by the IVF-ET technique. However, since IVF also makes it possible to observe the gametes and the fertilization process under the microscope, other infertility factors that may cause fertilization failures have also been indicated. Endometriosis, which is thought to cause problems with oocyte pick-up or transportation of the fertilized oocyte to the uterine cavity, has also been indicated for IVF. Although tubal factor infertility is the most popular indication for IVF, IVF indicated for endometriosis is gradually increasing in Japan. In 1989, the ratio was less than 10% of all IVF–ET treatment, but this reached 25% in 1992.

How successful is IVF–ET in patients with endometriosis? By comparison with tubal factor infertility, the IVF outcomes such as fertilization rate, cleavage rate and pregnancy rate in the patients with endometriosis were a little bit low but not significantly different (Table 1). Although IVF–ET is a useful tool for the treatment of infertile patients with endometriosis, the pregnancy and take-home-baby rates are not satisfactory. Thus, we have to make efforts to improve the success rate for patients with endometriosis on IVF–ET.

Although medical treatments for endometriosis have previously been performed

Table 1 IVF–ET outcomes in patients with endometriosis or tubal factor infertility (EMART Group, 1992–94)

	Endometriosis	Tubal factor
No. of patients	277	601
Patient age (years)	34.0 ± 0.8	33.0 ± 0.9
Duration of infertility (years)	6.1 ± 0.7	5.8 ± 0.7
No. of stimulation cycles	551	1191
No. of retrievals	538	1179
Fertilization rate	54.0%	61.3%
Cleavage rate	91.2%	95.1%
No. of embryo transfer cycles	449	999
Implantation rate	11.9%	11.0%
Pregnancy rate/ET	22.3%	24.5%
Abortion rate	23.0%	28.6%

using androgen or estrogen/progesterone, recently danazol and gonadotropin-releasing hormone analogs (GnRHa) have been used. Danazol is a synthetic steroid; this drug was synthesized in the early 1960s, and has been applied for the treatment of endometriosis since 1971[1]. Danazol exhibits mild progesterone and androgenic activities, and acts by a variety of mechanisms. It acts by binding to steroid hormone receptors[2], blocking the effects of gonadotropins on the ovary[3], binding to sex hormone-binding globulin with an increase of free testosterone[4] and blocking the luteinizing hormone (LH) surge[5]. Recently, it has been found that danazol has effects in improving some abnormal immunological situations[6,7]. To analyze the clinical effects of danazol pretreatment for patients with endometriosis on their IVF–ET outcomes, we carried out the following prospective study.

Materials and methods

The study involved ten university hospitals, at Akita, Yamagata, Gunma, Tokyo, Nagoya, Kyoto, Kinki, Tokushima, Fukuoka and Kumamoto. We used a common protocol for danazol pretreatment (see below) in IVF–ET. The study group was named EMART; this name consists of EM (endometriosis) and ART (assisted reproductive technology).

Patients

For this prospective study, 58 patients were selected. Forty-seven patients with endometriosis were indicated for IVF–ET. Thirty-two of these patients had received IVF–ET procedures previously, which had been unsuccessful. Eleven patients who were indicated for IVF for tubal factor infertility were also pretreated with danazol as a control for the study.

Danazol pretreatment and the IVF–ET procedure

Danazol (Tokyo Tanabe Co., Tokyo, Japan) 400 mg/day was administered to the patients on the IVF program for more than 12 weeks (Figure 1). Within 4 weeks after the danazol therapy, GnRHa (900 µg/day, Suprecur, Hoechst Japan Co., Tokyo, Japan; or 400 µg/day, Nasanyl, Yamanouchi Pharmaceutical Co., Tokyo, Japan) nasal spray administration was started, as the usual 'short' or 'long' protocol[8]. Human menopausal gonadotropin (hMG; Fertinom-P, Serono Japan Co., Tokyo, Japan; Pergonal and Humegon, Japan Organon Co., Tokyo, Japan; or Nikken 'HMG', Nikken-Kagaku Co., Tokyo, Japan) for ovarian hyperstimulation on IVF was performed as daily injections, initiated adjusting to the 'short' or 'long' protocol, and follicle growth was monitored by transvaginal ultrasound imaging and/or serum estradiol determinations. When the mature follicles were detected, human chorionic gonadotropin (hCG) was injected. About 36 h after the hCG injection, oocytes were retrieved transvaginally and inseminated. The oocytes and embryos were cultured in medium of Ham's F-10, α-minimum essential medium or human

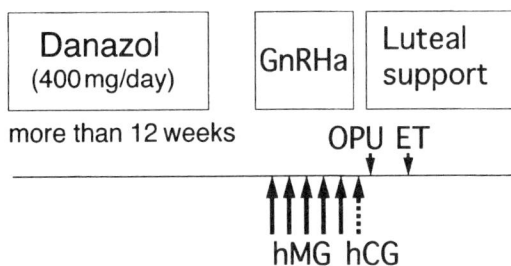

Figure 1 IVF–ET protocol with danazol pretreatment. GnRHa, gonadotropin-releasing hormone analog; hMG, human menopausal gonadotropin; hCG, human chorionic gonadotropin; OPU, oocyte pick-up; ET, embryo transfer

Table 2 Mean ± SD IVF–ET outcomes in danazol-pretreated patients with different indications

	Endometriosis (n = 47)	Tubal factor (n = 11)
Age (years)	33.0 ± 2.9	33.9 ± 2.9
Duration of infertility (years)	6.5 ± 3.1	6.1 ± 3.9
Total amount of hMG (IU)	2309 ± 1245	1950 ± 881
No. of retrieved oocytes	8.4 ± 6.7	8.1 ± 4.7
No. of fertilized oocytes	4.7 ± 3.4	3.8 ± 2.9
No. of transferred embryos	2.6 ± 1.3	2.4 ± 1.1
Grade of transferred embryo	1.8 ± 0.8	1.4 ± 0.5
Pregnancy rate	36% (17/47)	18% (2/11)

hMG, human menopausal gonadotropin

tubal fluid. After insemination, embryo transfer was performed using less than three embryos, 2 days after oocyte retrieval. Luteal support by hCG or progesterone administration was performed after embryo transfer and pregnancy was confirmed by detection of a gestational sac and fetal cardiac movement using ultrasound.

Evaluation of IVF–ET outcomes

Clinical IVF–ET parameters and outcomes such as ovarian response, number of retrieved oocytes, fertilization rate, embryo grade judged by scoring (grade 1 is the best grade, grade 3 the worst)[9], and pregnancy rate were evaluated.

All these procedures were performed after obtaining informed consent from the patients, and using the guidelines of the Japanese Society of Obstetrics and Gynecology.

Results

Parameters and outcomes of the danazol-pretreated IVF–ET

Although the patient profile, total amount of hMG injected, numbers of retrieved oocytes, fertilized oocytes and transferred embryos, and grades of transferred embryos in the patients with endometriosis were not different from those in the patients with tubal factor infertility, the pregnancy rates were clearly different between the two groups (Table 2). A 36% pregnancy rate was achieved in the patients with endometriosis, compared with only 18% in the tubal factor infertility patients.

Stage of endometriosis

To examine the relationship between stage of endometriosis and the effectiveness of IVF, 30 patients whose stage of endometriosis was evaluated using the revised American Fertility Society classification at laparoscopic examination or operation were analyzed (Table 3). There was no clear correlation between endometriotic stage and pregnancy rate.

Parameters and outcomes of IVF–ET with or without danazol pretreatment in individual patients

As described above, 32 patients had already received previous failed IVF–ET procedures.

Table 3 Pregnancy rates in different stages of endometriosis

Stage	No. of patients	No. of pregnancies (%)
I	4	1 (25%)
II	3	1 (33%)
III	12	7 (58%)
IV	11	2 (18%)
Total	30	11 (37%)

Table 4 Mean ± SD effects of danazol pretreatment in patients with previous failed IVF–ET

	Danazol-pretreated cycle	Previous cycle
Total amount of hMG (IU)	2453 ± 1234	2297 ± 1103
No. of retrieved oocytes	7.9 ± 6.9	8.3 ± 4.2
No. of fertilized oocytes	4.2 ± 2.7	4.4 ± 2.5
No. of transferred embryos	2.6 ± 1.3	2.5 ± 1.2
Grade of transferred embryo	1.9 ± 0.8	1.6 ± 0.7
Pregnancy rate	34% (10/29)	0% (0/29)

hMG, human menopausal gonadotropin

Since 29 patients had records of the previous IVF–ET attempt, the parameters of IVF–ET between the present danazol-pretreated IVF–ET and the previous usual IVF–ET were compared (Table 4). There were no significant differences in total amount of injected hMG, numbers of retrieved, fertilized and transferred oocytes, and grade of transferred embryo. However, 10 women became pregnant after the danazol pretreatment, and the pregnancy rate was 34%.

Parameters and outcomes of danazol-pretreated IVF–ET between pregnant and non-pregnant cases

The parameters and outcomes of the danazol-pretreated IVF–ET were compared between pregnant and non-pregnant cases (Table 5). Age and duration of infertility were not different, but the total amount of hMG and number of retrieved oocytes in pregnant cases were rather smaller than those in non-pregnant cases. Also, the transferred embryos were of a rather higher quality in the pregnant cases.

Table 5 IVF–ET parameters in pregnant and non-pregnant patients who received danazol pretreatment. Mean ± SD

	Pregnant ($n = 17$)	Non-pregnant ($n = 30$)
Age (years)	32.4 ± 3.2	33.3 ± 2.6
Duration of infertility (years)	6.4 ± 3.5	6.5 ± 2.9
Total amount of hMG (IU)	2104 ± 1198	2424 ± 1276
No. of retrieved oocytes	6.6 ± 3.7	9.4 ± 7.7
No. of fertilized oocytes	4.5 ± 2.3	4.8 ± 3.9
No. of transferred embryos	2.5 ± 0.9	2.7 ± 1.5
Grade of transferred embryo	1.6 ± 0.7	1.9 ± 0.8

hMG, human menopausal gonadotropin

Discussion

To improve the success rate of IVF–ET in patients with endometriosis, we designed this prospective study including pretreatment with danazol. As clinical IVF–ET parameters and outcomes, ovarian response, number of retrieved oocytes, fertilization rate, embryo grade and pregnancy rate were estimated. Through the present study, we can conclude that danazol pretreatment for the patients with endometriosis has a beneficial effect on their IVF–ET outcome, but not in the patients with tubal factor infertility. It has been reported that pretreatment using GnRHa as an 'ultra-long' protocol increases the pregnancy rate in IVF–ET of patients with endometriosis[10]. Since danazol is also a therapeutic drug for endometriosis, our results are consistent with this in that danazol improves the endometriotic problems such as oocyte pick-up or transportation of the fertilized oocyte. However, there was no clear correlation between endometriotic stage and pregnancy rate in the patients pretreated with danazol. Dmowski and colleagues[11] have also noted that the implantation rate in IVF–ET is comparable in women with and without endometriosis, regardless of the activity and stage of the disease. These findings suggest that danazol has therapeutic effects not only on endometriosis itself but also on other factors causing implantation failure.

We therefore have to ask why the danazol pretreatment is effective. In endometriosis, the associated autoimmune abnormalities are thought to induce fertilization and implantation failure. Gleicher and colleagues[12] reported that more than two-thirds of laparoscopically staged endometriosis patients exhibited evidence of abnormal polyclonal B cell activation, which resulted in an abnormal lupus anticoagulant and abnormal levels of the other autoantibodies. Moreover, the anatomical stage of endometriosis does not correlate with the incidence of infertility and with the risk of pregnancy losses, whereas a strong correlation with autoimmune abnormalities has been reported[13]. Taylor and associates[14] reported that the prevalence of autoantibodies is elevated in women with endometriosis compared with a control group. Ando and colleagues[15] also reported that 42.6% had endometriosis in the positive cases for antinuclear antibody, anti-DNA antibody and/or lupus anticoagulant, which was a higher proportion than that found in the negative cases in the patients who received IVF–ET.

Since it has been reported that danazol has some effects in improving the uterine environment from an immunological aspect[6,7], serum levels of immunoglobulins, complements and autoimmune antibodies were measured before and after treatment with danazol in the patients of the present study. Immunoglobulins and complements had tendencies to decrease and increase, respectively, but there were no significant changes. The levels of autoantibodies did not decrease through the danazol administration. These observations suggest that danazol cannot suppress the abnormal autoimmunity significantly.

By comparing the parameters and outcomes of the danazol-pretreated IVF–ET between pregnant and non-pregnant cases, even the smaller number of oocytes but with higher quality is more effective for IVF–ET. This result suggests that danazol is effective for improvement of oocyte quality by alteration of the intrafollicular microenvironment. To analyze this effect of danazol, concentrations of macrophage colony-stimulating factor, activin and follistatin were also measured in follicular fluid. However, no differences in the levels of these substances were observed between danazol-pretreated and non-treated groups.

Thus, to summarize the present study, danazol pretreatment is effective for the patients with endometriosis on IVF–ET, though the mechanism of danazol in improving implantation efficiency has yet to be elucidated.

Acknowledgments

We thank all the staff in each participating hospital for performing the IVF–ET procedures, and Tokyo Tanabe Co. for supporting this study.

References

1. Greenblatt, R.B., Dmowski, W.P., Mahesh, V.B. and Scholer, H.F.L. (1971). Clinical studies with an anti-gonadotropin, danazol. *Fertil. Steril.*, **22**, 102–12
2. Barbieri, R.L., Lee, H. and Ryan, K.J. (1979). Danazol binding to rat androgen, glucocorticoid, progesterone and estrogen receptors: correlation with biological activity. *Fertil. Steril.*, **31**, 182–6
3. Steingold, K.A., Lu, J.K.H., Judd, H.L. and Meldrum, D.R. (1986). Danazol inhibits steroidgenesis by human ovary *in vivo*. *Fertil. Steril.*, **45**, 649–54
4. Nilsson, B., Sodergard, R., Damber, M.G., Damber, J.E. and Von Schouler, B. (1983). Free testosterone levels during danazol therapy. *Fertil. Steril.*, **39**, 505–9
5. Wood, G.P., Wu, C.H., Flickinger, G.L. and Mikhail, G. (1975). Hormonal changes associated with danazol therapy. *Obstet. Gynecol.*, **45**, 302–4
6. El-Roeiy, A., Dmowski, W.P., Gleicher, N., Radwanska, E., Harlow, L., Binor, Z., Tummon, I. and Rawlins, R. (1988). Danazol but not gonadotropin-releasing hormone agonists suppresses autoantibodies in endometriosis. *Fertil. Steril.*, **50**, 864–71
7. Dmowski, W.P. (1990). Danazol: a synthetic steroid with diverse biological effects. *J. Reprod. Med.*, **35**, 69–75
8. MacNamee, M.C. and Brinsden, P.R. (1992). Superovulation strategies in assisted conception. In Brinsden, R.P. and Rainsbury, P.A. (eds.) *A Textbook of In Vitro Fertilization and Reproduction*, pp. 111–25. (New Jersey: Parthenon Publishing)
9. Cummins, J.M., Breen, T.M., Harrison, K.L., Shaw, J.M., Wilson, L.M. and Hennessey, J.F. (1986). A formula for scoring human embryo growth rates in *in vitro* fertilization: its value in predicting pregnancy and in comparison with visual estimates of embryo quality. *J. In Vitro Fertil. Embryo Transfer*, **3**, 284–95
10. Nakamura, K., Osawa, M., Kondo, I., Inagaki, S., Shibata, K., Narita, O., Suganuma, N. and Tomoda, Y. (1992). Menotropin stimulation after prolonged gonadotropin releasing hormone agonist pretreatment for *in vitro* fertilization in patients with endometriosis. *J. Assist. Reprod. Genet.*, **9**, 113–17
11. Dmowski, W.P., Friberg, J., Rana, N., Papierniak, C., Michalowska, J. and El-Roeiy, A. (1995). The effect of endometriosis, its stage and activity, and of autoantibodies on *in vitro* fertilization and embryo transfer success rates. *Fertil. Steril.*, **63**, 555–62
12. Gleicher, N., El-Roeiy, A., Confino, E. and Friberg, J. (1987). Is endometriosis an autoimmune disease? *Obstet. Gynecol.*, **70**, 115–22
13. Gleicher, N. (1994). The role of humoral immunity in endometriosis. *Acta Obstet. Gynecol. Scand.*, **159**, 15–17
14. Taylor, P.V., Maloney, M.D., Campbell, J.M., Skerrow, S.M., Nip, M.M.C., Parmar, R. and Tate, G. (1991). Autoreactivity in women with endometriosis. *Br. J. Obstet. Gynaecol.*, **98**, 680–4
15. Ando, T., Suganuma, N., Furuhashi, M., Asada, Y., Kondo, I. and Tomoda, Y. (1996). Successful glucocorticoid treatment for the patients with abnormal autoimmunity on *in vitro* fertilization and embryo transfer. *J. Assist. Reprod. Genet.*, **13**, 776–81

Section 10

GnRH antagonists

Antagonistic analogs of LHRH in oncology and gynecology

A.V. Schally, A.M. Comaru-Schally, D. Gonzalez-Barcena, T. Reissmann and J. Engel

Introduction

The discovery of luteinizing hormone-releasing hormone (LHRH) has had a major impact on medicine and has led to a variety of clinical uses of LHRH analogs in oncology and gynecology[1,2]. It has been demonstrated that repeated administration of large doses of superactive agonistic analogs of LHRH causes paradoxical inhibition of the pituitary–gonadal axis in animals and human beings[1-3]. The phenomena of downregulation of pituitary receptors for LHRH, desensitization of pituitary gonadotropes and inhibition of sex steroid levels by LHRH agonists are being used for treatment of endometriosis, uterine leiomyomas and benign prostatic hyperplasia[1,2]. Chronic administration of LHRH agonists is being utilized for therapy of hormone-dependent malignant neoplasms, especially prostate and breast cancer, ovarian cancer and endometrial carcinoma[1,2]. LHRH agonists are also applied for *in vitro* fertilization and embryo transfer (IVF-ET) procedures and for management of precocious puberty[2].

LHRH antagonists

Various experimental and clinical studies indicate that LHRH antagonists should also have major uses in gynecology and oncology[1,2]. Repeated administration of LHRH agonists is required to induce an inhibition of the pituitary–gonadal axis and reduction in the levels of sex steroids, but similar effects can be obtained after the first administration of LHRH antagonists[1,2]. The advantage of the antagonists is based on the fact that they inhibit luteinizing hormone (LH), follicle-stimulating hormone (FSH) and sex steroid secretion, from the start of the administration, and thus reduce the time of the onset of therapeutic effects. The use of antagonists would also avoid the temporary clinical 'flare-up' of the disease that can occur with the agonists[1,2].

Antagonistic analogs of LHRH were developed for contraception[1-4]. Modern antagonists possess modifications in positions 1, 2, 3, 6 an 10 and others. These antagonists act on the same receptor sites as LHRH and cause an immediate inhibition of the release of gonadotropins and sex steroids[1,2]. Since 1973, a series of potent LHRH antagonists has been synthesized and tested in animals and human beings[1-4]. Early antagonists were hydrophobic and active only in relatively large doses[1-7]. Subsequently, side-effects have been observed with hydrophilic LHRH antagonists having D-Arg in position 6[1-5]. In doses of 1.5 mg/kg administered subcutaneously, these antagonists caused a transient allergic reaction in rats (swollen tail, legs, face and ears), suggesting a local and general edema[1], most likely due to histamine release[1-6]. In preliminary human tolerance studies in Europe in women, a distinct erythema upon the skin at the site of the subcutaneous injection was observed in some cases after administration of D-Arginine antagonist ORG 30276 in doses of 0.5 mg[6]. This reaction was probably caused by histamine liberation. These allergenic side-effects of early LHRH

[Ac-D-Nal(2)1, D-Phe(4Cl)2,
D-Pal(3)3, D-Cit6, D-Ala10]LHRH

Acetyl-D-2-naphthylalanyl-D-4-chlorophenylalanyl-
D-3-pyridylalanyl-seryl-tyrosyl-D-citrullyl-leucyl-
arginyl-prolyl-D-alanine amide

Figure 1 The LHRH antagonist Cetrorelix

antagonists delayed clinical use of this class of analogs in humans[1,6].

Modern LHRH antagonists. Development of Cetrorelix

In order to eliminate the undesirable edematogenic effect of the LHRH antagonists containing basic D-amino acids at position 6, new analogues with D-ureidoalkyl amino acids such as D-Cit and D-Hci, at position 6 were synthesized in the laboratory of one of us (AVS) by solid-phase methods and tested in several *in vitro* and *in vivo* systems[7,8]. Among these new LHRH antagonists, [Ac-D-Nal(2)1, D-Phe(4Cl)2, D-Pal(3)3, D-Cit6, D-Ala10]LHRH (Cetrorelix, SB-75) (Figure 1), was shown to be one of the most powerful[8]. Cetrorelix inhibited LH release *in vitro* from superfused rat pituitaries at doses of 3–30 nmol/l and showed high binding affinity to membrane LHRH receptors in rat pituitaries and human breast cancers[8,9]. *In vivo*, Cetrorelix caused 100% inhibition of ovulation in cycling rats at a dose of 1.5 μg, and 2.5 μg suppressed LH levels in castrated male rats[8]. This peptide did not exert any edematogenic effects, even at a dose of 1.5 mg/kg[8,9]. Subsequently, Cetrorelix was synthesized both by classical and by solid-phase methods by ASTA Medica AG in Frankfurt/Main[9] and its safety profile was carefully studied[9]. In view of the absence of toxic effects, the LHRH antagonist Cetrorelix was tested clinically. Cetrorelix inhibited LH and FSH release in hypergonadotropic hypogonadal women at doses of 300–600 μg twice a day, and caused no allergic side-effects[10]. Inhibition of testosterone levels was obtained with Cetrorelix in normal men and in patients with advanced prostatic cancer[10,11]. Prolonged inhibition of serum testosterone (total and free) to castration levels was induced in patients with benign prostatic hyperplasia after subcutaneous administration of 500 μg of Cetrorelix every 12 h[11]. Other clinical studies with Cetrorelix are described below.

Development of sustained delivery systems of Cetrorelix

The development of sustained delivery systems for Cetrorelix should facilitate the clinical use of this powerful LHRH antagonist. Various batches of microcapsules of SB-75 in poly(D,L lactide-co-glycolide) (PLG) and other depot preparations were prepared and tested in rats[12–16]. Microparticles (microgranules) are prepared by cryogenic grinding and are not spherical like microcapsules[12–16]. We carried out extensive histological and immunochemical studies on the release of agonist [D-Trp6]LHRH and antagonist Cetrorelix from the microcapsules and microgranules[13]. Macrophages could be seen in the center of a microcapsule 4 days after the intramuscular injection[13], and 2 weeks after the injection of microcapsules of Cetrorelix, advanced decomposition of the matrix of microcapsules was noted. No foreign body reaction was seen[13]. These observations indicate that, contrary to previous views, the diffusion of the peptide analogs from the interior of the PLG matrix through aqueous channels is negligible, and does not play an important role in the release of the peptide from the sustained delivery systems[13]. The release of an insoluble peptide such as SB-75 pamoate through the aqueous channels in the microparticles would be even less likely. The peptides are liberated mainly by the biodegradation of the matrix. The intensity of the tissue reactions, especially macrophage activity, regulates the speed of this biodegradation[13]. The findings that the peptide release from the microcapsules or microparticles of PLG is controlled mainly by the speed of the biodegradation of the polymer matrix and that the diffusion of the peptides from the PGL is insignificant[13] are in accord with the work of other investigators. Recently other depot preparations of Cetrorelix pamoate have been developed, which may permit periodic administration[14].

Serum levels of SB-75, LH, FSH and testosterone were measured in rats injected with cetrorelix pamoate microcapsules or microgranules[15–17]. Levels of Cetrorelix in the serum of rats injected with microcapsules or microgranules containing 2.5–3.6 mg of the antagonist were significantly elevated for 70–90 days. Serum testosterone levels in these rats injected with these depot preparations were inhibited to castration levels for 70–164 days, and serum LH levels for 70–102 days[14–16]. Serum FSH levels were also suppressed. Testicular, ventral prostate and seminal vesicle weights in male rats treated with Cetrorelix depot were greatly decreased 30 days after injection[14–16]. A significant downregulation of the pituitary LHRH receptors in rats was produced after treatment with microcapsules or microgranules of Cetrorelix. This downregulation could be important clinically, since prolonged therapy should result in a powerful and long-lasting inhibition of the pituitary, and hence of gonadal function. Nevertheless, there was a complete recovery of the pituitary–gonadal axis in male and female rats 2–10 months after cessation of treatment with Cetrorelix[15–17].

Downregulation of pituitary LHRH receptors in rats by Cetrorelix

The binding characteristics of receptors for LHRH in membrane fractions from rat anterior pituitaries were investigated in rats after a single injection of 100 µg Cetrorelix[18]. To determine whether the treatment with Cetrorelix can affect the concentration of measurable LHRH binding sites, we used an *in vitro* method for desaturation of receptors based on chaotropic agents such as manganous chloride ($MnCl_2$) and ammonium thiocyanate (NH_4SCN)[18]. Receptor assays, following *in vitro* desaturation, demonstrated that pituitary LHRH receptors in rats were significantly downregulated for at least 72 h after administration of Cetrorelix[18]. The lowest receptor concentration was found 3–6 h after injection of Cetrorelix and a recovery in receptor number began within about 24 h. The downregulation of LHRH binding sites induced by SB-75 was accompanied by serum LH and testosterone suppression. Our results indicate that the LHRH antagonist Cetrorelix produces a marked downregulation of pituitary receptors for LHRH and not merely an occupancy of binding sites[18].

In another study, we treated male rats for 4 weeks with daily subcutaneous injections of Cetrorelix acetate or the LHRH agonist [D-Trp^6]LHRH[19]. Another group of rats received a single intramuscular injection of Cetrorelix pamoate depot, a sustained release formulation. An intravenous stimulation test with LHRH was performed after 4 weeks of treatment. To examine the effect of LHRH antagonist on the expression of the pituitary LHRH receptor gene, some of the rats injected with Cetrorelix pamoate depot were sacrificed after 2 weeks, and levels of LHRH receptor mRNA were determined by Northern blots[19]. LHRH-stimulated LH secretion at 30 min was suppressed by 90–96% in rats treated with Cetrorelix acetate or Cetrorelix pamoate depot. The concentration of pituitary receptors for LHRH fell by 69% in the [D-Trp^6]LHRH group, while the reduction in the Cetrorelix acetate or Cetrorelix pamoate depot groups was 77–82%[19]. Treatment with Cetrorelix pamoate depot led to a 75–83% decrease in the levels of LHRH receptor mRNA[19]. These results demonstrate that administration of the LHRH antagonist Cetrorelix in high doses causes an impairment of gonadotropin secretion and a marked decrease in the levels of LHRH receptors as well as in the expression of the LHRH receptor gene[19].

Prospective clinical applications of Cetrorelix and other LHRH antagonists

Clinical studies have demonstrated that various LHRH antagonists, including Detirelix[20,21], Ganirelix[22], Nal-Glu[23–26], antide[27] and Cetrorelix[10,11,28,29] strongly inhibit gonadotropin and sex steroid secretion in men and women. Gonzalez-Barcena and colleagues[10], Behre and colleagues[28] and Klingmuller and colleagues[29] investigated the effects of Cetrorelix in normal men. Cetrorelix significantly decreased serum levels of LH, FSH and testosterone[10,28,29] and appeared to be active in doses lower than those used with other antagonists such as Detirelix, Ganirelix, Nal-Glu and antide. Klingmuller and co-workers[29] indicated that Cetrorelix seems to be more potent than other antagonists such as Nal-Glu or Detirelix. Behre and associates[28] also reported that Cetrorelix, even in large doses of up to 5 mg, only occasionally caused minimal erythema, in contrast to the Nal-Glu antagonist that produces local side-effects[23,28].

In view of favorable clinical results with LHRH agonists in the treatment of prostate cancer, breast cancer, endometriosis, leiomyomas and precocious puberty as well as the demonstrated experimental efficacy of LHRH antagonists in animal models of prostate, ovarian and breast cancer, the clinical development of LHRH antagonists is progressing at a rapid pace. The advantage of the LHRH antagonists is due to the fact that they produce an inhibition of LH, FSH and sex steroid secretion immediately after administration[1,2], and thus achieve the desired therapeutic effects more rapidly than the agonists. The use of antagonistic analogs of LHRH for the treatment of prostate cancer and other conditions would avoid the transient stimulation of the release of gonadotropins and sex steroids that occurs initially in response to LHRH agonists, thus preventing the temporary clinical 'flare-up' of the disease[1,2]. The main applications of LHRH antagonists might be for the treatment of hormone-dependent malignancies such as prostate, breast, ovarian and endometrial cancer, as well as non-malignant conditions such as endometriosis, uterine leiomyomas and precocious puberty, in which the depression of the pituitary–gonadal function is desirable[1,2]. Antagonists such as Cetrorelix could also find an important application in the field of assisted reproductive technology (ART).

This review will now focus on specific applications. We will cite clinical investigations in the fields of gynecology and oncology as well as experimental studies performed with LHRH antagonists in various tumor models.

Assisted reproductive technology, in vitro fertilization and embryo transfer programs

LHRH agonists have been used in IVF-ET programs for more than a decade to prevent a premature rise in LH[2,30]. It has been demonstrated that Cetrorelix and Nal-Glu antagonist can postpone LH surges in normal women with regular ovulatory menstrual cycles[31,32]. Recently, several groups reported the successful use of Cetrorelix to prevent premature LH surges in women undergoing IVF-ET procedures[30,33–35]. In two of these studies, one or two injections of 3–5 mg of Cetrorelix on days 8–11 of the stimulation cycle with human menopausal gonadotropin (hMG) were reported to block LH surges in all the patients before a triggering of ovulation was achieved with human chorionic gonadotropin (hCG)[30,33]. A reduction in the dose of hMG was possible and the clinical pregnancy rate was stated to be satisfactory[30,33]. In another study, 1–3 mg of Cetrorelix was injected daily from day 7 until ovulation was induced by hCG[34,35]. A 50% reduction in the amount of hMG needed as compared to that required for a long protocol with LHRH agonists was noted. The number and quality of oocytes collected and the fertilization rate were comparable to those achieved with the 'long protocol' with LHRH agonists[34,35]. These results suggest a promising indication for Cetrorelix in the IVF protocols with a reduction in the costs of the assisted reproduction procedures.

Uterine leiomyomas (fibroids), endometriosis and other conditions

Many investigators have reported beneficial effects of LHRH agonists in the treatment of patients with leiomyomas[2]. It has been clearly demonstrated that the size of uterine leiomyomas could be reduced by long-term treatment with various LHRH agonists, because of the induction of a state of hypoestrogenism[2,36]. Overall results suggest that LHRH agonists may be used for medical management of uterine leiomyomas, as a primary therapy or as an adjunct to surgical myomectomy, particularly in those cases in which hysterectomy is not desirable, for instance in young patients who have not yet completed their families.

On the basis of the assumption that LHRH antagonists should achieve therapeutic effects more rapidly than the agonists, two groups evaluated different antagonistic analogs in patients with myomas[36,37]. Kettel and co-workers[36] reported regression of uterine leiomyomas in response to administration of the LHRH antagonist Nal-Glu[36]. Nal-Glu (50 μg/kg per day) was administered subcutaneously for 3 months to normally cycling women with symptomatic leiomyomas. Mean leiomyoma size decreased by more than 50% after 1 month of therapy. Serum levels of estradiol and estrone declined rapidly within 48 h and remained suppressed throughout treatment. Six patients became amenorrheic during therapy[36].

Gonzalez-Barcena and colleagues[37] administered Cetrorelix to 11 premenopausal women with symptomatic uterine myomas who had been candidates for hysterectomy. The mean age of the patients was 35 years and seven of them still desired to become pregnant. The initial dose of Cetrorelix was 5 mg subcutaneously twice a day for the first 2 days and thereafter 0.8 mg subcutaneously twice a day for at least 3 months[37]. Before the therapy with Cetrorelix, the mean uterine volume was 227.9 cm^3. Ten patients showed a progressive reduction in uterine volume to 139.2 cm^3 at 1 month and to 111.4 cm^3 at 3 months. One patient did not respond. All patients became amenorrheic and had hot flushes. After treatment with Cetrorelix a surgical myomectomy was performed in six women and one became pregnant[37]. The patients returned to normal menses 1 month after cessation of treatment. These results show that Cetrorelix produces a reduction in the uterine volume and that the decrease in the uterine vascularity facilitates the myomectomy, thus avoiding a hysterectomy[37]. The onset of the therapeutic effects of Cetrorelix is more rapid than that of LHRH agonists. LHRH antagonists appear to be promising for therapy of uterine leiomyomas. In addition, LHRH antagonists should be useful for the treatment of endometriosis. It is possible that Cetrorelix will also be beneficial in the treatment of polycystic ovarian disease (PCOD) and in the control of severe menometrorrhagia due to various clinical conditions such as abnormal hemostatic status.

Benign prostatic hypertrophy

Benign prostatic hypertrophy (BPH) affects a high proportion of men over 60 years of age and is a common cause of dysuria, incontinence and urinary tract obstruction[38,39]. BPH has also been considered to be a potentially precancerous lesion. Although surgical intervention is the standard treatment for BPH, some patients are not good candidates for prostatectomy. Consequently, a non-surgical treatment would be of great value, particularly for those men who are poor operative risks. The etiology of BPH is not completely clear, but much evidence indicates that prostatic tissue growth and prostate function are androgen dependent[38,39]. Dihydrotestosterone (DHT), a peripheral conversion product of testosterone, is the major nuclear androgen in sexual tissue. The prostate particularly is dependent upon DHT formation and receptor interaction. In addition to surgery, other forms of therapy for BPH include antiandrogens, the 5α-reductase inhibitor finasteride and α-adrenergic blockers. Since chronic administration of LHRH agonists or antagonists produces a reduction in circulating testosterone and DHT levels and decreases the concentration of tissue DHT, this appears to be a rational approach to therapy of BPH. It was previously reported that the LHRH agonist nafarelin acetate, given by subcutaneous daily injections for 6 months, reduced testosterone to castrate levels, decreased prostate size by 25% as measured by ultrasonography and improved urinary symptoms in men with BPH[38]. A similar shrinkage of the prostate and improvement in urinary flow occurred with the LHRH agonist leuprolide[39]. After the discontinuation of the therapy, the effects of the analogs were reversed.

The responses to the antagonistic analog Cetrorelix were evaluated in patients with BPH[11]. Cetrorelix was given subcutaneously at a dose of 500 μg every 12 h for 4 weeks to 11 patients with BPH presenting with prostatism and urinary outflow obstruction. There was a clear clinical improvement after the first week of SB-75 therapy which continued during the treatment[11]. Before therapy with SB-75, the serum levels of prostate-specific antigen (PSA) and acid phosphatase were elevated, but declined to normal values at 4 weeks. Initial serum testosterone levels were within normal limits, but during treatment with Cetrorelix they fell to castration values[11]. A decrease in serum LH and FSH levels was also found. Mean prostatic volume, assessed by ultrasonography, showed a significant decrease of 44%. In some patients, the reduction in prostatic volume was maintained for up to 11 months after therapy[11]. These results showed that Cetrorelix can be safely administered for prolonged periods of time. The rapid shrinkage of the prostate and improvement in obstructive symptoms of prostatism obtained with Cetrorelix suggests that the LHRH antagonists offer a therapeutic alternative in patients with BPH who are considered to be poor surgical risks.

Prostate cancer

Carcinoma of the prostate is one of the leading causes of death from cancer among men. The treatment of advanced prostate cancer is based upon its androgen dependence[1]. Endocrine therapy for carcinoma of the prostate includes orchidectomy and administration of estrogen or antiandrogens. The efficacy of palliation with agonistic analogs of LHRH in men with advanced prostate cancer was first demonstrated by Tolis and associates[40] in 1980–81. This new approach was based on the experimental work of Redding and Schally[41]. The study of Tolis and co-workers[40] and subsequent clinical trials[42–44] documented a fall in testosterone levels and marked subjective and objective improvement in patients with stage C or D prostate carcinoma after daily treatment with agonistic analogs, Decapeptyl, Buserelin, Leuprolide and Zoladex. Development of microcapsules and other sustained release formulations of LHRH agonists, that can be injected once a month, made the treatment of patients with prostate cancer even more convenient and more efficacious[45–47]. Clinical results accumulated to date indicate that therapy with agonists of LHRH is the preferred method of treatment for men with advanced prostate cancer. However, LHRH agonists alone or in combination with antiandrogens[42] will not prevent an eventual relapse[1]. The use of LHRH antagonists would avoid the temporary clinical 'flareup' of the disease that can occur with the agonists.

There is now much experimental and clinical evidence that LHRH antagonists can be used for the treatment of prostate cancer[1,11,48–52]. Early studies showed that an inhibition of growth of Dunning R3327 prostate cancer can be obtained in rats after treatment with microcapsules of the antagonist Cetrorelix[48]. When we treated nude mice bearing xenografts of human prostate adenocarcinoma PC-82 with the agonist [D-Trp[6]]LHRH or the antagonist Cetrorelix, we were able to demonstrate that in animals that received microgranules of the antagonist, there was a greater decrease in tumor weight and volume than were produced by the agonist[49]. Serum levels of testosterone were decreased by 90% in mice given the LHRH agonists and by 94% in response to cetrorelix[49]. Serum levels of PSA were likewise lower in mice treated with Cetrorelix[49]. We also showed that Cetrorelix inhibits the growth of androgen-independent human DU-145 and PC-3 prostate cancers transplanted into nude mice, probably through an effect on receptors for epidermal growth factor (EGF)[50].

Clinical studies with antagonist SB-75 in patients with prostate cancer demonstrated a marked clinical improvement parallel to lowering of serum testosterone levels to castration values[11,51,52]. In one study, the response to 500 μg SB-75 given every 12 h subcutaneously was evaluated in six prostatic cancer patients (two stage C and four stage D2)[11]. After the first week of therapy with Cetrorelix, there was a significant decrease in bone pain, relief in urinary outflow obstruction and reversal of the signs of prostatism. Subjective improvement continued during the following weeks of treatment and the patients no longer needed analgesics. The levels of PSA, acid and alkaline phosphatases gradually decreased, achieving nearly normal values at 6 weeks, and the serum testosterone level fell to castration values. In another study, 36 patients with prostate cancer, stage D, were treated with Cetrorelix[52]. Before therapy, all patients had elevated levels of PSA and most of them required high doses of potent analgesics for bone pain. Group I consisted of 16 patients with a mean age of 71.3 ± 1.8 years, who received 500 μg Cetrorelix subcutaneously twice a day for up to 37 months. During treatment, 13 of the 16 patients showed a clinical remission of prostate cancer, two did not respond and one remained stable[52]. Five patients in this group relapsed during the treatment with Cetrorelix. Group II included 20 patients with a mean age of 70.3 ± 1.7 years, who received initially a higher dose of Cetrorelix, 5 mg subcutaneously twice a day for the first 2 days and thereafter 800 μg subcutaneously twice a day for up to 20 months. Nineteen patients showed remission. One patient did not respond and three patients relapsed[52]. Before therapy, six patients (three each from groups I and II) were paraplegic, due to metastatic invasion of the spinal cord[51,52]. Five patients showed improvement of the neurological injury after the first week of therapy with Cetrorelix[51]. These studies show that Cetrorelix may be particularly useful for patients with prostate cancer and metastases to the brain, spinal cord, liver, bone marrow and other sites, in whom the LHRH agonists cannot be used as single drugs, because of the possibility of flare-up. Cetrorelix appears to be appropriate for the long-term therapy of prostate cancer.

Breast cancer

About 30% of breast cancers in women are estrogen dependent[53]. Various experimental and clinical studies suggest that analogs of LHRH might be useful for the treatment of estrogen-dependent breast cancer[1,2]. In clinical trials carried out so far, regression of tumor mass and disappearance of metastases in premenopausal and a small percentage of postmenopausal women with breast cancer treated with [D-Trp[6]]LHRH, Buserelin, Zoladex or Leuprolide have been reported[1,2,53–55]. The responses recorded in some postmenopausal patients suggest that LHRH agonists may have a direct antitumoral action[1]. These studies, including a large trial by Kaufmann and colleagues[54], support the view that LHRH agonists are efficacious for the treatment of premenopausal women with estrogen receptor positive (ER+) breast cancers[1,56].

The mechanism of the main effect of LHRH analogs is based on estrogen deprivation, but some direct antitumor effects of LHRH analogs on mammary carcinomas are also possible, since several groups found LHRH receptors in human breast cancers[1,57].

LHRH antagonists have been so far tested only in experimental models of breast cancer. In mice bearing MXT estrogen-dependent or -independent mammary adenocarcinomas, Cetrorelix administered in the form of microcapsules reduced tumor volume and tumor weight[58]. Histologically, the regressive changes in the treated tumors were characteristic of apoptosis (programmed cell death)[58]. In rats bearing DMBA-induced mammary carcinomas, cetrorelix in doses of 100–316 µg/kg per day also induced tumor regression[9]. Cetrorelix likewise inhibited tumor growth in nude mice bearing transplanted MCF-7 MIII human breast cancers[59]. The experimental findings indicate that Cetrorelix might be a possibly useful agent for the treatment of breast cancer.

Epithelial ovarian cancer

Epithelial ovarian cancer is the leading cause of death for women with gynecological cancers, and new therapeutic methods must be developed. Ovarian cancer may be dependent on LH and FSH, and suppression of the secretion of gonadotropins produced by LHRH analogs appears to inhibit the growth of ovarian tumors[1,2]. In addition, specific binding sites for LHRH have been found in samples of surgically removed human ovarian carcinomas and in EGF-21, EFO-27 and OV-1063 human ovarian cancer cell lines[60–62]. These receptors appear to mediate direct inhibitory effects of agonist [D-Trp6]LHRH or the antagonist Cetrorelix on proliferation of ovarian cell lines $in\ vitro$[61,62].

Previously, Parmar and colleagues[63,64] have treated patients with advanced ovarian carcinoma, who had relapsed following conventional treatment, with microcapsules of [D-Trp6]LHRH[63,64]. Some patients showed stabilization or partial remission. However, in a recent multicenter double-blind trial, no relevant beneficial effects of therapy with [D-Trp6]LHRH could be detected in patients with advanced epithelial ovarian cancer, who received standard surgical cytoreduction and cytotoxic chemotherapy[65].

Experimental results suggest that Cetrorelix inhibits growth of human OV-1063 epithelial ovarian cancers better than agonist [D-Trp6] LHRH and therefore may be more efficacious clinically[62]. In nude mice bearing xenografts of OV-1063 ovarian cancer, treatment with Cetrorelix inhibited tumor growth, reduced the number of EGF binding sites on tumor membranes and greatly decreased the levels of mRNA for EGF receptor[62,66]. Effects of SB-75 on EGF receptors might be related to inhibition of tumor growth. Our findings support the view that LHRH antagonists such as Cetrorelix could be considered for possible hormonal therapy of epithelial ovarian cancer[1,62,66].

Endometrial cancer

Endometrial carcinoma can be successfully treated with surgery or radiotherapy in most patients, but new methods are needed for advanced or relapsed cases. Endometrial carcinoma is estrogen dependent and might respond to therapy with LHRH analogs[1,2]. In addition, high-affinity receptors for LHRH have been found on the membranes of human endometrial cancers and HEC-1A and Ishikawa human endometrial cancer cell lines[67,68]. [D-Trp6]LHRH and Cetrorelix significantly inhibited the proliferation of both cell lines $in\ vitro$[68]. The functional role of receptors for LHRH in human endometrial carcinoma is not clear, but this finding provides an additional rationale for the use of therapeutic approaches based on LHRH analogs in this malignancy.

Other cancers

Exocrine pancreatic carcinomas and colorectal carcinomas may be sensitive to sex steroids[1]. Various observations indicate the presence of LHRH receptors in N-nitroso-bis(2-oxypropyl)amine (BOP)-induced hamster pancreatic carcinomas[69,70]. Tumor growth of BOP-induced pancreatic cancer in hamsters can be inhibited by treatment with Cetrorelix or agonist [D-Trp[6]]LHRH[69,70]. Cetrorelix also inhibited the growth of Mia PaCa-2 human pancreatic cell lines transplanted into nude mice.

The inhibitory effect of chronic treatment with LHRH analogs on pancreatic cancers might be explained by elimination of the stimulatory action of the sex steroids[69,70]. Nevertheless, LHRH agonists and antagonists could be envisioned only as possible adjuvants to other agents such as bombesin antagonist in the treatment of pancreatic and colorectal cancer[1].

effects on various tissues and tumors may also play a role. The advantage of the antagonists is based on the fact that they inhibit LH, FSH and sex steroid secretion from the start of the administration, and thus achieve rapid therapeutic effects. The use of antagonists avoids the temporary clinical flare-up of the disease which can occur with the agonists. Various endocrine-dependent or hormone-sensitive tumors can be treated with LHRH antagonists, and the use of sustained delivery systems will make the treatment more practical and efficacious. A successful utilization of Cetrorelix for treatment of androgen-dependent prostate cancer and BPH has been documented. Antagonists of LHRH might also be beneficial for the treatment of breast cancer. Work is in progress on the application of LHRH antagonists for treatment of ovarian and endometrial cancer. LHRH antagonists should also find important applications in the treatment of uterine leiomyomas and endometriosis, and in assisted reproductive technology.

Conclusions

Inhibition of the pituitary–gonadal axis forms the basis for gynecological and oncological applications of LHRH antagonists, but direct

Acknowledgements

Some experimental work described in this paper was supported by the Medical Research Service of the Veterans Affairs Department.

References

1. Schally, A.V. and Comaru-Schally, A.M. (1997). Hypothalamic and other peptide hormones. In Holland, J.F., Frei, E. III, Bast, R.C. Jr, Kufe, D.E., Morton, D.L. and Weichselbaum, R.R. (eds.) *Cancer Medicine*, 4th edn, pp. 1067–86. (Baltimore: Williams and Wilkins)
2. Schally, A.V. (1989). The use of LH-RH analogs in gynecology and tumor therapy. In Belfort, P., Pinotti, J.A. and Eskes, T.K.A.B. (eds.) *Advances in Gynecology and Obstetrics, General Gynecology*, vol. 6, pp. 3–20. (Carnforth, UK: Parthenon Publishing)
3. Vickery, B.H. (1986). Comparison of the potential for therapeutic utilities with gonadotrophin-releasing hormone agonists and antagonists. *Endocr. Rev.*, **7**, 115–24
4. Dutta, A.S. (1988). LH-RH antagonists. *Drugs Future*, **13**, 761–87
5. Coy, D.H., Horvath, A., Nekola, M.V., Coy, E.J., Erchegyi, J. and Schally, A.V. (1982). Peptide antagonists of LH-RH: large increases in antiovulatory activities produced by basic D-amino acids in the six position. *Endocrinology*, **110**, 1445–7
6. Debeljuk, L. and Schally, A.V. (1986). Antifertility effects of a potent LH-RH antagonist in male and female rats. *Int. J. Fertil.*, **31**, 284–92

7. Bajusz, S., Kovacs, M., Gazdag, M., Bokser, L., Karashima, T., Csernus, V.J., Janaky, T., Guoth, J. and Schally, A.V. (1988). Highly potent antagonists of luteinizing hormone-releasing hormone free of edematogenic effects. *Proc. Natl. Acad. Sci. USA*, **85**, 1637–41
8. Bajusz, S., Csernus, V.J., Janaky, T., Bokser, L., Fekete, M. and Schally, A.V. (1988). New antagonists of LHRH: II. Inhibition and potentiation of LHRH by closely related analogues. *Int. J. Peptide Prot. Res.*, **32**, 425–35
9. Reissmann, T.H., Engel, J., Kutscher, B., Bernd, M., Hilgard, P., Peukert, M., Szelenyi, I., Reichert, S., Gonzalez-Barcena, D., Nieschiag, E., Comaru-Schally, A.M. and Schally, A.V. (1994). Cetrorelix. *Drugs Future*, **19**, 228–37
10. Gonzalez-Barcena, D., Vadillo, B.M., Garcia, P.E., Guerra, A.L., Cardenas, C.I., Comaru-Schally, A.M. and Schally, A.V. (1994). Inhibition of luteinizing hormone, follicle-stimulating hormone and sex-steroid levels in men and women with a potent antagonist analog of luteinizing hormone-releasing hormone, Cetrorelix (SB-75). *Eur. J. Endocrinol.*, **131**, 286–92
11. Gonzalez-Barcena, D., Vadillo, B.M., Gomez, O.F., Fuentes, G.M., Cardenas, C.I., Graaf, S.A., Comaru-Schally, A.M. and Schally, A.V. (1994). Responses to the antagonistic analog of LH-RH (SB-75, Cetrorelix) in patients with benign prostatic hyperplasia and prostate cancer. *Prostate*, **24**, 84–92
12. Csernus, V.J., Szende, B., Groot, K., Redding, T.W. and Schally, A.V. (1990). Development of radioimmunoassay for a potent luteinizing hormone-releasing hormone antagonist; evaluation of serum levels after injection of [Ac-3-(2-naphthyl)-D-Ala^1,D-Phe(pCl)^2,3-(3-pyridyl)-D-Ala^3,D-Cit^6,D-Ala^{10}]LH-RH. *Arzneim. Forsch./Drug Res.*, **40**, 111–18
13. Csernus, V.J., Szende, B. and Schally, A.V. (1990). Release of peptides from sustained delivery systems (microcapsules and microparticles) *in vivo*: a histological and immunohistological study. *Int. J. Peptide Prot. Res.*, **35**, 557–65
14. Reissmann, T., Klenner, T., Deger, W., Hilgard, P., McGregor, G.P., Voigt, K. and Engel, J. (1996). Pharmacological studies with Cetrorelix (SB-75), a potent antagonist of luteinizing hormone-releasing hormone. *Eur. J. Cancer*, **32**, 1574–9
15. Bokser, L., Bajusz, S., Groot, K. and Schally, A.V. (1990). Prolonged inhibition of luteinizing hormone and testosterone levels in male rats with the luteinizing hormone-releasing hormone antagonist SB-75. *Proc. Natl. Acad. Sci. USA*, **87**, 7100–4
16. Pinski, J., Yano, T., Groot, K., Milovanovic, S. and Schally, A.V. (1992). Comparison of biological effects of a sustained delivery system and nonencapsulated LH-RH antagonist SB-75 in rats. *Peptides*, **13**, 905–11
17. Pinski, J., Yano, T., Szepeshazi, K., Groot, K. and Schally, A.V. (1993). Recovery of pituitary–gonadal function in male rats after long-term suppression induced by a single injection of microcapsules of LH-RH antagonist Cetrorelix (SB-75). *J. Androl.*, **14**, 164–9
18. Halmos, G., Schally, A.V., Pinsky, J., Vadillo-Buenfil, M. and Groot, K. (1996). Down-regulation of pituitary receptors for luteinizing hormone-releasing hormone (LH-RH) in rats by LH-RH antagonist Cetrorelix. *Proc. Natl. Acad. Sci. USA*, **93**, 2398–402
19. Pinski, J., Lamharzi, N., Halmos, G., Groot, K., Jungwirth, A., Vadillo-Buenfil, M., Kakar, S.S. and Schally, A.V. (1996). Chronic administration of the luteinizing hormone-releasing hormone (LH-RH) decreases gonadotrope responsiveness and pituitary LH-RH receptor messenger ribonucleic acid levels in rats. *Endocrinology*, **137**, 3430–6
20. Andreyko, J.L., Monroe, S.E., Marshall, L.A., Fluker, M.R., Nerenberg, C.A. and Jaffe, R.B. (1992). Concordant suppression of serum immunoreactive luteinizing hormone (LH), follicle-stimulating hormone, α subunit, bioactive LH, and testosterone in postmenopausal women by a potent gonadotropin releasing hormone antagonist (Detirelix). *J. Clin. Endocrinol. Metab.*, **74**, 399–405
21. Pavlou, S.N., Wakefield, G.B., Island, D.P., Hoffman, P.G., LePage, M.E., Chan, R.I., Nerenberg, C.A. and Kovacs, W.J. (1987). Suppression of pituitary–gonadal function by a potent new luteinizing hormone-releasing hormone antagonist in normal men. *J. Clin. Endocrinol. Metab.*, **64**, 931–6
22. Rabinovici, J., Rothman, P., Monroe, S.E., Nerenberg, C. and Jaffe, B. (1992). Endocrine effects and pharmacokinetic characteristics of a potent new gonadotropin-releasing hormone antagonist (Ganirelix) with minimal histamine-

releasing properties: studies in postmenopausal women. *J. Clin. Endocrinol. Metab.,* **75**, 1220–5

23. Pavlou, S.N., Wakefield, G., Schlechter, N.L., Lindner, J., Souza, K.H., Kamilaris, T.C., Konidaris, S., Rivier, J.E., Vale, W.W. and Toglia, M. (1989). Mode of suppression of pituitary and gonadal function after acute or prolonged administration of a luteinizing hormone-releasing hormone antagonist in normal men. *J. Clin. Endocrinol. Metab.,* **68**, 446–54

24. Jockenhovel, F., Bhasin, S., Steiner, B.S., Rivier, J.E., Vale, W.W. and Swerdloff, R.S. (1988). Hormonal effects of single gonadotropin-releasing hormone antagonist doses in men. *J. Clin. Endocrinol. Metab.,* **66**, 1065–70

25. Leal, J.A., Williams, R.F., Danforth, D.R., Gordon, K. and Hodgen, G.D. (1988). Prolonged duration of gonadotropin inhibition by a third generation GnRH antagonist. *J. Clin. Endocrinol. Metab.,* **67**, 1325–7

26. Matikainen, T., Ding, Y.-Q., Vergara, M., Huhtaniemi, I., Couzinet, B. and Schaison, G. (1992). Differing responses to plasma bioactive and immunoreactive follicle-stimulating hormone and luteinizing hormone to gonadotropin-releasing hormone antagonist and agonist treatments in postmenopausal women. *J. Clin. Endocrinol. Metab.,* **75**, 820–5

27. Bagatell, C.J., Conn, P.M. and Bremner, W.J. (1993). Single-dose administration of the gonadotropin-releasing hormone antagonist, Nal-Lys (antide) to healthy men. *Fertil. Steril.,* **60**, 80–5

28. Behre, H.M., Klein, B., Steinmeyer, E., McGregor, G.P., Voigt, K. and Nieschlag, E. (1992). Effective suppression of luteinizing hormone and testosterone by single doses of the new gonadotropin-releasing hormone antagonist Cetrorelix (SB-75) in normal men. *J. Clin. Endocrinol. Metab.,* **75**, 393–8

29. Klingmuller, D., Schepke, M., Enzweiler, C. and Bidlingmaier, F. (1993). Hormonal responses to the new potent GnRH antagonist Cetrorelix. *Acta Endocrinol.,* **128**, 15–18

30. Olivennes, F., Fanchin, R., Bouchard, P., de Ziegler, D., Taieb, J., Selva, J. and Frydman, R. (1994). The single or dual administration of the gonadotropin-releasing hormone antagonist Cetrorelix in an *in vitro* fertilization–embryo program. *Fertil. Steril.,* **62**, 468–76

31. Dubourdieu, S., Charbonnel, B., d'Acremont, M.-F., Carreau, S., Spitz, I.M. and Bouchard, P. (1994). Effect of administration of a gonadotropin-releasing hormone (GnRH) antagonist (Nal-Glu) during the periovulatory period: the luteinizing hormone surge requires secretion of GnRH. *J. Clin. Endocrinol. Metab.,* **78**, 343–7

32. Leroy, I., d'Acremont, M.F., Brailly-Tabard, S., Frydman, R., de Mouzon, J. and Bouchard, P. (1994). A single injection of a gonadotropin-releasing hormone (GnRH) antagonist (Cetrorelix) postpones the luteinizing hormone (LH) surge: further evidence for the role of GnRH during the LH surge. *Fertil. Steril.,* **62**, 461–7

33. Olivennes, F., Fanchin, R., Bouchard, P., Taieb, J., Selva, J. and Frydman, R. (1995). Scheduled administration of a gonadotrophin-releasing hormone antagonist (Cetrorelix) on day 8 of *in vitro* fertilization cycles: a pilot study. *Hum. Reprod.,* **10**, 1382–6

34. Diedrich, K., Diedrich, C., Santos, E., Zoll, C., Al-Hasani, S., Reissmann, T., Krebs, D. and Klingmuller, D. (1994). Suppression of the endogenous luteinizing hormone surge by the gonadotrophin-releasing hormone antagonist Cetrorelix during ovarian stimulation. *Hum. Reprod.,* **9**, 788–91

35. Reissmann, T., Felberbaum, R., Diedrich, K., Engel, J., Comaru-Schally, A.M. and Schally, A.V. (1995). Development and applications of LHRH antagonists in the treatment of infertility. *Hum. Reprod.,* **10**, 1974–81

36. Kettel, L.M., Murphy, A.A., Morales, A.J., Rivier, J., Vale, W. and Yen, S.S.C. (1993). Rapid regression of uterine leiomyomas in response to daily administration of gonadotropin-releasing hormone antagonist. *Fertil. Steril.,* **60**, 642–6

37. Gonzalez-Barcena, D., Perez, E., Cardenas, I., Fuentes, M., Macedo, M., Comaru-Schally, A.M. and Schally, A.V. (1996). Regression of uterine leiomyomas after the administration of the new LH-RH antagonist cetrorelix (SB-75). In *10th International Congress of Endocrinology (ICE '96),* June, San Francisco, abstr. P3-385, p. 851

38. Peters, C.A. and Walsh, P.C. (1987). The effect of nafarelin acetate, a luteinizing hormone-releasing hormone agonist, on benign prostatic hyperplasia. *N. Engl. J. Med.,* **317**, 599–604

39. Gabrilove, J.L., Levine, A.C., Kirschenbaum, A. and Droller, M. (1986). Effect of a GnRH analog (leuprolide) on benign prostatic hypertrophy. *J. Clin. Endocrinol. Metab.,* **64**, 1331–3

40. Tolis, G., Ackman, D., Stellos, A., Mehta, A., Labrie, F., Fazekas, A., Comaru-Schally, A.M. and Schally, A.V. (1982). Tumor growth inhibition in patients with prostatic carcinoma treated with luteinizing hormone-releasing agonists. *Proc. Natl. Acad. Sci. USA*, **79**, 1658–62
41. Redding, T.W. and Schally, A.V. (1981). Inhibition of prostate tumor growth in two rat models by chronic administration of D-Trp-6-LH-RH. *Proc. Natl. Acad. Sci. USA*, **78**, 6509–12
42. Crawford, E.D., Eisenberger, M.A., McLeod, D.G., Spaulding, J.T., Benson, R., Dorr, F.A., Blumenstein, B.A., Davis, M.A. and Goodman, P.J. (1989). A controlled trial of leuprolide with and without flutamide in prostatic carcinoma. *N. Engl. J. Med.*, **321**, 419–24
43. The Leuprolide Study Group (1984). Leuprolide versus diethylstilbestrol for metastatic prostate cancer. *N. Engl. J. Med.*, **311**, 1281–6
44. Sogani, P.C. and Fair, W.R. (1987). Treatment of advanced prostatic cancer. *Urol. Clin. North Am.*, **14**, 253–71
45. Ahmann, F.R., Citrin, D.L., deHaan, H.A., Guinan, P., Jordan, V.C., Kreis, W., Scott, M. and Trump, D.L. (1987). Zoladex: a sustained-release, monthly luteinizing hormone-releasing hormone analogue for the treatment of advanced prostate cancer. *J. Clin. Oncol.*, **5**, 912–17
46. Parmar, H., Lightman, S.L., Allen, L., Phillips, R.H., Edwards, L. and Schally, A.V. (1985). Randomised controlled study of orchidectomy vs long-acting D-Trp-6-LH-RH microcapsules in advanced prostatic carcinoma. *Lancet*, **2**, 1201–5
47. Sharifi, R., Soloway, M. and Leuprolide Study Group (1990). Clinical study of leuprolide depot formulation in the treatment of advanced prostate cancer. *J. Urol.*, **143**, 68–72
48. Korkut, E., Bokser, L., Groot, K. and Schally, A.V. (1991). Inhibition of growth of experimental Dunning R3327 rat prostate cancer with sustained delivery systems (microcapsules and microgranules) of an antagonist of luteinizing hormone-releasing hormone. *Proc. Natl. Acad. Sci. USA*, **88**, 844–8
49. Redding, T.W., Schally, A.V., Radulovic, S., Milovanovic, S., Szepehazi, K. and Isaacs, J. (1982). Sustained release formulation of LH-RH antagonists SB-75 inhibit proliferation and enhance the apoptotic cell death of human prostate carcinoma (PC-82) in male nude mice. *Cancer Res.*, **52**, 2538–44
50. Jungwirth, A., Galvan, G., Pinski, J., Halmos, G., Szepeshazi, K., Cai, R.-Z., Groot, K. and Schally, A.V. (1997). LH-RH antagonist Cetrorelix (SB-75) and bombesin antagonist RC-3940-II inhibit the growth of androgen-independent PC-3 prostate cancer in nude mice. *Prostate*, **33**, in press.
51. Gonzalez-Barcena, D., Vadillo, B.M., Cortez, M.A., Fuentes, G.M., Cardenas, C.I., Comaru-Schally, A.M. and Schally, A.V. (1995). Luteinizing hormone-releasing hormone antagonist Cetrorelix as primary single therapy in patients with advanced prostatic cancer and paraplegia due to metastatic invasion of spinal cord. *Urology*, **45**, 275–81
52. Gonzalez-Barcena, D., Schally, A.V., Comaru-Schally, A.M., Cortez-Morales, A., Vadillo-Buenfil, M. and Molina-Ayala, A. (1995). Treatment of patients with advanced prostate cancer with LHRH antagonist Cetrorelix. In Filicori, M. and Flamigni, C. (eds.) *Treatment with GnRH analogs: Controversies and Perspectives, Proceedings of a Satellite Symposium of the 15th World Congress on Fertility and Sterility*, pp. 139–44, September, Bologna. (Carnforth, UK: Parthenon Publishing)
53. Santen, R.J., Manni, A., Harvey, H. and Redmond, C. (1990). Endocrine treatment of breast cancer in women. *Endocr. Rev.*, **11**, 221–65
54. Kaufmann, M., Jonat, W., Kleeburg, U., Eirmann, W., Janicke, F., Hilfrich, J., Kreienberg, R., Albrecht, M., Weitzel, H.K., Schmid, H., Strunz, P., Schachner-Wunschmann, E., Bastert, G. and Maass, H. (1989). The German Zoladex trial group: goserelin, a depot gonadotropin releasing hormone agonist in the treatment of premenopausal patients with metastatic breast cancer. *J. Clin. Oncol.*, **7**, 1113–19
55. Plowman, P.N., Nicholson, R.I. and Walker, K.J. (1986). Responses in post-menopausal breast cancer with an LH-RH analog (ICI 118,630). *Eur. J. Cancer Clin. Oncol.*, **22**, 746–9
56. Walker, K.J., Walker, R.F., Turkes, A., Robertson, J.R.F., Blamey, R.W., Griffiths, K. and Nicholson, R.I. (1989). Endocrine effects of combination antioestrogen and LH-RH agonist therapy in premenopausal patients with advanced breast cancer. *Eur. J. Cancer Clin. Oncol.*, **25**, 651–4
57. Fekete, M., Wittliff, J.L. and Schally, A.V.

(1989). Characteristics and distribution of receptors for [D-Trp^6]-luteinizing hormone-releasing hormone, somatostatin, epidermal growth factor, and sex steroids in 500 biopsy samples of human breast cancer. *J. Clin. Lab. Anal.*, **3**, 137–47

58. Szende, B., Srkalovic, G., Groot, K., Lapis, K. and Schally, A.V. (1990). Growth inhibition of mouse MXT mammary tumor by the luteinizing hormone-releasing hormone antagonist SB-75. *J. Natl. Cancer Inst.*, **82**, 513–17

59. Yano, T., Pinski, J., Szepeshazi, K., Halmos, G., Radulovic, S., Groot, K. and Schally, A.V. (1994). Inhibitory effect of bombesin/gastrin releasing peptide (GRP) antagonist RC-3095 and LH-RH antagonist SB-75 on growth of MCF-7 MIII human breast cancer xenografts in athymic nude mice. *Cancer*, **73**, 1229–38

60. Emons, G., Pahwa, G.S., Brack, C., Sturm, R., Oberheuser, F. and Knuppen, R. (1989). Gonadotropin releasing hormone binding sites in human epithelial ovarian carcinomata. *Eur. J. Cancer Clin. Oncol.*, **25**, 215–21

61. Emons, G. and Schally, A.V. (1994). The use of luteinizing hormone releasing hormone agonsts and antagonists in gynaecological cancers. *Hum. Reprod.*, **7**, 1364–79

62. Yano, T., Pinski, J., Halmos, G., Szepeshazi, K., Groot, K. and Schally, A.V. (1994). Inhibition of growth of OV-1063 human epithelial ovarian cancer xenografts in nude mice by treatment with luteinizing hormone-releasing hormone antagonist SB-75. *Proc. Natl. Acad. Sci. USA*, **91**, 7090–4

63. Parmar, H., Phillips, R.H., Rustin, G., Hanham, I.W., Schally, A.V. and Lightman, S.L. (1988). Response to [D-Trp^6]LHRH (Decapeptyl) microcapsules in advanced ovarian cancer. *Br. Med. J.*, **296**, 1229

64. Parmar, H., Phillips, R.H., Rustin, G., Lightman, S.L. and Schally, A.V. (1988). Therapy of advanced ovarian cancer with D-Trp^6-LH-RH (decapetyl) microcapsules. *Biomed. Pharmacother.*, **42**, 531–48

65. Emons, G., Ortmann, O., Teichert, H.-M., Fassl, H.G., Löhrs, U., Kullander, S., Kauppila, A., Ayalon, D., Schally, A., Heinrich, C. and Oberheuser, F. (1996). Luteinizing hormone-releasing hormone agonist triptorelin in combination with cytotoxic chemotherapy in advanced epithelial ovarian cancer – a prospective double blinded randomized trial. *Cancer*, **78**, 1452–60

66. Shirahige, Y., Cook, C.B., Pinski, J., Halmos, G., Nair, R. and Schally, A.V. (1994). Treatment with luteinizing hormone-releasing hormone antagonist SB-75 decreases levels of epidermal growth factor receptor and its mRNA in OV-1063 human epithelial ovarian cancer xenografts in nude mice. *Int. J. Oncol.*, **5**, 1031–5

67. Srkalovic, G., Wittliff, J.L. and Schally, A.V. (1990). Detection and partial characterization of receptors for [D-Trp^6]-luteinizing hormone-releasing hormone and epidermal growth factor in human endometrial carcinoma. *Cancer Res.*, **50**, 1841–6

68. Emons, G., Schroder, B., Ortmann, O., Westphalen, S., Schulz, K.-D. and Schally, A.V. (1993). High affinity binding and direct antiproliferative effects of LH-RH agonists and antagonists in human endometrial cancer cell lines. *J. Clin. Endocrinol. Metab.*, **77**, 1458–64

69. Szende, B., Srkalovic, G., Schally, A.V., Lapis, K. and Groot, K. (1990). Inhibitory effects of analogs of luteinizing hormone-releasing hormone (LH-RH) and somatostatin on pancreatic cancers in hamsters: events which accompany tumor regression. *Cancer*, **65**, 2279–90

70. Szende, B., Srkalovic, G., Groot, K., Lapis, K. and Schally, A.V. (1990). Regression of nitrosamine-induced pancreatic cancers in hamsters treated with LH-RH antagonists or agonists. *Cancer Res.*, **50**, 3716–21

GnRH analogs in gynecology: agonists and antagonists

R. Felberbaum and K. Diedrich

Introduction

The disclosure of the neuroendocrine control of the menstrual cycle in adult women may be one of the most important challenges of the last three decades within gynecology. It has had a marked clinical impact on the treatment of hormonal disorders in gynecology and pediatrics, infertility treatment and oncology. As early as 1932 the German scientists Hohlweg and Junkmann postulated an active sexuality center situated over the pituitary gland as the organ with a direct stimulatory effect on the ovaries[1]. In 1952 it was shown that the stimulatory activity of the anterior pituitary gland depended on hypothalamic function, revealing a neural control mechanism[2–4]. The hypothalamus is the super-ordinate organ, releasing gonadotropin-releasing hormone (GnRH) in a pulsatile manner. GnRH is a peptide composed of ten amino acid residues; its existence was postulated by Green and Harris in 1947 and it was first isolated and characterized in 1971 by two independent groups, after they had competed against each other for 10 years. Schally and Guillemin were awarded the Nobel prize for their pioneering work in 1977[5–7]. Figure 1 shows the amino acid sequence of native GnRH. GnRH is secreted by the neural cells of the nucleus arcuatus in the mediobasal portion of the hypothalamus. The axons in these neurons are in intimate contact with the vessels of the hypothalamic–pituitary portal vein system. The pulsatile release of GnRH by the hypothalamic neurons causes the gonadotropic cells of the pituitary gland, which make up about 10% of its cell mass, to release the gonadotropins follicle-stimulating hormone

```
1    2    3    4    5    6    7    8    9    10
pGlu - His - Trp - Ser - Tyr - Gly - Leu - Arg - Pro - Gly-NH2
```

Figure 1 Amino acid sequence of native GnRH

(FSH) and luteinizing hormone (LH), also in a pulsatile fashion. FSH and LH in turn control follicular maturation and gonadal sexual steroid biosynthesis. Circulating GnRH is short-lived, with a plasma half-life of 2–5 min, due to a rapid enzymatic degradation by peptidases. These preferentially interact with the peptide bonds in position 6 of the molecule. This short half-life ensures that the hypothalamic pulses of GnRH are recognized as single events by the pituitary receptors. The extraordinary importance of this mechanism with regard to the maintenance of normal ovarian function was recognized in 1978. At that time it was shown that GnRH, when given continuously, caused a decrease in LH and FSH levels, followed by an arrest of follicular maturation as well as of sexual steroid biosynthesis[8].

The spontaneous activity of the so-called hypothalamic pulse generator is modulated by a variety of neurotransmitters (e.g. noradrenaline, γ-amino butyric acid (GABA), dopamine, serotonin), neuropeptides (e.g. neuropeptide Y, proenkephaline, prodynorphin, corticotropin-releasing hormone), endogenous opioids (β-endorphin) and steroids such as estradiol, progesterone and testosterone. In humans the frequency of pulses is between 70 and 90 min. Once the serum concentration of FSH rises above an individual threshold level, a cohort of follicles in both ovaries is recruited for further development[9]. Normally this elevation of FSH starts in the late luteal phase of the biphasic cycle and is maintained until the early follicular phase of the subsequent cycle. The recruitment of the cohort is terminated on cycle day 3, when selection of the dominant follicle occurs. This phase is characterized by an exponential rise in the level of serum estradiol, followed by a fall in the levels of FSH and LH, due to a negative feedback mechanism. After serum estradiol reaches preovulatory serum concentrations of about 150–500 pg/ml, a sudden and pronounced increase in LH occurs, due to a positive feedback mechanism, and this results in the induction of ovulation about 10–12 h after the LH maximum[10].

GnRH/GnRH-receptor interaction

GnRH binds to specific transmembrane receptors in the gonadotropic cells. These represent about 10% of the total weight of the anterior pituitary gland. In general, they can produce LH as well as FSH, but the ratio of these hormones is dependent on the stage of the cycle. Both the synthesis and the liberation of LH and FSH are regulated by GnRH. When the GnRH receptor is occupied, complexes are formed by microaggregation of the GnRH receptors. These complexes seem to be the basis for the action of GnRH. Their importance is emphasized by the fact that it is possible to convert a GnRH antagonist into a potent agonist by the use of 'double-linked' antibodies[11]. In addition to microaggregation, binding to the GnRH receptor on the surface of a gonadotropic cell leads to a change in the receptor conformation itself. These changes induce the calcium-dependent release of gonadotropins, a process involving many other second messengers such as phospholipids, diacyl glycerol, protein kinase C, inositol phosphates, arachidonic acid, leukotrienes and cyclic adenosine monophosphate (cAMP)[12]. After the binding of GnRH to its receptors, the complex formed is internalized and degraded, although internalization is not necessary for the liberation of the gonadotropins. The number of GnRH receptors is subject to physiological alteration, showing a progressive decrease in the elderly and during lactation and an increase after ovariectomy[13].

GnRH agonists

After the amino acid sequence of GnRH had been successfully isolated and analyzed, it was possible by modification of the molecular structure of this decapeptide to obtain analog compounds with agonistic effects[14–16]. The modifications introduced into the sequence affected mainly positions 6 and 10, and it was found that changes in both positions resulted in cumulative effects on the potency[17]. Table 1 shows the amino acid sequences of GnRH agonists currently used. These compounds have a 100–200 times higher binding affinity for the GnRH receptors than the native molecule. The agonists were originally designed to enhance their affinity for the GnRH receptors of the gonadotropic cells as well as their duration of action. This made them more resistant against enzymatic digestion, and, after a short period of stimulation of FSH and LH secretion (the so-called 'flare-up'), led to a reduction of GnRH receptors on the cell membrane of the gonadotropic cells. The flare-up effect leads within 12 h to a five-fold increase of basic serum levels of FSH and about a 10-fold increase in the basic serum concentrations of LH, while the estradiol concentrations are elevated about four-fold[18]. As a result of the subsequent reduction in number of GnRH receptors, a paradoxical suppression of pituitary gonadotropin synthesis and liberation occurs. After a period of about 14–21 days of constant impact from GnRH agonists, the pituitary gland becomes completely desensitized and refractory to a GnRH stimulus. Clearly, the degradation of the agonist/receptor complexes by lysosomal enzymes cannot be compensated

Table 1 Amino acid sequences of native gonadotropin-releasing hormone (GnRH) and its currently used agonistic analogs

	1	2	3	4	5	6	7	8	9	10
GnRH	pGlu	His	Trp	Ser	Tyr	Gly	Leu	Arg	Pro	Gly-NH$_2$
Buserelin	1	2	3	4	5	D-Ser	7	8	9	Ethylamide
Goserelin	1	2	3	4	5	D-Ser	7	8	9	Az-Gly
Leuprorelin	1	2	3	4	5	D-Leu	7	8	9	Ethylamide
Triptorelin	1	2	3	4	5	D-Trp	7	8	9	Gly-NH$_2$
Nafarelin	1	2	3	4	5	D-Nal(2)	7	8	9	Gly-NH$_2$

by the normal receptor turnover and, in addition, post-receptor mechanisms are uncoupled. Decreased levels of LH and FSH result in the arrest of follicular development. This fall in gonadotropins is followed by a fall in sex steroids to the castrate range. These phenomena represent the basis for the clinical use of GnRH agonists. When the treatment is stopped, resumption of pituitary gonadotropin secretion usually begins within 2 weeks, while full restoration of ovarian function takes place in about 6 weeks[19]. Currently, agonists can be administered by daily subcutaneous injection or nasal spray, or can be formulated as depot preparations for monthly injections.

Clinical indications for the use of GnRH agonists

GnRH agonists have become well established compounds wherever an iatrogenically induced, fully reversible and limited castration of the patient is desired. This is useful in the treatment of sexual steroid-dependent benign diseases such as precocious puberty, endometriosis, uterine fibroids, malignancies such as sexual steroid-receptor-positive breast cancer and prostatic cancer and in controlled ovarian hyperstimulation within assisted reproductive techniques. Regarding ovarian cancer, the situation is not yet clear. The administration of GnRH agonists as part of the so-called decapeptyl study has produced no therapeutic benefit (Table 2).

Table 2 Clinical indications for GnRH analogs: agonists and antagonists

Uterine fibroma
Endometriosis
Precocious puberty
Assisted reproduction techniques
Estrogen receptor-positive breast cancer in the premenopausal woman
Prostatic cancer

Ovarian cancer?
Endometrial cancer?

Uterine fibroids and endometriosis

Myomas are the most frequent benign tumors in women of reproductive age. Among women entering menopause after the age of 50, about 40% develop myomas. Internationally, uterus myomatosus is the most frequent indication for gynecological surgery. GnRH pretreatment has become a standard procedure in patients with larger myomas who are scheduled for a fertility-preserving operation, in those with hemoglobin-reducing hypermenorrhea and in those requiring a hysteroscopic ablation of submucosal fibroids. Therapy is efficient and reduces the size of the myomas by about 50% within 3 months[20]. In the case of endometriosis GnRH agonists as well as danazol have been proven to be efficient therapeutic tools within the 'three step concept' (primary operation, medical treatment, second-look operation). All symptoms of endometriosis can be relieved by long-term treatment with GnRH agonists for about 6 months[21].

Metastatic breast cancer

During the last 10 years GnRH agonists have been proven to achieve an objective response of about 40% in premenopausal and about 10% in postmenopausal women with metastatic breast cancer[22]. Patients with estrogen receptor-positive breast cancer showed an objective response more frequently than patients with receptor-negative tumors[23]. Nevertheless, appreciable response rates in estrogen receptor-poor patients have also been described[24].

Side-effects of GnRH agonist therapy

The side-effects of long-term GnRH agonist therapy cannot be neglected. Hot flushes occur in about 80%, headaches in about 30%, nausea and dizziness in about 20%. Furthermore, younger women are at risk for development of osteoporosis. Loss of bone mass is reported at 3.4–7.4% after 6 months of continuous therapy, for instance in the case of severe endometriosis[25,26].

GnRH agonists within controlled ovarian hyperstimulation

The occurrence of premature LH surges is a main reason for a relatively low efficacy of ovarian stimulation by human menopausal gonadotropin (hMG) in *in vitro* fertilization (IVF) programs. In addition, these LH surges have a negative impact on the quality of the oocytes and embryos and subsequently on the rate of pregnancy[27]. By introducing the GnRH agonists into the stimulation protocols of programs using assisted reproduction techniques (ART), an improved synchronization of follicular maturation and an important reduction of premature luteinization to less than 2% could be achieved[28]. While the 'flare protocols' (short protocol and ultrashort protocol) try to harvest the initial flare-up effect for follicular stimulation, the so-called long protocol aims at desensitizing the pituitary before hMG stimulation starts. For this purpose the GnRH agonist is administered either daily subcutaneously or transnasally or in the form of a subcutaneous or intramuscular depot preparation from the mid-luteal phase or early follicular phase. The advantage of starting medication in the mid-luteal phase is that the flare-up coincides with the physiological rise in gonadotropins. By 14 days after the initiation of GnRH agonist treatment, it can be assumed that the hypothalamic–pituitary axis has essentially been decoupled.

Stimulation begins with 2 ampules of hMG daily on days 1, 2 and 3. On days 4–7 the patient receives 3 ampules of hMG daily and, from day 8 on, regular measurements of estradiol and LH are taken along with transvaginal ultrasound measurements of the follicles. As soon as one or preferably several follicles measuring 20 mm are identified, and the estradiol level increases to about 300–500 pg/ml per follicle larger than 17 mm, 10 000 IU of human chorionic gonadotropin (hCG) are administered intramuscularly. Follicular puncture monitored by transvaginal sonography is performed 36 h later. The timing of the puncture has become fully calculable under this regime and can be managed in relation to clinical necessities as well as patients' wishes (Figure 2). The long protocol synchronizes follicle maturation and makes it possible to select a larger number of follicles or oocytes for IVF than the other protocols. Regarding pregnancy rates, retrospective studies have shown a significant benefit for patients treated according to the long protocol compared with those treated by a 'flare protocol'[29]. In prospective studies pregnancy rates were also higher after long-protocol stimulation (25.7% vs. 16.6%), but these differences were not significant[30] (Table 3). The long protocol is

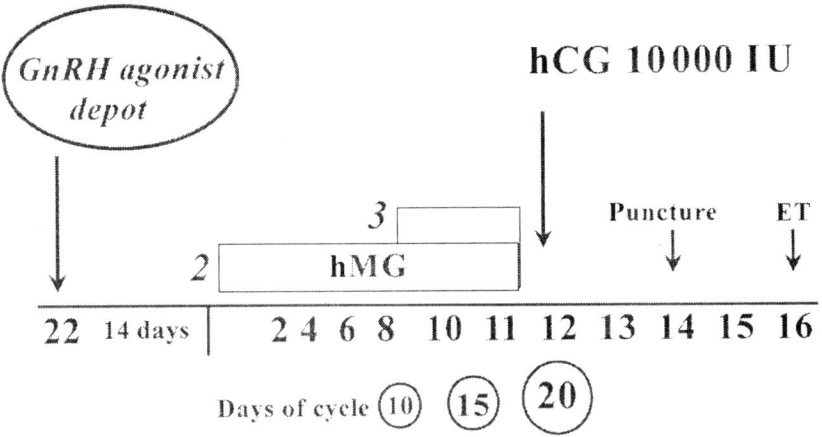

Figure 2 Controlled ovarian hyperstimulation with hMG and GnRH agonist treatment: the 'long' protocol. ET, embryo transfer

Table 3 GnRH agonists in IVF: prospective studies (long vs. short protocol)

References	hMG (ampules)		Embryos (n)		Pregnancy rate (%)	
	Short	Long	Short	Long	Short	Long
Hedon[38]	27.3	36.5	2.9	4	12.8	37.5
Zorn[39]	20.5	39.5	1.8	2.3	25.3	26.6
Remorgida[40]	23.7	31.7	—	—	34.7	36.4
Tan et al.[30]	24	27	1	3	16.6	25.7
Pados[41]	27.9	37.7	4	6.3	19.4	25.8

most used at present for controlled ovarian hyperstimulation. However, it has the disadvantage of a long treatment period until desensitization occurs, as well as of relatively high costs, due to an increased requirement for hMG[31].

GnRH antagonists

The pharmacological mode of action of the GnRH antagonists is completely different. Instead of 'down-regulation' and desensitization a classic competitive blockade of the GnRH receptors on the cell membrane of the gonadotropic cells takes place. Without any intrinsic activity of these compounds the 'flare-up effect' is completely avoided. The antagonists block the receptors and inhibit their microaggregation, and the post-receptor mechanisms are not initiated. Within 8 h suppressed serum concentrations of LH can be achieved[32].

It was shown that a short application of the antagonist Nal-Glu in the mid-cycle phase of healthy women with normal cycles was able to avoid the mid-cycle LH peak and, because of this, spontaneous ovulation[33]. The first generation of GnRH antagonists caused important problems due to allergic reactions, which inhibited their clinical introduction, but Cetrorelix, as a representative of the youngest generation of these compounds, seems to avoid these disturbances. It is now used in clinical phase II and III studies[34].

Cetrorelix was introduced in our IVF program to examine whether it was possible to avoid premature LH surges and to lower the interference with the hypothalamic–hypophyseal–ovarian axis, which would resemble a more physiological approach of treatment.

A total of 35 patients, all suffering from tubal infertility with no other observed infertility factors, were treated with hMG, starting on day 2. From day 7 until induction of

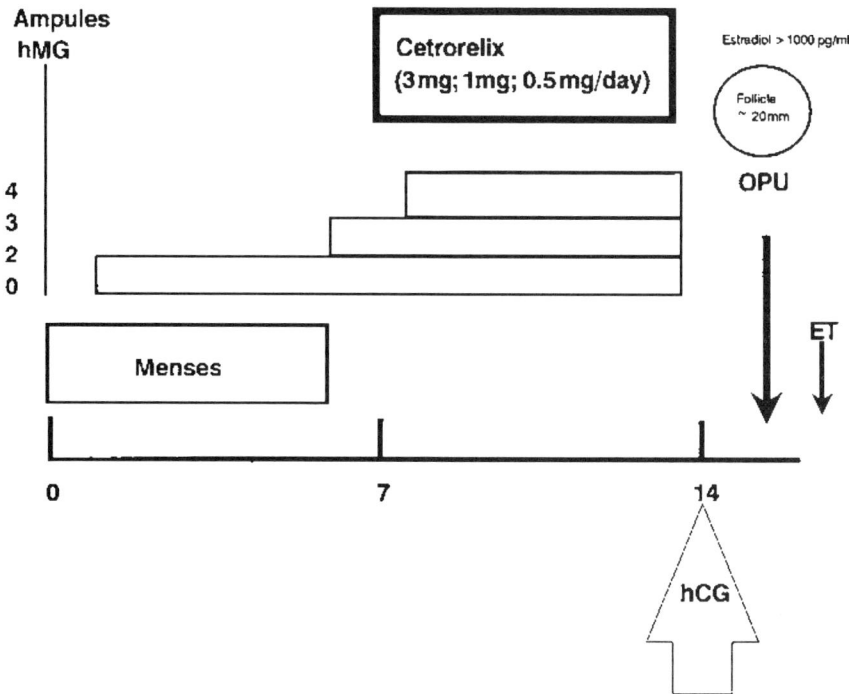

Figure 3 Controlled ovarian hyperstimulation with hMG and concomitant GnRH antagonist treatment (Cetrorelix) in different dosages: the 'Lübeck protocol'. OPU, ovum pick-up; ET, embryo transfer

ovulation by hCG, 12 patients were treated with 3 mg/day Cetrorelix subcutaneously. As no premature LH surge was observed, 12 patients received 1 mg/day Cetrorelix and another 11 patients received 0.5 mg/day Cetrorelix. When estradiol values and sonographic findings indicated satisfactory follicular maturation, hCG was administered (Figure 3: the 'Lübeck protocol'). Oocyte pick-up, IVF and embryo transfer were carried out as usual at our IVF center. During the treatment cycles blood samples were drawn daily for measurement of estradiol, progesterone, LH and FSH.

No premature LH surge was observed. The mean courses of FSH and LH in the three different dosage groups were quite similar, with a profound suppression of LH (Figure 4). Estradiol concentrations reflected satisfactory follicular maturation, with a higher increase of estradiol levels in the group treated with 0.5 mg/day Cetrorelix. The fertilization rates of the recovered oocytes were 45.3% in the 3-mg group, 53.2% in the 1-mg group and 67.7% in the 0.5-mg group. In the 3-mg group, 106 oocytes were retrieved and 30 embryos replaced after IVF. Of these, 36.7% were considered 'excellent' by microscopic–morphological criteria. In the 1-mg group, 94 oocytes were retrieved and 28 embryos replaced, and 53.6% of them were judged 'excellent'. In the 0.5-mg group, 27 of 127 retrieved oocytes were replaced as embryos after IVF, and 37% were 'excellent' (Table 4). The average use of hMG ampules was 30, 27 and 26, respectively. Thus, 0.5 mg/day Cetrorelix proved to be sufficient to avoid the premature LH surge during controlled ovarian hyperstimulation. The ovarian response to stimulation by hMG under this dosage seemed to be slightly more sensitive than in patients treated with higher dosages of antagonists. Regarding fertilization rates and the use of hMG, the lower dosage was the most favorable[35].

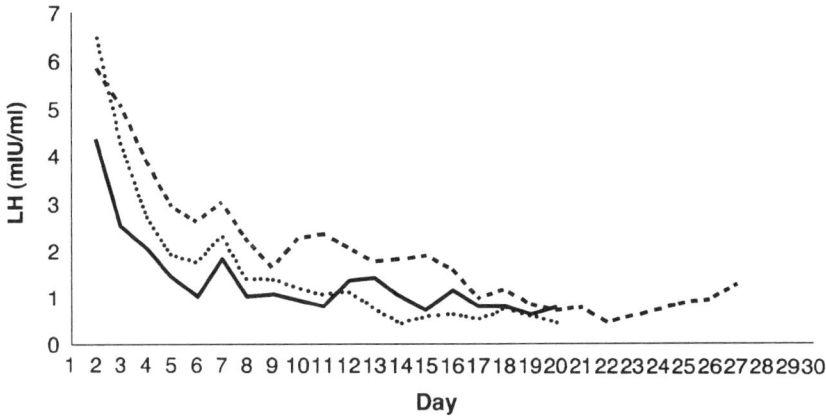

Figure 4 Mean serum levels of luteinizing hormone (LH) under controlled ovarian hyperstimulation with hMG and concomitant GnRH antagonist treatment (Cetrorelix) in different dosages: 0.5 mg (unbroken line); 1 mg (dotted line); and 3.0 mg (dashed line)

Table 4 Controlled ovarian stimulation with hMG and concomitant GnRH antagonist treatment (Cetrorelix) in different dosages

	3 mg	1 mg	0.5 mg
No. of oocytes	106	94	127
Fertilization rate (%)	45.3	53.2	67.7
No. of embryos	30	28	27
'Excellent' embryos (%)	36.7	53.6	37

GnRH antagonists and uterine fibroids

Without any doubt most of our clinical experience with GnRH antagonists has been gained within assisted reproduction techniques. The only clinical indication for which we are able to present our own and recent data is the uterine fibroid. In 1993, for the first time, reduction of uterine fibroids by daily administration of the GnRH antagonist Nal-Glu was reported, achieving a shrinkage rate of 50% within 3 months, and avoiding any flare-up effect[36]. Since August 1995 we have been provided by the ASTA-Medica AG (Frankfurt/Main-Germany) with the first depot preparation of a GnRH antagonist ever used for this clinical indication. The Cetrorelix-pamoat microparticle formulation is an amorphous compound with microparticles in a range between 80 and 120 μm, which, due to their low solubility, produce the slow release effect after intramuscular administration. By a two-times administration of 60 mg of this compound followed by another 60 mg or 30 mg after 3 or 4 weeks, depending on the degree of sexual steroid suppression (< 50 pg/ml), we were able to suppress gonadotropin secretion as well as estradiol concentrations for about 6–8 weeks, achieving a mean shrinkage rate of the volume of the leading fibroids of about 35% (Figures 5 and 6). No 'flare-up', as in the case of GnRH agonists, was observed[37]. This could be an important advantage, as the 'flare-up effect' cannot be in favor of a sex steroid-dependent disease.

Conclusions

GnRH agonists are valuable pharmaceutical tools for the therapy of sex steroid-dependent diseases and for controlled ovarian hyperstimulation. However, from what is known today, the advantages of GnRH antagonists are most evident, in our opinion. Suitable sustained delivery systems and the GnRH antagonists with sufficient oral bioavailability represent the present and future of these important compounds.

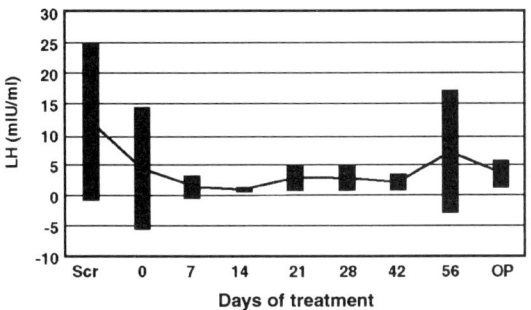

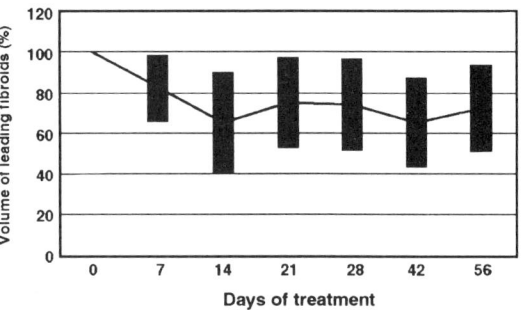

Figure 5 Mean serum levels of luteinizing hormone (LH) and SEM under Cetrorelix-depot treatment for 8 weeks in case of uterus myomatosus. Scr, screening; OP, day of operation

Figure 6 Mean shrinkage rate of the leading fibroids volume under Cetrorelix-depot treatment of 8 weeks in case of uterus myomatosus

References

1. Hohlweg, W. and Junkmann, K. (1932). Die hormonal-nervöse Regulierung der Funktion des Hypophysenvorderlappens. *Klin. Wochenschr.*, **11**, 321–3
2. Harris, G.W. and Jacobsohn, D. (1952). Functional grafts of the anterior pituitary gland. *Proc. R. Soc.*, **139**, 263–76
3. Martini, L., Fraschini, F. and Motta, M. (1968). Neural control of anterior pituitary functions. *Rec. Prog. Horm. Res.*, **24**, 429–39
4. Schally, A.V., Arimura, A., Bowers, C.Y., Kastin, A.J., Sawano, S. and Redding, T.W. (1968). Hypothalamic neurohormones regulating anterior pituitary function. *Rec. Prog. Horm. Res.*, **24**, 497–581
5. Green, J.D. and Harris, G.W. (1947). The nervovascular link between the neurohypophysis and adenohypophysis. *J. Endocrinol.*, **5**, 136–46
6. Burgus R., Butcher, M. and Amoss, M. (1972). Primary structure of the ovine hypothalamic luteinizing hormone-releasing factor (LFR). *Proc. Natl. Acad. Sci. USA*, **69**, 278–82
7. Matsuo, H., Baba, Y., Nair, R.M.G., Arimura, A. and Schally, A.V. (1971). Structure of porcine LH and FSH releasing factor. I. The proposed amino acid sequence. *Biochem. Biophys. Res. Commun.*, **43**, 1334–9
8. Knobil, E. (1980). The neuroendocrine control of the menstrual cycle. *Rec. Prog. Horm. Res.*, **36**, 53–88
9. Hillier, S.G. (1994). Current concepts of the role of FSH and LH in folliculogenesis. *Hum. Reprod.*, **9**, 188–91
10. Diedrich, K., Al-Hasani, S., Van der Ven, H., Diedrich, C. and Krebs, D. (1990). In vitro Fertilisation und Embryotransfer. In Diedrich, K. (ed.) *Neue Wege in Diagnostik und Therapie der Sterilität*, p. 169. (Stuttgart: Enke Verlag)
11. Blum, J.J. and Conn, P.M. (1982). Gonadotrophin-releasing hormone stimulation of luteinizing hormone release: a ligand–receptor–effector model. *Proc. Natl. Acad. Sci. USA*, **79**, 7307–11
12. Kiesel, L. and Runnenbaum, B. (1993). Gonadotropin-releasing Hormon und Analog – Physiologie und Pharmakologie. *Gynäkol. Geburtsh. Rundsch.*, **32**, 22–30
13. Clayton, R.N. and Catt, K.J. (1981). Gonadotropin-releasing hormone receptors: characterization, physiological regulation and relationship to reproductive function. *Endocr. Rev.*, **2**, 186–209
14. Koch, Y., Baram, T., Hazum, E. and Fridkin, M. (1977). Resistance to enzymatic degradation of LH-RH analogs processing increased biological activity. *Biochem. Biophys. Res. Commun.*, **74**, 488–92
15. Clayton, R.N. and Catt, K.J. (1980). Receptor binding affinity of gonadotrophin-releasing hormone analogs: analysis by radio ligand receptor assay. *Endocrinology*, **106**, 1154–9

16. Schally, A.V., Comaru-Schally, A.M. and Hollander, V. (1993). Hypothalamic and other peptide hormones. In Hollander, J.R., Frei, E. and Bast, R.C. (eds.) *Cancer Medicine*, 3rd edn, p. 827. (Philadelphia: Lea & Febiger)
17. Coy, D.H., Horvath, A., Nekola, M.V., Coy, E.J., Ercheigyi, J. and Schally, A.V. (1982). Peptide antagonists of LH-RH: large increases in antiovulatory activities produced by basic D-amino acids in the six position. *Endocrinology*, **110**, 1445–7
18. Lemay, A., Maheux, R., Faure, N., Jean, C. and Fazekas, A.T.A. (1984). Reversible hypogonadism induced by a luteinizing hormone-releasing hormone (LH-RH) agonist (Buserelin) as a new therapeutic approach for endometriosis. *Fertil. Steril.*, **41**, 863–71
19. Gordon, K. and Hodgen, G.D. (1993). Evolving role of gonadotrophin-releasing hormone antagonists. *Trends Endocrinol. Metab.*, **3**, 259–63
20. Healy, D.L. and Vollenhoven, B.J. (1992). The role of GnRH agonists in the treatment of uterine fibroids. *Br. J. Obstet. Gynaecol.*, **99**(Suppl. 7), 23–6
21. Franssen, A.M., Zijlstra, J.A., Kauer, F.M., Rolland, R. and Chadha, D.R. (1989). Endometriosis: treatment with the gonadotropin-releasing hormone agonist buserelin. *Fertil. Steril.*, **51**, 401–8
22. Klijn, J.G.M. (1992). LH-RH agonist in treatment of metastatic breast cancer: ten years experience. In *LH-RH Agonists and Antagonists. Recent Results in Cancer Research*, Vol. 124, pp. 75–90. (Berlin: Springer Verlag)
23. Dixon, A.R., Robertson, J.F.R., Jackson, L., Nicholson, R.I., Walker, K.J. and Blamay, R.W. (1990). Goserelin (Zoladex) in premenopausal advanced breast cancer: duration of response and survival. *Br. J. Cancer*, **62**, 868–70
24. Kaufmann, M., Jonat, W., Klieberg, U., Eiermann, W., Jänicke, F., Hilfrich, J., Kreinberg, R., Albrecht, M., Weitzel, H.K., Schmid, H., Stunz, P., Schachner-Wünschmann, E., Bastert, G., Maas, H. and German Zoladex Trial Group (1989). Goserelin, a depot gonadotrophin-releasing hormone agonist in the treatment of premenopausal patients with metastatic breast cancer. *J. Clin. Oncol.*, **7**, 1113–19
25. Uemura, T., Mohri, J., Osada, H., Suzuki, N., Katagiri, N. and Minaguchi, H. (1994). Effect of gonadotropin-releasing hormone agonist on the bone mineral density of patients with endometriosis. *Fertil. Steril.*, **62**, 246–50
26. Matta, W., Shaw, R.W., Hesp, R. and Evans, R. (1988). Reversible trabecular bone density loss following induced hypooestrogenism with GnRH-analog Buserelin in premenopausal women. *Clin. Endocrinol.*, **29**, 45–51
27. Stanger, J.D. and Yovich, J.L. (1985). Reduced *in vitro* fertilization of human oocytes from patients with raised basal luteinizing hormone levels during the follicular phase. *Br. J. Obstet. Gynecol.*, **92**, 385–93
28. Diedrich, K., Diedrich, C., Santos, E., Zoll, C., Al-Hasani, S., Reissmann, T. and Krebs, D. (1994). Suppression of the endogenous luteinizing hormone surge by the gonadotrophin-releasing hormone antagonist Cetrorelix during ovarian stimulation. *Hum. Reprod.*, **9**, 788–91
29. De Mouzon, J., Belaisch-Allart, J., Cohen, J., Dubuisson, J.B., Guichard, A., Parinaud, J., Bachelot, A. and Chalais, J.J. (1988). Dossier FIVNAT, Analyse des resultats 1987. Stimulations. *Contracept. Fertil. Sexual.*, **16**, 599–615
30. Tan, S.L., Kingsland, C. and Campbell, S. (1990). The use of buserelin in *in-vitro* fertilization – a comparison between the long and short protocols of administration (Abstr. 107). *Gynecol. Endocrinol.*, **4**
31. Ron-El, R., Herman, A., Golan, A., Nachum, H., Soffer, Y. and Caspi, E. (1991). Gonadotropins and combined gonadotropin-releasing hormone agonist-gonadotropins protocol in a randomized prospective study. *Fertil. Steril.*, **55**, 574–8
32. Sommer, L., Diedrich, K. and Klingmüller, D. (1993). Effects of the GnRH antagonist Cetrorelix in normal women. *Gynecol. Endocrinol.*, **7**, 2
33. Ditkoff, E.C., Cassidenti, D.L., Paulson, R.J., Sauer, M.V., Wellington, L.P., Rivier, J., Yen, S.S.C. and Lobo, R.A. (1991). The gonadotrophin-releasing hormone antagonist (Nal-Glu) acutely blocks the luteinizing hormone surge but allows for resumption of folliculogenesis in normal women. *Am. J. Obstet. Gynecol.*, **165**, 1811–17
34. Reissmann, T., Felberbaum, R., Diedrich, K., Engel, J., Comaru-Schally, A.M. and Schally, A.V. (1995). Development and applications of luteinizing hormone-releasing hormone antagonists in the treatment of infertility: an overview. *Hum. Reprod.*, **10**, 1974–81

35. Felberbaum, R., Reissmann, T., Zoll, C., Al-Hasani, S., Küpker, W., Diedrich, C. and Diedrich, K. (1995). Fertilization rate and amount of human menopausal gonadotrophin needed in controlled ovarian hyperstimulation under low-dose gonadotrophin-releasing hormone antagonist treatment (Abstr. 2). *Hum. Reprod.*, **10**, 8
36. Kettel, M., Murphy, A.A., Morales, A.J., Rivier, J. Vale, W. and Yen, S.C.C. (1993). Rapid regression of uterine leiomyomas in response to daily administration of gonadotrophin-releasing hormone antagonist. *Fertil. Steril.*, **60**, 642–6
37. Felberbaum, R., Riethmüller-Winzen, H., Germer, U., Bauer, O., Zoll, C., Schill, T., Heise, S., Gehl, B., Siebert-Weigel, M., Reissmann, T., Küpker, W., Vollersen, E., Diedrich, C. and Diedrich, K. (1996). Administration of a slow-release formulation of the GnRH antagonist Cetrorelix (SB-75) in patients with uterine fibroma to undergo surgery: first clinical results (Abstr. 1). *Hum. Reprod.*, **11**, 75
38. Hedon, B., Arnal, F., Basor, E., Boulot, P., Huet, J.M., Fries, N., Deschamps, F., Cristol, P. and Humeau, C. (1988). Comparison randomisée protocole long-protocole court dans les stimulations de l'ovaire en association avec un agoniste de la GnRH en vue de fécondation in vitro. *Contr. Fertil. Sex.*, **16**, 624–7
39. Zorn, J.R., Barata, M., Brami, Ch., Epelboin, S., Nathan, C., Papageorgiou, G., Quantin, P., Rolet, F., Svale, M., Boyer, P., Guichar, A., Cedard, L., Comaru-Schally A.M. and Schally, A.V. (1988). Ovarian stimulation for *in vitro* fertilization combining administration of gonadotropin and blockade of the pituitary with D-Trp6-LHRH microcapsules: pilot studies with two protocols. *Hum. Reprod.*, **3**, 235–9
40. Remorgida, V., Anserini, P., Crose, S., Costa, M., Ferraiolo, A., Centonze, A., Gaggero, G. and Capitanio, G.L. (1989). The duration of pituitary suppression by means of intranasal gonadotropin hormone-releasing-hormone analogue administration does not influence the ovarian response to gonadotropin stimulation and success rate in a gamete intrafallopian transfer (GIFT) program. *J. In Vitro Fertil. Embryo Trans.*, **6**, 76–80
41. Pados, G., Tarlatzis, B.C., Bontis, J., Lagos, S., Papadimas, J., Spanos, E. and Mantalenakis, S. (1991). Ovarian stimulation with buserelin/HMG/HCG: prospective study of short vs long protocol. *7th Annual Meeting of the ESHRE*, Paris, 28–30 June, pp. 364–5

Future possibilities for endometriosis treatment with GnRH antagonists

E.W. Bergink and H.J.T. Coelingh Bennink

Introduction

Several million women from different ethnic and social groups suffer from endometriosis as a 'benign' gynecological disease that can manifest itself in variable forms ranging from severe complaints to asymptomatic disease. The prevalence of endometriosis in women who consult their physician for pelvic pain, dysmenorrhea, menometrorrhagia, dyspareunia and/or infertility varies because of differences in the nature of the complaints, differences in diagnostic procedures and differences in the interpretation of such procedures.

Most of these women are of reproductive age but endometriosis has also been detected in adolescents and in postmenopausal women on hormonal replacement therapy. Endometriosis in a silent and asymptomatic form has been detected in women at reproductive age undergoing tubal ligation; variable prevalences of 3–43%[1] and 1–7%[2] have been found. Endometriosis in some minimal form might develop every now and then in all women[3] and as a disease might affect approximately 1 in 15 women of reproductive age[4], up to 25% of those with subfertility and up to 80% of women with dysmenorrhea[5].

The symptomatic patient presents herself with the classic complaints of chronic pelvic pain, dysmenorrhea, menometrorrhagia, dyspareunia and/or infertility. The diagnosis of endometriosis needs to be confirmed by procedures such as laparoscopy (preferentially) or explorative laparotomy. If during the surgical diagnostic intervention ectopic endometriotic lesions and adhesions in the pelvic and abdominal cavity are found, they can be removed by laser techniques. Biopsies of the obviously affected and suspected sites should be collected during this procedure for histological examination[6,7]. Staging based on laparoscopic findings is carried out according to the classification proposed by the American Fertility Society (AFS) in 1979[8], with a revision in 1985[9]: stage I (minimal); stage II (mild); stage III (moderate); and stage IV (severe). With the present state-of-the-art surgical treatment, estimates of the cumulative recurrence rate of symptoms are 14% and 40% at 3 and 5 years, respectively[10]. After hormonal treatment the retreatment rate is 15–22% of patients after a 1-year follow-up[11].

The etiology of endometriosis and its underlying cause have never been firmly established; however, it is strongly believed that retrograde menstruation or lymphatic flow from the uterus to the ovary are causative factors for the appearance of endometrial tissue in the pelvic and abdominal domain[1]. Furthermore, immunological factors may play an as yet unidentified but important role[1]. Genetically, endometriosis appears to be a multifactorially inherited risk[1].

The immune dysfunction to the ectopic endometrial implants is characterized by a defect in natural killer cell activity, a decrease in T-cell cytotoxicity and the presentation of antigens differing from eutopic endometrial tissue[12].

The growth and maintenance of the ectopic, as well as of the eutopic, endometrial tissue is hormonally responsive and estrogen dependent. However, in addition to sex steroid hormones, a host of growth factors, such as epidermal growth factor, transforming growth factors and platelet-derived growth factor also play a role[12]. Furthermore, interleukin-1β concentrations in peritoneal fluid are increased particularly in stage I and II endometriosis, whereas the messenger RNA of interleukin-1β and that of the interleukin-1 receptor antagonist are expressed in peritoneal macrophages from patients with endometriosis[13]. Cell adhesion molecules, the family of integrins, have been implicated in the development of endometriosis[14]. Very recently, vascular endothelial growth factor (VEGF; vascular permeability factor) has been identified in secretory endometrium, and has been shown to increase in an *in vitro* endometrial cell culture when estradiol or medroxyprogesterone acetate was added[15].

No markers in blood, urine or peritoneal fluid have been identified as yet which can assist, with high clinical sensitivity, in the diagnosis and in the follow-up (recurrence) of endometriosis. Cancer antigen-125 (CA-125) levels in blood during menstruation may be helpful in establishing recurrence of endometriosis, but not for diagnostic purposes[16]. A progesterone-induced endometrial protein (PP14, also called glycodelin), as well as CA-125, is secreted by ectopic endometrial tissue; superficial pelvic endometrial explants secrete mainly towards the peritoneal fluid compartment, while deeply infiltrating endometriosis mainly secretes towards the blood compartment[17]. However, the clinical sensitivity of PP14 as a marker appears to be only 36%, with a clinical specificity of 87%[17]. VEGF levels in peritoneal fluid from endometriosis patients (AFS stages III and IV) were significantly higher than those in women without or with AFS stage I or II endometriosis[15].

An interesting observation is that the serum or peritoneal fluid from patients with endometriosis inhibits the development of the mouse embryo *in vitro*[18,19]. Stage I and II patients were investigated in the serum study[19]. The nature of the inhibiting factor is unknown, but these results demonstrate the direct relation between endometriosis and subfertility.

Treatment

Once the diagnosis of endometriosis has been confirmed, the clinician has the option of surgical treatment (usually done at the same session as first-look laparoscopy in cases of stage I and II endometriosis) or medical treatment which can also be applied prior to surgery especially in cases of severe endometriosis to reduce vascularization and nodular size[20]. In minimal or mild cases, endometriosis may be considered a non-disease[3,20], and an 'expectant management' should be followed. The goal of the treatment of endometriosis as a progressive disease[21] should be to eliminate the lesions and to treat pain and subfertility. Medical management has consisted, from the late 1950s[22] until the end of the 1980s, of steroid(-like) hormones which suppress the cyclicity of endogenous estrogen levels and/or antagonize the effects of estradiol[1]. For that purpose oral contraceptives (continuous treatment with low-dose combination oral contraceptives), progestins, danazol and, more recently, anti-progestins or partial anti-progestins (such as gestrinone[1] and mifepristone[23]) have been used with reasonable to good success during treatment. Alleviation of pain, return of eumenorrhea and improvement of fecundity after stopping the medication in the more advanced stages were observed. In many instances the drug of choice has been danazol. Although effective, the hormonal treatment does not cure the disease, whereas in addition to estrogen deficiency, other (androgenic) side-effects have been associated with danazol[1].

At the end of the 1980s, gonadotropin-releasing hormone (GnRH) agonists were investigated for the treatment of endometriosis, since these produced a decrease of luteinizing hormone (LH) and follicle-stimulating hormone (FSH) to low or undetectable levels and consequently also of the sex steroid hormone levels. It is important to note that this effect is preceded by an increase in the levels of gonadotropins and sex steroid hormones,

Table 1 Structural formulae of native gonadotropin-releasing hormone and its agonist and antagonist analogs. Only the amino acids which differ from the native hormone are indicated

Analog name	Peptide position									
	1	2	3	4	5	6	7	8	9	10
Native	pGlu	His	Trp	Ser	Tyr	Gly	Leu	Arg	Pro	GlyNH$_2$
Agonists										
Buserelin						D-Ser				pro-ethylamide
Goserelin						D-Ser				AzGly
Leuprorelin						D-Leu				pro-ethylamide
Nafarelin						D-Nal				
Triptorelin						D-Trp				
Antagonists										
Antide	D-Nal	D-Phe	D-Pal	NicLys		D-NicLys		Lys(iPr)		D-Ala
Azaline-B	D-Nal	D-Phe	D-Pal	Phe		D-Phe		Lys(iPr)		D-Ala
Cetrorelix	D-Nal	D-Phe	D-Pal			D-Cit				D-Ala
Ganirelix	D-Nal	D-Phe	D-Pal			D-hArg		hArg		D-Ala
Nal-Glu	D-Nal	D-Phe	D-Pal	Arg		D-Glu				D-Ala
Ramorelix*	D-Nal	D-(Cl)-Phe	D-Trp	Tyr(o-sugar)		D-Ser				AzGly

D-Ala, D-alanine; AzGly, azaglycine; D-Cit, D-citrulline; D-Glu, D-glutamic acid; D-hArg, D-homoarginine; hArg, homoarginine; D-Leu, D-leucine; Lys(iPr), lysine isopropyl; D-Nal, (2-naphthyl)-D-alanine; D-NicLys, D-nicotinyl lysine; D-Pal, (3-pyridyl)-D-alanine; D-Phe, D-phenylalanine; D-(Cl)-Phe, D-chlorophenylalanine; D-Ser, D-serine; D-Trp, D-tryptophane; Tyr(o-sugar), Tyrosine (o-sugar); *development has been discontinued

due to an initial stimulation observed before the down-regulation of GnRH receptors[24].

GnRH *antagonists* have been synthesized successfully. Of the many hundreds of compounds prepared, at least six of them have been tested clinically, and five are now in clinical trials for the assessment of their effectiveness in artificial reproductive techniques (e.g. *in vitro* fertilization), gynecological cancers and other cancers (Table 1). The effectiveness of GnRH antagonists for the regression of uterine leiomyomas has been established[25]. However, thus far the efficacy of these drugs in the medical treatment of endometriosis still needs to be tested[26].

GnRH agonists and GnRH antagonists

Gonadotropin releasing hormone is a decapeptide which can be chemically modified for (super-)agonistic activity. It appears that position 6 (glycine in the natural peptide) plays a pivotal role and that position 10 (glycinamide in the natural peptide) can be changed to ethylamide. At position 6, D-amino acids can be introduced, such as D-serine, D-tryptophane, D-leucine and D-Nal (2-naphthyl-D-alanine) (Table 1). It should be noted that the other eight amino acids found in the naturally occurring compound should not be changed, in order to maintain agonistic properties.

When administered to an animal or human volunteers, these agonistic compounds are continuously present in the bloodstream and thereby will continuously activate the GnRH receptors of the pituitary gonadotrophs. This is in contrast to the natural, physiological situation, where GnRH is released episodically, with approximately one pulse every 90 min, for optimal response of the pituitary in manufacturing and releasing LH and FSH. The receptors have therefore been shown to be continuously occupied by the agonist with consequent down-regulation of the receptor content of the gonadotrophs[24]. Shortly after administration of the agonist the blood concentrations of LH and FSH will rise sharply, with a concomitant increase in the concentration of estradiol (flare-up phenomenon). The long-term effect, usually observed 1–3 weeks after administration, is the suppression of serum LH and FSH and a resulting decrease of sex steroid concentrations. It should be noted that at the stage of down-regulation, exogenous (and endogenous) GnRH are without effect. This effect of agonists on GnRH receptors is different from that of antagonists. Unlike agonists, GnRH antagonists do not induce down-regulation of the GnRH receptor[27,28]. Following the administration of antagonists, GnRH receptors continue to be present and responsive and a competitive binding to the receptor and biological activity have been observed following administration of exogenous GnRH to monkeys[27], and to patients treated with GnRH antagonists[28].

In addition to these central actions of GnRH agonists and antagonists, direct effects on peripheral tissues have also been found, such as an autocrine/paracrine role for GnRH analogs in endometrial and myometrial tissue[29,30]. The clinical relevance of these direct effects on the growth of endometriotic tissue as well as on the estrogen production by the ovaries needs to be established.

Following the publication of the primary structure of porcine GnRH in 1971[31], and the subsequent synthesis and clinical testing of synthetic agonists[32,33], the activities of the first competitive antagonist of GnRH were being reported by 1972[34]. The chemical synthesis of subsequent series of antagonists proved difficult but feasible[32,35]. The natural decapeptide was changed at five to seven positions (Table 1); it should be noted that in the antagonists the positions 4 (serine), 7 (leucine) and 9 (proline) are conserved. Hundreds of compounds have been made and many of them have satisfactory or excellent antagonistic properties as measured by anti-ovulatory activity in a rat model. However, histamine-like reactions and edema[36] were usually observed, and these compounds therefore were not useful for application in human volunteers. Moreover, 'gelling' could occur when the compounds were injected in the form of depot preparations or in other formulations containing relatively high dosages. Hydrophobicity of the so-called first- and second-generation GnRH antagonists seems to be the most likely explanation for these effects.

Nowadays, so-called 'third-generation' antagonists have been synthesized that show only minimal histamine-release properties and, after proper pharmaceutical formulation, no 'gelling' occurs. It should also be noted that some of the agonists have been associated with a minimal histamine release. The minimal histamine-release property and greatly reduced 'gelling' property are most likely the results of (a) reduced hydrophobicity, (b) the protection of the basic groups of the side-chains, and (c) the introduction of various chemical groups in positions 5, 6 and/or 8. Consequently, solubility of these substituted compounds has been improved, and acceptable pharmaceutical formulations have been developed. The following compounds (Table 1) are now in clinical trials or have been in trials for various intended indications: Nal-Glu, cetrorelix, ganirelix, antide, azaline B and ramorelix.

With the present data on dose-finding in humans, it can be concluded that the daily dose required for an antagonist is approximately 5–10 times that of the dose required for an agonist to suppress sex steroid levels adequately. This dose is approximately 2–5 mg/day for the antagonist and 0.4–0.8 mg/day for the agonist. Much of the success of the clinical application(s) of antagonists will depend on an adequate and well-designed pharmaceutical formulation and/or presentation form. Presently aqueous solutions of antagonists have been prepared for subcutaneous administration, as well as for depot preparations.

Clinical outcome of medical treatment of endometriosis with agonists

The clinical results of several comparative trials with agonists and other hormonal treatments of endometriosis (mainly danazol) have been reported[11,37–41]. Such multicenter double-blind comparative studies have been performed in Europe[40] as well as in the USA[38]. A review appeared in 1993[42] on the trials with agonists between 1982 and 1993; it was concluded that the treatment of symptomatic endometriosis with GnRH agonists is efficacious. In comparison with danazol, equivalent improvement was observed based on subjective and objective findings. The author observed that the side-effects of GnRH agonist therapy would make it more acceptable for general use. The treatment period with agonists is usually 6 months.

As mentioned above, there are as yet no published results demonstrating efficacy of GnRH antagonists for the treatment of endometriosis[26]. However, it has already been reported that a continuous daily treatment with the GnRH antagonist Nal-Glu in patients with symptomatic leiomyomas results in a rapid decline in gonadal steroids within 48 h and a decrement (as observed after 1 month of treatment) in leiomyoma size[25]. An important difference between the efficacy of the agonists versus the antagonists is the rapidity with which the latter produce a decline in blood levels of gonadotropins and especially a decline in the levels of the sex steroid hormones. With the antagonist, such a decline in LH levels can be observed within 8 h of administration, whereas with the agonist an increase is observed within the same period[43].

Whether the dose regimen for the antagonists can be adapted to a lower dose than that required for a maximum suppression of sex steroid levels, to a lower frequency of administration or to a reduced treatment period, needs to be established.

Dosage

The primary goal of medical treatment with GnRH analogs in women is to achieve a state of hypoestrogenism (i.e. serum estradiol levels of about 30 pmol/l or less) or that of relatively low estrogen levels as observed in the early follicular phase of the normal menstrual cycle (i.e. around 100 pmol/l). This latter concentration, the so-called 'estradiol target', has been advocated by Barbieri[44]. Very low estradiol levels (hypoestrogenism) will adversely affect bone turnover and women will experience hot flushes, whereas relatively 'high' estradiol levels (e.g. 200 pmol/l or above) are expected to activate the endometriotic tissue.

Treatment with antagonists could produce fixed and predetermined blood levels of estradiol in patients with endometriosis since their effects are expected to be fast. Such a treatment will depend on the formulation, the number of dosages to be administered and on the cumulative half-life in blood of the antagonists.

Side-effects

The major drawbacks of all presently used medical (hormonal) treatments are summarized in Table 2. Most patients experience 'hot flushes'; this phenomenon appears to be dependent on the estradiol levels in blood, i.e. the number of flushes will greatly diminish above 100 pmol/l. Complaints of vaginal dryness with agonist medication are frequent, and decreased libido is noted less frequently, as are complaints of acne, depression and emotional liability. Complaints of headaches are substantial, and complaints of nausea are sporadic[11].

Bone resorption is increased and bone formation impaired. The result is bone loss in the spine or hip as measured by dual-energy X-ray absorptiometry or by quantitative computerized tomography[45]. The loss of bone appears to be recovered after discontinuation

Table 2 Occurrence of adverse side-effects in medical treatment of endometriosis. Numbers in parentheses are the literature references

	Treatment	
	Danazol	Agonists
Hypoestrogenic state or low estrogen levels		
Bone mineral density loss	no change (44)	↓, 5–12% (44, 45)
		↓, 0–6% (44, 45)
Cardiovascular changes		
HDL	↓, 35% (38)	↑, 20% (38)
	↓, 45–50% (51)	no change (52)
		↓, 10% (44)
LDL	↑, 20% (38)	no change (38)
	↑, 10–30% (52)	no change (52)
Hot flushes	70% (38, 39)	90% (38, 39, 50)
		7% (49)
Headache	9–50% (49)	9–65% (49)
Libido loss	9–52% (49)	10–66% (49)
Vaginal dryness	6–29% (49)	18–71% (49)
Depression/emotional lability	5–44% (49)	7–50% (49)
Biochemistry		
SHBG	↓ (44)	
Free testosterone	↑ (44)	
SGOT	↑ (38, 39)	no change (38, 39)
	↑, 40–100% (11)	↑, 15–40% (11)
LDH	↑, < 20% (11)	↑, < 20% (11)
Alkaline phosphatase		↑, 14–25% (53)
PAI		↓, 25% (53)
Fibrin		↓, 35% (53)
Hemoglobin		↑, 80% (50)
Hematocrit		↑, 50% (50)
Serum ferritin		↑, 80–200% (50)
Total iron binding capacity		↓, 15% (53)
General		
Body weight	↑, 50% (38)	no change (39)
	↑, 3–10% (41)	no change (11)
Blood pressure	↑ (41)	no change (11)

↑, increase in parameter; ↓, decrease in parameter; HDL, high-density lipoprotein; LDL, low-density lipoprotein; SHBG, sex hormone binding globulin; SGOT, serum glutamate-oxalacetate transaminase; LDH, lactate dehydrogenase; PAI, plasminogen activator inhibitor; agonists used in the studies (38, 39, 11, 49): nafarelin, intranasal; (41, 44): not specified; (45, 52): different agonists; (51): goserelin depot; (53): depot goserelin, intranasal nafarelin and s.c. and intranasal buserelin

of the drug; the cause for concern is that some patients do not return to their pre-medication bone density[45].

The danger of excessive bone loss as a result of medical treatment was understood early, at the time of clinical trials. The concept of 'add-back' was applied, i.e. to administer, together with the agonist regimen, protective agents for bone loss, e.g. norethisterone, norethindrone, medroxyprogesterone acetate and the bisphosphonate ethindronate plus extra calcium[45], or even a combined add-back regimen with an estrogen administered concomitantly with a progestogen[46,47]. A substantial reduction in bone loss could be achieved. Add-back therapy with tibolone (Livial®, Organon, The Netherlands), a compound with mixed estrogenic, progestogenic and androgenic properties, prevented bone loss whilst at the same time the therapeutic effects of the agonist treatment remained unaffected[48].

The changes in blood biochemistry after agonist administration may or may not be explained on the basis of low estrogen levels. Liver enzymes such as serum glutamate-oxalacetate transaminase (SGOT) or lactate dehydrogenase (LDH) are increased in a small number of patients, and alkaline phosphatase levels increase, possibly due to the increased bone turnover. The coagulation system appears to be affected, with plasminogen activation inhibitor levels in blood decreasing by 25% and fibrin levels by 35%[49]. Hemoglobin, hematocrit, serum ferritin and serum iron all increase, while the total iron binding capacity is decreased[50].

During the flare-up stage of agonist medication, vaginal bleeding and exacerbation of hormone-sensitive disease may occur. A word of caution is warranted if the patient has (submucous) leiomyomata next to the endometriosis; pelvic pain may increase during the first few weeks of treatment with agonists until the down-regulation has settled. A special case has been reported[51] of a patient with ileocecal endometriosis who was preoperatively treated with an agonist. During the flare-up period of treatment she developed intestinal obstruction which required major surgery.

With the regimen presently used to treat endometriosis with GnRH agonists, the effect of low estrogen levels persists for 4–5 weeks after cessation of the therapy; ovarian function is restored after a (median) time of 9 weeks. Possibly with differing regimens of treatment with GnRH antagonists, the time for restoration of ovarian function may be shorter. The clinical outcomes of future trials for the treatment of endometriosis with GnRH antagonists will determine their usefulness.

Conclusions

Endometriosis is a so-called 'benign' gynecological disease with a high prevalence, approximately 3–7% in the female population of reproductive age; for the same age group, but in the sub-population of women with subfertility and/or pain, the prevalence ranges between 20 and 90%.

The treatment of endometriosis by means of GnRH agonist medication now seems firmly established. By their nature, agonists induce a flare-up of gonadotropins and concomitant sex steroid hormone levels; this effect lasts for approximately 1–3 weeks. Thereafter, the pituitary gonadotropins are switched off, as are the sex steroid hormones. Many of the side-effects of agonist medication, i.e. 'hot flushes' and increased bone turnover, can be explained on the basis of the resulting low estrogen levels.

The future possibilities for using antagonists instead of agonists for the treatment of this condition are manifold: there is no flare-up period with the antagonists and the consistent suppression of the gonadotropins is immediate (within 24 h). Different regimens of antagonist treatment should be explored to find out whether there is an optimal window for estrogen levels by which the endometriotic lesions are put into quiescence, whilst at the same time the adverse effects on bone metabolism and other estrogen deficiency symptoms such as hot flushes can be minimized. Much will depend on the quality of the pharmaceutical formulation for a particular antagonist which is to be used for the adjunctive management of endometriosis.

Acknowledgements

The authors gratefully acknowledge the expert information and advice given by Dr F. de Haan and Mr B. Raaben. The authors also gratefully acknowledge Dr R.M. Lequin, at Diagnostics Consultancy (Therametry), Eindhoven, The Netherlands, for preparation of the drafts of this manuscript.

References

1. D'Hooghe, T.M. and Hill, J.A. (1996). Endometriosis. In Berek, J.S., Adashi, E.Y. and Hillard, P.A. (eds.) *Novak's Gynecology*, 12th edn., Ch. 26, pp. 887–914. (Baltimore: Williams & Wilkins)
2. Barbieri, R.L. (1990). Etiology and epidemiology of endometriosis. *Am. J. Obstet. Gynecol.*, **162**, 565–7
3. Evers, J.L.H. (1996). Do all women have endometriosis? Presented at the *Vth World Congress on Endometriosis*, Yokohama, October, Abstract 0–1
4. Olive, D.L. and Schwartz, L.B. (1993). Endometriosis. *N. Engl. J. Med.*, **328**, 1759–69
5. Evers, J.L.H. (1996). Silent endometriosis. Reflections on epidemiology. Presented at the *Vth World Congress on Endometriosis*, Yokohama, October, Abstract 0–45
6. Nisolle, M., Paindaveine, B., Bourdon, A., Berliere, M., Casanas-Roux, F. and Donnez, J. (1990). Histologic study of peritoneal endometriosis in infertile women. *Fertil. Steril.*, **53**, 984–8
7. Cornillie, F.J., Oosterlynk, D., Lauweryns, J.M. and Koninckx, P.R. (1990). Deeply infiltrating pelvic endometriosis: histology and clinical significance. *Fertil. Steril.*, **53**, 978–83
8. The American Fertility Society (1979). Classification of endometriosis. *Fertil. Steril.*, **32**, 633–4
9. The American Fertility Society (1985). Revised American Fertility Society classification of endometriosis. *Fertil. Steril.*, **43**, 351–2
10. Wheeler, J.M. and Malinak, L.R. (1983). Recurrent endometriosis: incidence, management and prognosis. *Am. J. Obstet. Gynecol.*, **146**, 247–53
11. The Nafarelin European Endometriosis Trial Group (1992). Nafarelin for endometriosis: a large-scale danazol-controlled trial of efficacy and safety, with 1-year follow-up. *Fertil. Steril.*, **57**, 514–22
12. Olive, D.L. (1992). Endometriosis: advances in understanding and management. *Curr. Opin. Obstet. Gynecol.*, **4**, 380–7
13. Mori, H., Sawairi, M., Nakagawa, M., Itoh, N., Wada, K. and Tamaya, T. (1992). Expression of interleukin-1(IL-1)beta messenger ribonucleic acid (mRNA) and IL-1 receptor antagonist mRNA in peritoneal macrophages from patients with endometriosis. *Fertil. Steril.*, **57**, 535–42
14. Lessey, B.A., Castelbaum, A.J. and Sawin, S.J. (1994). Aberrant integrin expression in the endometrium of women with endometriosis. *J. Clin. Endocrinol. Metab.*, **79**, 643–9
15. Shifren, J.L., Tseng, J.F., Zaloudek, C.J., Ryan, I.P., Meng, Y.G., Ferrara, N., Jaffe, R.B. and Taylor, R.N. (1996). Ovarian steroid regulation of vascular endothelial growth factor in the human endometrium: implications for angiogenesis during the menstrual cycle and in the pathogenesis of endometriosis. *J. Clin. Endocrinol. Metab.*, **81**, 3112–18
16. Masahashi, T., Matsuzawa, K., Ohsawa, M., Narita, O., Asai, T. and Ishihara, M. (1988). Serum CA-125 levels in patients with endometriosis: changes in CA-125 levels during menstruation. *Obstet. Gynecol.*, **72**, 328–31
17. Koninckx, P.R., Riitinen, L., Seppala, M. and Cornillie, F.J. (1992). CA-125 and placental protein 14 concentrations in plasma and peritoneal fluid from women with deeply infiltrating pelvic endometriosis. *Fertil. Steril.*, **57**, 523–30
18. Morcos, R.N., Gibbons, W.E. and Findley, W.E. (1985). Effect of peritoneal fluid on *in vitro* cleavage of 2-cell mouse embryos: possible role in infertility associated with endometriosis. *Fertil. Steril.*, **44**, 678–83
19. Damewood, M.D., Hesla, J.S., Schlaff, W.D., Hubard, M., Gearhart, J.D. and Rock, J.A. (1990). Effect of serum from patients with minimal to mild endometriosis on mouse embryo development *in vitro*. *Fertil. Steril.*, **54**, 917–20
20. Koninckx, P.R., Oosterlynck, D., D'Hooghe, T.M. and Meuleman, C. (1994). Deeply infiltrating endometriosis is a disease whereas mild endometriosis could be considered a non-disease. *Ann. NY Acad. Sci.*, **734**, 333–41
21. Koninckx, P.R., Meuleman, C., Demeyer, S., Lesaffre, E. and Cornillie, E.J. (1991). Suggestive evidence that pelvic endometriosis is a progressive disease, whereas deeply infiltrating endometriosis is associated with pelvic pain. *Fertil. Steril.*, **55**, 759–65
22. Kistner, R.W. (1958). The use of progestins in the treatment of endometriosis. *Am. J. Obstet. Gynecol.*, **75**, 264–78

23. Kettel, L.M., Murphy, A.A., Morales, A.J., Ulmann, A., Baulieu, E.E. and Yen, S.S.C. (1996). Treatment of endometriosis with the antiprogesterone mifepristone (RU486). *Fertil. Steril.*, **65**, 23–8
24. Yenn, S.S.C. (1991). The hypothalamic control of pituitary hormone secretion. In Yenn, S.S.C. and Jaffe, R.B. (eds.) *Reproductive Endocrinology*, pp. 65–104. (Philadelphia: Saunders)
25. Kettel, L.M., Murphy, A.A., Morales, A.J., Rivier, J., Vale, W. and Yenn, S.S.C. (1993). Rapid regression of uterine leiomyomas in response to daily administration of gonadotropin-releasing hormone antagonist. *Fertil. Steril.*, **60**, 642–6
26. Coelingh Bennink, H.J.T. (1996). Potential clinical applications of GnRH antagonists. In Filicori, M. and Flamigni, C. (eds.) *Treatment with GnRH Analogues: Controversies and Perspectives*, pp. 77–80. (New York and London: Parthenon Publishing)
27. Gordon, K., Williams, R.F., Danforth, D.R. and Hodgen, G.D. (1990). A novel regimen of gonadotropin-releasing hormone (GnRH) antagonist plus pulsatile GnRH: controlled restoration of gonadotropin secretion and ovulation induction. *Fertil. Steril.*, **154**, 1140–5
28. Olivennes, F., Fanchin, R., Bouchard, P., Taieb, J., and Frydman, R. (1996). Triggering of ovulation by a gonadotropin-releasing hormone (GnRH) agonist in patients pretreated with a GnRH antagonist. *Fertil. Steril.*, **66**, 151–3
29. Srkalovic, G., Wittliff, J.L. and Schally, A.V. (1990). Detection and partial characterization of receptor for (D-Tryp6)-luteinizing hormone-releasing hormone and epidermal growth factor in human endometrial carcinoma. *Cancer Res.*, **50**, 1841–6
30. Chegini, N., Rong, H., Dou, Q., Kipersztok, S. and Williams, R.S. (1996). Gonadotropin-releasing hormone (GnRH) and GnRH receptor gene expression in human myometrium and leiomyomata and the direct action of GnRH analogs on myometrial smooth muscle cells and interaction with ovarian steroids *in vitro*. *J. Clin. Endocrinol. Metab.*, **81**, 3215–21
31. Matsuo, H., Baba, Y., Nair, R.M., Arimura, A. and Schally, A.V. (1971). Structure of the porcine LH- and FSH-releasing hormone. I. The proposed amino-acid sequence. *Biochem. Biophys. Res. Commun.*, **43**, 1334–9
32. Karten, M.J. and Rivier, J.E. (1986). Gonadotropin-releasing hormone analog design. Structure-function studies towards the development of agonists and antagonists: rationale and perspective. *Endocr. Rev.*, **7**, 44–66
33. Nillius, S.J., Berquist, C. and Wide, L. (1978). Inhibition of ovulation in women by chronic treatment with a stimulatory LRH-analogue – a new approach to birth control? *Contraception*, **17**, 537–45
34. Vale, W., Grant, G., Rivier, J., Monahan, M., Amoss, M., Blackwell, R., Burgus, R. and Guillemin, R. (1972). Synthetic polypeptide antagonists of the hypothalamic luteinizing hormone releasing factor. *Science*, **176**, 933–4
35. Janecka, A., Janecki, T., Bowers, C. and Folkers, K. (1994). The structural features of effective antagonists of the luteinizing hormone releasing hormone. *Amino Acids*, **6**, 111–30
36. Rivier, J., Porto, J., Rivier, C.L., Perrin, M., Corrigan, A. and Hook, W.A. (1986). New effective gonadotropin-releasing hormone antagonists with minimal potency for histamine release *in vitro*. *J. Med. Chem.*, **29**, 1846–51
37. Buttram, V.C., Reiter, R.C. and Ward, S. (1985). Treatment of endometriosis with danazol: report of a 6-year prospective study. *Fertil. Steril.*, **43**, 353–60
38. Henzl, M.R., Corson, S.L., Moghissi, K., Buttram, V.C., Berquist, C. and Jacobson, J. (1988). Administration of nasal nafarelin as compared with oral danazol for endometriosis/the nafarelin study group. *N. Engl. J. Med.*, **318**, 485–9
39. Henzl, M.R. and Kwei, L. (1990). Efficacy and safety of nafarelin in the treatment of endometriosis. *Am. J. Obstet. Gynecol.*, **162**, 570–4
40. Kennedy, S.H., Williams, I.A., Brodribb, J., Barlow, D.H. and Shaw, R.W. (1990). A comparison of nafarelin acetate and danazol in the treatment of endometriosis. *Fertil. Steril.*, **53**, 998–1003
41. Barbieri, R.L. (1990). Comparison of the pharmacology of nafarelin and danazol. *Am. J. Obstet. Gynecol.*, **162**, 581–5
42. Emmi, A.M. (1993). The use of GnRH agonists in the medical therapy of endometriosis in the women with pain. *Semin. Reprod. Endocrinol.*, **11**, 119–26
43. Diedrich, K. and Felberbaum, R. (1996). Use of LHRH-analogues in gynecology. Presented at the *Vth World Congress on Endometriosis*, Yokohama, October, Abstract 0–148

44. Barbieri, R.L. (1993). Gonadotropin-releasing hormone agonists: treatment of endometriosis. *Clin. Obstet. Gynecol.*, **36**, 636–41
45. Gallagher, J.C. (1993). Effect of gonadotropin-releasing hormone agonists on bone metabolism. *Semin. Reprod. Endocrinol.*, **11**, 201–8
46. Friedman, A.J. and Hornstein, M.D. (1993). Gonadotropin releasing hormone agonist plus estrogen–progestin 'add-back' therapy for endometriosis-related pelvic pain. *Fertil. Steril.*, **60**, 236–41
47. Howell, R., Edmonds, D.K., Dowsett, M., Crook, D., Lees, B. and Stevenson, J.C. (1995). Gonadotrophin-releasing hormone analogue (goserelin) plus hormone replacement therapy for the treatment of endometriosis: randomised controlled trial. *Fertil. Steril.*, **64**, 474–81
48. Lindsay, P.C., Shaw, R.W., Coelingh Bennink, H.J. and Kicovic, P. (1996). The effect of add-back treatment with tibolone (Livial) on patients treated with the gonadotrophin-releasing hormone agonist triptorelin (Decapeptyl). *Fertil. Steril.*, **65**, 342–8
49. Shaw, R.W. (1992). The role of GnRH analogues in the treatment of endometriosis. *Br. J. Obstet. Gynaecol.*, **99** (Suppl. 7), 9–12
50. Miller, R.M. and Frank, R.A. (1992). Zoladex (goserelin) in the treatment of benign gynecological disorders: an overview of safety and efficacy. *Br. J. Obstet. Gynaecol.*, **99** (Suppl. 7), 37–41
51. Hall, L.H., Malone, J.M. and Ginsburg, K.A. (1995). Flare-up of endometriosis induced by gonadotropin-releasing hormone agonist leading to bowel obstruction. *Fertil. Steril.*, **64**, 1204–6
52. Burry, K.A., Patton, P.E. and Illingworth, D.R. (1989). Metabolic changes during medical treatment of endometriosis: nafarelin acetate versus danazol. *Am. J. Obstet. Gynecol.*, **160**, 1454–61
53. Quagliarello, J. (1993). Safety of GnRH agonists: short-term side-effects and cyst formation. *Semin. Reprod. Endocrinol.*, **11**, 112–18

Development of an LHRH antagonist

T. Uemura, H. Minaguchi, H. Mori and Y. Taketani

Introduction

Since the structure of luteinizing hormone-releasing hormone (LHRH) was determined in 1971 by Schally and colleagues[1], many LHRH analogs have been synthesized and developed. While five LHRH agonists are now clinically available as therapeutic agents for sex hormone-related disorders, the clinical use of LHRH antagonists has been hindered by their edematogenic reactions due to histamine release[2-4]. Cetrorelix, one of a new group of LHRH antagonists synthesized by Schally and colleagues, however, has not produced any serious adverse drug reactions in animal and clinical studies[5-11], and has shown therapeutic potential for female and male indications, e.g. controlled ovulatory induction, benign prostatic hyperplasia and prostate cancer[5,6,10,11].

In Japan, clinical development of Cetrorelix was started in April 1995 and a phase I single rising dose study and multiple dose study were conducted to investigate the tolerability, endocrinological effects and pharmacokinetic profile of Cetrorelix in healthy premenopausal women.

Phase I single rising dose study

Subjects and methods

During the period from April 1995 to March 1996, a phase I single rising dose study of Cetrorelix was conducted in 15 healthy premenopausal women at doses of 1, 3 and 5 mg. Subjects were accrued under the eligibility criteria which included an age between 30 and 45 years, stable menstrual cycle length between 24 and 35 days, normal ovarian function judged from basal body temperature and endocrinological data at screening, no desire to have a child, maintenance of contraception during the study period, and informed consent.

In the first five subjects, 1 mg of the drug (four subjects) or placebo (one subject) was administered into the subcutaneous adipose tissue of the lower abdomen on one day during days 6–10 of the menstrual cycle. After confirming safety at 1 mg, including the observation of menstruation recurrence after dosing, administration at 3 mg was performed in another five subjects (including one placebo), followed by administration at 5 mg in the same manner after confirming safety at 3 mg.

Pharmacokinetics

In pharmacokinetic analysis (Figure 1), mean maximum concentration (C_{max}) and area under the curve (AUC) values at 1 mg were 9.6 ng/ml and 257 ng h/ml, respectively, and those at 3 mg were 31.5 ng/ml and 657 ng h/ml, respectively, showing dose-dependent increases in these pharmacokinetic parameters. However, the C_{max} and AUC values at 5 mg were 37.3 ng/ml and 594 ng h/ml, respectively, not correlating with the dose escalation from 3 mg to 5 mg. At all three doses, the plasma drug levels decreased to below the detection limit of 1 ng/ml 1 week after dosing.

Adverse drug reaction

Mild local reactions, such as erythema, were found at injection sites in all subjects, though

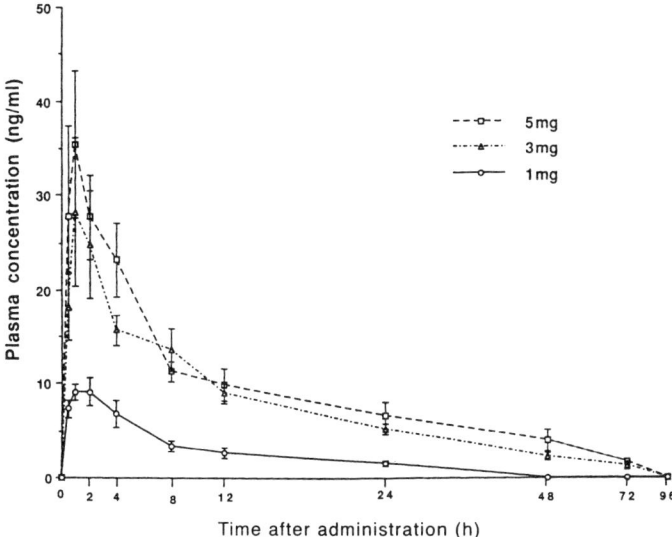

Figure 1 Plasma concentrations of Cetrorelix in healthy women ($n = 4$) after single subcutaneous administration at various doses. Values are given as means ± SE

they were milder in placebo cases. These local reactions appeared approximately 15 min after dosing and disappeared within 2 h. Dose dependency was not found in the intensity and frequency of the local reactions among the three doses. Systemic reactions observed were mainly mild and transient symptoms attributable to decrease in serum estrogen levels, such as vaginal bleeding, discharge and low back pain. Some of the subjective symptoms were also found in the placebo cases. In the 3 and 5 mg groups, the length of the menstrual cycle tended to be prolonged in the treatment cycle, though this returned to the length equivalent to that of the pretreatment cycle in the next menstrual cycle. The single subcutaneous administration of Cetrorelix was therefore well tolerated at the dose levels of 1, 3 and 5 mg.

Endocrinological effects

Serum luteinizing hormone (LH), follicle-stimulating hormone (FSH) and estradiol levels were suppressed immediately after dosing at all the dose levels (Figure 2). The suppression of serum LH and estradiol levels was dose-dependent in degree and duration between 1 and 3 mg, but not significantly different between 3 and 5 mg. At 3 and 5 mg, mean serum estradiol levels reached a nadir approximately 2 days after dosing and were kept suppressed to under 50 pg/ml for more than 6 days. Progesterone levels were continuously suppressed until 7–14 days after dosing but showed rapid increase thereafter (Figure 2). No changes attributable to Cetrorelix administration were found for serum prolactin, thyroxine (T4) and cortisol levels.

Phase I multiple dose study

Subjects and methods

A phase I multiple dose study at 3 mg was started in July 1996 and is now in the follow-up period after dosing. Four healthy premenopausal women were accrued with the same eligibility criteria as in the single dose study. Subcutaneous administration of Cetrorelix at

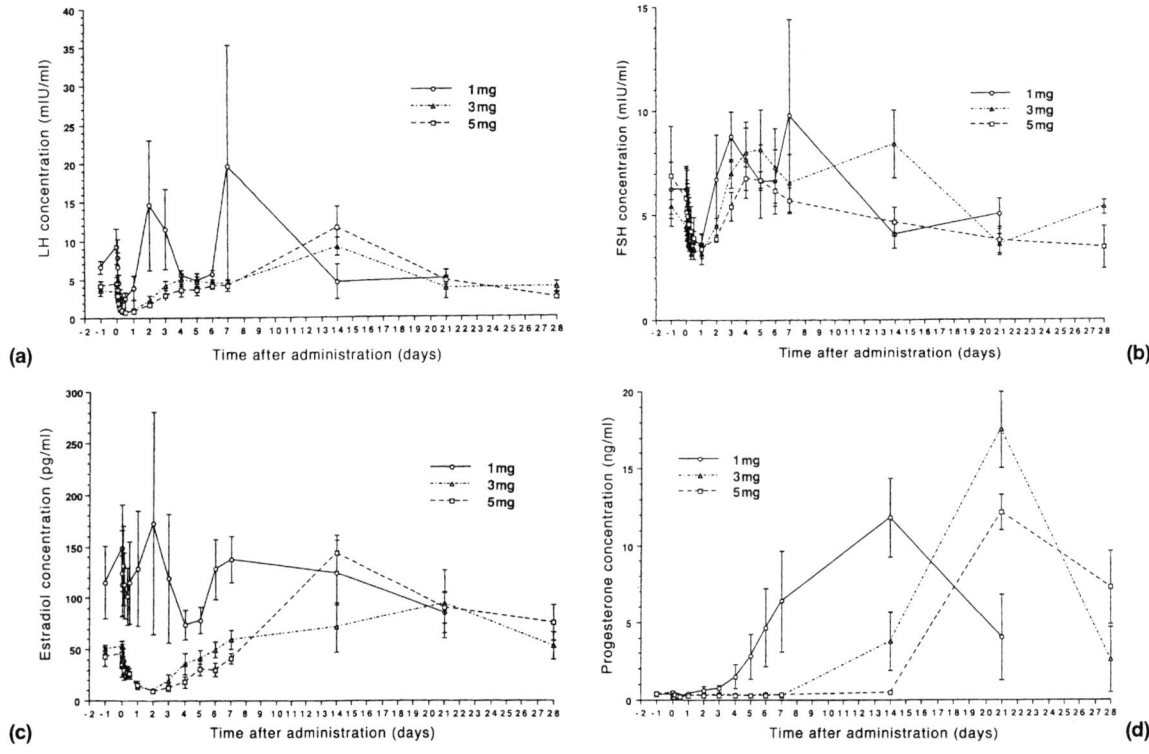

Figure 2 (a) Serum luteinizing hormone (LH), (b) serum follicle-stimulating hormone (FSH), (c) serum estradiol and (d) serum progesterone levels in healthy premenopausal women ($n = 4$) after single subcutaneous administration of Cetrorelix at various doses. Values are given as means ± SE

3 mg was repeated three times; the first dosing was conducted between days 2 and 5 of the menstrual cycle, followed by the second and third dosing at weekly intervals.

Pharmacokinetics

Cetrorelix was eliminated from the blood within 1 week of each administration and no drug accumulation in the blood was found during the multiple administration (Figure 3). The C_{max} values were thought to be equivalent to those in a single administration of 3 mg.

Adverse drug reaction

Local reactions observed were mild and transient, showing no difference in type and intensity from those found in the single dose study. Systemic reactions were the same in type but less frequent in comparison with those in the single administration, and no vaginal bleeding was found. In addition, no unknown adverse effects were observed. Thus, good tolerability was confirmed in the weekly administration of 3 mg.

Endocrinological effect

Suppression of serum LH, FSH and estradiol levels immediately after the first dosing was almost equivalent in degree and duration to that in the single dose study at 3 and 5 mg, but the nadir values of serum LH and estradiol gradually increased after the second and third dosing (Figure 4). In two of the four subjects, estradiol levels were suppressed to under 50 pg/ml for most of the period from

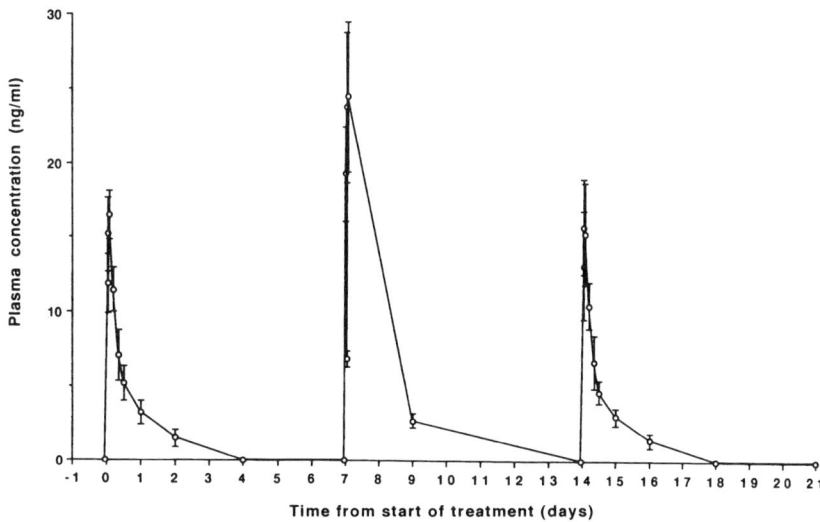

Figure 3 Plasma concentrations of Cetrorelix in healthy women ($n = 4$) during weekly subcutaneous administration at 3 mg. Values are given as means ± SE

the time immediately after the first dosing until 14 days after the final dosing. Serum progesterone levels were continuously suppressed to the levels of the follicular period until the third dosing, but showed rapid increase thereafter.

Discussion and conclusion

In the phase I single and multiple dose studies performed in healthy premenopausal women, good tolerability was confirmed in single administration at 1, 3 and 5 mg and in multiple administration at 3 mg. The local reactions, such as erythema and itching, found in these studies were mild and transient and no such serious edematogenic reactions as reported for LHRH antagonists of earlier generations were observed. In multiple administration, no vaginal bleeding was observed, though slight prolongation of the menstrual period was found in one case, and other systemic adverse effects attributable to the decrease in estrogen levels were shown to be less frequent than in single administration at 3 mg. This was thought to be possibly due to the earlier timing of the first dosing in multiple administration (one case each on day 2 and day 3 and two cases on day 5 of the menstrual cycle) than that of the single administration (two cases on day 6 and one case each on day 7 and day 8).

In the multiple dose study at 3 mg, Cetrorelix suppressed serum estradiol levels to under 50 pg/ml during most of the period from the time immediately after the first dosing until 14 days after the final dosing in two of the four cases. Considering that estrogen-dependent gynecological disorders often become ameliorated in menopause, and that suppression of serum estrogen levels to menopausal levels, e.g. to under 50 pg/ml, has been indicated in the treatment of such gynecological disorders, weekly administration of Cetrorelix at the dose of 3 mg or higher is expected to show therapeutic effects against estrogen-dependent disorders such as myoma. The nadir values of serum LH and estradiol gradually increased after the second and third dosing and this may suggest a hormonal counter-regulation of the hypothalamus–pituitary axis. Rapid increase of progesterone levels found 7–14 days after the

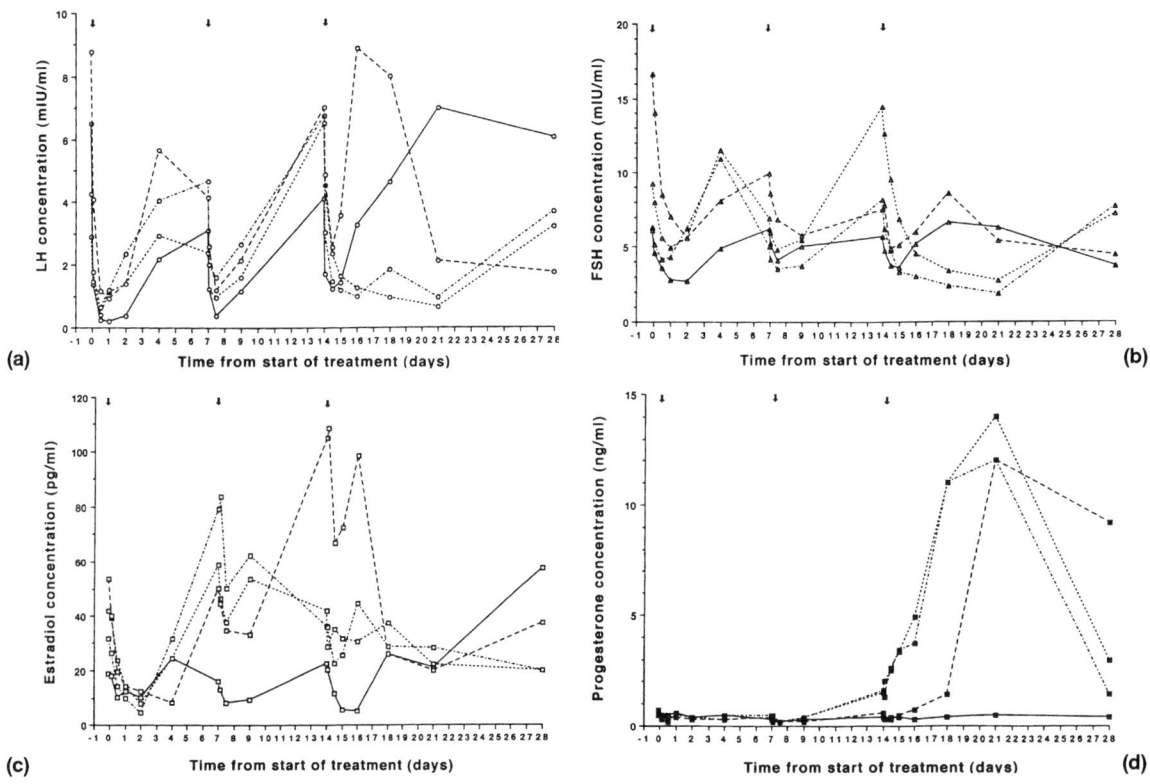

Figure 4 (a) Serum luteinizing hormone (LH), (b) serum follicle-stimulating hormone (FSH), (c) serum estradiol and (d) serum progesterone levels in individual healthy premenopausal women ($n = 4$) during weekly subcutaneous administration of Cetrorelix at 3 mg. Each administration is indicated by an arrow

single administration and the first dosing in multiple administration suggests the occurrence of ovulation. This may indicate that suppressed endocrinological function can immediately be normalized after the suppressive effects of the drug become insufficient.

The results obtained in these phase I single and multiple dose studies suggest that Cetrorelix has the desirable characteristics of an LHRH antagonist, in comparison with LHRH agonists, such as producing rapid and controllable suppression of serum gonadotropin and sex hormone levels without showing flare-up effects. Thus Cetrorelix is thought worthy of further clinical investigation for sex hormone-dependent gynecological disorders.

References

1. Schally, A.V., Nair, R.M.G., Redding, T.W. and Arimura, A. (1971). Isolation of the luteinizing hormone and follicle-stimulating hormone-releasing hormone from porcine hypothalami. *J. Biol. Chem.*, **246**, 7230–6

2. Schmidt, F., Sundaram, K., Thau, R.B. and Bardin, C.W. (1984). (Ac-D-Nal(2)1, 4FD-Phe2, D-TRP3, D-Arg6)LHRH, a potent antagonist of LHRH, produces transient edema and behavioral changes in rats. *Contraception*, **29**, 283–9

3. Phillips, A., Hahn, D.W., McGuire, J.L., Ritchie, D., Capetola, R.J., Bowers, C. and Folkers, K. (1988). Evaluation of the anaphylactoid activity of a new LHRH antagonist. *Life Sci.*, **43**, 883–8
4. Hahn, D.W., McGuire, J.L., Vale, W.W. and Rivier, J. (1985). Reproductive/endocrine and anaphylactoid properties of an LH-RH-antagonist, ORF-18260 (Ac-DNal1(2), 4FDPhe2, D-TRP3, D-Arg6)-GnRH. *Life Sci.*, **37**, 505–14
5. Gonzalez-Barcena, D., Buenfil, M.V., Procel, E.G., Guerra-Arguero, L., Cornejo, I.C., Comaru-Schally, A.M. and Schally, A.V. (1994). Inhibition of luteinizing hormone, follicle-stimulating hormone and sex-steroid levels in men and women with a potent antagonist analog of luteinizing hormone-releasing hormone, Cetrorelix (SB-75). *Eur. J. Endocrinol.*, **3**, 286–92
6. Gonzalez-Barcena, D., Vadillo-Buenfil, M., Gomez-Orta, F., Garcia, M.F., Cardenas-Cornejo, I., Graef-Sanchez, A., Comaru-Schally, A.M. and Schally, A.V. (1994). Responses to the antagonistic analog of LH-RH (SB-75, Cetrorelix) in patients with benign prostatic hyperplasia and prostatic cancer. *Prostate*, **24**, 84–92
7. Hermann, M.B., Britta, K., Elke, S., Gerard, P.M., Karlheinz, V. and Eberhard, N. (1992). Effective suppression of luteinizing hormone and testosterone by single doses of the new gonadotropin-releasing hormone antagonist cetrorelix (SB-75) in normal men. *J. Clin. Endocrinol. Metab.*, **75**, 393–8
8. Klingmüller, D., Schepke, M., Enzweiler, C. and Bidlingmaier, F. (1993). Hormonal responses to new potent GnRH antagonist Cetrorelix. *Acta Endocrinol.*, **128**, 15–18
9. Sommer, L., Zanger, K., Dyong, T., Dorn, C., Luckhaus, J., Diedrich, K. and Klingmüller, D. (1994). Seven-day administration of the gonadotropin-releasing hormone antagonist Cetrorelix in normal cycling women. *Eur. J. Endocrinol.*, **131**, 280–5
10. Diedrich, K., Diedrich, C., Santos, E., Zoll, C., Al-Hasanil, S., Reissmann, T., Krebs, D. and Klingmüller, D. (1994). Suppression of the endogenous luteinizing hormone surge by the gonadotropin-releasing hormone antagonist Cetrorelix during ovarian stimulation. *Hum. Reprod.*, **9**, 788–91
11. Olivennes, F., Taieb, J., Fanchin, R., Selva, J., Bouchard, P., Frydman, R. and De Ziegler, D. (1994). The single or dual administration of the gonadotropin-releasing hormone antagonist Cetrorelix in an *in vitro* fertilization-embryo transfer program. *Fertil. Steril.*, **3**, 468–76

Section 11

In vitro fertilization

The place of *in vitro* fertilization in the treatment of endometriosis-related infertility

J.L. Pouly, M. Canis, L. Janny, P. Vye-Pouly, R. Zambrano, H. Laurichesse, R. Botroshvilli and C. Boyer-Medeville

Introduction

In endometriosis-related infertility, various treatments are available: surgery (laparotomy or laparoscopy), suppressive medical therapy (danazol, progestins or gonadotropin-releasing hormone (GnRH) analogs), expectant management, other medical therapy (ovarian stimulators) and assisted reproductive technologies (ART). Numerous manuscripts have been published on each of these treatments, but manuscripts comparing ART with one other therapeutic modality are rare[1,2]. It seems that we are the first to propose a strategy[3] based on results of different therapeutic modalities.

Initial management (excluding ART)

ART is still not considered as first-line therapy in endometriosis-related infertility[4]. In a previous paper[3] we attempted a synthesis of the literature on a comparison between ART and other therapies. Even though numerous points are still controversial, we can reach the following conclusions:

(1) At any American Fertility Society (AFS) stage of endometriosis, surgical treatment provides better results than medical suppressive therapy[5];

(2) In stages 1 or 2, surgery is not deleterious, compared to expectant management;

(3) In opposition, there is some doubt that medical suppressive therapy can be deleterious[5];

(4) Postoperative therapy does not improve the results of surgery;

(5) Results of surgery are unrelated to the AFS stage;

(6) Surgery can be performed by laparoscopy (with or without laser) or with pseudomicrosurgical techniques by laparotomy. The results of both methods seem to be equivalent[5,6]; and

(7) The postoperative conception rate per cycle is improved by the use of ovulation stimulators (clomifene, human menopausal gonadotropin (hMG) or follicle-stimulating hormone (FSH))[7].

For all these reasons it has become more and more evident that the first-line therapy should be laparoscopic surgery, which can be performed at the same time as the diagnosis.

Surgical treatment

Analysis of the results of surgery can be made from two standpoints: what are the results, and are there any predictive data?

Results of surgical treatment

Faced with partial series, selected series, doubtful series, imprecise results (a pregnancy does not mean a delivery), etc., it is impossible to have a clear grasp of the actual results. One can estimate that the delivery rate in an unselected series is roughly 40% per patient. This aspect will certainly be reported in other parts of this book, or the reader can refer to a recent paper that we have published on this point[3].

Predictive data of surgical treatment

Some of the data have been known for a long time, such as the presence of extensive adhesions mainly in cases of tubal involvement[8]. This has been confirmed by more recent publications[9]. Numerous publications have demonstrated that the results are independent of the AFS stage, or the presence and size of endometriomas.

In a retrospective 133-patient continuous series of endometriosis-related infertility treated by laparoscopic surgery, we attempted to elucidate the predictive data. No patient was excluded. The overall delivery rate was 37%[10]. We concluded that the factors not influencing the results were the following: AFS stage, presence and size of endometrioma, association with medical suppressive treatment and quality of the surgical treatment (complete or not). Factors negatively influencing the results were the following: tubal adhesions or blockage, age over 38 years, duration of infertility mainly over 7 years and sperm quality. For this last point, precise results are reported in Table 1. The results were dramatically poor in cases of frozen donor-sperm insemination. In cases of sperm abnormalities (numbers $< 20 \times 10^6$, motility $< 20\%$, or teratospermia $> 70\%$), overall results were lowered, but this was only significant in AFS stage 1 or 2. To our knowledge, there has never been any other publication on this point.

We also found that the second treatment provided better results than the first. As it was a retrospective series and, in the second surgery group most of the initial treatment was performed in other hospitals, often by poorly experienced surgeons, we thought that this conclusion was doubtful. Recently Pagidas and colleagues[2], in a retrospective non-randomized series, have clearly shown that second treatment gets poor results, much lower than those obtained with one attempt at *in vitro* fertilization (IVF).

All the data found in our retrospective study were confirmed by a prospective study, to be published later on.

Table 1 Delivery rate based on sperm quality and AFS stage in the 1987–89 series

Sperm	Normal	Abnormal	FDSI
n	80	38	15
All stages	52.5	18.4	0
Stage 1	57.8*	7.1*	0
Stage 2	54.5*	12.5*	0
Stage 3	44.0†	2.5†	0
Stage 4	55.5†	37.5†	0

FDSI, frozen donor sperm insemination; *$p < 0.05$; †NS

Cumulative delivery rate

The last important point of the results was the cumulative delivery rate curve. In a former series[11] we showed that most of the deliveries were obtained in the first 18 months. These data were confirmed by Nezhat and co-workers[12], and were also found in our series of 1987–89 and 1990–93. The results of the cumulative delivery rate for the 1987–89 series are shown in Figure 1.

ART and endometrosis-related infertility

ART cannot be reviewed simply. Various techniques are available (IVF, gamete intra-Fallopian transfer (GIFT), zygote intra-Fallopian transfer (ZIFT), etc.), ovarian hyperstimulation is obtained with different

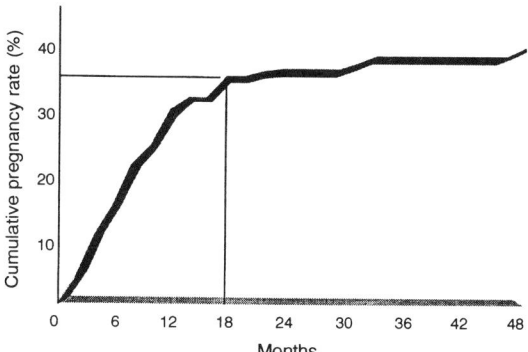

Figure 1 Cumulative intrauterine pregnancy rate observed after laparoscopic treatment in the series of 1987–89

Table 2 Comparison of IVF vs. GIFT (%) (personal series 1987–90)

	IVF ($n = 158$)	GIFT ($n = 75$)	Statistics
Transfer	77.8	100	
Implantation/OPU	32.9	28.0	
Clinical pregnancy/OPU	31.0	21.3	
Deliveries/OPU	27.2	18.6	$p = 0.17$

OPU, ovum pick-up

protocols and ART may be preceded by 'preparation' treatments. Opinions on results are divergent, as are the conclusions drawn from the series on the etiopathogenesis of endometriosis-related infertility.

Which technology?

The main discussion arises between IVF and GIFT. From 1987 to 1990 we were using both procedures in a non-randomized, non-controlled mode. From these cases, a comparison can be made (Table 2). The difference in the delivery rate per attempt (27.2% for IVF vs. 18.6% for GIFT) was not significant ($p = 0.17$), but it seemed to us non-ethical to continue with a more traumatic method that was not better than IVF.

In the literature, four series have been reported. Yovich and Matson[13] and Krasnow and Berga[14] concluded that GIFT was superior to IVF; three concluded the opposite[15–17]. Guzick and colleagues[17] thought that endometriosis impaired the results of GIFT and suggested using IVF rather than GIFT for endometriosis-related infertility. In our opinion, those studies in favor of IVF are much more convincing than those that reported poor IVF results.

On the other hand, Johns[18], Surrey and Hill[19] and Gindoff and co-workers[20] had advocated the use of GIFT at the same time as laparoscopic treatment of endometriosis. In our experience, the results of GIFT were not impaired by this association of procedures, but the quality of laparoscopic surgery was poor and its results dramatically low. Johns[18] and Gindoff and colleagues[20] have concluded that GIFT was not impaired by concomitant surgery, but they do not give clear reports of the results of surgical treatment. Only Surrey and Hill[19] assert that the surgery results were good in terms of pregnancy, but curiously this paper was published in a surgical journal and not in a reproductive or gynecological journal.

Which ovarian stimulation?

The protocols using hMG or FSH after hypophysis desensitization with GnRH agonists (long protocol) are now the 'gold-standard' regimen for ovarian hyperstimulation in IVF. As GnRH agonists are a transitory treatment of endometriosis, it is possible that they could also improve the results of IVF. In our experience from 1987 to 1990, the comparison between the long protocol (112 ovum pick-up (OPU)) and clomiphene plus hMG (46 OPU) in cases of endometriosis-related infertility showed that the transfer rate was higher with the long protocol (81.2% vs. 60.9%; $p < 0.05$), but the delivery rate per OPU was not significantly different (28.6% vs. 23.9%; $p = 0.20$). On the other hand, it was in the cases of endometriosis-related infertility that the difference between the two protocols was the largest. We decided to use GnRH analogs in all cases of endometriosis after 1990. In the literature, three series have found a superiority of the long protocol over the protocol without analogs[16,21,22], and no series has been published proving the opposite. Therefore, it seems logical to prefer the long protocol in this IVF indication.

Previous treatment

Endometriosis is a slow recurrent disease even after surgical or medical treatment. It affects fertility in various ways that we will not discuss here. Some of them, such as antispermatozoid effects, are eliminated by IVF, but some could persist until the OPU or after the transfer, and therefore it seems advisable to shorten the delay between the end of the treatment and the IVF. In our experience from 1987 to 1990[10], we found that the delivery rate per OPU was 50% when this delay was shorter than 6 months, 33.3% when it was 6–12 months, 29% when it was 12–18 months and 20% when this delay was over 18 months. Moreover, we found that the results were better when the last treatment was with GnRH agonists rather than laparoscopic surgery (28.9% vs. 21.5%; $p = 0.07$).

However, in a non-randomized series, Dicker and co-workers[23] found that the results of IVF in cases of endometriosis-related infertility were largely improved when IVF was performed at the end of several months' administration of GnRH analogs (ultralong protocol). Since this initial publication, Dicker and co-workers[24] have published a randomized series confirming these data. This was also found in a non-randomized series in GIFT by Remorgida and colleagues[25] and in IVF by Marcus and Edwards[26] and Nakamura and associates[27]. Chedid and co-workers[17], however, did not find any difference between the ultralong protocol and the long protocol. Moreover, they found that, for stages 1 and 2, the best embryos were obtained with the long protocol rather than the ultralong protocol (66.5% vs. 54.3%), but they did not find any difference in stages 3 and 4. Nevertheless, it was a retrospective study and it seems to be the only one not to have found an improvement.

One can question whether it is a specific effect of GnRH agonists or an effect of a recent treatment of endometriosis. Based on the series of Aboulghar and co-workers[28] and Dicker and colleagues[29], both having shown that puncture of endometriomas previous to IVF improved the results, it can be speculated that the most important effect is the treatment of endometriosis and that the easiest method for temporary suppression of endometriosis is the administration of GnRH analogs, as they act on any sites in this widespread disease. Nevertheless, a specific effect of a long pre-treatment with GnRH agonists (unrelated to endometriosis treatment) cannot be ruled out.

Results of IVF in cases of endometriosis-related infertility

During the early days of IVF, endometriosis-related infertility was considered as a poor indication for IVF[30,31], mainly in comparison with tubal infertility. Fewer oocytes, poor oocyte quality, low fertilization rates and a low implantation rate were the main complaints. During the last few years, ideas have largely changed, and endometriosis-related infertility is more and more considered to be one of the good indications for IVF.

In our experience (Table 3), endometriosis-related infertility appears as the best 'main' indication. It provided better results than in cases of tubal infertility (25.3% delivery/OPU vs. 21.2%; $p < 0.05$), better than in cases of male infertility (25.3% delivery/OPU vs. 17.0%; $p < 0.01$) and similar to those obtained in cases of idiopathic infertility (25.3% delivery/OPU vs. 22.3%; NS).

In a review of the recent series published in the literature (Table 4), it appears that delivery rates over 25% per OPU are frequent, but

Table 3 Comparison of IVF results (1987–95) for endometriosis, tubal infertility, pure male infertility and idiopathic infertility

	Endometriosis	Tubal	Male	Idiopathic
OPU (n)	589	1554	481	376
Oocytes (mean ± SD)	10.05 ± 6.9	9.24†† ± 6.3	10.88†† ± 6.7	9.5†† ± 6.2
Fertilization (%)	45.1	52.6*	26.6†	49.1*
Transfers (%)	81.1	85.6**	58.9*	79.9††
Transferred embryos (mean ± SD)	2.73 ± 1.14	3.02 ± 1.19‡	2.60 ± 1.18††	2.68 ± 1.09††
Clinical pregnancy/OPU (%)	30.9	27.5**	21.4†	25.8††
Clinical pregnancy/transfer (%)	38.0	32.1‡	36.3††	32.3††
Delivery/OPU	25.3	21.2**	17.0‡	22.3††
Delivery/transfer	31.2	24.8‡	29.0††	28.0††
Implantation ratio‡‡ (%)	14.9	11.4*	15.9††	13.9††

OPU, ovum pick-up. All statistical comparisons were made vs. the endometriosis group:
*$p < 0.001$; †$p < 0.0001$; ‡$p < 0.01$; **$p < 0.05$; ††NS. ‡‡, Newborn/transferred embryos

that a comparison with results in cases of tubal infertility are divergent.

Is there some specificity of IVF in cases of endometriosis?

There have been numerous publications underlining the specificity of IVF in case of endometriosis-related infertility. Unfortunately, they are often divergent, so the conclusions must be considered as doubtful. Personal experience, use of different ovarian hyperstimulation regimens and short series are the main causes of these differences of opinion.

In our series (Table 3), we found that the number of harvested oocytes was similar in cases of endometriosis to other indications, that the fertilization rate was reduced compared to tubal infertility and to idiopathic infertility, that the transfer rate was lower than in cases of tubal infertility but similar to idiopathic infertility, that the delivery rate per transfer was higher in cases of endometriosis compared to tubal infertility but similar to those obtained among the male infertility group and the idiopathic infertility group, and that the implantation ratio (newborn per transferred embryos) was similar to those found among the idiopathic infertility group or in case of male infertility and much higher than in the tubal infertility group.

Molloy and associates[30] and Oehninger and co-workers[32] found that fewer oocytes were recovered, but Geber and colleagues[33], like many other authors, found no difference. For Geber and colleagues[33], the fertilization rate was similar in endometriosis compared to tubal infertility, but for Harlow and co-workers[34] there was a major drop in the fertilization rate in cases of endometriosis-related infertility. Geber and colleagues[33] found no difference in the implantation rate in comparison with that in tubal infertility, but for Olivennes and co-workers[21], this rate was decreased in cases of endometriosis compared to tubal infertility. For Tanbo and co-workers it was better in 1990[15] and similar in 1995[35]. For us, it has been improved.

In our opinion the most interesting paper was published by Pellicer and co-workers[36] with a triple analysis: tubal infertility vs. endometriosis-related infertility, oocyte donation results according to the origin of the oocytes (endometriosis or not) and oocyte donation results according to the destination of the oocytes (endometriosis or not). They demonstrated that the main problem in endometriosis seems to come from the poor quality of oocytes, giving poor quality embryos with a

Table 4 Results of large series of IVF in cases of endometriosis-related infertility

Authors	OPU (n)	Pregnancies/OPU (%)	Pregnancies/transfer (%)	Deliveries/OPU (%)	Tubal (%)
Olivennes et al.[21]	314	33.1	35.9	27.7	34.1
Dmowski et al.[39]	119	26.1	29.2	21.8	17.8
Geber et al.[33]	129	34.1	40.0	27.9	29.2
Chedid et al.[16]	114	39.4		27.7*	—
Tanbo et al.[15]	42	38.1	45.7	33.3	
Check et al.[46]	105	23.8		22.9	32.0
Curtis et al.[47]	92	14.1	18.1		15.3
Nakamura et al.[27]	32	53.1	53.1	43.7	—
Remorgida et al.[25]	55	40		29.1	
Dicker et al.[24]	99	14.1	18.9		
Marcus and Edwards[26]	177	28.4		15.8	
Our series	589	31.4	38.0	25.3	21.2

OPU, number of ovum pick-ups in cases of endometriosis-related infertility (ERI); Pregnancies/OPU, clinical pregnancies per OPU in cases of ERI; Pregnancies/transfer, clinical pregnancies per transfer in cases of ERI; Deliveries/OPU, deliveries per OPU in cases of ERI; Tubal, deliveries per OPU in cases of tubal infertility; *IVF + ZIFT + GIFT

lower *in vitro* development ability at day 3 after OPU. In a paper to be published in the future, we will confirm these data through a randomized co-culture series of tubal infertility and endometriosis-related infertility: the percentage of embryos reaching the blastocyst stage was lowered in cases of endometriosis vs. tubal infertility (30.5% vs. 39.5%).

What data influence the results of IVF?

Here again, ideas are divergent. The stage of endometriosis was reported to have a negative impact on the results[30,32,37], but in recent studies the authors did not find any difference[21,33,38]. In our experience there has been no relationship between stage and results, but a tendency to obtain the best results in the more severe cases.

Olivennes and colleagues[21] and we ourselves[10] did not find any difference based on the presence and size of endometriomas. That is at least partially in opposition to Aboulghar and co-workers[28] and Dicker and colleagues[29], who recommended the drainage of these cysts.

Dmowski and co-workers[39] reported that the administration of corticosteroids could improve the IVF results among endometriosis patients having some biological evidence of autoimmune troubles.

Finally, in the analysis of our series, no data seemed to have special influence, except those that are well known in IVF such as age, sperm values and duration of infertility.

Are the results of IVF equivalent at each attempt? This is a highly controversial point, because of patients' rejection or patients' drop-out. In our experience, as in those of IVF units having high results (overall delivery rate per OPU over 20%), the best results are obtained during the first attempts, and these decrease slowly with the range of the OPU. Thereafter, it is extremely hazardous to draw a theoretical delivery rate per patient after *n* attempts from an overall delivery rate per OPU.

Cumulative delivery rate

Analysis of IVF results cannot be limited to the delivery rate per OPU. Cumulative

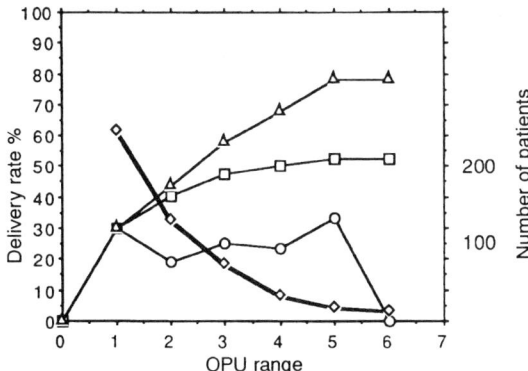

Figure 2 Results of IVF in a 245-patient cohort: number of patients treated for each attempt range (diamonds); delivery rate for each attempt range (circles); real cumulative delivery rate per patient (CDRP) after each attempt range (squares); and theoretical CDRP after each attempt range (triangles)

delivery rate per patient (CDRP) is a more accurate measure to check the efficacy of this treatment, as the patients can be submitted to several attempts[6,40]. CDRP can be expressed in two different ways. We have described these in a previous paper on tubal infertility[41]. The theoretical CDRP is the most commonly used. It gives the percentage of patients that should have delivered after n attempts, if no patients had dropped out. IVF is a stressful and expensive treatment, and many patients stop by themselves for psychological or financial reasons. Even in our unit, where the first four attempts of IVF are free of charge for the patients, 20% of the non-pregnant patients drop out after each attempt. That leads to a small number of patients submitted to more than four attempts. This observation in our series was also made in all the other published series[40–44].

The definition of the real CDRP is the ratio of patients that have delivered after a delay that was large enough for them to have been submitted to n attempts (for example: 24 months and four attempts). The difference between real and theoretical CDRP increases with time (or potential attempts).

We give figures from our experience among 245 patients who started IVF from 1987 to 1994 and were suffering from endometriosis-related infertility. In September 1996, only 129 patients (real CDRP 52.7%) had delivered (at least once) or were pregnant, but the theoretical CDRP was 78.4% after six IVF attempts. The difference came from the large drop-out rate. An illustration of these data is provided in Figure 2.

Nevertheless, in our experience, the patients suffering from endometriosis were those that reached the highest real and theoretical CDRP.

The place of ART in the management of endometriosis-related infertility

Proposition for a logical management of endometriosis-related infertility

From all these data, we proposed a system of management of endometriosis-related infertility[3] (Figure 3). Laparoscopic surgery is the first step in any case, except for severe and inflammatory cases that can be managed with suppressive medical treatment before a 'second' operative laparoscopy. Thereafter, patients can be divided into two groups. When the fertility prognosis appears poor (tubal involvement, massive adhesions, age over 38, duration of infertility over 7 years, association of male infertility with minimal or mild stages, requirement of frozen donor sperm use), IVF is indicated rapidly and must be preceded by 3 months' administration of GnRH analogs, at least in moderate and severe cases. In the other cases, expectant management is proposed for a period of 6 months. Later on, ovarian stimulation is proposed for 6–9 months. Then, in persistent infertility, IVF is proposed after a 3-month period of pretreatment with GnRH agonists.

Results of this management

Basic results The management that we have defined was proposed for all the patients

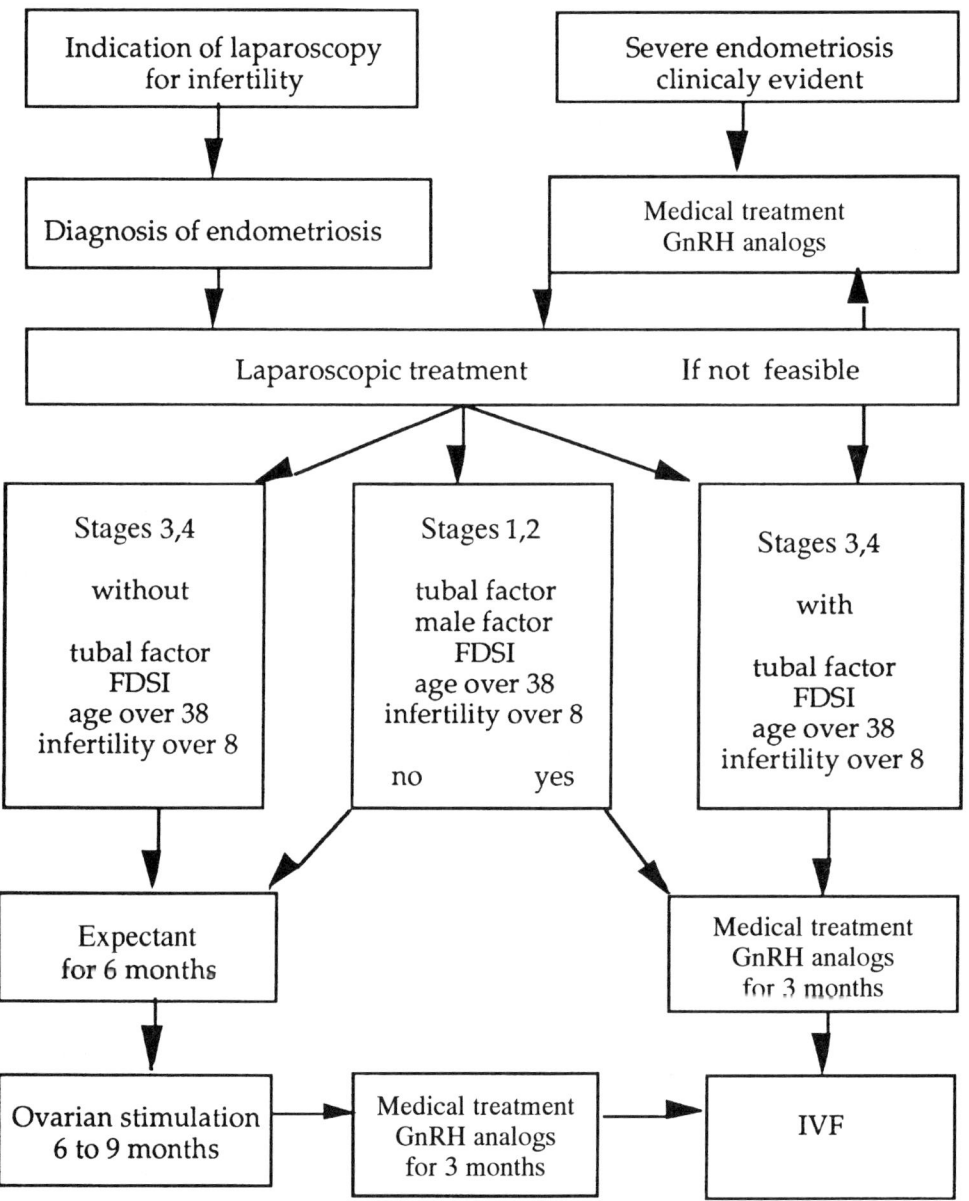

Figure 3 Proposed management of endometriosis-related infertility. FDSI, frozen donor sperm insemination

treated during the period 1991–93, but did not include the ovarian stimulation that was added after the beginning of 1994. The 3-months' pretreatment with analogs was advised to the patients, but not imposed.

The series included 242 patients and no exclusion was made, except for the patients who were completely lost to follow-up immediately after the laparoscopic treatment (27 patients). Endometriosis-related infertility was defined as the association of infertility over 18 months and any type of endometriosis, without respect to any other infertility causes. A 'final' result was observed in June 1996.

According to our management schedule, 25 patients were directly referred to IVF and 217 were managed on the other arm.

With the laparoscopic treatment we obtained 82 clinical pregnancies that resulted in 71 deliveries. This represents a real delivery rate of 29.3% (71/242) for all the patients or 32.7% (71/217) for only these patients for whom the surgical procedure offered some chance.

These results show that 171 patients should have been taken in charge in IVF: 25 immediately and 146 after failures of surgery. In fact only 130 went to the IVF unit (76%); financial considerations cannot explain this drop, as the first four IVF attempts were fully reimbursed by the French Social Security (State Medical Insurance). After IVF, 70 patients (53.8%) delivered (at least once). This ratio is in fact the real CDRP after four attempts. Because of the short duration and our experience of the patients' behavior, we expect that this will probably increase to 57%. The theoretical CDRP (after four attempts) in this series was 72%. More precise results on this series will be published later on.

Presentation of the results Different statistical presentations of this series can be made.

The more pessimistic result is that 141/242 patients (58.3%) had delivered at least once: 71 after laparoscopic treatment and 70 after IVF (49.6%).

An ultra-optimistic presentation can be made: 32.7% of the patients delivered after laparoscopic treatment (only considering the patients having a chance after surgery). Among the remaining, 72% should have delivered after four IVF attempts, representing 48.5% of the complete group $((1-0.327) \times 72\% = 48.5\%)$. And the final results would be 81.2% (32.7% + 48.5% = 81.2%).

In spite of the large difference between these two extreme presentations, it is obvious that the place of IVF is major in the management of endometriosis-related infertility. In the first, IVF represented 49.6% of the deliveries and in the second, 59.5%.

Discussion

To define the place of ART in endometriosis-related infertility, it is mandatory to take into account several other points, such as:

(1) Financial considerations;

(2) Risk of multiple pregnancies; and

(3) Ethical considerations.

Financial considerations

The cost-effectiveness ratio is becoming more and more important in medicine. However, in comparison of two extremely different treatments, it can be dramatically different from one country to another.

The estimated cost of IVF ranges from US$2500 (Australia) to US$12 000 (USA). The difference mainly comes from two points: the price of hMG (or FSH) (US$12 per ampule in France to US$60 in the USA), and from the mean size of the IVF centers (1000 OPU per year in Australia vs. less than 100 in the USA).

On the other hand, IVF is largely paid for by the state health system in countries such as Israel, Australia or France and not at all in others such as the USA or Germany. Therefore, the logical scientific management can be disturbed by these considerations, making IVF too expensive or too cheap for the patients.

Prices of surgery are certainly not so divergent, but there again the access to expert laparoscopist surgeons differs from one country to another and even from one city to another.

The risk of multiple pregnancies

In any IVF series or register, the multiple delivery rate ranges from 20 to 35% and the triplet (or more) pregnancy rate ranges from 2 to 6%. This has a major economic impact, as neonatal care required by these 'multiple' babies has a cost higher than the direct cost of IVF[45]. Nowadays, no one knows what the sociological impact will be of such a large number of people having one or more twin brothers or sisters. Moreover, it is evident that the risk of family breakdown (e.g. divorce, depression, desertion) is dramatically increased in cases of triplets or quadruplets. That is certainly the largest disadvantage of current ART. However, this risk is much lower with conventional treatment.

Ethical and sociological considerations

Access to ART can also be limited by personal, ethical, legal or religious considerations that we will not develop here. Finally, it is clear that the ratio of IVF per inhabitant, even in well developed countries (to eliminate the cost problem), diverges from 1 to 10. For instance, the estimated number of IVF (or ICSI) attempts was roughly the same in France and the USA in the year 1994 (32 000) for a respective population of 60 and 270 million (comparative ratio 1:0.222). For 1989, Kenny[37] reported 11 047 IVF or GIFT attempts in Australia (17×10^6 inhabitants; ratio 650 procedures for 10^6 people) and 22 583 IVF or GIFT treatments in the USA (270×10^6 inhabitants; ratio 84 procedures for 10^6 people), representing a comparative ratio of 1:0.129. One can easily understand that such a large difference has a direct influence on the scientific management of endometriosis-related infertility.

Conclusion

It is evident that IVF has a major place in endometriosis-related infertility. For a long time, laparoscopy should remain the first-line therapy. IVF will be recommended in cases of poor prognosis after surgery and after failures.

Our proposal of management is based on personal experience and literature analysis. Only multicenter cohort studies will permit a more precise definition of when IVF must be proposed. That will require a high co-operation between IVF biologist and reproductive surgeons whose role must be complementary[2] and not opposed[1].

References

1. Soliman, S., Daya, S., Collins, J. and Jarrell, J. (1993). A randomized trial of *in vitro* fertilization versus conventional treatment for infertility. *Fertil. Steril.*, **59**, 1239–44
2. Pagidas, K., Falcone, T., Hemmings, R. and Miron, P. (1996). Comparison of reoperation for moderate (stage III) and severe (stage IV) endometriosis-related infertility with *in vitro* fertilization–embryo transfer. *Fertil. Steril.*, **65**, 791–5
3. Pouly, J.L., Drolet, J., Canis, M., Boughazine, S., Mage, G., Bruhat, M.A. and Wattiez, A. (1996). Laparoscopic treatment of symptomatic endometriosis. *Hum. Reprod.*, (Suppl.) in press
4. Shushan, A, Eisenberg, V.H. and Schenker, J.G. (1995). Subfertility in the era of assisted reproduction: changes and consequences. *Fertil. Steril.*, **64**, 459–69
5. Adamson, G.D. and Pasta, D.J. (1994). Surgical treatment of endometriosis-associated infertility: metaanalysis compared with survival analysis. *Am. J. Obstet. Gynecol.*, **171**, 1488–505
6. Hull, M.G.R. (1992). Infertility treatment: effectiveness of conventional and assisted conception methods. *Hum. Reprod.*, **7**, 785–96
7. Kemmann, E., Ghazi, D., Corsan, G. and Bohrer, M.K. (1993). Does ovulation stimulation improve fertility in women with minimal/mild endometriosis after laser laparoscopy? *Int. J. Fertil.*, **38**, 16–21
8. Kistner, R.W. (1975). Management of endometriosis in the infertile patients. *Fertil. Steril.*, **26**, 1151–60
9. Canis, M., Pouly, J.L., Wattiez, A., Manhes, H., Mage, G. and Bruhat, M.A. (1992). Incidence of bilateral adnexal disease in severe

endometriosis (revised American Fertility Society, stage IV). Should a stage V be included in the American Fertility Society classification? *Fertil. Steril.*, **57**, 691–2
10. Chassagnard, F. (1990). External endometriosis. Results of laparoscopic treatment of endometriosis in pain and in infertile patients. Indication and results for IVF in endometriosis. Thèse Medicale Clermont Ferrand
11. Pouly, J.L., Manhes, H., Mage, G., Canis, M. and Bruhat, M. (1986). Laparoscopic treatment of endometriosis. In Bruhat, M. and Canis, M. (eds.) *Endometriosis*, p. 91. (Basel: Karger)
12. Nezhat, C., Crowgey, S. and Nezhat, F. (1989). Videolaseroscopy for the treatment of endometriosis associated with infertility. *Fertil. Steril.*, **51**, 237–40
13. Yovich, J.L. and Matson, P.L. (1990). The influence of infertility etiology on the outcome of IVF-ET and GIFT treatments. *Int. J. Fertil.*, **35**, 26–33
14. Krasnow, J.S. and Berga, S.L. (1993). Endometriosis and gamete intrafallopian transfer. *Assist. Reprod. Rev.*, **3**, 121–8
15. Tambo, T., Dale, P.O. and Abyholm, T. (1990). Assisted fertilization in infertile women with patent Fallopian tubes. A comparison of in-vitro fertilization, gamete intra-Fallopian transfer and tubal embryo stage transfer. *Hum. Reprod.*, **5**, 266–70
16. Chedid, S., Camus, M., Smitz, J., Van Steirteghern, A.C. and Devroey, P. (1995). Comparison among different ovarian stimulation regimens for assisted procreation procedures in patients with endometriosis. *Hum. Reprod.*, **10**, 2406–11
17. Guzick, D.S., Yao, Y.A.S., Berga, S.L., Krasnow, J.S., Stovall, D.W., Kubik, C.J. and Zeleznik, A.J. (1994). Endometriosis impairs the efficacy of gamete intrafallopian transfer: results of a case–control study. *Fertil. Steril.*, **62**, 1186–91
18. Johns, D.A. (1991). Clomiphene citrate-induced gamete intrafallopian transfer with diagnosis and operative laparoscopy. *Fertil. Steril.*, **56**, 311–13
19. Surrey, J. and Hill, D.L. (1994). Treatment of endometriosis by carbon dioxide laser during gamete intrafallopian transfer. *Am. J. Coll. Surg.*, **179**, 440–2
20. Gindoff, P.R., Hall, J.L., Nelson, L.M. and Stillman, R.J. (1990). Efficacy of assisted reproductive technology during diagnostic and operative infertility laparoscopy. *Obstet. Gynecol.*, **75**, 299–301
21. Olivennes, F., Feldberg, D., Liu, H.-C., Cohen, J., Moy, F. and Rosenwaks, Z. (1995). Endometriosis: a stage by stage analysis – the role of *in vitro* fertilization. *Fertil. Steril.*, **64**, 392–8
22. Oehninger, S., Brzyski, R.G., Muasher, S.J., Acosta, A.A. and Jones, G.S. (1989). In-vitro fertilization and embryo transfer in patients with endometriosis: impact of a gonadotrophin releasing hormone agonist. *Hum. Reprod.*, **4**, 541–4
23. Dicker, D., Goldman, G.A., Ashkenazi, J., Feldberg, D., Voliovitz, I. and Goldman, J.A. (1990). The value of pre-treatment with gonadotrophin releasing hormone (GnRH) analogue in IVF-ET therapy of severe endometriosis. *Hum. Reprod.*, **5**, 418–20
24. Dicker, D., Goldman, J.A., Levy, T., Feldberg, D. and Ashkenazi, J. (1992). The impact of long-term gonadotropin-releasing hormone analogue treatment on preclinical abortions in patients with severe endometriosis undergoing *in vitro* fertilization–embryo transfer. *Fertil. Steril.*, **57**, 597–600.
25. Remorgida, V., Anserini, P., Croce, S., Costa, M., Ferraiolo, A. and Capitanio, G.L. (1990). Comparison of different ovarian stimulation protocols for gamete intrafallopian transfer in patients with minimal and mild endometriosis. *Fertil. Steril.*, **53**, 1060–3
26. Marcus, F. and Edwards, R.G. (1994). High rate of pregnancy after long term down regulation of women with severe endometriosis. *Am. J. Obstet. Gynecol.*, **171**, 812–17
27. Nakamura, K., Oosawa, M., Kondou, I., Inagaki, S., Shibata, H., Narita, O., Suganuma, N. and Tomoda, Y. (1992). Menotropin stimulation after prolonged gonadotropin releasing hormone agonist pretreatment for *in vitro* fertilization in patients with endometriosis. *J. Assist. Reprod. Genet.*, **9**, 113–17
28. Aboulghar, M.A., Mansour, R.T., Serour, G.I. and Rizk, B. (1991). Ultrasonic transvaginal aspiration of endometriotic cysts: an optional line of treatment in selected cases of endometriosis. *Hum. Reprod.*, **6**, 1408–10
29. Dicker, D., Goldman, J.A., Feldberg, D., Ashkenazi, J. and Levy, T. (1991). Transvaginal ultrasonic needle-guided aspiration of endometriotic cysts before ovulation induction for

in vitro fertilization. *J. In Vitro Fertil. Embryo Transf.*, **8**, 286–9

30. Molloy, D., Martin, M., Speirs, A. *et al.* Performance of patients with a 'frozen pelvis' in an *in vitro* fertilization program. *Fertil. Steril.*, **47**, 450–5

31. Barri, P.N., Pintado, J.M., Sanfeliu, F., Coroleu, B., Martinez, F. and Veiga, A. (1988). IVF performance of patients with endometriosis. *Prog. Obstet. Gynecol.*, **31**, 305–8

32. Oehninger, S., Acosta, A.A., Kreiner, D., Muasher, S.J., Jones, H.W. Jr and Rosenwaks, Z. (1988). *In vitro* fertilization and embryo transfer (IVF/ET): an established and successful therapy for endometriosis. *J. In Vitro Fertil. Embryo Transf.*, **5**, 249–56

33. Geber, S., Paraschos, T., Atkinson, G., Margara, R. and Winston, R.M.L. (1995). Results of IVF in patients with endometriosis: the severity of the disease does not affect outcome, or the incidence of miscarriage. *Hum. Reprod.*, **10**, 1507–11

34. Harlow, C.R., Cahill, D.J., Maile, L.A., Talbot, W.M., Mears, J., Wardle, P.G. and Hull, M.G.R. (1996). Reduced preovulatory granulosa cell steroidogenesis in women with endometriosis. *J. Clin. Endocrinol. Metab.*, **81**, 426–9

35. Tanbo, T., Omland, A., Dale, P.O. and Abyholm, T. (1995). *In vitro* fertilization/embryo transfer in unexplained infertility and minimal peritoneal endometriosis. *Acta Obstet. Gynecol. Scand.*, **74**, 539–43

36. Pellicer, A., Oliveira, N., Ruiz, A., Remohi, J. and Simon, C. (1995). Exploring the mechanism(s) of endometriosis-related infertility: an analysis of embryo development and implantation in assisted reproduction. *Hum. Reprod.*, **10** (Suppl. 2), 91–7

37. Kenny, D.T. (1995). *In vitro* fertilisation and gamete intrafallopian transfer: an integrative analysis of research, 1987–1992. *Br. J. Obstet. Gynaecol.*, **102**, 317–25

38. Tummon, I.S., Colwell, K.A., Mackinnon, C.J., Nisker, J.A. and Yuzpe, A.A. (1991). Abbreviated endometriosis-associated infertility correlates with *in vitro* fertilization success. *J. In Vitro Fertil. Embryo Transf.*, **8**, 149–53

39. Dmowski, W.P., Rana, N., Michalowska, J., Friberg, J., Papierniak, C. and El-Roeiy, A. (1995). The effect of endometriosis, its stage and activity, and of autoantibodies on *in vitro* fertilization and embryo transfer success rates. *Fertil. Steril.*, **63**, 555–62

40. Tan, S.L., Royston, P., Campbell, S., Jacobs, H.S., Betts, J., Mason, B. and Edwards, R.G. (1992). Cumulative conception and livebirth rates after *in-vitro* fertilisation. *Lancet*, **339**, 1390–4

41. Pouly, J.L., Janny, L., Pouly-Vye, P., Boyer, C., Canis, M., Bassil, S., Chapron, C., Zambrano, R., Moussali, F., Boucher, D. and Bruhat, M.A. (1995). Cumulative delivery rate after *in vitro* fertilization for tubal infertility. *Ref. Gynecol. Obstet.*, **3** (Special Issue), 224–30

42. Alsalili, M., Yuzpe, A., Tummon, I., Parker, J., Martin, J., Daniel, S., Rebel, M. and Nisker, J. (1995). Cumulative pregnancy rate and pregnancy outcome after *in vitro* fertilization: > 5000 cycles at one centre. *Hum. Reprod.*, **10**, 470–4

43. Chardon, C., Boulieu, D., Rochet, Y., Payan, F. and Ayzac, L. (1992). Sterilite d'origine tubaire. Quel traitement proposer: FIV ou chirurgie? *Rev. Fr. Gynecol. Obstet.*, **87**, 355–60

44. Check, J.H., Lurie, D., Callan, C., Baker A. and Benfer, K. (1994). Comparison of the cumulative probability of pregnancy after *in vitro* fertilization–embryo transfer by infertility factor and age. *Fertil. Steril.*, **61**, 257–61

45. Callahan, T.L., Hall, J.E., Ettner, S.L., Christiansen, C.L., Greene, M.F. and Crowley, W.F. (1994). The economic impact of multiple-gestation pregnancies and the contribution of assisted reproduction techniques to their incidence. *N. Engl. J. Med.*, **331**, 244–9

46. Check, J.H., Lurie, D., O'Shaughnessy, A. and Dietterich, C. (1995). The relationship of endometriosis to endometrial sonographic studies prior to administration of human chorionic gonadotrophin in patients undergoing *in-vitro* fertilization and embryo transfer. *Hum. Reprod.*, **10**, 938–41

47. Curtis, P., Jackson, A., Bernard, A. and Shaw, R.W. (1993). Pretreatment with gonadotrophin releasing hormone (GnRH) analogue prior to *in vitro* fertilisation for patients with endometriosis. *Eur. J. Obstet. Gynecol. Reprod. Biol.*, **52**, 211–16

Assisted reproductive technologies, endometriosis and decision making

I.S. Tummon, B. Bany and J. Martin

Rational use of assisted reproductive technologies for patients with endometriosis-associated infertility depends on accurate information about both the treated and untreated prognosis. The purpose of this review is to scrutinize decision making regarding endometriosis-associated infertility and assisted reproduction.

The untreated prognosis for endometriosis-associated infertility

Endometriosis has a strong negative effect on the likelihood of live birth[1]. Collins and co-workers studied a cohort of 312 untreated couples with endometriosis-associated infertility followed for up to 7 years[1]. Using a proportional hazards analysis the effect of a diagnosis of endometriosis was an overall negative multiplication factor of 0.4 on the prognosis for live birth. Cumulative live birth rates were higher in the less severe subgroup of endometriosis (Figure 1). The 95% confidence limits of severe/moderate endometriosis did not overlap the confidence limits of unexplained infertility. Left untreated, severe/moderate endometriosis had a cumulative 36-month fecundity of only 5%. Minimal/mild endometriosis had an intermediate position with confidence intervals overlapping both other diagnostic groups.

The prognosis for endometriosis-associated infertility treated with assisted reproduction techniques

Evidence of effective therapy requires more than knowledge of the untreated natural

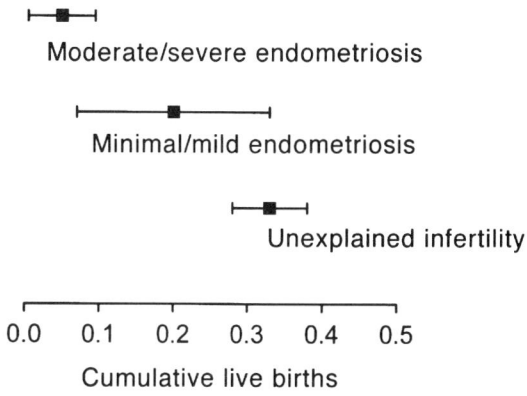

Figure 1 Prognosis without treatment: cumulative live births at 36 months (with confidence limits) (adapted from reference 1)

history of endometriosis-associated infertility. The best quality evidence of effective therapy is based on randomized, controlled trials. If treatment is effective, then relative risks of treatment are consistent in a series of randomized clinical trials. Relative risks are significant when their confidence intervals do not cross unity.

There is a paucity of randomized controlled trials of *in vitro* fertilization for endometriosis-associated infertility. In the single randomized trial of *in vitro* fertilization compared to no treatment the relative risk of pregnancy cannot be calculated due to small sample size ($n = 21$)[2]. Early treatment with *in vitro* fertilization resulted in pregnancy in five of 15 (33%) women compared to none of six (0%) women randomized to 6 months of waiting.

Decisions about the place of assisted reproduction techniques for refractory endometriosis-associated infertility must be made with lesser degrees of evidence.

Controlled ovarian hyperstimulation/intrauterine insemination

Analysis of the subset of women with endometriosis studied by Nulsen and co-workers[3] showed combined ovarian hyperstimulation and intrauterine insemination with greater fecundity (relative risk 5.3, confidence interval 1.1–22.5) than intrauterine insemination alone[3].

Analysis of the subset of women with endometriosis studied by Chaffkin and co-workers[4] in a non-randomized trial found marginal benefit of combining intrauterine insemination to controlled ovarian hyperstimulation. Combined treatment gave a relative risk of pregnancy of 2.1 (confidence interval 0.7–6.1) compared to controlled ovarian hyperstimulation alone. It is concluded that controlled ovarian hyperstimulation is the more potent component of combined controlled ovarian hyperstimulation and intrauterine insemination for endometriosis-associated infertility.

Meta-analysis of 962 cycles of controlled ovarian hyperstimulation and intrauterine insemination with a primary diagnosis of endometriosis was performed by Peterson and co-workers[5]. Aggregate pregnancy rates per cycle were 0.13 (confidence interval 0.04–0.23) for minimal/mild endometriosis and 0.08 (confidence interval 0–0.27) for moderate/severe endometriosis. The authors of the meta-analysis acknowledged the difficulty in performing cost analysis and that differences between patient groups may have accounted for their conclusions.

Evolution of *in vitro* fertilization

General advances

Comprehensive assessment of subfertility before assisted reproduction takes advantage of improved diagnosis of ovarian reserve[6] and sperm function[7-11]. Knowledge of gamete reserve permits more rational use of assisted reproduction and allows better selection of treatment. For instance, severe sperm defects are more properly treated by intracytoplasmic sperm injection, while occult defects in ovarian reserve can be detected prior to the performance of futile treatment[6]. Rational decision making for endometriosis-associated infertility depends on accurate laparoscopic assessment of pelvic deformity.

Poor results for moderate/severe endometriosis prior to 1990

During the laparoscopic oocyte retrieval era of *in vitro* fertilization the outlook for pregnancy was compromised for women with moderate/severe endometriosis-associated infertility[11]. In a report representative of the era, Oehninger and co-workers indicated the relative risk of ongoing pregnancy (per cycle started) was 4.4 (confidence interval 0.98–20.1) for minimal/mild endometriosis compared to moderate/severe endometriosis[11]. Reduced ovarian access was one factor associated with the poorer prognosis of moderate/severe endometriosis compared to minimal/mild disease. After laparoscopic retrieval was superseded by transvaginal retrieval, *in vitro* fertilization became effective treatment for moderate and severe stages of endometriosis-associated infertility[12] (Figure 2).

Improved results using contemporary techniques for in vitro *fertilization*

Transvaginal oocyte retrieval and gonadotropin-releasing hormone (GnRH) agonist are standard therapy for *in vitro* fertilization[13]. Analysis of reports published in 1995 for moderate/severe endometriosis indicates pregnancy rates that are not reduced compared to minimal/mild endometriosis[14–16] (Table 1).

Improved aggregate results do not mean that the untreated fertility capacity in all stages of endometriosis is the same, only that use of a complex, costly technique, *in vitro* fertilization, can be effective in overcoming subfertility.

Assisted reproductive technologies and endometriosis

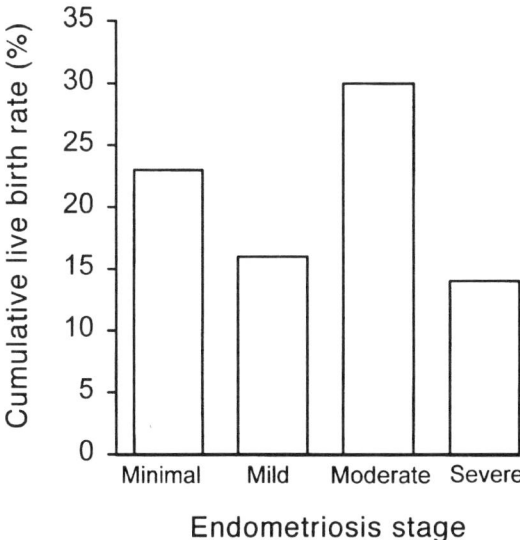

Figure 2 Cumulative live births after three cycles in 240 patients, by endometriosis revised American Fertility Society stage (from reference 12)

Table 1 *In vitro* fertilization for endometriosis-associated infertility

	Pregnancies/number of cycles	
Reference	Minimal/mild endometriosis	Moderate/severe endometriosis
Geber et al.[14]	29/100	15/29
Olivennes et al.[15]	43/132	37/104
Dmowski et al.[16]	22/89	9/30
Total	94/321 (29%)	61/163 (37%)

All studies are retrospective cohort studies using gonadotropin-releasing hormone agonists and transvaginal oocyte retrieval, and were published in 1995

In 1990, the last year in which the Society for Assisted Reproductive Technology categorized results by diagnostic category, there was no diminution of results for *in vitro* fertilization performed for a primary diagnosis of endometriosis compared to other diagnostic categories[17].

Gamete intrafallopian transfer *or* in vitro *fertilization?*

With a primary diagnosis of endometriosis, data in the 1989 United States registry showed that gamete intrafallopian transfer produced a relative risk for pregnancy per cycle of 6.0 (confidence interval 4.8–7.4) compared to *in vitro* fertilization[17]. Treatment was not allocated randomly and differences between patient groups may have accounted for different results. In the only randomized, controlled comparison of gamete intrafallopian transfer and *in vitro* fertilization, pregnancy rates were not different[18]. However, the subjects had a diagnosis of idiopathic infertility and it may be inappropriate to apply this lack of difference to endometriosis.

In a case–control study of gamete intrafallopian transfer by Guzick and co-workers[19] the presence of endometriosis was associated with a reduced likelihood of birth (relative risk 0.67, confidence interval 0.47–0.97) compared to no endometriosis. The authors speculated that *in vitro* fertilization may bypass an unfavorable peritoneal environment and that gamete intrafallopian transfer does not protect against a potentially unfavorable environment.

How successful is in vitro *fertilization?*

Life table analysis was used to analyze a series of 5000 *in vitro* fertilization cycles at one center. No negative relationship of endometriosis compared to other diagnostic categories was found[20] (Figure 3).

Life table analysis assumes that probability of pregnancy in those not continuing treatment is the same as for those who continue treatment. This assumption may be quite invalid. During and after treatment prognostic information is deliberately and aggressively sought[6–11]. With accurate information individuals with the best prognosis can be advised to accept treatment, while poor prognostic cases are advised to discontinue treatment.

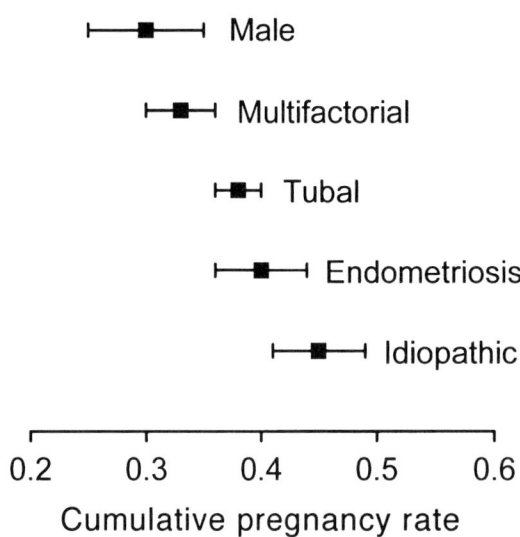

Figure 3 Cumulative pregnancy rates after three cycles in 4598 patients (with confidence limits), by diagnosis (from reference 20)

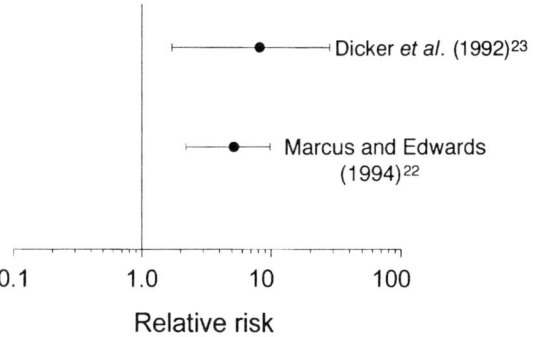

Figure 4 Relative risk of pregnancy per cycle (with confidence limits), comparing pretreatment to no pretreatment

Life table analysis may be falsely optimistic in its estimation of results. Acknowledging this limitation, life table analysis remains the conventional method for assessing *in vitro* fertilization success and comparing results from different centers.

An integrative analysis of 39 000 cycles of *in vitro* fertilization and gamete intrafallopian transfer concluded that minimal/mild endometriosis treated with either form of assisted reproduction had a higher rate of clinical pregnancy than other causes of infertility[21].

Medical pretreatment before *in vitro* fertilization

Medical pretreatment before *in vitro* fertilization is of uncertain benefit. Trials of medical treatment prior to *in vitro* fertilization have not included strict randomization[22,23] (Figure 4). Although medical pretreatment is popular in some centers and 95% confidence intervals of these two trials do not cross unity, the reader is cautioned that the trials were not random comparisons. The value of GnRH agonist pretreatment for endometriosis-associated infertility before assisted reproduction is uncertain.

Endometriomata

Endometriomata and complex cysts associated with moderate and severe endometriosis are amenable to a variety of technical approaches during treatment with *in vitro* fertilization. Descriptive reports of successful management include no treatment[24], transvaginal aspiration[25] and re-operation[26]. It is the experience of the authors that individualized treatment depending on the size and location of endometriomata, the rapidity of their recurrence and previous experience with oocyte retrieval is most appropriate.

Re-operation

Pagidas and co-workers retrospectively studied women undergoing re-operation for moderate/severe endometriosis and compared them to a concurrent group undergoing *in vitro* fertilization but with a prior history of surgical reduction of moderate/severe endometriosis[26]. The authors performed life table analysis. Re-operation was not recommended for asymptomatic women with prior surgical reduction of moderate/severe endometriosis. The relative risk of live birth was 1.6 (confidence interval 0.5–6.4) with one cycle of *in vitro* fertilization compared to re-operation and follow-up with a mean of 19 months (range 1–43). The authors concluded that a single cycle of *in vitro* fertilization is an effective alternative to re-operation.

Conclusions

Improved prognosis for moderate/severe endometriosis treated by in vitro *fertilization*

Untreated moderate/severe endometriosis has a poor prognosis for live birth[1]. Accurate diagnosis and staging of endometriosis is therefore a prerequisite to rational therapy for endometriosis-associated infertility. Prior to 1990, *in vitro* fertilization for moderate/severe endometriosis showed diminished results compared to minimal/mild endometriosis[11]. However, aggregate results published in 1995 of *in vitro* fertilization for moderate/severe endometriosis showed no diminution of pregnancy rates (Table 1).

Role of assisted reproduction

Endometriosis is a negative prognostic factor for live birth[1]. Surgery is primary therapy for endometriosis while assisted reproduction is a secondary approach for multifactorial infertility or infertility refractory to surgical reduction of endometriosis. To overcome the poor fecundity associated with endometriosis a more intrusive use of assisted reproduction for patients with endometriosis compared to those without endometriosis may be required. A hierarchy of assisted reproductive procedures are available. Choice of procedure remains empirical with a principle of ascending intrusion from least to most complex potentially effective treatment.

When assisted reproduction is chosen, controlled ovarian hyperstimulation and intrauterine insemination is the usual first approach. For determined individuals with minimal/mild endometriosis whose condition is refractory to less intrusive treatment and those with major anatomic deformity *in vitro* fertilization may be required.

References

1. Collins, J.A., Burrows, E.A. and Willan, A.R. (1995). The prognosis for live birth among untreated infertile couples. *Fertil. Steril.*, **64**, 22–8
2. Soliman, S., Daya, S., Collins, J. and Jarrell, J. (1993). A randomized trial of *in vitro* fertilization versus conventional treatment for infertility. *Fertil. Steril.*, **59**, 1239–44
3. Nulsen, J.C., Walsh, S., Dumez, S. and Metzger, D.A. (1993). A randomized and longitudinal study of human menopausal gonadotropin with intrauterine insemination in the treatment of infertility. *Obstet. Gynecol.*, **82**, 780–6
4. Chaffkin, L., Nulsen, J.C., Luciano, A.A. and Metzger, D. (1991). A. A comparative analysis of the cycle fecundity rates associated with combined human menopausal gonadotropin (hMG) and intrauterine insemination (IUI) versus either hMG or IUI alone. *Fertil. Steril.*, **55**, 252–7
5. Peterson, C.M., Hatasaka, H.H., Jones, K.P., Pouson, A.M., Carrell, D.T. and Urry, R.L. (1994). Ovulation induction with gonadotropins and intrauterine insemination compared with *in vitro* fertilization and no therapy: a prospective, non-randomized, cohort study and meta analysis. *Fertil. Steril.*, **62**, 535–44
6. Martin, J.S.B., Nisker, J.A., Tummon, I.S., Daniel, S.A.J., Auckland, J.L. and Feyles, V. (1996). Future *in vitro* fertilization pregnancy potential of women with variably elevated day 3 follicle stimulating hormone levels. *Fertil. Steril.*, **65**, 1238–40
7. Tummon, I.S., Yuzpe, A.A., Daniel, S.A.J. and

Deutsch, A. (1991). Total acrosin activity correlates with fertility potential after fertilization in vitro. *Fertil. Steril.*, **56**, 933–8

8. Clarke, G.N., Elliott, P.J. and Smaila, C. (1985). Detection of sperm antibodies in semen using the immunobead test: a survey of 813 consecutive patients. *Am. J. Reprod. Immunol. Microbiol.*, **7**, 118–23

9. Lopata, A., Patullo, M.J., Chang, A. and James, B. (1976). A method for collecting motile spermatozoa from human semen. *Fertil. Steril.*, **27**, 677–84

10. Kruger, T.F., Acosta, A.A., Simmons, K.F., Swanson, R.J., Matta, J.F. and Oehninger, S. (1988). Predictive value of abnormal sperm morphology in *in vitro* fertilization. *Fertil. Steril.*, **48**, 112–17

11. Oehninger, S., Acosta, A.A., Kreiner, D., Muasher, S.J., Jones, H.W. Jr and Rosenwaks, Z. (1988). *In vitro* fertilization and embryo transfer (IVF/ET): an established and successful therapy for endometriosis. *J. In Vitro Fertil. Embryo Transfer*, **5**, 249–56

12. Tummon, I.S., Colwell, K.A., Mackinnon, C.J., Nisker, J.A. and Yuzpe, A.A. (1991). Abbreviated endometriosis-associated infertility correlates with *in vitro* fertilization success. *J. In Vitro Fertil. Embryo Transfer*, **8**, 149–53

13. Hughes, E.G., Fedorkow, D.M., Daya, S., Sagle, M.A., Van de Koppel, P. and Collins, J.A. (1992). The routine use of gonadotropin-releasing hormone agonist prior to *in vitro* fertilization and gamete intrafallopian transfer: a meta-analysis of randomized, controlled trials. *Fertil. Steril.*, **58**, 888–96

14. Geber, S., Paraschos, T., Atkinson, G., Margara, R. and Winston, R.M. (1995). Results of IVF in patients with endometriosis: the severity of the disease does not affect outcome, or the incidence of miscarriage. *Hum. Reprod.*, **10**, 1507–11

15. Olivennes, F., Feldberg, D., Liu, H.C., Cohen, J., Moy, F. and Rosenwaks, Z. (1995). Endometriosis: a stage by stage analysis – the role of *in vitro* fertilization. *Fertil. Steril.*, **64**, 392–8

16. Dmowski, W.P., Rana, N., Michalowska, J., Friberg, J., Papierniak, C. and el Roeiy, A. (1995). The effect of endometriosis, its stage and activity, and of autoantibodies on *in vitro* fertilization and embryo transfer success rates. *Fertil. Steril.*, **63**, 555–62

17. The American Fertility Society (1991). *In vitro* fertilization–embryo transfer (IVF-ET) in the United States: 1989 results from the IVF-ET registry. *Fertil. Steril.*, **55**, 14–23

18. Leeton, J., Rogers, P., Caro, C., Healy, D. and Yates, C. (1987). A controlled study between the use of gamete intrafallopian transfer (GIFT) and *in vitro* fertilization and embryo transfer in the management of idiopathic and male infertility. *Fertil. Steril.*, **48**, 605–8

19. Guzick, D.S., Yao, Y.A.S., Berga, S.L., Krasnow, J.S., Stovall, D.W., Kubik, C.J. and Zelenik, A.J. (1994). Endometriosis impairs the efficacy of gamete intrafallopian transfer results of a case–control study. *Fertil. Steril.*, **62**, 1186–91

20. Alsalili, M., Yuzpe, A., Tummon, I., Parker, J., Martin, J., Nisker, J, Daniel, S. and Rebel, M. (1995). Cumulative pregnancy rates and pregnancy outcome after *in vitro* fertilization: five thousand cycles at one centre. *Hum. Reprod.*, **10**, 470–4

21. Kenny, D. (1995). *In vitro* fertilisation and gamete intrafallopian transfer: an integrative analysis of research, 1987–92. *Br. J. Obstet. Gynaecol.*, **102**, 317–25

22. Marcus, S.F. and Edwards, R.G. (1994). High rates of pregnancy after long-term down-regulation of women with severe endometriosis. *Am. J. Obstet. Gynecol.*, **17**, 812–17

23. Dicker, D., Goldman, J.A., Levy, T., Feldberg, D. and Ashkenazi, J. (1992). The impact of long-term gonadotropin-releasing hormone analogue treatment on preclinical abortions in patients with severe endometriosis undergoing *in vitro* fertilization–embryo transfer. *Fertil. Steril.*, **57**, 597–600

24. Stewart, E.A., Jackson, K.V., Friedman, A.J., Rein, M.S., Fox, J.H. and Hornstein, M.D. (1992). The effect of baseline complex ovarian cysts on *in vitro* fertilization outcome. *Fertil. Steril.*, **57**, 1274–8

25. Dicker, D., Goldman, J.A., Feldberg, D., Ashkenazi, J. and Levy, T. (1991). Transvaginal ultrasonic needle-guided aspiration of endometriotic cysts before ovulation induction for *in vitro* fertilization. *J. In Vitro Fertil. Embryo Transfer*, **8**, 286–9

26. Pagidas, K., Falcone, T., Hemmings, R. and Miron, P. (1996). Comparison of reoperation for moderate (stage III) and severe (stage IV) endometriosis-related infertility with *in vitro* fertilization–embryo transfer. *Fertil. Steril.*, **65**, 791–5

In vitro fertilization in patients with endometriosis

62

H. Saito, K. Nakahara, T. Saito, M. Ito, N. Ohta, T. Takahashi, N. Tezuka, N. Sakai and M. Hiroi

Introduction

In vitro fertilization and embryo transfer (IVF-ET) has been employed for various infertility causes including tubal factor, male factor and unexplained infertility. Patients with endometriosis have also been treated by IVF-ET with good success rates. However, when compared with other infertility causes, the rate of pregnancy in patients with endometriosis is not constant among reporters. Kenny[1] reported that women with endometriosis (stage I or II) achieved higher rates of clinical pregnancy than patients with other causes of infertility. Meanwhile there are reports that the number of transferred embryos in each cycle and the implantation rates per transfer were similar in tubal factor, male factor, unexplained infertility and endometriosis[2–5]. Moreover, there are reports that endometriosis patients have a poor IVF outcome in terms of reduced pregnancy rate per cycle, reduced pregnancy rate per transfer and reduced implantation rate[6,7]. Endometriosis may have various effects on each stage of reproduction including follicle development in the ovary, oocyte–sperm interaction in the Fallopian tube, development of preimplantation embryos in the Fallopian tube and embryo–endometrium interaction in the uterus.

During the process of oogenesis in mammals a limited number of follicles continue to develop while the majority become atretic[8]. Follicular atresia was recently found to be associated with apoptosis in various kinds of animals: chickens, pigs[8], rats[9] and so on. Apoptosis is a physiological process resembling mitosis which leads in a controlled fashion to cell death. It is triggered by changes in levels of specific physiological stimuli. The term apoptosis is applied to a group of characteristic structural and molecular events that distinguish this type of cell death from necrosis, where a group of cells dies simultaneously[10]. Apoptosis always occurs in a single cell surrounded by viable cells. In tissues such as liver, gastroduodenal mucosa and ovaries[8,9], apoptosis plays an important physiological role in maintaining tissue homeostasis[11].

These changes are recognized under the light microscope as pyknosis of nuclei, decrease in cell volume, extraordinary surface convolutions and the explosion of the cell into cytoplasmic fragments containing condensed chromatin[11]. The incidence of apoptotic bodies has been applied as a morphological marker for physiological cell renewal in the liver and gastroduodenal mucosa[8], as a biomarker for regression of liver hyperplasia[12] and for prognosis of patients with neoplasms such as non-Hodgkin's lymphoma[13], prostatic intraepithelial neoplasm and prostatic cancer[14]. Based on these observations, the incidence of apoptotic bodies in membrana granulosa was used to examine ovarian function in an IVF program.

In this study we examined the characteristics of patients with endometriosis in an IVF-ET program including the day of oocyte collection, endometrial thickness, the number of follicles developed, the number of oocytes retrieved, fertilization rate, the number of fertilized oocytes/cycle, embryo transfer rate, pregnancy rate and ongoing pregnancy rate. Based on apoptosis observations in other kinds of cells, the incidence of apoptotic bodies in granulosa cells was also examined to determine the effects of endometriosis on follicle development in the ovary during the IVF program.

Materials and methods

Infertility patients undergoing *in vitro* fertilization (4005 cycles in total) were treated with a combination of gonadotropin-releasing hormone agonist (GnRHa) (buserelin acetate, Hoechst Japan, Tokyo, Japan), human menopausal gonadotropin (hMG) (Humegon®, Organon, Oss, The Netherlands; Pergogreen®, Serono, Tokyo, Japan; Fertinorm®, Serono) and human chorionic gonadotropin (hCG) (hCG Mochida®, Mochida Pharmaceuticals, Tokyo, Japan; Profasi®, Serono). GnRHa (600 μg/day) was administered nasally from the midluteal phase of the previous menstrual cycle or from the first day of the menstrual cycle to the last day of hMG treatment. hMG (150–300 IU/day, intramuscularly) was administered on cycle day 3 and stopped on the day when the mean diameter of the second largest follicle exceeded 16 mm. hCG was administered on the day that hMG was stopped. Oocyte aspiration was performed transvaginally, 34 h after the hCG injection. Thereafter, oocyte–cumulus complexes were incubated for 4 h at 37 °C before insemination. Human tubal fluid (HTF)[15] culture media were used as sperm wash, insemination media and growth media. The HTF culture media were supplemented with heat-inactivated patient preovulatory serum or heat-inactivated human plasma at a concentration of 10% by volume.

Semen samples were washed twice centrifugally with HTF media. Swim-up sperm were collected for insemination after 30 min. Prior to insemination, the most mature oocyte cumulus complex from each patient was identified and divided mechanically into an oocyte portion and a cumulus cell-matrix portion using two 26-gauge needles. The cumulus cells and cumulus matrix portion were transferred into HTF media and then used as culture media for fertilized oocytes or used for analysis of the incidence of apoptotic bodies. After 14 h following insemination with 1×10^5/ml motile sperm, fertilization was confirmed by the presence of two pronuclei. Fertilized oocytes were each placed in the cumulus cells and cumulus matrix in growth media. After 48 h following oocyte aspiration, embryos which had developed to the two to eight cell stage were transferred into a uterus through the uterine cervix. Progesterone and/or hCG supplement was administered during the luteal phase.

Granulosa cell fixation and quantification of apoptotic bodies

Aspirated follicular fluid was transferred into tissue culture dishes (Falcon 3002, Becton Dickinson Co., Lincoln Park, NJ, USA). Oocyte–cumulus cell complexes were isolated under a dissecting microscope (SZH-ILLB, Olympus, Tokyo, Japan) using × 10–20 magnifications, and put into an organ tissue culture dish (Falcon 3037, Becton Dickinson Co.) with HTF medium. The oocyte–cumulus cell complexes were classified into two groups: complexes with a large, loose cumulus and distinct corona radiata were judged as mature, and complexes with a small, dense cumulus and opaque corona radiata were defined as immature[16]. The mural granulosa cell masses were put into another dish with HTF medium. After the oocytes had been isolated mechanically from the cumulus cell masses using 26-gauge needles, the cumulus cell masses were transferred into a different organ culture dish. Hyaluronidase (Sigma, St. Louis, MO, USA), 0.1% weight/volume, in human tubal fluid medium was added to the dishes containing cumulus cell masses or mural granulosa cell masses (0.05% by volume of final concentration). Both cell masses were then pipetted thoroughly for 10 min, placed on a glass slide, and fixed with 4% neutral buffered formaline for 15 min. This process was completed within an hour of follicle aspiration to avoid post-aspiration cell death. After fixation, the slides were washed with phosphate-buffered saline three times, and the nuclei of the cells were stained with 0.5 μg/ml Hoechst 33258® (fluorescence dye, Wako, Osaka, Japan), with 5% DABCO (1,4-diazabiccyclo-2,2,2-octane, Sigma) in 90% glycerol/10% 0.2 mol/l Na_2HPO_3. The DABCO blocked the bleaching effect of the fluorescence and allowed the slides to be re-checked within a few weeks. Apoptotic bodies were revealed as cytoplasmic fragments containing condensed chromatin or fragments of condensed chromatin when examined by fluorescence microscopy. The apoptotic bodies were identified and counted among 1000 granulosa cells chosen at random, at × 1000 magnification.

Statistical analysis

The data are presented as the mean ± SEM. Statistical methods included the *t*-test, the Wilcoxon test, the Kruskal–Wallis test, the Dunn *post hoc* test and the Mann–Whitney U-test.

Results

The patients with endometriosis had a thicker endometrium than those with other causes of infertility. When the figures per cycle for each parameter were examined, the number of follicles developed, the number of oocytes harvested, and the number of mature oocytes were smaller in the endometriosis patients than in the other patients. The numbers of fertilized oocytes were fewer in the endometriosis patients than in those with tubal factor and unexplained infertility, and greater than in those with male factor infertility (Table 1). The percentages of mature oocytes/total oocytes, fertilized oocytes/total oocytes, and transferred embryos/fertilized oocytes showed no statistical differences between the groups. The pregnancy rate (pregnancy/embryo transferred cycle) and birth rate (delivery/embryo transferred cycle) also did not show statistical differences between the groups (Table 1).

The incidence of apoptotic bodies of mural granulosa cells in the endometriosis patients was higher than that in the patients with other infertility factors. The incidence of apoptotic bodies of cumulus cells in the patients with endometriosis was also significantly higher than that in the other patients (Table 2).

Discussion

In the outcome of IVF treatment, the endometriosis patients showed various results. Kenny[1] reported that women with endometriosis (stage I or II) achieved a higher rate of clinical pregnancy than patients with other causes of infertility. But several authors have reported that no different outcome could be observed between tubal factor infertility and endometriosis[2–5,17]. Meanwhile, there have been reports that endometriosis patients show poor pregnancy results[6,7,18,19]. Our results show that there is no statistical difference in pregnancy rate between endometriosis patients and patients with other causes of infertility.

In assessing these reports, the ovulation induction method and the treatment prior to ovulation induction should be considered. Ovulation induction with gonadotropin-releasing hormone agonist (GnRHa) causes a dramatic improvement in the total number of oocytes retrieved, oocytes transferred per cycle, and the pregnancy rate[20]. Treatment with GnRHa prior to IVF treatment is variable in the suppression of active diseases, and achieves good outcomes[17,21–23]. Transvaginal ultrasonic needle-guided aspiration of the endometrioma prior to IVF treatment results in a significantly higher number of oocytes being recovered, subsequently more embryos being transferred, and a significantly higher clinical pregnancy rate per cycle[24].

In the present study, short and long protocols of GnRHa were employed in all patients. This may improve to some extent the ovarian

Table 1 Various parameters related to the different causes of infertility. Values are presented as means ± SEM or as percentages

	Cause of infertility			
Parameter	Endometriosis	Tubal factor	Male factor	Unexplained
Total treated cycles	529	1320	1159	1007
Age (years)	33.5 ± 0.2	33.1 ± 0.2	33.5 ± 0.2	33.7 ± 0.2
Endometrium thickness**	10.1 ± 0.1	9.6 ± 0.1	9.9 ± 0.1	9.7 ± 0.1
No. of follicles developed/cycle**	2.4 ± 0.1	2.9 ± 0.1	3.1 ± 0.1	2.7 ± 0.1
Cycle day of operation	13.3 ± 0.3	12.5 ± 0.1	12.2 ± 0.1	12.6 ± 0.2
No. of oocytes retrieved/cycle**	3.0 ± 0.1	4.2 ± 0.1	4.7 ± 0.1	4.4 ± 0.1
No. of mature oocytes/cycle**	2.6 ± 0.1	3.4 ± 0.1	3.8 ± 0.1	3.6 ± 0.1
No. of oocytes fertilized/cycle**	2.0 ± 0.1	2.5 ± 0.1	1.7 ± 0.1	2.3 ± 0.1
Total no. of oocytes retrieved	1530	5336	5316	4355
Total no. of mature oocytes	1162	3944	4019	3323
% of total oocytes	75.9%	73.9%	75.6%	76.3%
Total no. of fertilized oocytes	833	2837	1411	1962
% of total oocytes	54.4%	53.2%	26.5%	45.1%
No. of embryo transfer cycles	364	981	595	694
% of total cycles	68.8%	74.3%	51.3%	68.9%
No. of pregnancy cycles	71	150	90	120
% of embryo transfer cycles	19.5%	15.3%	15.1%	17.3%
No. of deliveries	49	93	63	72
% of embryo transfer cycles	13.5%	9.5%	10.6%	10.4%

**$p < 0.01$, endometriosis compared with the other factors

Table 2 The incidence of apoptotic bodies of mural granulosa cell masses and cumulus cell masses, related to the different infertility factors. Values are given as means ± SEM

	Incidence of apoptotic bodies		
Infertility factors	No. of patients	Mural granulosa cell masses	Cumulus cell masses
Tubal	39	0.79 ± 0.10†	0.17 ± 0.02
Endometriosis	15	1.21 ± 0.23†	0.32 ± 0.03‡
Male	38	1.11 ± 0.17†	0.22 ± 0.04
Unexplained	37	0.79 ± 0.11†	0.22 ± 0.04

†$p < 0.001$ compared with cumulus cell masses in each group;
‡$p < 0.05$ compared with cumulus cell masses in other groups

circumstances in the endometriosis patients during ovulation induction; oocyte quality may be improved, and consequently no significant difference was observed in pregnancy rates and delivery rates between the endometriosis patients and the patients with other causes of infertility.

The actual number of follicles developed in the patients with endometriosis was smaller than that in the other patients. Regarding the number of oocytes harvested, the number of mature oocytes and the number of fertilized oocytes, the same tendency was observed. This implies that the ovarian circumstances for follicle development in the patients with endometriosis were disturbed to some extent, even though GnRHa was used for ovulation induction.

It takes several months for a primary follicle to develop into a secondary follicle. Several months of GnRHa therapy is therefore needed to preserve follicle development from the effects of endometriosis. Because the administration of GnRHa in our study did not cover the entire cycle of follicle development, smaller numbers of follicles may have developed when compared to the patients with other causes of infertility.

Apoptosis has been reported to play a key role in follicle development and atresia[25]. Apoptosis in the ovary is induced by androgens, GnRH and its analog, whereas it is blocked or inhibited by FSH, hCG, LH and estrogen[25]. The presence of apoptotic cells in atretic follicles is associated with decreased levels of aromatase mRNA and a significant decrease in follicular fluid estrogen concentration[26].

In this study the incidence of apoptotic bodies in the patients with endometriosis was higher than that in the other infertile patients. This implies that in the ovary of a patient with endometriosis, more follicles are going to be atretic than in the ovaries of other infertile patients. This would mean that smaller numbers of follicles develop in the endometriosis patient, even when exogenous gonadotropins are administered.

In summary, a smaller number of follicles developed in endometriosis patients than in patients with other causes of infertility, and consequently the numbers of oocytes harvested and fertilized were also smaller. The incidence of apoptotic bodies in the granulosa cells of the patients with endometriosis was higher than that in the other infertile patients. This phenomenon may explain why a smaller number of follicles developed in the endometriosis patients.

References

1. Kenny, D.T. (1995). *In vitro* fertilization and gamete intrafallopian transfer: an integrative analysis of research, 1987–1992. *Br. J. Obstet. Gynaecol.*, **102**, 317–25
2. Geber, S., Paraschos, T., Atkinson, G., Margara, R. and Winston, R.M. (1995). Results of IVF in patients with endometriosis: the severity of the disease does not affect outcome, or the incidence of miscarriage. *Hum. Reprod.*, **10**, 1507–11
3. Olivennes, F., Feldberg, D., Liu, H.C., Cohen, J., Moy, F. and Rosenwaks, Z. (1995). Endometriosis: a stage-by-stage analysis – the role of *in vitro* fertilization. *Fertil. Steril.*, **64**, 392–8
4. Dmowski, W.P., Rana, N., Michalowska, J., Friberg, J., Papierniak, C. and el-Roeiy, A. (1995). The effect of endometriosis, its stage and activity, and of autoantibodies on *in vitro* fertilization and embryo transfer success rates. *Fertil. Steril.*, **63**, 555–62
5. Pagidas, K., Falcone, T., Hemmings, R. and Miron, P. (1996). Comparison of reoperation for moderate (stage III) and severe (stage IV) endometriosis-related infertility with *in vitro* fertilization–embryo transfer. *Fertil. Steril.*, **65**, 791–5
6. Simon, C., Gutierrez, A., Vidal, A., de los Santos, M.J., Tarin, J.J., Remohi, J. and Pellicer, A. (1994). Outcome of patients with endometriosis in assisted reproduction; results from *in vitro* fertilization and oocyte donation. *Hum. Reprod.*, **9**, 725–9
7. Matson, P.L. and Yovich, J.L. (1986). The treatment of infertility associated with endometriosis by *in vitro* fertilization. *Fertil. Steril.*, **46**, 432–4
8. Tilly, J.L., Kowalski, K.I.N., Johnson, A.L. and Hsueh, A.D. (1991). Involvement of apoptosis in ovarian follicle atresia and postovulatory regression. *Endocrinology*, **129**, 2799–801
9. Palumbo, A. and Yeh, J. (1994). *In situ* localization of apoptosis in the rat ovary during follicle atresia. *Biol. Reprod.*, **51**, 888–95
10. Kerr, J.F.R., Wyllie A.H. and Currie, A.R. (1972). Apoptosis: a basic biological phenomenon with wide-ranging implications in tissue kinetics. *Br. J. Cancer*, **26**, 239–57
11. Benedetti, A., Mancini, R., Marucci, L., Paolucci, F., Jezequel, A.M. and Orlandi, F. (1990). Quantitative study of apoptosis in normal rat gastroduodenal mucosa. *J. Gastroenterol. Hepatol.*, **5**, 369–74
12. Bursch, W., Taper, H.S., Lauer, B. and Schulte-Hermann, R. (1985). Quantitative histological and histochemical studies on the occurrence and stages of controlled cell death (apoptosis) during regression of rat liver

hyperplasia. *Virchows Arch. (Cell Pathol.),* **50**, 153–66
13. Leoncini, L., Del Vecchio, M.T., Megha, T., Barbini, P., Galieni, P. and Pileri, S. (1993). Correlation between apoptotic and proliferative indices in malignant non-Hodgkin's lymphoma. *Am. J. Pathol.,* **142**, 755–63
14. Wheeler, T.M., Rogers, E., Aihara, M., Scardino, P.T. and Thompson, T.C. (1994). Apoptotic index as a biomarker in prostatic intraepithelial neoplasma (PIN) and prostatic cancer. *J. Cell Biol.,* **19**, 202–7
15. Oqinn, P., Warnes, G.M., Kern, J.F. and Kirby, C. (1984). Culture factors in relation to the success of human *in vitro* fertilization and embryo transfer. *Fertil. Steril.,* **41**, 202–9
16. Saito, H. and Hiroi, H. (1986). Correlation between the follicular gonadotropin inhibitor and the maturity of the ovum–corona–cumulus complex. *Fertil. Steril.,* **46**, 66–72
17. Curtis, P., Jackson, A., Bernard, A. and Shaw, R.W. (1993). Pretreatment with gonadotropin releasing hormone (GnRH) analogue prior to *in vitro* fertilization for patients with endometriosis. *Eur. J. Obstet. Gynecol. Reprod. Biol.,* **52**, 211–16
18. Oehninger, S., Acosta, A.A., Kreiner, D., Muasher, S.J., Jones, H.W. Jr and Rosenwaks, Z. (1988). *In vitro* fertilization and embryo transfer (IVF/ET): an established and successful therapy for endometriosis. *J. In Vitro Fertil. Embryo Transfer,* **5**, 249–56
19. Wardle, P.G., Mitchell, J.D., McLaughlin, E.A., Ray, B.D., McDermott, A. and Hull, M.G. (1985). Endometriosis and ovulatory disorder: reduced fertilization *in vitro* compared with tubal and unexplained infertility. *Lancet,* **2**, 236–9
20. Oehninger, S., Brzski, R.G., Muasher, S.J., Acosta, A.A. and Jones, G.S. (1989). *In vitro* fertilization and embryo transfer in patients with endometriosis: impact of a gonadotropin releasing hormone agonist. *Hum. Reprod.,* **4**, 541–4
21. Dicker, D., Goldman, J.A., Levy, T., Feldberg, D. and Ashkenazi, J. (1992). The impact of long-term gonadotropin-releasing hormone analogue treatment on preclinical abortions in patients with severe endometriosis undergoing *in vitro* fertilization–embryo transfer. *Fertil. Steril.,* **57**, 597–600
22. Dicker, D., Goldman, G.A., Ashkenazi, J., Feldberg, D., Voliovitz, I. and Goldman, J.A. (1990). The value of pre-treatment with gonadotropin releasing hormone (GnRH) analogue in IVF-ET therapy of severe endometriosis. *Hum. Reprod.,* **5**, 418–20
23. Damewood, M.D. (1989). The role of the new reproductive technologies including IVF and GIFT in endometriosis. *Obstet. Gynecol. Clin. North. Am.,* **16**, 179–91
24. Dicker, D., Goldman, J.A., Feldberg, D., Ashkenazi, J. and Levy, R. (1991). Transvaginal ultrasonic needle-guided aspiration of endometriotic cysts before ovulation induction for *in vitro* fertilization. *J. In Vitro Fertil. Embryo Transfer,* **8**, 286–9
25. Chun, S.Y., Billig, H., Tilly, J.L., Furuta, I., Tsafriri, A. and Hsueh, A.J. (1994). Gonadotropin suppression of apoptosis in cultured preovulatory follicles: mediatory role of endogenous insulin-like growth factor I. *Endocrinology,* **135**, 1845–53
26. Tilly, J.L., Kowalskim, K.I., Schomberg, D.W. and Hsueh, A.J. (1992). Apoptosis in atretic ovarian follicles is associated with selective decreases in messenger ribonucleic acid transcripts for gonadotropin receptors and cytochrome P450 aromatase. *Endocrinology,* **131**, 1670–6

The role of assisted reproductive techniques in endometriosis

63

S.C. Ng and S. Chew

Introduction

Subfertility is a frequent problem encountered in patients with endometriosis. While the incidence of endometriosis in women of reproductive age has been estimated to be between 2 and 10%[1,2], the incidence of endometriosis in subfertile women undergoing laparoscopy or laparotomy has been reported to range from 20 to 50%[3–5]. With the advent of assisted reproductive techniques, more subfertile patients with endometriosis are being treated with these procedures. It has been reported that patients with endometriosis refractory to medical or surgical treatment currently account for 7–35% of cases undergoing *in vitro* fertilization (IVF) procedures[6,7]. In this review, we will examine the role of IVF and gamete intrafallopian transfer (GIFT) in subfertile patients with pelvic endometriosis.

Extensive work investigating the cause of subfertility in women with endometriosis has been done in the last decade. Various mechanisms have been proposed to explain the association between endometriosis and infertility (Table 1). How then may IVF improve the fertility of women with endometriosis? The role of IVF in patients with extensive adhesions and tubal blockage because of endometriosis is obvious. However, even in the absence of mechanical damage, IVF may correct a variety of factors, such as abnormal ovum pick-up and altered embryo transport that have been implicated in low fecundity in endometriosis. As IVF is conducted under strict laboratory conditions, the gametes are protected, during the process of fertilization, from a potentially hostile peritoneal environment associated with endometriosis. Furthermore, controlled ovarian hyperstimulation during the IVF cycle and the luteal phase support after embryo transfer may also correct ovulatory dysfunction and luteal phase defects that may be contributory to infertility in endometriosis.

Table 1 Proposed mechanisms for infertility in endometriosis

Adhesions (Ohtsuka[8])
Tubal dysfunction (Drake *et al.*[9], Badawy *et al.*[10])
Impaired oocyte pick-up (Suginami *et al.*[11])
Ovulatory dysfunction (Marik and Hulka[12], Pittaway *et al.*[13])
Altered immune response (Meek *et al.*[14], Steele *et al.*[15])
Intraperitoneal inflammation (Haney *et al.*[16,17])
Implantation defects (Simon *et al.*[18])
Spontaneous abortions (Groll[19])

Indications

Subfertile patients with all stages of endometriosis have been treated with IVF, but timing of the procedure depends on the severity of disease, patient age and duration of subfertility. For minimal or mild endometriosis, the consensus seems to be that IVF or GIFT treatment be recommended only after at least 2 years of infertility[20]. In patients with severe endometriosis and tubal blockage, IVF should be expedited and treatment recommended within 1–2 years following unsuccessful medical or surgical treatment[21].

Does endometriosis affect the outcome of *in vitro* fertilization?

To answer this question, we have reviewed the literature to determine whether endometriosis does indeed affect oocyte recovery rates, fertilization rates, embryo quality, pregnancy and miscarriage rates.

Endometriosis and oocyte recovery

Chillik and colleagues[22], in an analysis of 39 IVF cycles in patients with a past history of endometriosis, found that there was a significant decrease in the total number of oocytes recovered laparoscopically in patients with severe endometriosis compared to those with mild/moderate disease. This difference was reported to be due mainly to technical difficulties at the time of laparoscopic oocyte retrieval because of adhesions and endometriomas in patients with severe endometriosis. Oehninger and colleagues[23], in a 6-year review of 136 patients who underwent 280 IVF cycles, found that patients with moderate/severe endometriosis also had a lower laparoscopic oocyte recovery rate when compared with cases with minimal/mild endometriosis. Matson and Yovich[24] also reported a significantly lower number of oocytes obtained in patients with grade III/IV endometriosis compared to cases with tubal factor infertility. However, they attributed this to a reduced number of follicles available for aspiration rather than to a lower recovery rate per follicle. With the advent of transvaginal ultrasound-guided oocyte recovery, the technical difficulties associated with laparoscopic oocyte recovery in severe endometriosis are now a thing of the past. More recent data[25-27] have also shown no associated reduction in the number of follicles with stimulation or decreased recovery rate per follicle in all stages of endometriosis.

Effect of endometriosis on fertilization rate

Wardle and colleagues[28] were the first to report that fertilization rates per oocyte were significantly reduced in patients with endometriosis (27% per oocyte) compared to cases with tubal disease (52% per oocyte). They attributed this finding to the fact that their patients had untreated endometriosis at the time of laparoscopic oocyte recovery. A later report by the same investigators[29] confirmed the reduced fertilization rates in women with untreated endometriosis. Mills and associates[30] also reported a significantly lower fertilization rate (48%) in 67 women with endometriosis as compared with a 65% fertilization rate in 198 patients with tubal or unexplained infertility. However, other workers has observed comparable fertilization rates in endometriosis and other infertility categories as well as no relationship between the severity of endometriosis and the percentage of oocytes fertilized (mild endometriosis 56–86%; severe endometriosis 46–90%; tubal infertility 56–80%; and unexplained infertility 53–67%)[18,22,24-27,31-33]. Thus, on balance, the present literature seems to suggest that the fertilization rate in IVF is not influenced by early or advanced endometriosis.

Embryo cleavage, implantation and transfer

Chillik and colleagues[22] analyzed 39 IVF cycles in infertile patients with endometriosis and reported that the presence or severity of endometriosis did not appear to affect embryo cleavage rates. Oehninger and Rosenwaks[32] conducted a 6-year review of IVF cycles carried out in the Jones Institute of Reproductive Medicine because of endometriosis. They found that the presence or degree of endometriosis did not affect embryo cleavage rates. Simon and colleagues[18] compared 78 IVF patients with tubal infertility and 59 IVF patients with endometriosis and reported a lower implantation rate in all stages of endometriosis (5.6–6.9%) compared to tubal

Table 2 Data showing an effect of endometriosis on IVF pregnancy rates

Study	No. of patients/IVF cycles	Pregnancy rate per cycle (%)		
		Mild endometriosis	Severe endometriosis	Control (tubal infertility)
Yovich et al.[36]	not stated	—	9.1	23.3
O'Shea et al.[37]	—/54	—	4	10
Chillik et al.[22]	26/39	60	7	33
Matson and Yovich[24]	97/149	13	4	18
Yovich and Matson[25]	96/154	13	3	14
Simon et al.[18]	59/96	14.2	12.1	34.4
Kenny[35]	review	38	11	20

infertility (13.4%). They also analyzed the results of their oocyte donation program according to the origin of the oocytes donated and reported that patients who received embryos derived from endometriotic ovaries had a significantly reduced implantation rate as compared with the other infertility groups. The authors concluded that infertility in endometriosis patients may be related to the oocytes, which produce embryos with a decreased ability to implant. However, these results were based on a retrospective analysis of different infertile populations and there were only a limited number of patients in the endometriosis group. Furthermore, Geber and colleagues[33], in a large study comparing 129 IVF cycles for endometriosis and 1136 IVF cycles for tubal factor infertility, reported no significant differences in implantation rates for IVF carried out for tubal factor infertility (23.4%) and endometriosis (21.8%).

Endometriosis and IVF pregnancy rates

Various authors[22,27,30,34] have reported IVF pregnancy rates in subfertile patients with minimal/mild endometriosis that were comparable with those for women with tubal factor or unexplained infertility. Chillik and colleagues[22] actually reported IVF pregnancy rates for mild endometriosis that were higher (60%) compared to the control group of IVF patients with tubal disease (33%). Kenny[35], in an analysis of IVF results (1987–92) in the English literature reported that women with endometriosis (stage I or II) actually achieved higher IVF pregnancy rates than patients with other causes (tubal, idiopathic) of infertility. However, the same author also reported a reduced overall IVF pregnancy rate for women with stage III or IV endometriosis (11%) compared to patients with tubal factor infertility (20%). Other investigators[18,22,24,25,36,37] have also reported lower IVF pregnancy rates with severe endometriosis (Table 2).

However, more recent data[27,33,39,40] consistently show no effect of endometriosis, regardless of stage, on IVF pregnancy rates (Table 3). Several publications from large national registers[6,41,42] have also reported similar IVF pregnancy rates for women with endometriosis when compared with other causes of infertility. Still, these results should be interpreted with caution as these registers often include patients with varying grades of disease, undergoing diverse stimulation regimens in different centers. Furthermore, the use of IVF in patients with endometriosis seems to result in favorable cumulative pregnancy and live birth rates[43,44]. Tan and colleagues[43] reported a 47% cumulative pregnancy rate after five treatment cycles in endometriotic patients, which was comparable

Table 3 Data showing no effect of endometriosis on IVF pregnancy rates

		Pregnancy rate per cycle (%)			
Study	No. of patients/cycles	Endometriosis (all stages)	Mild endometriosis	Severe endometriosis	Tubal infertility
Mahadevan et al.[31]	—/14	15	—	—	11.5
Jones et al.[38]	11/20	30	—	—	19
Oehninger and Rosenwaks[32]	136/280	—	16.7	20	22.3
Inoue et al.[39]	309/476	31	31	30*	27*
Dmowski et al.[27]	84/119	—	26	25*	25*
Geber et al.[33]	140/182	40	35	35*	45*
Olivennes et al.[40]	147/236	34	32	46	36

*Pregnancy rates per transfer

to cumulative pregnancy rates in tubal (52%) and unexplained (56%) infertility. Alsalili and associates[44] analyzed the cumulative pregnancy rates in a series of 5209 IVF cycles over a 10-year period in an Ontario IVF center. They reported a cumulative pregnancy rate, following six cycles, of 60% for endometriosis which was comparable to cumulative pregnancy rates for tubal (55%) and idiopathic (65%) infertility.

On balance, the current literature therefore seems to suggest that IVF pregnancy rates are not affected by the presence or severity of endometriosis. Furthermore, cumulative pregnancy rates after IVF are not reduced in patients with endometriosis when compared with other infertility categories.

Endometriosis and miscarriage rates

In an initial study by Oehninger and colleagues[23], a significantly higher miscarriage rate was reported in moderate/severe endometriosis (71%) compared to minimal/mild disease (36.9%). However, a later study by the same group[32], as well as reports by other authors[26,33], has shown no increase in miscarriage rates in women with all stages of endometriosis undergoing IVF.

Role of pretreatment of endometriosis before IVF

Wardle and colleagues[29], in a prospective trial, treated endometriotic patients with danazol (400–800 mg/day) or gestrinone (2.5 mg twice weekly) for 6–9 months. They reported that pretreated patients had better IVF fertilization, implantation and pregnancy rates (21%) compared to the untreated patients (15%), and similar IVF pregnancy rates compared to patients with tubal factor infertility (23%).

In a semi-randomized prospective trial[45], 84 patients with stage III or IV endometriosis were recruited, and 35 patients were down-regulated for 2–7 months (with one subcutaneous implant of 3.6 mg goserelin per month) prior to IVF. They reported higher IVF pregnancy rates (42.8%), especially in patients in whom IVF was performed during the fourth month of down-regulation. The pregnancy rate in the control group (patients with severe endometriosis given routine IVF treatment using ultrashort or short gonadotropin-releasing hormone agonist regimens) was 12.7%. The authors concluded that higher pregnancy rates might be achieved with IVF after long-term down-regulation in women with extensive endometriosis. Dicker and colleagues[46] studied 31 patients with stage III or IV endometriosis who had failed to conceive with previous IVF attempts. Suppression with intranasal buserelin for 6 months prior to IVF resulted in a 35% pregnancy rate per transfer in patients who had previously failed IVF treatment. In another study by the same authors[47], involving 67 patients with severe endometriosis referred for IVF, 35 were randomized to receive a 6-month pretreatment course of down-regulation with Decapeptyl (Organon). The authors reported that the group with gonadotropin-releasing hormone (GnRH) agonist treatment prior to IVF had significantly higher clinical pregnancy rates per cycle (25%) compared to the group without GnRH agonist pretreatment (4%).

However, a 6-month course of GnRH agonist prior to IVF is costly and not without its side-effects. Some workers[48] have therefore examined the role of a 6-week pretreatment course of GnRH agonist prior to IVF. Curtis and colleagues[48] analyzed 92 IVF cycles in patients with endometriosis (37 cycles in minimal/mild disease and 55 cycles in moderate/severe endometriosis). All endometriosis patients had a minimum of 6 weeks of GnRH treatment (intranasal buserelin) prior to superovulation therapy. They reported similar IVF pregnancy rates (per transfer) of 17.7% for tubal infertility, 17.2% for patients with minimal/mild endometriosis, and 18.6% for women with moderate/severe endometriosis. However, other authors[26] have failed to report any association between prior therapy of endometriosis and improved IVF pregnancy rates.

These conflicting results only highlight the urgent need for proper prospective and randomized trials to determine the role of pretreatment of endometriosis in improving IVF results.

Aspiration of endometriomas before IVF

Endometriomas may affect IVF outcome by interfering with oocyte recovery. They may also interfere with normal follicular and oocyte maturation, resulting in poorer quality of oocytes retrieved. Dicker and colleagues[49], in a study involving 41 patients with endometriomas who had failed previous IVF cycles, carried out transvaginal aspiration of the endometriomas prior to restarting IVF. They reported significantly higher numbers of oocytes retrieved, more embryos replaced and pregnancy rates per cycle of 24%. Thus in patients with severe endometriosis undergoing IVF, aspiration of endometriomas prior to ovulation induction could enhance the chances of success.

Role of GIFT in endometriosis

Gamete intrafallopian transfer may be useful in subfertile patients with minimal to mild endometriosis, without tubal involvement. The GIFT procedure may bypass the hostile peritoneal environment associated with endometriosis, while utilizing the normal site of fertilization in the ampullary portion of the Fallopian tube. Asch and associates[50] reported the results of 800 patients treated with GIFT from ten centers worldwide. They found that the highest pregnancy rates (38%) were actually achieved in infertile patients with endometriosis. Hulme and colleagues[51] published data on 59 GIFT cycles in 46 patients with minimal to moderate endometriosis. The clinical pregnancy rates per cycle for patients with endometriosis were higher (30.5%) than those for all GIFT cycles (23.7%). Other authors[52], in a review of seven studies in which GIFT procedures were carried out in patients with endometriosis, reported a pregnancy rate of 23.7%.

However, there are concerns that GIFT pregnancy rates may be impaired in patients with endometriosis as compared with those without endometriosis. Guzick and colleagues[53], in a case–control study, compared the results of 114 GIFT procedures in women with endometriosis with 214 GIFT procedures in a control group of patients without endometriosis. They reported a GIFT pregnancy rate of 32.5% in the endometriosis group and 47.2% in the control group. Although it was concluded that GIFT pregnancy rates were significantly lower in patients with endometriosis than in matched controls, the authors did concede that their pregnancy rate of 32.5% in patients with endometriosis was well within the range of what one might expect from a GIFT procedure. Furthermore, other authors[54] have reported that there are no differences in the rate of spontaneous abortions among the different stages of endometriosis following GIFT.

Conclusion

In vitro fertilization and gamete intrafallopian transfer are effective procedures for subfertile patients with endometriosis. However, timing of the procedure depends on the severity of disease, patient age and duration of infertility. Current literature seems to suggest that the presence and severity of endometriosis does not adversely affect the outcome of IVF.

However, the role of medical therapy prior to IVF requires further evaluation with well-designed randomized prospective trials.

References

1. Schifrin, B.S., Erez, S. and Moore, J.G. (1973). Teenage endometriosis. *Am. J. Obstet. Gynecol.*, **116**, 973–80
2. Barbieri, R.L. (1990). Etiology and epidemiology of endometriosis. *Am. J. Obstet. Gynecol.*, **162**, 565–7
3. Gruppo italiano per lo studio dell'endometriosi (1994). Prevalence and anatomical distribution of endometriosis in women with selected gynaecological conditions: results from a multicentric Italian study. *Hum. Reprod.*, **9**, 1158–62
4. Wheeler, J.M. (1989). Epidemiology of endometriosis-associated infertility. *J. Reprod. Med.*, **34**, 41–6
5. Williams, T.J. and Pratt, J.H. (1977). Endometriosis in 1000 consecutive celiotomies: incidence and management. *Am. J. Obstet. Gynecol.*, **129**, 245–50
6. HFEA (1993). *Human Fertilization and Embryology Authority. Annual Report*, pp. 17–24. (London: HFEA)
7. Damewood, M.D. (1989). The role of the new reproductive technologies including IVF and GIFT in endometriosis. *Obstet. Gynecol. Clin. North. Am.*, **16**, 179–91
8. Ohtsuka, N. (1980). Study on pathogenesis of adhesions in endometriosis. *Nippon Sanka Fujinka Gakkai Zasshi*, **32**, 1758–60
9. Drake, T.S., O'Brien, W.F. and Ramwell, P.W. (1981). Peritoneal fluid thromboxane B2 and 6-keto-prostaglandin F2 in endometriosis. *Am. J. Obstet. Gynecol.*, **140**, 401–4
10. Badawy, S.Z.A., Marshall, L. and Gabal, A.A. (1982). The concentration of 13,14-dihydro-15-keto-prostaglandin F2 and prostaglandin E2 in peritoneal fluid of infertile patients with and without endometriosis. *Fertil. Steril.*, **38**, 166–70
11. Suginami, H., Yano, K., Watanabe, K. and Matsuura, S. (1986). A factor inhibiting ovum capture by the oviductal fimbriae present in peritoneal fluid. *Fertil. Steril.*, **46**, 1140–6
12. Marik, J. and Hulka, J. (1978). Luteinized unruptured follicle syndrome: a subtle case of infertility. *Fertil. Steril.*, **29**, 270–4
13. Pittaway, D.E., Maxson, W., Daniell, J., Herbert, C. and Wentz, A.C. (1983). Luteal phase defects in infertility patients with endometriosis. *Fertil. Steril.*, **39**, 712–13
14. Meek, S.C., Hodge, D.D. and Musich, J.R. (1988). Autoimmunity in infertile patients with endometriosis. *Am. J. Obstet. Gynecol.*, **158**, 1365–73
15. Steele, R.W., Dmowski, W.P. and Marmer, D.J. (1984). Immunologic aspects of human endometriosis. *Am. J. Reprod. Immunol.*, **6**, 33–6
16. Haney, A.F., Muscato, J.I. and Weinberg, J.F. (1981). Peritoneal cell populations in infertility patients. *Fertil. Steril.*, **35**, 696–8
17. Haney, A.F., Jenkins, S. and Weinberg, J.F. (1991). The stimulus responsible for the peritoneal fluid inflammation observed in infertile women with endometriosis. *Fertil. Steril.*, **56**, 408–13
18. Simon, C., Gutierrez, A., Vidal, A., de los Santos,

M.J., Tarin, J.J., Remohi, J. and Pellicer, A. (1994). Outcome of patients with endometriosis in assisted reproduction: results from *in vitro* fertilization and oocyte donation. *Hum. Reprod.*, **9**, 725–9
19. Groll, M. (1984). Endometriosis and spontaneous abortion. *Fertil. Steril.*, **41**, 933–5
20. Hull, M.G.R. (1994). Effectiveness of infertility treatments: choice and comparative analysis. *Int. J. Gynaecol. Obstet.*, **47**, 99–108
21. Amso, N.N. (1995). Role of assisted reproduction in endometriosis. In Shaw, R.W. (ed.) *Endometriosis, Current Understanding and Management*, pp. 282–95. (Oxford: Blackwell Science)
22. Chillik, C.F., Acosta, A.A., Garcia, J.E., Perera, S., Van Uem, J.F.H.M. and Rosenwaks, Z. (1985). The role of *in vitro* fertilization in infertile patients with endometriosis. *Fertil. Steril.*, **44**, 56–61
23. Oehninger, S., Acosta, A.A. and Kreiner, D. (1988). *In vitro* fertilization and embryo transfer (IVF/ET): an established and successful therapy for endometriosis. *J. In Vitro Fertil. Embryo Transfer*, **5**, 249–56
24. Matson, P.L. and Yovich, J.L. (1986). The treatment of infertility associated with endometriosis by *in vitro* fertilization. *Fertil. Steril.*, **46**, 432–4
25. Yovich, J.L. and Matson, P.L. (1990). The influence of infertility etiology on the outcome of IVF-ET and GIFT treatments. *Int. J. Fertil.*, **35**(1), 26–33
26. Tummon, I.S., Colwell, K.A., MacKinnon, C.J., Nisker, J.A. and Yuzpe, A.A. (1991). Abbreviated endometriosis-associated infertility correlates with *in vitro* fertilization success. *J. In Vitro Fertil. Embryo Transfer*, **81**, 149–53
27. Dmowski, P.W., Rana, N., Friberg, J. and Papierniak, C. (1995). Effect of endometriosis, its stage and activity, and of autoantibodies on *in vitro* fertilization and embryo transfer success rates. *Fertil. Steril.*, **63**(3), 555–62
28. Wardle, P.G., McLaughlin, E.A., McDermott, A., Mitchell, J.D., Ray, B.D. and Hull, M.G.R. (1985). Endometriosis and ovulatory disorder: reduced fertilisation *in vitro* compared with tubal and unexplained infertility. *Lancet*, **2**, 236–9
29. Wardle, P.G., Foster, P.A., Mitchell, J.D., McLaughlin, E.A., Skyes, J.A.C., Corrigan, E., Hull, M.G.R., Ray, B.D. and McDermott, A. (1986). Endometriosis and IVF: effect of prior therapy. *Lancet*, **1**, 276–80
30. Mills, M.S., Eddowes, H.A., Cahill, D.J., Fahy, U.M., Abuzeid, M.I.M. and McDermott, A. (1992). A prospective controlled study of *in vitro* fertilization, gamete intrafallopian transfer and intrauterine insemination combined with superovulation. *Hum. Reprod.*, **7**, 490–4
31. Mahadevan, M.M., Trounson, A.D. and Leeton, J.F. (1983). The relationship of tubal blockage, infertility of unknown cause, suspected male infertility, and endometriosis to success of *in vitro* fertilization and embryo transfer. *Fertil. Steril.*, **40**, 755–62
32. Oehninger, S. and Rosenwaks, Z. (1990). *In vitro* fertilization and embryo transfer: an established and successful therapy for endometriosis. *Prog. Clin. Biol. Res.*, **323**, 319–35
33. Geber, S., Paraschos, T., Atkinson, G., Margara, R. and Winston, R.M.L. (1995). Results of IVF in patients with endometriosis: the severity of the disease does not affect outcome, or the incidence of miscarriage. *Hum. Reprod.*, **10**, 1507–11
34. Sharma, V., Riddle, A., Mason, B.A., Pampiglioni, J. and Campbell, S. (1988). An analysis of factors influencing the establishment of a clinical pregnancy in an ultrasound-based ambulatory *in vitro* fertilization program. *Fertil. Steril.*, **49**, 468–78
35. Kenny, T.D. (1995). *In vitro* fertilization and gamete intrafallopian transfer: an integrative analysis of research. *Br. J. Obstet. Gynaecol.*, **102**, 317–25
36. Yovich, J.L., Yovich, J.M. and Tuvik, A.I. (1985). *In vitro* fertilization for endometriosis. *Lancet*, **2**, 552
37. O'Shea, R.T., Chen, C. and Weiss, T. (1985). Endometriosis and *in vitro* fertilization. *Lancet*, **2**, 723
38. Jones, H.W., Acosta, A., Andrews, M.C., Garcia, J.E., Jones, G.S., Mayer, J., McDowell, J.S., Rosenwaks, Z., Sandow, B.A., Veeck, L.L. and Wilkes, C.A. (1984). Three years of *in vitro* fertilization at Norfolk. *Fertil. Steril.*, **42**, 826–34
39. Inoue, M., Kobayashi, Y., Honda, I., Awaji, H. and Fujii, A. (1992). The impact of endometriosis on the reproductive outcome of infertile patients. *Am. J. Obstet. Gynecol.*, **167**(1), 278–82
40. Olivennes, F., Feldberg, D., Liu, H.C., Cohen, J., Moy, F. and Rosenwaks, Z. (1996). Endometriosis: a stage by stage analysis – the role of *in vitro* fertilization. *Fertil. Steril.*, **64**, 392–8

41. Medical Research International, Society for Assisted Reproductive Technology, American Fertility Society (1990). *In vitro* fertilization – embryo transfer in the United States: 1988 results from the IVF-ET registry. *Fertil. Steril.*, **53**, 13–20
42. Medical Research International, Society for Assisted Reproductive Technology, American Fertility Society (1991). *In vitro* fertilization – embryo transfer (IVF-ET) in the United States: 1989 results from the IVF-ET registry. *Fertil. Steril.*, **55**, 14–23
43. Tan, S.L., Royston, P. and Campbell, S. (1992). Cumulative conception and livebirth rates after *in vitro* fertilization. *Lancet*, **339**, 1390–4
44. Alsalili, M., Yuzpe, A., Tummon, I., Parker, J., Martin, J., Daniel, S., Rebel, M. and Nisker, J. (1995). Cumulative pregnancy rates and pregnancy outcome after *in vitro* fertilization: > 5000 cycles at one centre. *Hum. Reprod.*, **10**, 470–4
45. Marcus, S.F. and Edwards, R.G. (1994). High rates of pregnancy after long-term down-regulation of women with severe endometriosis. *Am. J. Obstet. Gynecol.*, **171**, 812–17
46. Dicker, D., Goldman, G.A. and Ashkenazi, J. (1990). The value of pre-treatment with gonadotrophin releasing hormone (GnRH) analogue in IVF-ET therapy of severe endometriosis. *Hum. Reprod.*, **5**, 418–20
47. Dicker, D., Goldman, J.A., Levy, T., Feldbert, D. and Ashkenzai, J. (1992). The impact of long-term gonadotropin-releasing hormone analogue treatment on preclinical abortions in patients with severe endometriosis undergoing *in vitro* fertilization–embryo transfer. *Fertil. Steril.*, **57**, 597–600
48. Curtis, P., Jackson, A., Bernard, A. and Shaw, R.W. (1993). Pretreatment with gonadotrophin releasing hormone (GnRH) analogue prior to *in vitro* fertilisation for patients with endometriosis. *Eur. J. Obstet. Gynecol. Reprod. Biol.*, **52**, 211–16
49. Dicker, D., Goldman, J.A., Feldbert, D., Ashkenzai, J. and Levy, T. (1991). Transvaginal ultrasonic needle-guided aspiration of endometriotic cysts before ovulation induction for *in vitro* fertilization. *J. In Vitro Fertil. Embryo Transfer*, **8**, 286–9
50. Asch, R.H., Balmaceda, J.P., Cittadini, E., Figueroa-Casa, P., Gomel, V. and Hohl, M.K. (1988). Gamete intrafallopian transfer. International cooperative study of the first 800 cases. *Ann. NY Acad. Sci.*, **541**, 722–7
51. Hulme, V.A., van der Merwe, J.P. and Kruger, T.F. (1990). Gamete intrafallopian transfer as treatment for infertility associated with endometriosis. *Fertil. Steril.*, **53**, 1095–6
52. Mahmood, T.A. and Templeton, A. (1990). Pathophysiology of mild endometriosis: review of literature. *Hum. Reprod.*, **5**, 765–84
53. Guzick, D.S., Yao, Y.A.S., Berga, S.L., Krasnow, J.S., Stovall, D.W., Kubik, C.J. and Zeleznik, A.J. (1994). Endometriosis impairs the efficacy of gamete intrafallopian transfer: results of a case–control study. *Fertil. Steril.*, **62**, 1186–91
54. Craft, I. and Brinsden, P. (1989). Alternatives to IVF: the outcome of 1071 first GIFT procedures. *Hum. Reprod.*, **4** (Suppl.), 29–36

Index

abortion, in endometriosis 83
adenomyosis
  apoptosis 92–7
  role of MMPs 210–15
  surgery 290–1
adenomyotic nodule, rectovaginal septum 25–41
adhesions 283
  in infertility 254
  and pregnancy rate 304, 305–6, 307–8
adnexal mass, laparoscopy 274
adolescent endometriosis 21–6
Allen-Masters syndrome 52
American Association of Gynecologic Laparoscopists (AAGL) 283
American Fertility Society (AFS)
  revised classification 28–9, 53, 239–40, 244–7
    251, 252–5, 304, 316
  staging 18–19, 42–3, 60, 329, 443, 444, 457
  videolaparoscopy results 271–2
American Society for Reproductive Medicine (ASRM) 320
anesthesia, local, for office microlaparoscopy 309–10
animal models
  baboon 58–9
  nude mice 98–103
  rats 402–3
  SCID mice 98–103
antibody, immunostaining 93–4
apoptosis 92–7, 461–5
appendectomy 278
appendix, endometriosis, treatment 278
aromatase inhibitor, YM511 339–44
assisted reproductive technologies (ART) 352, 404,
  443, 444–6, 449–51, 467–74
  infertility prognosis 455–60
autoantibodies, effect on embryo implantation 123–31

benign prostatic hypertrophy (BPH) 405–6
bladder, laparoscopy 282
bone loss 428–30
bowel endometriosis
  operative laparoscopy 277–8
  resection 279–80
breast cancer 407–8
  metastatic, GnRH agonist therapy 417
buserelin, intranasal 471

cadherins 17–18, 232
Canadian Fertility and Andrology Society 271
cancer antigen-125 (CA-125) 425
cavitational ultrasonographic surgical aspirator (CUSA) 282
cell adhesion molecules (CAMs)
  integrin family 216
  in pathogenesis of endometriosis 231–6

cell(s)
  adhesion 17
  proliferation in endometriosis 69, 70–2
  proliferation scores 72
Cetrorelix 402–4
  clinical studies 434–7
Cetrorelix-depot therapy 421
chromosome abnormalities 161
cysts
  chocolate 35
    pregnancy rates after laparoscopic procedures 307
  ovarian, laparoscopy 274–5
  ovarian endometrial 33–4
cytokeratin
  expression 169, 170–1
  in FbEM-1 cells 161
cytokines
  assays 330
  and endometrial cell growth 329
  as endometrial tissue function modulators 107–8
  inflammatory 132–3
  in peritoneal fluid 144–8
danazol 329–30, 425, 470
  action analysis 381–5
  action model 384
  in autoimmune disorders 153
  cell growth effect 381–2
  effect
    on estrogen receptor levels 386–91
    on estrogen receptor-mediated transcriptional activity 383–4
    on IVF–ET 392–7
    on MAPK activity 382–3
  and IVF–ET outcomes 392–7
  side-effects 429
depot formulation 360–4
diaphragm, laparoscopy 282
DNA, synthesis study 86
dysmenorrhea 75–6
  after RU486 336
  uterine hypercontractility 80

EMART 393
embryo cleavage rates 468
embryo implantation, autoantibody effect 123–31
embryo transfer see in vitro fertilization-embryo transfer
endometrial glands and stroma 38, 44
endometrioma
  aspiration before IVF 471
  in infertility 254
  laparoscopy 275
  ovarian 33–4
    histogenesis 42–9
    outcomes 367

wall biopsy 44
treatment before IVF 458
endometriosis
  'activity' 243–4
  in baboons 58–65
  deep 50–7, 244
  diagnosis 310–11
  evolution 30
  groups 368
  and infertility 216–24
  pathology 15–16
  patient age 18
  physiology 14
  prevalence 50–1
  progression 19
  staging system 242–3, 250
endometriosis protein-I (Endo-I) 107, 108–9, 111–15
endometriosis protein-II (Endo-II) 107, 108–9, 111–15
Endometriosis Study Group 259, 261
endometriosis-derived cell line (FbEM-1)
  chromosome abnormalities 161
  cytochemical characteristics 159–60
  establishment 157–64
  growth curve 160
  phenotype 159
endometrium 69–74
  cancer 408
  cell proliferation 69, 70–2
endoscopy, and videolaparoscopy 271–88
epidermal growth factor (EGF) 85, 86–8, 90
  in endometriotic tissues 181–2
  receptor 174–5
  receptor change 89
estradiol
  GnRH response 355
  leuprorelin depot dose effects 374
estrogen receptor (ER) 38–9, 165–6
  gene transcription rate 389
  monocyte expression 386–8
estrogen receptor (ER) mRNA
  degradation rate 389
  levels with danazol 386, 389–90
  monocyte expression 388–9

FbEM-1 cells see endometriosis-derived cell line
fertilization
  peritoneal macrophage impairment 122
  rate in endometriosis 468
fibrin/fibrinolytic system 231–2
fibroblast growth factor (FGF) 175–6
fibroids
  Cetrorelix-pamoat microparticle formulation 420
  GnRH agonist therapy 416–7
  and LHRH antagonists 405
FOATI classification 259–60, 261–7
follicle-stimulating hormone (FSH) 352
  changes with leuprorelin depot 373
  leuprorelin depot effects 372
follicular atresia 461

gamete intrafallopian transfer (GIFT) 444, 445–6, 457
  role 471–2

genitourinary tract
  evaluation 280–1
  implants 281
glandular cells, electron micrograph 94–6
glucuronide, levels after RU486 335
GnRH
  agonists 348, 350, 353, 358, 415, 416–8, 426–7
    clinical outcome 428–30
    in ovarian stimulation 445–6
    potency 354
    side-effects 429
    type and formulation 354–6
  agonists in IVF 462–5, 471
  amino acid sequence 414
  analogs 349, 351–3, 357–9, 414–23
    clinical indications 416
  antagonists 348–9, 353, 418–20
    endometriosis therapy 424–33
  receptor activation model 350
  type development 347
GnRH/GnRH-receptor interaction 415
gonadotropin, GnRH response 355
gonadotropin-releasing hormone see GnRH
goserelin 470
granulosa cells 462–3, 464–5
growth factors
  cell proliferative effect 90–1
  in endometriotic tissues 181–2
  gene expression 86–9, 174–80
  in inflammation 132–3
  in proliferative regulation 85–91
  roles 91

heat shock proteins (HSPs) 149–54
hemorrhage 294
hepatocyte growth factor (HGF) 191–9
  mitogenic effects 195
  secretion 197
histology, ovarian cyst 44–5, 46
hormone therapy 307
human chorionic gonadotropin (hCG) 349, 462
hysterectomy 293–5
  laparoscopic 272–3, 303

ICAM-1 28–9, 30–1, 32
  expression in endometrial cells 225–30
IGFBP-3 181–5, 187
  mitogenic fragments in peritoneal fluid 183–4
  mitogenic and proteolytic activities 184–6
imaging diagnosis 24–5
immune system, and endometriosis 107–17, 128–9
immunocytochemistry, leukocytes 139
immunology, endometrial 118–19
immunosuppression 62
in vitro fertilization (IVF)
  costs 451
  for endometriosis-associated infertility 457
  ethical and sociological considerations 452
  evolution 456–8
  GnRH agonists 418
  for infertility 443–54
  multiple pregnancy risk 451–2
  pregnancy rates in endometriosis 469–70
  results 446, 447–8, 449

success rate 457–8
vs. GIFT 445
in vitro fertilization–embryo transfer (IVF–ET) 123, 126–8
    effects of danazol 392–7
    outcomes 393
    patient characteristics 461–6
infertility
    classification 255–7
    endometriosis-associated, treatment guidelines 315–22
      expectant management' 325–8
      trials results 327
    IVF role 443–54
    laparoscopic management 303–8
    laser laparoscopy *vs.* placebo 297–302
    and macrophages 120–2
    mechanisms in endometriosis 467
    office microlaparoscopy for evaluation 312–13
    parameters 464
    and peritoneal inflammation 132–7
    possible mediators 134–5
    preoperative medical treatment (PMT) 305-7
    risk-benefit decision 327
    TNF-α, peritoneal concentrations 331
    treatment comparisons 318
    tubal factor 392, 463, 467–71
    untreated, prognosis 455, 459
inflammation
    role in infertility 132–7
    sources 132
insulin-like growth factor (IGF)/IGF binding protein-3 *see* IGFBP-3
integrins 17
    and endometrium 217, 218–19
    family of 232
intercellular adhesion molecule-1 *see* ICAM-1
interleukin-1 (IL-1) 386–7
interleukin-1β 110–11, 425
interleukin-6
    effects on blastocyst formation 146
    in peritoneal fluid 329–32
    peritoneal fluid levels 146
interleukin-8
    effects on cell proliferation 147
    peritoneal fluid levels 146

Japanese Society of Obstetrics and Gynecology 394

keratinocyte growth factor (KGF) 85, 88

laparoscopic surgery, for infertility 303–8
laparoscopy
    see also microlaparoscopy, office
    complications 282–3
    treatment results 245
laser laparoscopy *vs.* placebo 297–302
lesions, incidence by site 29, 30
leukocyte adhesion molecule (LFA-1) 225, 228
leukocytes 138–43
    population 139, 140–1
leuprolide 360–4
    with surgical treatment 365–9

leuprorelin 357, 358
    amino acid sequence 416
    dose improvements 375–6
    dose-related effects 370-7
    patient usefulness assessment 377
life-table analysis 326
lipopolysaccharide (LPS) 108–13
Lübeck protocol 419
lupus anti-coagulant syndrome (LACS) 126
luteinizing hormone (LH), serum changes with depot leuprorelin 370–1
luteinizing hormone-releasing hormone (LHRH)
    analog development 347–53
    antagonist development 434–9
    antagonistic analogs 401–13

macrophage colony-stimulating factor (M-CFS) receptor 386–7
macrophages
    effect on embryonic development *in vitro* 121
    effect of *in vitro* fertilization 121
    and infertility 120–2
    peritoneal 16–17
Mantel-Haenszel estimate 316, 319
matrix metalloproteinases (MMPs) 201–2, 204–7
    in adenomyosis 210–15
    expression model 204–6
    regulation by TGF-β 206
mechanical signal acquisition 81
    uterine pressure 82–3
medical treatment, effects 329–33
menstrual pain *see* dysmenorrhoea
menstruation
    in history 3–5
    retrograde 61, 69
metaplasia theory 45, 48
MHC class I 118–19
microlaparoscopy
    office
      see also laparoscopy
      under local anesthesia 309–14
mifepristone *see* RU486
miscarriage 470
mitogens and insulin-like growth factor (IGF) 181–90
mRNA
    basic fibroblast growth factor 176
    EGF receptor 174–5
Müllerian malformations 22
myomectomy, laparoscopic 273

natural killer (NK) cells 118
    binding to stromal cells 227
nerve fibers, distribution 77
nude mice, transplanted human endometrium 98–103

oocyte recovery 468
oophorectomy, laparoscopic 274–5, 291–2, 303
ovary
    chocolate-colored fluid cysts 35
    endometrioma 33–4
      histogenesis 42–9
    epithelial cancer 408
    GnRH agonist hyperstimulation 417–18

GnRH antagonist hyperstimulation 419
hyperstimulation 444–6, 467
hyperstimulation/intrauterine insemination 456
remnant laparoscopy 276
tumour laparoscopy 274–5
ovulation induction 463
ovulation stimulators, conception rate improvement 443
ovum capture inhibitor (OCI) 133
ovum pick-up (OPU) 445–6, 447–8

pain
   after RU486 336
   chronic pelvic 246–7
   classification 255
   endometriotic 75
   laser laparoscopy *vs.* placebo 297–302
   office microlaparoscopy 311–12
   symptom scores 360–1, 363
'pain memory' 300
peritoneal cavity, defense systems 16–17
peritoneal excision 289–90
peritoneal fluid
   cytokine levels 329, 332
   increase 16
   interferon-6 concentrations 331–2
peritoneal macrophages 386
peritoneum
   endometriosis 244
      laparoscopy 276
   ovarian, adhesion classification 256
platelet-derived growth factor (PDGF) 85, 88
postoperative fever 294
pouch of Douglas, laparovaginal surgery 292–3
pregnancy
   after laparoscopic surgery 304
   rate
      with adhesions 304, 305–6, 307–8
      after laparoscopic treatment 445, 449
      after surgery 44
      by treatment group 317
   treatment comparisons 321
presacral neurectomy, laparoscopy 276–7
progesterone 200–2
progesterone receptors (PR) 38–9, 165–6, 167–9
   in FbEM-1 cells 161
prostaglandin E2 (PGE2), production 76
prostaglandin F 300
prostaglandins
   nociceptive stimulus 77–8
   and pain 75
   radioimmunoassay 76
prostate cancer 406–7
proteases, secretion by endometrial cells 186–7
proteolysis products 17

rectovaginal adenomyosis 37
rectovaginal endometriosis
   complications 37
   technical aspects 36
rectovaginal septum
   adenomyotic nodule 35–41
   endometriosis 35–6, 37–41
   videolaparoscopy 279

rectum, endometriosis, videolaparoscopy 279
recurrent endometriosis 290
reflux implantation theory 15
reproduction, peritoneal fluid adverse effects 133–4
reproductive autoimmune failure syndrome 126
reproductive tract, development 6–12
retrograde menstruation 61, 69
Rokitansky-Kuster-Hauser syndrome 48
Royal Australian College of Gynaecologists 294
RU486 334–8

Sampson hypothesis 61, 80
SCID mice, transplanted human endometrium 98–103
severe combined immunodeficiency *see* SCID
Society for Assisted Reproductive Technology 457
sperm, for IVF 462
sperm insemination, frozen donor (FDSI) 444, 450
sperm toxicity, peritoneal fluid types 134
stromal cells, growth factors secretion 182–3
stromal fibroblasts 11
surgery
   radical laparoscopic 289–96
   repeated 458–9
surgical staging 242–3

tissue inhibitor of metalloproteinase-1 (TIMP-1) 112–15
'TOP' classification 255
transforming growth factor-α (TGF-α) 85, 133, 175, 181–2
transforming growth factor-β (TGF-β) 176–7
   expression 204–7, 204
   radioreceptor assay 203, 204
   treatment studies 18–19
tumor necrosis factor (TNF) 386
tumor necrosis factor-α (TNF-α) 330, 332

ureter, obstructed 281–2
uterus
   bleeding with leuprorelin depot administration 372
   contractability 80–4
   evolution 5–12
   nerve ablation 300
   receptivity defects 219–20

vascular cell adhesion molecule-1 (VCAM-1) 228
vascular endothelial growth factor (VEGF) 177, 181
videolaparoscopy 271–88
vimentin, expression 169, 170–2

YM511 339–44
   cell growth inhibition 340
   estradiol concentrations 343
   plasma concentration profiles 341–2

zygote 10
zygote intra-Fallopian transfer (ZIFT) 444